# Advances in Mental Health Research

# Advances in Mental Health Research

## Implications for Practice

EDITED BY

JANET B. W. **WILLIAMS**, DSW

KATHLEEN **ELL**, DSW

WITH A FOREWORD BY

STEVEN E. **HYMAN**, MD

*Director, National Institute of Mental Health*

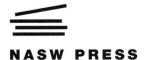

## NASW PRESS

National Association of Social Workers

Washington, DC

*Josephine A.V. Allen, PhD, ACSW,* President
*Josephine Nieves, MSW, PhD,* Executive Director

**Jane** Browning, *Director of Member Services and Publications*

**Paula** Delo, *Executive Editor*

**Christina** A. Davis, *Senior Editor*

**Christine** Cotting, UpperCase Publication Services, *Project Manager*

**Patricia** Borthwick and Elizabeth Reynolds, *Copy Editors*

**Caroline** Polk, *Proofreader*

**Bernice** Eisen, *Indexer*

**Chanté** Lampton, *Acquisitions Associate*

**Heather** Peters, *Editorial Secretary*

First printing, April 1998
Second printing, September 1998
Third printing, January 2001

© 1998 by the NASW Press

**Library of Congress Cataloging-in-Publication Data**

Advances in mental health research / edited by Janet B.W. Williams,
  Kathleen Ell.
    p.   cm.
  Includes bibliographical references and index.
  ISBN 0-87101-291-X (pbk. : alk. paper)
    1. Mental health—Research.  2. Mental health services—Research.
  3. Psychology, Pathological—Research.  I. Williams Janet B. W.,
  1947– .  II. Ell, Kathleen Obier, 1940– .
  RA790.5.A345   1998
  616.89—dc21                     98-11120
                                       CIP

Printed in the United States of America

Dedicated to

K  E  N  N  E  T  H        L  U  T  T  E  R  M  A  N

A N D     J  U  A  N       R  A  M  O  S

for their enduring commitment to excellent care for all

people with mental illness and for their vigorous and unwavering support of

infrastructure development to advance social work research and research training.

This book is proof that their efforts have brought forth sweet fruit.

# Contents

# Foreword

Research conducted over the past several decades has contributed greatly to the nature, breadth, and efficacy of interventions available for treating severe mental illness, and research now underway promises significant further enhancements in the near future. Yet, in sharp contrast, the quality of care typically provided to people with severe mental illnesses does not reflect the dramatic expansion of our knowledge about the brain and behavior and, in turn, of our refinement of scientifically based diagnostic and therapeutic capacities.

The gap between what is known and what is practiced undermines the credibility of all clinical mental health services providers and presents the research community with an urgent challenge: To be more effective in communicating the results of research and thus to help frontline clinicians provide state-of-the-art care to patients through the course of illness.

One source of disparity between what currently is known and what is practiced is the relative infrequency of research exposure or experience in clinical training for all of the core mental health professions. This volume, published by the National Association of Social Workers (NASW) with funding from the National Institute of Mental Health (NIMH) in recognition of the Institute's 50th anniversary, is an important step toward redressing this disparity.

Social work as a discipline has had a significant presence within NIMH since the Institute's beginning in the late 1940s. That presence continues today at the policy level and, to a lesser but important extent, in research. Through the 1970s, the profession of social work related to the Institute primarily through service-related and clinical training programs. Two decades ago, almost every school of social work in the country had an NIMH training grant, and the Institute annually provided 1,500 or more clinical training stipends to social work students. Today, although the focus of NIMH has shifted decisively away from clinical training and onto scientific research, maintaining and nurturing our long relationship with social work remains in the best interest of people with mental illness and of NIMH. With the membership of the NASW exceeding 155,000, more than half of whom are involved in mental health services delivery, strengthening the links between the research mission of NIMH and the interest and expertise of social workers is critical.

Over five decades, NIMH has played a critical role in supporting and conducting research and then in moving that research out of the realms of description and speculation and into the realms of neuroscience and clinical practice. It is now commonly held that mental illnesses are disorders of the brain that can be understood in terms of well-characterized neural and neuropathologic processes. Although much remains to be learned, we must not forget that even as we exploit powerful new molecular and cellular tools, our ultimate goals cannot be reductionist. The symptoms and signs of disorders such as affective illnesses, anxiety disorders, attention deficit disorder, schizophrenia, and others affect human beings at the levels of behavior and subjective experience. It is vitally important that we understand human behavior, cognition, and emotion; how these become altered with mental illness; and how we can translate our knowledge into improved clinical interventions.

Thanks to our increasingly strong research base, the most important message that I have to convey, in my role as Institute director, is simple and straightforward: Mental illnesses are real brain disorders that can be diagnosed with precision and for which effective treatments exist. Appropriate treatment can make an extraordinary difference in the lives of people who have these severe disorders. Although I sometimes feel I repeat myself, it seems that every time I deliver this message (whether to legislators, to general medical audiences, to research colleagues, or even to mental health advocates) the light goes on in someone's eyes.

*Advances in Mental Health Research: Implications for Practice,* edited by Janet B. W. Williams and Kathleen Ell, links research to treatment in a direct and understandable manner. The goals of NIMH-sponsored research are more effective diagnosis, treatment and, eventually, prevention of mental disorders. With each advance, the science of our field is having an increasingly immediate and greater impact on how we diagnose and treat mental disorders. Information drawn from many basic disciplines makes clear that all brain activity (and, in turn, the onset of mental disorders and their treatment) reflects the impact of disparate environmental influences on genetic and molecular processes. This insight argues strongly for NIMH's support of research on matters of profound interest to the discipline of social work. We must seek research opportunities that will establish connections across disciplines and levels, even as we continue research within single levels of analysis, including the molecular, cellular, circuits, integrative functions, organism, and psychosocial context levels, and we must be energetic in translating the knowledge we acquire into new and effective treatments and improved service delivery systems.

The first implication of an emphasis on basing clinical practice on an empirical scientific foundation is obvious: To remain relevant and accountable, all mental health clinicians must be able to read, interpret, and understand the potential for research in its applications to clinical practice. A second implication is that not only must social workers know about mental illness research, but that increasing numbers of social workers also ought to consider seeking careers or roles in research.

The need to improve the lives of people with mental disorders makes it imperative that all professionals in the field share and benefit from the insights and knowledge of others. *Advances in Mental Health Research* is an important contribution toward that end.

STEVEN E. HYMAN, MD

*Director*
*National Institute of Mental Health*

# Preface

Social workers are strategically positioned to provide the full range of preventive, treatment, and rehabilitative mental health services in today's rapidly changing health and human services systems. Social work practitioners provide a very large proportion of mental health services within the formal mental health care system and across the spectrum of health and human services. They also compose a significant proportion of the administrative personnel who manage public and private mental health services agencies. Health and social services systems are increasingly held accountable for the human and cost outcomes produced by their services. These intersecting factors spurred the development of this book, which is aimed at providing social workers (and other health care practitioners) with a readily accessible and practitioner-relevant resource on advances in mental health research for diverse populations and service systems.

The National Institute of Mental Health commissioned us to prepare this volume to commemorate the 50th anniversary of the signing of the National Mental Health Act. The book is divided into two major sections: "Research on Psychopathology" and "Mental Health Treatment and Services Research." The chapters discuss recent findings that we hope will enhance the extent to which social work practice is based on empirical data and sound knowledge.

The ultimate purpose of research and of social work is to help people solve and deal with complex and difficult human problems—including mental illnesses. Children, adolescents, adults, and families have a right to the most effective treatment and services that can be provided. The purposes of research, and of this book, are to help individuals, families, and communities in need make use of what is known and to challenge all of us to help in developing and applying the knowledge we need to help people.

We would like to thank the chapter authors and other professional colleagues who have supported this effort to further the extent to which social work contributes to research and bases its practice and education on sound empirical knowledge. We would also like to thank our families for supporting us through the many hours we spent putting this volume together.

JANET B. W. WILLIAMS, DSW
KATHLEEN ELL, DSW

# Research on Psychopathology

# The Epidemiology of Mental Disorders

Ronald C. Kessler, Jamie M. Abelson, and Shanyang Zhao

*Epidemiology* is the study of the distribution and correlates of illness in the population. *Descriptive epidemiology* is concerned with the distribution of illness onset and course. *Analytic epidemiology* is concerned with the use of nonexperimental data to elucidate causal processes involved in illness onset and course. *Experimental epidemiology* is concerned with the development and evaluation of interventions aimed at modifying risk factors to prevent illness onset or to modify illness course. Most epidemiologic studies of psychiatric disorders are either descriptive or analytic. Experimental epidemiologic studies are for the most part limited to preventive interventions for children (for reviews, see Dryfoos, 1990; Hamburg, 1992), although there also are a small number of experimental epidemiologic studies of high-risk adults (for example, Howe, Caplan, Foster, Lockshin, & McGrath, 1995; Price & Vinokur, 1995). See Rothman (1986) for an in-depth introduction to epidemiology overall and Tsuang, Tohen, and Zahner (1995) for an in-depth introduction to psychiatric epidemiology.

Although descriptive psychiatric epidemiologic studies comparing admission and discharge rates to and from asylums were carried out as early as the 17th century, it was not until the early 19th century that analytic epidemiologic studies of psychiatric disorders began to appear (Hunter & Macalpine, 1963). The latter consistently documented associations that were interpreted as showing that environmental stresses, especially stresses associated with poverty, can lead to psychiatric disorders. However, most of these early studies were hampered by the fact that they either focused on treatment statistics or assessed disorders in the community by using key informants such as physicians and clergy rather than direct assessment. These research design features led to confounding of information about illness prevalence with information about help-seeking and labeling, resulting in the underestimation of the prevalence of clinically significant psychiatric disorders.

Portions of this chapter have previously appeared in the *Encyclopedia of Mental Health* (H. Friedman, ed.), San Diego: Academic Press, 1998; *Sociology of Mental Health and Illness* (A. V. Horwitz and T. L. Scheid, eds.), New York: Cambridge University Press, in press; and *Treatment Strategies for Patients with Psychiatric Comorbidity* (S. Wetzler and W. C. Sanderson, eds.), New York: John Wiley & Sons, 1997.

The preparation of this chapter was supported by National Institute of Mental Health grants R01-MH46376, R01-MH49098, K05-MH00507, and T32-MH16806.

The end of World War II brought with it the beginning of modern psychiatric epidemiology. Evidence of widespread emotional problems in selective service recruits before the war and concerns about traumatic stress reactions in the wake of the war led to widespread concern about the prevalence and distribution of psychiatric disorders. A number of local and national surveys were carried out to study these matters. Unlike prewar studies, though, these new surveys were based on direct interviews with representative community samples.

The earliest of these postwar surveys were either carried out by clinicians or used lay interview data in combination with record data as input to clinician evaluations of caseness. In later studies, clinician judgment was abandoned in favor of less expensive, self-report symptom-rating scales that assigned each respondent a score on a continuous dimension of nonspecific psychological distress. Controversy surrounded the use of these screening scales from the onset, focusing on such things as item bias, insensitivity, restriction of symptom coverage, and the arbitrariness of decisions regarding the selection of caseness thresholds (for example, Dohrenwend & Dohrenwend, 1965; Seiler, 1973). Nonetheless, they continued to be the mainstay of community psychiatric epidemiology through the 1970s due to the combination of three factors. First, they were much less expensive to administer than clinician-based interviews. Second, compared with dichotomous clinician caseness judgments, continuous measures of distress dealt directly with the actual constellations of signs and symptoms that exist in the population rather than with the classification schemes imposed on these constellations by the committees that created the official diagnoses in the *Diagnostic and Statistical Manual of Mental Disorders* (DSM) of the American Psychiatric Association (APA). Third, the clinician-based diagnostic interviews available during this period did not have good psychometric properties when administered in community samples (Dohrenwend, Yager, Egri, & Mendelsohn, 1978).

However, there also were disadvantages of working with distress measures. Perhaps the most important of these was that there was nothing in the measures themselves that allowed researchers to discriminate between people who did and did not have clinically significant psychiatric problems. This discrimination was important for making social policy decisions regarding such things as the number of people in need of mental health services. Researchers who worked with measures of nonspecific psychological distress dealt with this problem by developing rules for classifying people with scores above a certain threshold as psychiatric cases (for example, Radloff, 1977). The precise cutpoints were usually based on statistical analyses that attempted to discriminate optimally between the scores of patients in psychiatric treatment and those of people in a community sample. However, as noted above, considerable controversy surrounded the decision of exactly where to specify cutpoints. Dichotomous diagnostic measures, in comparison, allowed this sort of discrimination to be made directly based on an evaluation of diagnostic criteria and were preferable if all else was equal. All else was not equal, however, during the first three decades after World War II. Diagnostic interviews were less than optimal because a lack of agreement existed on appropriate research diagnostic criteria and an absence of valid instruments for carrying out research diagnostic interviews.

It was not until the 1970s that the field was able to move beyond this controversy with the establishment of clear research diagnostic criteria (Feighner, Robins, & Guze, 1972) and the development of systematic research diagnostic interviews aimed at operationalizing these criteria (Endicott & Spitzer, 1978). The early interviews of this type required administration by clinicians; the interviews yielded rich data but had limited use in epidemiologic surveys because of the high costs associated with large-scale use of clinicians as interviewers. The majority of interviewers in these studies were clinical social workers. It is unsurprising, in light of the high costs and logistic complications of mounting a large-field operation using professionals of this sort as interviewers, that only a handful of such studies were carried out, were small (for example, Weissman & Myers, 1978), were based on samples that were not representative of the general population (for example, Kendler, Neale, Kessler, Heath, & Eaves, 1992), or were outside the United States in countries where the costs of clinician interviewing are much lower (for example, Dohrenwend, Levav, Shrout, & Schwartz, 1992).

Two responses to this situation occurred in the late 1970s. The first was the refinement of two-stage screening methods, in which an inexpensive first-stage screening scale can be administered by a lay interviewer to a large community sample and followed with more expensive, second-stage clinician-administered interviews for the subsample of initial respondents who screen positive along with a small subsample of those who screen negative (Newman, Shrout, & Bland, 1990). The hope was that two-stage screening would substantially reduce the costs of conducting clinician-administered community epidemiologic surveys. However, problems associated with reduced response rates resulting from the requirement of respondents participating in two interviews and the increased administrative costs associated with logistic complications in this design prevented it from being used widely in community surveys. It continues to be used in surveys of captive populations, however, such as schoolchildren in classrooms.

The second response was the development of research diagnostic interviews that could be administered by lay interviewers. The first instrument of this type was the Diagnostic Interview Schedule (DIS) (Robins, Helzer, Croughan, & Ratcliff, 1981), which was developed with support from the National Institute of Mental Health (NIMH) for use in the Epidemiologic Catchment Area (ECA) Study (Robins & Regier, 1991). Several other interviews, most of them based on the DIS, have been developed. The most widely used of these is the World Health Organization's (WHO, 1990) Composite International Diagnostic Interview (CIDI).

The remainder of this chapter will provide a selective overview of the results regarding the descriptive epidemiology of psychiatric disorders in the United States based on recent surveys that have used the DIS or CIDI to study the prevalence and correlates of DSM-III (APA, 1980) or DSM-III-R (APA, 1987) disorders. The focus will be on *lifetime prevalence*, the proportion of a population who have experienced a particular disorder at some time in their lives, and *recent prevalence*—the proportion of a population who have experienced an episode of a particular disorder over some specified recent interval of time such as the past month or the past year. Some indirect information also will be reported on *incidence*—the proportion of the subpopulation without a history of a particular disorder who have a first onset over some specified interval of time—in the presentation of age of onset curves. The latter provide a graph of the cumulative population prevalences of disorders over the life course. For a more detailed discussion of these and other commonly used descriptive statistics in psychiatric epidemiology, see Zahner, Hsieh, and Fleming (1995). Although a thorough discussion of analytic psychiatric epidemiology is beyond the scope of this review, a brief sketch of current issues in this area also is included in a later section of the chapter.

## Data Sources

The need for general population data on the prevalence of mental illness was recognized two decades ago in the report of the President's Commission on Mental Health and Illness (1978). It was impossible to undertake such a survey at that time because of the absence of a structured research diagnostic interview capable of generating reliable psychiatric diagnoses in general population samples. As noted above, NIMH, recognizing this need, funded the development of the DIS (Robins et al., 1981), a research diagnostic interview that could be administered by trained interviewers who are not clinicians. The DIS was first used in the ECA study, a landmark study that interviewed over 20,000 respondents in a series of five community epidemiologic surveys (Robins & Regier, 1991). The ECA has been the main source of data in the United States on the prevalence of psychiatric disorders and utilization of services for these disorders for the past decade (Bourdon, Rae, Locke, Narrow, & Regier, 1992; Regier et al., 1993; Robins, Locke, & Regier, 1991) and is a major source of data for the review presented in this chapter.

General population reliability and validity studies of the DIS were not carried out until after the completion of the ECA data collection (Anthony et al., 1985; Helzer et al., 1985), and the results of these methodological studies showed generally low agreement between DIS classifications and the classifications independently made by clinical reinterviewers. Questions have been raised about the accuracy of the ECA results based on these methodological studies (for example, Parker, 1987; Rogler, Malgady, & Tryon, 1992). However, other analysts have noted that the validity problems in the DIS are concentrated among respondents who either fall just short of meeting criteria or just barely meet criteria and that the errors from false positives and false negatives tend to balance to produce fairly accurate total population prevalence estimates (Robins, 1985). Although this observation provides no assurance that the different errors are counterbalanced in all important segments of the population (Dohrenwend, 1995), the documentation that this is true in the population as a whole suggests that the ECA results yield useful overall prevalence data.

Another important limitation of the ECA Study for purposes of providing representative data is that it was carried out in only five areas in the country: New Haven, Connecticut; Baltimore; Durham, North Carolina; St. Louis; and Los Angeles. Although the ECA investigators used after-the-fact weighting to combine these local data into a consolidated data file that was representative of the country as a whole on the distribution of age, sex, and race, no attempt was made to adjust the sample for the distributions of such important variables as socioeconomic status or health insurance coverage. Furthermore, it was impossible to apply any type of weighting or adjustment procedure to compensate for the fact that all five ECA sites were in urban areas that contained large, university-based hospitals. Because the interviews were conducted entirely within the metropolitan areas containing these hospitals, the results reveal nothing about areas of the country that have low access to specialty mental and addictive services, including rural areas that are not contiguous to a major metropolitan area. Of the U.S. population, 20 percent live in such areas.

This problem was addressed when NIMH funded the National Comorbidity Survey (NCS) (Kessler, McGonagle, et al., 1994), a household survey of more than 8,000 respondents ages 15 to 54 that was carried out in a widely dispersed (174 counties in 34 states) sample designed to be representative of the entire United

States. The NCS interview used a modified version of the DIS known as the CIDI (Robins et al., 1988). The CIDI expands the DIS to include diagnoses based on DSM-III-R (APA, 1987) criteria as well as the International Classification of Diseases (ICD-10) (WHO, 1990). WHO field trials of the CIDI have documented adequate reliability and validity for all diagnoses. (For a review, see Wittchen, 1994.) However, most of the WHO field trials were carried out in clinical samples. Previous research has shown that the estimated accuracy of diagnostic interviews is greater in clinical samples than in general population samples (Dohrenwend et al., 1978). Therefore, the same caution regarding diagnostic accuracy as noted above is needed in interpreting the results of the NCS.

Some assistance in evaluating the magnitude of the potential problems with the diagnoses based on the structured lay interviews in the ECA and NCS can be obtained by comparing those results with findings from the small number of modern epidemiologic surveys mentioned earlier in this chapter. Some of those surveys have used semistructured research diagnostic interviews such as the Structured Clinical Interview for DSM-III-R (SCID) (Spitzer, Williams, Gibbon, & First, 1990), administered by clinical interviewers either in an entire community sample or in a second-stage subsample of a larger community sample that was selected to overrepresent possible cases. The fact that these studies are few in number and generally based on small samples that are not entirely representative of the population makes it impossible to aggregate their results to generate an accurate portrait of the prevalence of mental illness in the U.S. population. Nonetheless, we refer to these studies in several places in the following review in an effort to provide a rough external comparison with the results based on the lay interview diagnoses obtained in the ECA and NCS surveys.

A final point regarding data sources concerns diagnostic coverage. Almost all the diagnoses are Axis I disorders in the DSM-III and DSM-III-R diagnostic systems. Not all Axis I disorders are covered in these surveys. However, the most commonly assessed Axis I disorders are mood disorders (major depression, dysthymia, and mania), anxiety disorders (generalized anxiety disorder, panic disorder, phobia, obsessive–compulsive disorder, and posttraumatic stress disorder), addictive disorders (alcohol abuse and dependence and drug abuse and dependence), and nonaffective psychoses (schizophrenia, schizophreniform disorder, schizoaffective disorder, delusional disorder, and brief reactive psychosis). Axis II disorders, which include the personality disorders and mental retardation, are generally not covered, although antisocial personality disorder (ASPD) and some measures of cognitive impairment are often assessed. The absence of information on personality disorders other than ASPD is a major omission but was necessitated by the fact that valid structured diagnostic interview methods to assess personality disorders did not exist at the time these surveys were carried out. That situation is changing rapidly, however, because several groups are working to develop measures of personality disorders that are appropriate for use in general population surveys (for example, Lenzenweger, Loranger, Korfine, & Neff, 1997; Pilkonis et al., 1995), and we can anticipate, based on this work, that future large-scale epidemiologic surveys will include comprehensive evaluations of personality disorders. For now, though, our review of evidence regarding the prevalences of personality disorders other than ASPD has to rely on the results of a small number of surveys from around the world that have been carried out using one of the recently developed assessment methods.

## Lifetime and Recent Prevalences of Axis I DSM-III-R Disorders

We focus on results from the NCS, because it is the only nationally representative survey in the United States to have assessed the prevalences of a broad range of DSM-III-R disorders. As described in more detail elsewhere (Kessler, McGonagle, et al., 1994), the NCS is based on a national household sample of 8,098 respondents ages 15 to 54, including a supplemental sample of students living in group housing, the largest segment of the population that is not in the household population. The results in Table 1-1 show NCS/DSM-III-R prevalence estimates for the lifetime and 12-month disorders assessed in the core NCS interview. The prevalence estimates are presented without exclusions for DSM-III-R hierarchy rules.

The most common psychiatric disorders assessed by the NCS are major depression and alcohol dependence. A total of 17.1 percent of respondents reported a history of a major depressive episode in their lifetimes, and 10.3 percent had had an episode in the past 12 months. A total of 14.1 percent have a lifetime history of alcohol dependence, and 7.2 percent continued to be dependent in the past 12 months. The next most common disorders are social and simple phobias, with lifetime prevalences of 13.3 percent and 11.3 percent, respectively, and 12-month prevalences of 7.9 percent and 8.8 percent, respectively. As a group, addictive disorders and anxiety disorders are somewhat more prevalent than mood disorders. Approximately one in every four respondents reported a lifetime history of at least one addictive disorder, and a similar number reported a lifetime history of at least one anxiety disorder. Approximately one in every five respondents reported a lifetime history of at least one mood disorder. Anxiety disorders as a group were considerably more likely to occur in the 12 months prior to interview (19.3 percent) than either addictive disorders (11.3 percent) or mood disorders (11.3 percent), suggesting that anxiety disorders are more chronic than either addictive disorders or mood disorders. The prevalences of other NCS disorders are much lower. Antisocial personality disorder, which was assessed only on a lifetime basis, was reported by 2.8 percent of respondents, while schizophrenia and other nonaffective psychoses (NAP) were found among 0.5 percent of respondents. It is important to note that the diagnosis of NAP was based on clinical reinterviews using the SCID rather than on the lay CIDI interviews. As documented elsewhere (Kendler, Gallagher, Abelson, & Kessler, 1996), the prevalence estimate for nonaffective psychoses based on the CIDI was considerably higher but was found to have low validity when judged in comparison with the clinical reappraisals.

A total of 49.7 percent of the sample reported a lifetime history of at least one NCS/DSM-III-R disorder and 30.9 percent had one or more disorders in the 12 months prior to the interview. Although there is no meaningful sex difference in these overall prevalences, sex differences exist in prevalences of specific disorders. Consistent with previous research (Bourdon et al., 1992; Robins et al., 1981; Robins et al., 1991), men are much more likely to have addictive disorders and ASPD than women are, whereas women are much more likely to have mood disorders (with the exception of mania, for which there is no sex difference) and anxiety disorders than men are. The data also show, consistent with a trend found in the ECA (Keith, Regier, & Rae, 1991) that women in the household population are more likely to have nonaffective psychoses than men.

It is instructive to compare these NCS results with the results of the earlier ECA study. As noted above, the ECA was carried out in five communities in the United

TABLE 1-1

## Lifetime and 12-Month Prevalences of CIDI/DSM-III-R Disorders in the NCS

| DISORDER | MALE | | | | FEMALE | | | | TOTAL | | | |
|---|---|---|---|---|---|---|---|---|---|---|---|---|
| | LIFETIME | | 12-MONTH | | LIFETIME | | 12-MONTH | | LIFETIME | | 12-MONTH | |
| | % | SE | % | SE | % | SE | % | SE | % | SE | % | SE |
| I. Mood disorders | | | | | | | | | | | | |
| Major depression | 12.7 | 0.9 | 7.7 | 0.8 | 21.3 | 0.9 | 12.9 | 0.8 | 17.1 | 0.7 | 10.3 | 0.6 |
| Dysthymia | 4.8 | 0.4 | 2.1 | 0.3 | 8.0 | 0.6 | 3.0 | 0.4 | 6.4 | 0.4 | 2.5 | 0.2 |
| Mania | 1.6 | 0.3 | 1.4 | 0.3 | 1.7 | 0.3 | 1.3 | 0.3 | 1.6 | 0.3 | 1.3 | 0.2 |
| Any mood disorder | 14.7 | 0.8 | 8.5 | 0.8 | 23.9 | 0.9 | 14.1 | 0.9 | 19.3 | 0.7 | 11.3 | 0.7 |
| II. Anxiety disorders | | | | | | | | | | | | |
| Generalized anxiety disorder | 3.6 | 0.5 | 2.0 | 0.3 | 6.6 | 0.5 | 4.3 | 0.4 | 5.1 | 0.3 | 3.1 | 0.3 |
| Panic disorder | 2.0 | 0.3 | 1.3 | 0.3 | 5.0 | 1.4 | 3.2 | 0.4 | 3.5 | 0.3 | 2.3 | 0.3 |
| Social phobia | 11.1 | 0.8 | 6.6 | 0.4 | 15.5 | 1.0 | 9.1 | 0.7 | 13.3 | 0.7 | 7.9 | 0.4 |
| Simple phobia | 6.7 | 0.5 | 4.4 | 0.5 | 15.7 | 1.1 | 13.2 | 0.9 | 11.3 | 0.6 | 8.8 | 0.5 |
| Agoraphobia | 3.5 | 0.4 | 1.7 | 0.3 | 7.0 | 0.6 | 3.8 | 0.4 | 5.3 | 0.4 | 2.8 | 0.3 |
| Posttraumatic stress disorder | 4.8 | 0.6 | 2.3 | 0.3 | 10.1 | 0.8 | 5.4 | 0.7 | 7.6 | 0.5 | 3.9 | 0.4 |
| Any anxiety disorder | 22.6 | 1.2 | 13.4 | 0.7 | 34.3 | 1.8 | 24.7 | 1.5 | 28.7 | 0.9 | 19.3 | 0.8 |
| III. Addictive disorders | | | | | | | | | | | | |
| Alcohol abuse | 12.5 | 0.8 | 3.4 | 0.4 | 6.4 | 0.6 | 1.6 | 0.2 | 9.4 | 0.5 | 2.5 | 0.2 |
| Alcohol dependence | 20.1 | 1.0 | 10.7 | 0.9 | 8.2 | 0.7 | 3.7 | 0.4 | 14.1 | 0.7 | 7.2 | 0.5 |
| Drug abuse | 5.4 | 0.5 | 1.3 | 0.2 | 3.5 | 0.4 | 0.3 | 0.1 | 4.4 | 0.3 | 0.8 | 0.1 |
| Drug dependence | 9.2 | 0.7 | 3.8 | 0.4 | 5.9 | 0.5 | 1.9 | 0.3 | 7.5 | 0.4 | 2.8 | 0.3 |
| Any addictive disorder | 35.4 | 1.2 | 16.1 | 0.7 | 17.9 | 1.1 | 6.6 | 0.4 | 26.6 | 1.0 | 11.3 | 0.5 |
| IV. Other disorders | | | | | | | | | | | | |
| Antisocial personality | 4.8 | 0.5 | — | — | 1.0 | 0.2 | — | — | 2.8 | 0.2 | — | — |
| Nonaffective psychosis[a] | 0.3 | 0.1 | 0.2 | 0.1 | 0.7 | 0.2 | 0.4 | 0.1 | 0.5 | 0.1 | 0.3 | 0.1 |
| V. Any NCS disorder | 51.2 | 1.6 | 29.4 | 1.0 | 48.5 | 2.0 | 32.3 | 1.6 | 49.7 | 1.2 | 30.9 | 1.0 |

NOTES: All disorders are operationalized using DSM-III-R criteria ignoring diagnostic hierarchy rules. Mania has been redefined based on methodological refinements described by Kessler, Rubinow, Holmes, Abelson, & Zhao (1997). Agoraphobia is defined here with or without panic. It was defined with or without panic in Kessler, McGonagle, et al. (1994). Posttraumatic stress disorder was not reported in Kessler, McGonagle, et al. (1994) because the disorder was assessed only in the Part II NCS sample. Nonaffective psychosis is redefined based on methodological refinements described by Kendler, Gallagher, Abelson, & Kessler (1996). SE = standard error; NCS = National Comorbidity Survey.

[a]Nonaffective psychosis = schizophrenia, schizophreniform disorder, schizoaffective disorder, delusional disorder, and atypical psychosis.

SOURCE: Adapted from Kessler, R. C., McGonagle, K. A., Zhao, S., Nelson, C. B., Hughes, M., Eshleman, S., Wittchen, H-U., & Kendler, K. S. (1994). Lifetime and 12-month prevalence of DSM-III-R psychiatric disorders in the United States: Results from the National Comorbidity Survey, *Archives of General Psychiatry, 51*, 8–19. Copyright 1994, American Medical Association.

States, and the results were subsequently combined and weighted to the population distribution of the United States on the cross-classification of age, sex, and race in an effort to make national estimates (Regier et al., 1993). To the extent that this poststratification succeeded in adjusting for the lack of representativeness of the local samples, it should be possible to make valid comparisons between the ECA and NCS results. A limitation in doing this is that the ECA was based on an unrestricted age range of adults, whereas the NCS was based on the 15 to 54 age range. Another limitation is that the ECA diagnoses were based on DSM-III criteria (APA, 1980), whereas the NCS diagnoses were based on DSM-III-R criteria (APA, 1987). These two diagnostic systems differ substantially in a number of respects. To resolve these problems, collaborative ECA–NCS comparative analyses have been carried out in which subsamples in the 18 to 54 age range in both samples were compared using common measures that operationalize DSM-III criteria, which can be reconstructed from the NCS data, although DSM-III-R criteria cannot be reconstructed from the ECA data. The as yet unpublished results show a great deal of consistency between the two surveys, both in the prevalences of individual disorders and in the overall prevalence of having any disorder (Regier et al., in press).

## Personality Disorders

Although the concept of personality disorder can be traced back to the beginnings of 19th-century psychiatry (for a review, see Tyrer, Casey, & Ferguson, 1991), it has only recently become the subject of epidemiologic research because standardized diagnostic criteria became available for the first time with the ICD-9 (WHO, 1977) and DSM-III (APA, 1980) classification systems. Unfortunately, it has proved to be difficult to develop reliable and valid measures of personality disorders (Perry, 1992; Zimmerman, 1994). Furthermore, there are a number of differences between the ICD and DSM systems (Blashfield, 1991) as well as substantial changes within each system in recent revisions (Morey, 1988) that add to the complexity of synthesizing the available epidemiologic evidence.

All classification schemes recognize three broad clusters of personality disorder, each defined by a series of traits that must be manifest habitually in a number of life domains to qualify as a disorder: (1) the odd cluster (for example, paranoid or schizoid personality disorders), (2) the dramatic cluster (for example, histrionic or borderline personality disorders), and (3) the anxious cluster (for example, avoidant or dependent personality disorders). A recent comprehensive international review of the epidemiology of personality disorders found only four fairly small community studies that assessed personality disorders in all three of these clusters using valid assessment methods (de Girolamo & Reich, 1993). These four studies yielded consistent lifetime prevalence estimates for overall personality disorders ranging from 10.3 percent to 13.5 percent. Caution is needed in interpreting these results, however, because previous research has shown that prevalence estimates vary substantially depending on whether, as in these surveys, full diagnostic criteria for personality disorders are required or respondents are counted if they manifest some traits of personality disorders on dimensional scales (Kass, 1985).

A number of community surveys have included assessments of one or more specific personality disorders without attempting to assess the full range of personality disturbances. By far the most commonly studied of these has been ASPD, which is characterized by persistent evidence of "irresponsible and antisocial behavior beginning in childhood or early adolescence and continuing into adulthood" (APA, 1987).

Irritability, aggressiveness, persistent reckless behavior, promiscuity, and the absence of remorse about the effects of their behavior on others are cardinal features of ASPD. A number of epidemiologic surveys, including both the ECA and NCS, have found lifetime prevalences of ASPD averaging about 1 percent among women and 4 percent to 5 percent among men (de Girolamo & Reich, 1993; Merikangas, 1988). Much less is known about the prevalences of other individual personality disorders, although the available evidence suggests that none of them alone has a prevalence greater than about 2 percent in the general population (de Girolamo & Reich, 1993; Merikangas, 1988; Weissman, 1993).

## Comorbidity

An important observation about the results in Table 1-1 is that the sum of the individual prevalence estimates across the disorders in each row consistently exceeds the prevalence of having any disorder in the last row. This means that there is a good deal of comorbidity among these disorders. For example, whereas the 49.7 percent lifetime prevalence in the total NCS sample means that 50 respondents out of every 100 in the sample reported a lifetime history of at least one disorder, a summation of lifetime prevalence estimates for the separate disorders shows that these 50 people reported a total of 102 lifetime disorders. This comorbidity is important for understanding the distribution of psychiatric disorders in the United States (Kessler, 1995). Although it is beyond the scope of this chapter to delve into the many types of comorbidity in the population, some aggregate results are important to review.

The results presented in Table 1-2 document that comorbidity is important in understanding the distribution of psychiatric disorders among people ages 15 to 54 in the United States. These results also provide an empirical rationale for more detailed examination of particular types of comorbidity. The four horizontal rows of Table 1-2 represent the number of lifetime disorders reported by respondents. The

TABLE **1-2**

### Concentration of Lifetime and 12-Month CIDI/DSM-III-R Disorders among People with Lifetime Comorbidity in the NCS

| NO. OF LIFETIME DISORDERS | PROPORTION OF SAMPLE | | PROPORTION OF LIFETIME DISORDERS | | PROPORTION OF 12-MONTH DISORDERS | | PROPORTION OF RESPONDENTS WITH SEVERE 12-MONTH DISORDERS[a] | |
|---|---|---|---|---|---|---|---|---|
| | % | SE | % | SE | % | SE | % | SE |
| 0 | 52.0 | 1.1 | — | — | — | — | — | — |
| 1 | 21.0 | 0.6 | 20.6 | 0.6 | 17.4 | 0.8 | 2.6 | 1.7 |
| 2 | 13.0 | 0.5 | 25.5 | 1.0 | 23.1 | 1.0 | 7.9 | 2.1 |
| 3 or more | 14.0 | 0.7 | 53.9 | 2.7 | 58.9 | 1.8 | 89.5 | 2.8 |

NOTES: The 52 percent with no lifetime disorder is inconsistent with the 51.2 percent with any disorder reported in Table 1-1 because NCS Part II disorders were excluded from the calculations in Table 1-2. SE = standard error; NCS = National Comorbidity Survey.

[a]Severe 12-month disorders = active mania, nonaffective psychoses, or active disorders of other types that either required hospitalization or created severe role impairment.

SOURCE: Kessler, R. C., McGonagle, K. A., Zhao, S., Nelson, C. B., Hughes, M., Eshleman, S., Wittchen, H-U., & Kendler, K. S. (1994). Lifetime and 12-month prevalence of DSM-III-R psychiatric disorders in the United States: Results from the National Comorbidity Survey. *Archives of General Psychiatry, 51,* 8–19. Copyright 1994, American Medical Association.

set of disorders considered here is somewhat smaller than in Table 1-1, accounting for the fact that 52 percent of respondents are estimated as never having any NCS/DSM-III-R disorder (which means that 48 percent are estimated to have one or more such disorders, which is smaller than the 49.7 percent in Table 1-1), 21 percent as having one, 13 percent as having two, and 14 percent as having three or more disorders.

Only 21 percent of all the lifetime disorders occurred in respondents with a lifetime history of just one disorder. This means that the vast majority of lifetime disorders in this sample (79 percent) are comorbid disorders. Furthermore, an even greater proportion of 12-month disorders occurred in respondents with a lifetime history of comorbidity. It is particularly striking that close to six out of every 10 (58.9 percent) 12-month disorders and nearly nine out of 10 (89.5 percent) severe 12-month disorders occurred to the 14 percent of the sample with a lifetime history of three or more disorders. These results show that whereas a history of some psychiatric disorder is common among people ages 15 to 54 in the United States, the major burden of psychiatric disorders in this sector of society is concentrated in a group of people with high comorbidity, who constitute about one-sixth of the population.

Given this evidence, it is of some interest to learn more about detailed patterns of comorbidity. The ECA investigators were the first to do this in a community sample. They documented that comorbidity is widespread; over 54 percent of ECA respondents with a lifetime history of at least one DSM-III psychiatric disorder were found to have a second diagnosis as well. Fifty-two percent of people with lifetime alcohol abuse received a second diagnosis, and 75 percent of people with lifetime drug abuse had a second diagnosis (Robins et al., 1991). Compared with respondents with no mental disorder, respondents with a lifetime history of at least one mental disorder had a relative-odds of 2.3 of having a lifetime history of alcohol abuse or dependence and a relative-odds of 4.5 of some other drug use disorder (Regier et al., 1990). Similar results were found in the NCS. Fifty-six percent of the respondents with a lifetime history of at least one DSM-III-R disorder also had one or more other disorders (Kessler, 1995). Fifty-two percent of respondents with lifetime alcohol abuse or dependence also had a lifetime mental disorder, whereas 36 percent had a lifetime illicit drug use disorder. Fifty-nine percent of the respondents with a lifetime history of illicit drug abuse or dependence also had a lifetime mental disorder and 71 percent had a lifetime alcohol use disorder.

The results in Table 1-3 show the proportions of people having each lifetime NCS/DSM-III-R disorder who reported at least one other lifetime disorder. Lifetime comorbidity is the norm, with proportions ranging from a low of 62.1 percent for alcohol abuse to a high of 99.4 percent for mania. The average proportion of comorbidity among disorders is 86.6 percent. This does not mean that 86.6 percent of people with one or more lifetime disorders have comorbidity, though, as those with comorbidity are counted multiple times in Table 1-3. Instead, 59.8 percent of the people who ever had one of the disorders considered in the NCS also had one or more other disorders.

Data on lifetime comorbidities of specific pairs of disorders in the NCS are reported in Table 1-4. Results are shown in the form of odds-ratios (ORs), statistics that describe the relationship between two disorders as the odds of having disorder A in patients who have disorder B, divided by the odds of having disorder A in patients who do not have disorder B. An OR of 1.0 means that there is no relationship between the two disorders, whereas an OR greater than 1.0 means that there is a positive relationship, and an OR less than 1.0 means that there is a negative

TABLE **1-3**

## Lifetime Comorbidity among NCS/DSM-III-R Disorders

| DISORDER | PROPORTION OF PEOPLE WITH LIFETIME COMORBIDITY AMONG THOSE HAVING THE DISORDER | |
|---|---|---|
| | % | SE |
| I. Mood disorders | | |
| Major depression | 83.1 | 2.2 |
| Dysthymia | 91.3 | 1.8 |
| Mania | 99.4 | 0.6 |
| Any mood disorder | 82.2 | 2.1 |
| II. Anxiety disorders | | |
| Generalized anxiety disorder | 91.3 | 1.5 |
| Panic disorder | 92.2 | 1.9 |
| Social phobia | 81.0 | 1.5 |
| Simple phobia | 83.4 | 1.5 |
| Agoraphobia | 87.3 | 2.9 |
| Posttraumatic stress disorder | 81.0 | 3.3 |
| Any anxiety disorder | 74.1 | 1.5 |
| III. Addictive disorders | | |
| Alcohol abuse | 62.1 | 2.6 |
| Alcohol dependence | 80.6 | 2.4 |
| Illicit drug abuse | 89.0 | 2.6 |
| Illicit drug dependence | 95.7 | 2.0 |
| Any addictive disorder | 73.3 | 1.3 |
| IV. Other disorders | | |
| Antisocial personality | 96.2 | 1.0 |
| Nonaffective psychosis | 93.0 | 4.4 |
| V. Any NCS disorder | 59.8 | 1.2 |

NOTES: All disorders are operationalized using DSM-III-R criteria ignoring diagnostic hierarchy rules. SE = standard error; NCS = National Comorbidity Survey.

SOURCE: Kessler, R. C. (1997). The prevalence of psychiatric comorbidity. In S. Wetzler & W. C. Sanderson (Eds.), *Treatment strategies for patients with psychiatric comorbidity.* Copyright © 1997 John Wiley & Sons. Reprinted by permission of John Wiley & Sons. Inc.

relationship. A more detailed discussion of ORs is presented by Hillis and Woolson (1995). Diagnostic hierarchy rules were not used in making these calculations so as to avoid artificially deflating estimates of comorbidity. The exceptions are substance abuse and dependence, which are defined in such a way as to be mutually exclusive.

As shown in Table 1-4, all but four of the 118 ORs are greater than 1.0. This means that there is a positive association between the lifetime occurrences of almost every pair of disorders considered here. However, there is a great deal of variation in the size of the ORs. It is conceivable that this variation is due to random error. To determine whether this is the case, a comparison was made between the ORs presented here and ORs obtained by reanalyzing data from the ECA study. This comparison found a rank-order correlation between the two sets of ORs of 0.79 (Kessler, 1995), which demonstrates that the variation in ORs is systematic rather than random.

Several patterns related to this variation are worthy of note. First, one would expect that the relative sizes of the ORs would show the disorders of a single type to

## Lifetime Comorbidities (Odds-Ratios) between Pairs of NCS/DSM-III-R Disorders

| DISORDER | MOOD DISORDERS | | | ANXIETY DISORDERS | | | | | | SUBSTANCE USE DISORDERS | | | | OTHER DISORDERS | |
|---|---|---|---|---|---|---|---|---|---|---|---|---|---|---|---|
| | MD | DD | MA | GAD | PD | SOC | SIM | AG | PTSD | AA | AD | DA | DD | CD | AAB |
| I. Mood disorders | | | | | | | | | | | | | | | |
| Major depression (MD) | | | | | | | | | | | | | | | |
| Dysthymia (DD) | 14.4* | | | | | | | | | | | | | | |
| Mania (MA) | 18.0* | 8.2* | | | | | | | | | | | | | |
| II. Anxiety disorders | | | | | | | | | | | | | | | |
| Generalized anxiety disorder (GAD) | 9.7* | 13.6* | 10.4* | | | | | | | | | | | | |
| Panic disorder (PD) | 7.0* | 5.2* | 11.0* | 12.3* | | | | | | | | | | | |
| Social phobia (SOC) | 3.6* | 3.2* | 4.6* | 3.8* | 4.8* | | | | | | | | | | |
| Simple phobia (SIM) | 4.5* | 3.4* | 10.1* | 4.9* | 7.9* | 7.8* | | | | | | | | | |
| Agoraphobia (AG) | 4.8* | 3.1* | 7.9* | 5.8* | 11.9* | 7.1* | 8.7* | | | | | | | | |
| Posttraumatic stress disorder (PTSD) | 5.3* | 5.1* | 6.4* | 3.9* | 3.9* | 2.8* | 3.8* | 4.2* | | | | | | | |
| III. Addictive disorders | | | | | | | | | | | | | | | |
| Alcohol abuse (AA) | 0.9 | 0.9 | 0.9 | 0.8 | 1.0 | 1.2 | 1.3* | 1.0 | 0.7* | | | | | | |
| Alcohol dependence (AD) | 2.7* | 3.0* | 7.0* | 2.7* | 2.0* | 2.2* | 2.1* | 1.7* | 2.6* | — | | | | | |
| Drug abuse (DA) | 1.7* | 1.4 | 1.1 | 1.5 | 1.6 | 1.2 | 1.1 | 0.9 | 1.6* | 5.8* | 3.8* | | | | |
| Drug dependence (DD) | 2.8* | 3.0* | 7.2* | 3.8* | 3.8* | 2.6* | 2.5* | 2.9* | 4.0* | 2.3* | 11.9* | — | | | |
| IV. Other disorders | | | | | | | | | | | | | | | |
| Conduct disorder (CD) | 1.9* | 2.0* | 5.8* | 1.8* | 1.6* | 2.1* | 1.8* | 1.9* | 2.2* | 2.0* | 5.6* | 2.6* | 5.3* | | |
| Adult antisocial behavior (AAB) | 2.4* | 3.0* | 7.3* | 3.6* | 2.2* | 2.9* | 2.5* | 2.6* | 3.5* | 1.8* | 10.7* | 2.8* | 13.7* | 13.9* | |
| Nonaffective psychosis | 7.0* | 4.2* | 12.3* | 6.1* | 7.0* | 3.0* | 2.5* | 4.0* | 5.1* | 1.1 | 3.3* | 1.2 | 5.4* | 2.6* | 9.3* |

NOTES: All disorders are operationalized using DSM-III-R criteria ignoring diagnostic hierarchy rules. NCS = National Comorbidity Survey.

*p = 0.05, two-tailed test.

SOURCE: Kessler, R. C. (1997). The prevalence of psychiatric comorbidity. In S. Wetzler & W. C. Sanderson (Eds.), *Treatment strategies for patients with psychiatric comorbidity*. Copyright © 1997 John Wiley & Sons, Inc. Reprinted by permission of John Wiley & Sons. Inc.

be more strongly related to each other than to disorders of another type. This is generally true. For example, mood disorders are strongly related to other mood disorders. However, the strength of these pairwise associations among mood disorders is generally stronger than within the anxiety disorders, with an average OR of 13.5 for mood disorders, compared with 6.2 for anxiety disorders. Second, most mood and anxiety disorders are strongly related to each other. In fact, pairwise associations between a mood disorder and an anxiety disorder (averaging 6.6) are generally stronger than between two anxiety disorders. Third, despite a substantial clinical literature pointing to the importance of comorbidity between mood disorders and addictive disorders (for example, Allen & Frances, 1986; Penick, Powell, Liskow, & Jackson, 1988) and between anxiety disorders and addictive disorders (for example, Chambless, Cherney, Caputo, & Rheinstein, 1987; Roy et al., 1991), they are among the weakest comorbidities in the table (averaging 2.4).

One of the main purposes of investigating comorbid disorders is to help refine definitions of syndromes and diagnoses. With this in mind, it is important to recognize that some of the strongest ORs in the table are associated with clusters that are generally recognized as disorders in their own right. The largest OR is between major depression and mania, a conjunction that represents bipolar disorder. Another strong OR is between mania and nonaffective psychosis, a conjunction that is part of the definition of schizoaffective disorder. There also are a number of strong ORs that are linked to discussions in the clinical literature of heretofore unrecognized disorders. For example, the suggestion has been made that comorbidity between major depression and mania is often due to a phasic panic–depressive illness characterized by panic, depressive, and mixed anxious–depressive phases (Akiskal, 1986). This possibility is consistent with the finding of a strong OR between panic and depression in the table.

## Ages of Onset

The ECA and NCS studies both collected retrospective data on the ages of first onset of each lifetime disorder. They were consistent in showing that simple and social phobia have a much earlier age of onset than the other disorders considered here (Burke, Burke, Rae, & Regier, 1991; Magee, Eaton, Wittchen, McGonagle, & Kessler, 1996), with simple phobia often beginning during middle or late childhood and social phobia during late childhood or early adolescence. Substance abuse was found to have a typical age of onset during the late teens or early 20s. A substantial proportion of people with lifetime major depression and dysthymia also reported that their first episode occurred before age 20. Some other disorders, such as generalized anxiety disorder and mania, had later ages of onset, but the most striking overall impression from the data as a whole is that most psychiatric disorders have first onsets early in life.

Given the importance of comorbidity, a related question concerns which disorders in comorbid sets have the earliest ages of onset. The results in the first column of Table 1-5 show that there is considerable variation across disorders in the probability of being the first lifetime disorder. Simple phobia, social phobia, alcohol abuse, and conduct disorder are the only four disorders considered here where the majority of lifetime cases are temporally primary in this way. In general, anxiety disorders are most likely to be temporally primary, with 82.8 percent of NCS respondents having one or more anxiety disorders reporting that one of these was their first lifetime disorder compared with 71.1 percent of those with conduct disorder, 43.8 percent of

TABLE **1-5**

**Percent and Distribution of Temporally Primary NCS/DSM-III-R Disorders**

| DISORDER | PERCENT TEMPORALLY PRIMARY AMONG THOSE HAVING THE DISORDER | | DISTRIBUTION OF TEMPORALLY PRIMARY DISORDER | |
|---|---|---|---|---|
| | % | SE | % | SE |
| I. Mood disorders | | | | |
| Major depression | 41.1 | 2.7 | 13.4 | 0.9 |
| Dysthymia | 37.7 | 3.1 | 4.8 | 0.5 |
| Mania | 20.2 | 6.0 | 0.7 | 0.2 |
| Any mood disorder | 43.8 | 2.4 | 16.4 | 0.9 |
| II. Anxiety disorders | | | | |
| Generalized anxiety disorder | 37.0 | 2.9 | 3.6 | 0.4 |
| Panic disorder | 23.3 | 3.2 | 1.6 | 0.2 |
| Social phobia | 63.1 | 2.0 | 16.0 | 0.9 |
| Simple phobia | 67.6 | 2.7 | 14.5 | 1.0 |
| Agoraphobia | 45.2 | 4.0 | 5.9 | 0.7 |
| Posttraumatic stress disorder | 52.1 | 3.0 | 7.5 | 0.7 |
| Any anxiety disorder | 82.8 | 1.3 | 45.3 | 1.4 |
| III. Addictive disorders | | | | |
| Alcohol abuse | 57.0 | 2.3 | 10.2 | 0.6 |
| Alcohol dependence | 36.8 | 3.1 | 9.9 | 0.6 |
| Illicit drug abuse | 39.7 | 3.0 | 3.4 | 0.3 |
| Illicit drug dependence | 20.8 | 2.5 | 3.0 | 0.3 |
| Any addictive disorder | 48.1 | 1.6 | 24.5 | 1.0 |
| IV. Other disorders | | | | |
| Conduct disorder | 71.1 | 2.0 | 17.7 | 1.0 |
| Adult antisocial behavior | 14.0 | 1.8 | 1.4 | 0.2 |
| Nonaffective psychosis | 28.8 | 5.6 | 0.4 | 0.1 |

NOTES: All disorders are operationalized using DSM-III-R criteria ignoring diagnostic hierarchy rules. SE = standard error; NCS = National Comorbidity Survey.

SOURCE: Kessler, R. C. (1997). The prevalence of psychiatric comorbidity. In S. Wetzler & W. C. Sanderson (Eds.), *Treatment strategies for patients with psychiatric comorbidity.* Copyright © 1997 John Wiley & Sons. Reprinted by permission of John Wiley & Sons. Inc.

those with a mood disorder, and 48.1 percent of those with a substance use disorder. Results in the third column of the table show the percentage of overall respondents who reported each disorder as temporally primary. Once again anxiety disorders are more likely to be temporally primary (45.3 percent of all lifetime cases) than are mood disorders (16.4 percent), substance use disorders (24.5 percent), or other disorders (19.5 percent).

## Utilization of Services

Only a minority of those with a lifetime NCS/DSM-III-R disorder (42.0 percent) reported ever obtaining professional treatment for their problems. The proportions treated in the mental health specialty sector (26.2 percent) or in a substance abuse treatment setting (8.4 percent) are even smaller. Only about one-fifth of respondents who reported an episode of a disorder during the year before interview obtained any professional treatment during that year, and only about half of those people were seen in a mental or addictive disorders specialty setting. These results are consistent with those of the ECA study (Regier et al., 1993) and suggest that there is considerable unmet need for services. It is worth noting, however, that strong relationships exist between the of number and severity of disorders and the probability of obtaining professional help.

## Social Consequences

The recent debates concerning the place of mental health coverage in health care reform has led to a new interest on the part of psychiatric epidemiologists in the social consequences of psychiatric disorders. A number of recent studies of this issue have documented that psychiatric disorders have substantial personal costs for the people who experience them as well as for their families and communities in terms of both finances (Kessler, Foster, Saunders, & Stang, 1995) and role functioning (Rhode, Lewinsohn, & Seeley, 1990; Wells et al., 1989; Wohlfarth, van den Brink, Ormel, Koeter, & Oldehinkel, 1993). Data from the ECA showed that people with psychiatric disorders have considerably more work loss days than others (Broadhead, Blazer, George, & Kit, 1990; Johnson, Weissman, & Klerman, 1992), a result replicated in the NCS (Kessler & Frank, 1997). NCS analyses also showed that early-onset psychiatric disorders are strongly related to subsequent teenage childbearing, school dropout, marital instability, and long-term financial adversity (Kessler et al., 1995; Kessler et al., 1997; Kessler & Forthofer, in press). These results document hidden societal costs of psychiatric disorders not only in the indirect sense of threats to our ability to maintain an educated and well-functioning citizenry and work force but also in the direct sense that the outcomes documented here are associated with increased use of entitlement programs, such as unemployment and welfare, which are paid for by all taxpayers. These costs need to be taken into consideration in policy evaluations of the societal cost–benefit ratio of comparing providing mental health treatment irrespective of ability to pay with the costs of failing to do so.

## Analytic Epidemiology

In analytic epidemiology, the ultimate interest is in pinpointing potentially modifiable risk factors that can be subjected to experimental evaluation to develop interventions for prevention or amelioration of disease outcomes. Analytic epidemiology is such a fertile research arena that no single chapter could provide a thorough overview of contemporary research. However, several broad themes can be detected and critical works cited to provide a road map for the reader who is interested in pursuing a more in-depth investigation of this literature. Three of these themes are mentioned here, concerning the effects of stress, stress-modifiers, and genetic predisposition.

The first of these broad themes involves the intuition that stressful life experiences play a part in bringing about the onset of many psychiatric disorders. A useful recent overview of research on this theme can be found in *Does Stress Cause Psychiatric Illness?* edited by Carolyn Mazure (1995). Part of the research on this theme is concerned with the long-term effects of exposure to childhood adversities on adult psychopathology (for example, Kendler, Davis, & Kessler, 1997). Another part is concerned with the triggering effects of adult stressful life events on episode onsets of recurrent disorders (for example, Kessler, 1995). Still another part is concerned with the effects of exposure to chronic role-related stresses on such widely documented associations as the higher prevalence of depression among women than men (for example, McGrath, Keita, Strickland, & Russo, 1990) and the higher prevalence of most psychiatric disorders among lower- than among middle-class people (Dohrenwend et al., 1992).

Although this research consistently shows that stress is significantly related to psychiatric disorder, it also finds that a substantial proportion of people who are exposed to even the most severe types of stress do not develop clinically significant psychiatric problems as a result of this exposure. This observation has led to a second dominant theme in analytic psychiatric epidemiology, one that emphasizes the importance of individual differences in vulnerability to stress. Active lines of research exist on a number of presumed stress modifiers, including social support (Kessler, Kendler, Heath, Neale, & Eaves, 1992), appraisal and coping processes (Taylor & Aspinwall, 1996), social identities (Burke, 1996), and personality (Gilbert & Connolly, 1991). Much of the currently active work on interventions for stress-related psychiatric disorders operates by attempting to manipulate these sorts of stress modifiers. A third dominant theme is that genetic factors play an important part in most common psychiatric disorders, a finding that has been clearly and consistently documented in a number of epidemiologic studies based on either twin or adoption designs (Kendler et al., 1995; Tsuang & Farone, 1990). Population genetic studies of psychiatric disorders estimate such things as the proportion of variance in disorders from genetic factors (for example, Kendler et al., 1992) and the extent to which genetic variation operates as a stress modifier (for example, Kessler, Kendler, Heath, Neale, & Eaves, 1994).

## Conclusion

Psychiatric disorders are highly prevalent in the general population. Although no truly comprehensive assessment of all Axis I and Axis II disorders has been carried out in a general population sample, it is almost certainly the case that such a study would find that the majority of the population has experienced at least one of these disorders. Although such a result might initially seem remarkable, it is actually easy to understand. The DSM classification system is very broad. It includes a number of disorders that are usually self-limiting and not severely impairing. It should be no more surprising to find that half the population has had one or more of these disorders than to find that the vast majority of the population has had the flu or measles or some other common physical malady at some time in their life.

The more surprising result is that although many people have been touched by mental illness at some time in their lives, the major burden of psychiatric disorder in the population is concentrated in the relatively small subset of people who are highly comorbid. This means that a pile-up of multiple disorders is the most important defining characteristic of serious mental illness, a result that points to the previously underappreciated importance of research on the primary prevention of secondary disorders (Kessler & Price, 1993). It also means that epidemiologic information about the prevalences of individual disorders is much less important than information on the prevalences of functional impairment, comorbidity, and chronicity. This realization has led to a recent interest in functional impairment in the changes in diagnostic criteria in DSM-IV (APA, 1994). This same emphasis also can be seen in the emphasis of NIMH's National Advisory Mental Health Council (1993) on what they defined as "severe and persistent mental illness" (SPMI) and the emphasis of the Substance Abuse and Mental Health Service Administration (1993) on what they defined as "serious mental illness" (SMI). Joint methodological analyses of the ECA and NCS suggest that the one-year prevalences of DSM-III-R SPMI and SMI are approximately 3 percent and 6 percent, respectively, compared with one-year prevalences of any DSM-III-R disorder in excess of 30 percent (Kessler et al., 1996). It is likely that epidemiologic research on adult mental disorders over the next decade will focus on these serious and severe disorders rather than on overall prevalence. To the extent that the prevalences of particular disorders are emphasized in this work, it will likely be to study the underlying pathologies associated with ongoing impairment in functioning. An increased interest in the part played by personality disorders in the creation of ongoing role impairment is likely to emerge over the next decade in light of recent advances in conceptualization and measurement (Loranger, Sartorius, & Janca, 1996). There also is going to be a considerable expansion of research on the epidemiology of child and adolescent disorders, a topic that has not been covered in this chapter, because new initiatives have not yet advanced far enough to be reviewed here.

# References

Akiskal, H. S. (1986). Mood disturbances. In G. Winokur & P. Clayton (Eds.), *The medical basis of psychiatry* (pp. 365–379). Philadelphia: W. B. Saunders.

Allen, M. H., & Frances, R. J. (1986). Varieties of psychopathology found in patients with addictive disorders: A review. In R. E. Meyer (Ed.), *Psychopathology and addictive disorders* (pp. 17–38). New York: Guilford Press.

American Psychiatric Association. (1980). *Diagnostic and statistical manual of mental disorders* (3rd ed.). Washington, DC: Author.

American Psychiatric Association. (1987). *Diagnostic and statistical manual of mental disorders* (3rd ed., rev.). Washington, DC: Author.

American Psychiatric Association. (1994). *Diagnostic and statistical manual of mental disorders* (4th ed.). Washington, DC: Author.

Anthony, J. C., Folstein, M., Romanoski, A. J., Von Korff, M. R., Nestadt, G. R., Chahal, R., Merchant, A., Brown, C. H., Shapiro, S., Kramer, M., & Gruenberg, E. M. (1985). Comparison of the lay Diagnostic Interview Schedule and a standardized psychiatric diagnosis: Experience in eastern Baltimore. *Archives of General Psychiatry, 42,* 667–675.

Blashfield, R. K. (1991). An American view of the ICD-10 personality disorders. *Acta Psychiatrica Scandinavica, 82,* 250–256.

Bourdon, K. H., Rae, D. A., Locke, B. Z., Narrow, W. E., & Regier, D. A. (1992). Estimating the prevalence of mental disorders in U.S. adults from the Epidemiologic Catchment Area Study. *Public Health Report, 107,* 663–668.

Broadhead, W. E., Blazer, D. G., George, L. K., & Kit, T. C. (1990). Depression, disability days, and days lost from work in a prospective epidemiologic survey. *JAMA, 264,* 2524–2528.

Burke, K. C., Burke, J. D., Rae, D. S., & Regier, D. A. (1991). Comparing age of onset of major depression and other psychiatric disorders by birth cohorts in five U.S. community populations. *Archives of General Psychiatry, 48*, 789–795.

Burke, P. J. (1996). Social identities and psychosocial stress. In H. B. Kaplan (Ed.), *Psychosocial stress: Perspectives on structure, theory, life-course, and methods* (pp. 141–174). San Diego: Academic Press.

Chambless, D. L., Cherney, J., Caputo G. D., & Rheinstein, B. J. (1987). Anxiety disorders and alcoholism. *Journal of Anxiety Disorders, 1*, 24–40.

de Girolamo, G., & Reich, J. H. (1993). *Epidemiology of mental disorders and psychosocial problems: Personality disorders.* Geneva: World Health Organization.

Dohrenwend, B. P. (1995). The problem of validity in field studies of psychological disorders—revisited. In M. T. Tsuang, M. Tohen, & G.E.P. Zahner (Eds.), *Textbook in psychiatric epidemiology* (pp. 3–22). New York: John Wiley & Sons.

Dohrenwend, B. P., & Dohrenwend, B. S. (1965). The problem of validity in field studies of psychological disorder. *Journal of Abnormal Psychology, 70*, 52–69.

Dohrenwend, B. P., Levav, I., Shrout, P. E., & Schwartz, S. (1992). Socioeconomic status and psychiatric disorders: The causation selection issue. *Science, 255*, 946–952.

Dohrenwend, B. P., Yager, T. J., Egri, G., & Mendelsohn, F. S. (1978). The psychiatric status schedule (PSS) as a measure of dimensions of psychopathology in the general population. *Archives of General Psychiatry, 35*, 731–739.

Dryfoos, J. G. (1990). *Adolescents at risk.* New York: Oxford University Press.

Endicott, J., & Spitzer, R. (1978). A diagnostic interview: The Schedule for Affective Disorders and Schizophrenia. *Archives of General Psychiatry, 35*, 837–844.

Feighner, J. P., Robins, E., & Guze, S. B. (1972). Diagnostic criteria for use in psychiatric research. *Archives of General Psychiatry, 26*, 57–63.

Gilbert, D. G., & Connolly, J. J. (1991). *Personality, social skills, and psychopathology: An individual differences approach.* New York: Plenum Press.

Hamburg, D. A. (1992). *Today's children: Creating a future for a generation in crisis.* New York: Random House.

Helzer, J. E., Stoltzman, R. K., Farmer, A., Brockington, I. F., Plesons, D., Singerman, B., & Works, J. (1985). Comparing the DIS with a DIS/DSM-III–based physician reevaluation. In W. W. Eaton & L. G. Kessler (Eds.), *Epidemiologic field methods in psychiatry* (pp. 285–308). Orlando, FL: Academic Press.

Hillis, S. L., & Woolson, R. F. (1995). Analysis of categorical data: Use of the odds ratio as a measure of association. In M. T. Tsuang, M. Tohen, & G. E. P. Zahner (Eds.), *Textbook in psychiatric epidemiology* (pp. 55–80). New York: John Wiley & Sons.

Howe, G. W., Caplan, R. D., Foster, D., Lockshin, M., & McGrath, C. (1995). When couples cope with job loss. A research strategy for developing preventative interventions. In L. R. Murphy, J. J. Hurrell, S. L. Sauter, & G. P. Keita (Eds.), *Job stress interventions* (pp. 131–158). Washington, DC: American Psychological Association.

Hunter, R., & Macalpine, I. (Eds.). (1963). *Three hundred years of psychiatry.* Oxford, England: Oxford University Press.

Johnson, J., Weissman, M. M., & Klerman, G. L. (1992). Service utilization and social morbidity associated with depressive symptoms in the community. *JAMA, 267*, 1478–1483.

Kass, F. (1985). Scaled ratings of DSM-III personality disorders. *American Journal of Psychiatry, 142*, 627–630.

Keith, S. J., Regier, D. A., & Rae, D. S. (1991). Schizophrenic disorders. In L. N. Robins & D. A. Regier (Eds.), *Psychiatric disorders in America: The Epidemiologic Catchment Area Study* (pp. 33–52). New York: Free Press.

Kendler, K. S., Davis, C. G., & Kessler, R. C. (1997). The familial aggregation of common psychiatric and substance use disorders in the National Comorbidity Study: A family history study. *British Journal of Psychiatry, 170,* 541–548.

Kendler, K. S., Gallagher, T. J., Abelson, J. M., & Kessler, R. C. (1996). Lifetime prevalence, demographic risk factors and diagnostic validity of nonaffective psychosis as assessed in a U.S. community sample: The National Comorbidity Survey. *Archives of General Psychiatry, 53,* 1022–1031.

Kendler, K. S., Neale, M. C., Kessler, R. C., Heath, A. C., & Eaves, L. J. (1992). A population based twin study of major depression in women: The impact of varying definitions of illness. *Archives of General Psychiatry, 49,* 257–266.

Kendler, K. S., Walters, E. E., Neale, M. C., Kessler, R. C., Heath, A. C., & Eaves, L. J. (1995). The structure of the genetic and environmental risk factors for six major psychiatric disorders in women. *Archives of General Psychiatry, 52,* 374–383.

Kessler, R. C. (1995). Epidemiology of psychiatric comorbidity. In M. T. Tsuang, M. Tohen, & G.E.P. Zahner (Eds.), *Textbook in psychiatric epidemiology* (pp. 179–197). New York: John Wiley & Sons.

Kessler, R. C., Berglund, P. A., Foster, C. L., Saunders, W. B., Stang, P. E., & Walters, E. E. (1997). The social consequences of psychiatric disorders: II. Teenage parenthood. *American Journal of Psychiatry, 154,* 1405–1411.

Kessler, R. C., Berglund, P. A., Zhao, S., Leaf, P. J., Kouzis, A. C., Bruce, M. L., Friedman, R. M., Grosser, R. C., Kennedy, C., Kuehnel, T. G., Laska, E. M., Manderscheid, R. W., Narrow, B., Rosenbeck, R. A., Santoni, T. W., & Schneier, M. (1996). The 12-month prevalence and correlates of serious mental illness (SMI). In R. W. Manderscheid & M. A. Sonnenschein (Eds.), *Mental health, United States, 1996* (pp. 59–70). Washington, DC: U.S. Government Printing Office.

Kessler, R. C., & Forthofer, M. S. (in press). The effects of psychiatric disorders on family formation and stability. In J. Brooks-Gunn & M. Cox (Eds.), *Family risk and resilience: The roles of conflict and cohesion.* New York: Cambridge University Press.

Kessler, R. C., Foster, C. L., Saunders, W. B., & Stang, P. E. (1995). Social consequences of psychiatric disorders, I: Educational attainment. *American Journal of Psychiatry, 152,* 1026–1032.

Kessler, R. C., & Frank, R. G. (1997). The impact of psychiatric disorders on work loss days. *Psychological Medicine, 27,* 861–873.

Kessler, R. C., Kendler, K. S., Heath, A., Neale, M. C., & Eaves, L. J. (1992). Social support, depressed mood, and adjustment to stress: A genetic epidemiologic investigation. *Journal of Personality and Social Psychology, 62,* 257–272.

Kessler, R. C., Kendler, K. S., Heath, A., Neale, M. C., & Eaves, L. J. (1994). Perceived support and adjustment to stress in a general population sample of female twins. *Psychological Medicine, 24,* 317–334.

Kessler, R. C., McGonagle, K. A., Zhao, S., Nelson, C. B., Hughes, M., Eshleman, S., Wittchen, H-U., & Kendler, K. S. (1994). Lifetime and 12-month prevalence of DSM-III-R psychiatric disorders in the United States: Results from the National Comorbidity Survey. *Archives of General Psychiatry, 51,* 8–19.

Kessler, R. C., & Price, R. H. (1993). Primary prevention of secondary disorders: A proposal and agenda. *American Journal of Community Psychology, 21,* 607–634.

Kessler, R. C., Rubinow, D. R., Holmes, C., Abelson, J. M., & Zhao, S. (1997). The epidemiology of DSM-II-R bipolar I disorder in a general population survey. *Psychological Medicine, 37,* 1079–1089.

Lenzenweger, M. F., Loranger, A. W., Korfine, L., & Neff, C. (1997). Detecting personality disorders in a non-clinical population: Application of a two-stage procedure for case identification. *Archives of General Psychiatry, 54,* 345–351.

Loranger, A. W., Sartorius, N., & Janca, A. (Eds.). (1996). *Assessment and diagnosis of personality disorders: The International Personality Disorder Examination (IPDE).* New York: Cambridge University Press.

Magee, W. J., Eaton, W. W., Wittchen, H-U., McGonagle, K. A., & Kessler, R. C. (1996). Agoraphobia, simple phobia, and social phobia in the National Comorbidity Survey. *Archives of General Psychiatry, 53,* 159–168.

Mazure, C. M. (Ed.). (1995). *Does stress cause psychiatric illness?* Washington, DC: American Psychiatric Press.

McGrath, E., Keita, G. P., Strickland, B. R., & Russo, N. F. (1990). *Women and depression: Risk factors and treatment issues.* Washington, DC: American Psychological Association.

Merikangas, K. R. (1988). Epidemiology of DSM-III personality disorders. In R. Michels & J. O. Cavenar, Jr. (Eds.), *Psychiatry* (Vol. 3, pp. 1–16). Philadelphia: Lippincott.

Morey, L. C. (1988). Personality disorders in DSM-III and DSM-III-R: Convergence, coverage and internal consistency. *American Journal of Psychiatry, 145,* 573–577.

National Advisory Mental Health Council. (1993). Health care reform for Americans with severe mental illness. *American Journal of Psychiatry, 150,* 1447–1465.

Newman, S. C., Shrout, P. E., & Bland, R. C. (1990). The efficiency of two-phase designs in prevalence surveys of mental disorders. *Psychological Medicine, 20,* 183–193.

Parker, G. (1987). Editorial: Are the lifetime prevalence estimates in the ECA study accurate? *Psychological Medicine, 17,* 275–282.

Penick, E. C., Powell, B. J., Liskow, B. I., & Jackson, J. O. (1988). The stability of coexisting psychiatric syndromes in alcoholic men after one year. *Journal of Studies on Alcohol, 49,* 395–405.

Perry, J. S. (1992). Problems and considerations in the valid assessment of personality disorders. *American Journal of Psychiatry, 149,* 1645–1653.

Pilkonis, P. A., Heape, C. L., Proiette, J. M., Clark, S. W., McDavid, J. D., & Pitts, T. E. (1995). The reliability and validity of two structured diagnostic interviews for personality disorders. *Archives of General Psychiatry, 52,* 1025–1033.

President's Commission on Mental Health and Illness. (1978). *Report to the President from the President's Commission on Mental Health, Volume 1.* Washington, DC: U.S. Government Printing Office.

Price, R. H., & Vinokur, A. D. (1995). Supporting career transitions in a time of organizational downsizing: The Michigan JOBS Program. In M. London (Ed.), *Employees, careers and job creation: Developing growth-oriented human resource strategies and programs* (pp. 191–209). San Francisco: Jossey-Bass.

Radloff, L. S. (1977). The CES-D Scale: A self-report depression scale for research in the general population. *Applied Psychology Measurement, 1,* 385–401.

Regier, D. A., Farmer, M. E., Rae, D. A., Locke, B. Z., Keith, B. J., Judd, L. L., & Goodwin, F. K. (1990). Comorbidity of mental health disorders with alcohol and other drug abuse. *JAMA, 264,* 2511–2518.

Regier, D. A., Kaelber, C. T., Rae, D. S., Farmer, M. E., Knauper, B., Kessler, R. C., & Norquist, G. S. (in press). Limitations of diagnostic criteria and assessment instruments for mental disorders: Implications for research and policy. *Archives of General Psychiatry.*

Regier, D. A., Narrow, W. E., Rae, D. S., Manderscheid, R. W., Locke, B. Z., & Goodwin, F. K. (1993). The de facto U.S. Mental and Addictive Disorders Service System: Epidemiologic Catchment Area prospective 1-year prevalence rates of disorders and services. *Archives of General Psychiatry, 50,* 85–94.

Rhode, P., Lewinsohn, P., & Seeley, J. (1990). Are people changed by the experience of having an episode of depression? A further test of the scar hypothesis. *Journal of Abnormal Psychology, 99,* 264–271.

Robins, L. N. (1985). Epidemiology: Reflections on testing the validity of psychiatric interview. *Archives of General Psychiatry, 42,* 918–924.

Robins, L. N., Helzer, J. E., Croughan, J. L., & Ratcliff, K. S. (1981). National Institute of Mental Health Diagnostic Interview Schedule: Its history, characteristics and validity. *Archives of General Psychiatry, 38,* 381–389.

Robins, L. N., Locke, B. Z., & Regier, D. A. (1991). An overview of psychiatric disorders in America. In L. N. Robins & D. A. Regier (Eds.), *Psychiatric disorders in America: The Epidemiologic Catchment Study* (pp. 328–366). New York: Free Press.

Robins, L. N., & Regier, D. A. (1991). *Psychiatric disorders in America: The Epidemiologic Catchment Area Study.* New York: Free Press.

Robins, L. N., Wing, J., Wittchen, H., Helzer, J. E., Babor, T. F., Burke, J. D., Farmer, A., Jablenski, A., Pickens, R., Regier, D. A., Sartorius, N., & Towle, L. H. (1988). The Composite International Diagnostic Interview: An epidemiologic instrument suitable for use in conjunction with different diagnostic systems and in different cultures. *Archives of General Psychiatry, 45,* 1069–1077.

Rogler, L. H., Malgady, R. G., & Tryon, W. W. (1992). Evaluation of mental health: Issues of memory in the Diagnostic Interview Schedule. *Journal of Nervous and Mental Disease, 180,* 215–222.

Rothman, K. J. (1986). *Modern epidemiology.* Boston: Little, Brown.

Roy, A., DeJong, J., Lamparski, D., Adinoff, B., George, T., Moore, V., Garnett, D., Kerich, M., & Linnoila, M. (1991). Mental disorders among alcoholics: Relationship to age of onset and cerebrospinal fluid neuropeptides. *Archives of General Psychiatry, 48,* 423–427.

Seiler, L. H. (1973). The 22-item scale used in field studies of mental illness: A question of method, a question of substance, and a question of theory. *Journal of Health and Social Behavior, 14,* 252–264.

Spitzer, R. L., Williams, J.B.W., Gibbon, M., & First, M. B. (1990). *Structured Clinical Interview for DSM-III-R, Patient edition (SCID-P), Version 1.0.* Washington, DC: American Psychiatric Press.

Substance Abuse and Mental Health Service Administration. (1993). Final notice establishing definitions for (1) children with a serious emotional disturbance, and (2) adults with a serious mental illness. *Federal Register, 58,* 29422–29425.

Taylor, S. E., & Aspinwall, L. G. (1996). Mediating and moderating processes in psychosocial stress: Appraisal, coping, resistance, and vulnerability. In H. B. Kaplan (Ed.), *Psychosocial stress: Perspectives on structure, theory, life-course, and methods* (pp. 71–110). San Diego: Academic Press.

Tsuang, M. T., & Farone, J. V. (1990). *The genetics of mood disorders.* Baltimore: Johns Hopkins University Press.

Tsuang, M. T., Tohen, M., & Zahner, G.E.P. (Eds.). (1995). *Textbook in psychiatric epidemiology.* New York: John Wiley & Sons.

Tyrer, P., Casey, P., & Ferguson, B. (1991). Personality disorder in perspective. *British Journal of Psychiatry, 159,* 463–471.

Weissman, M. M. (1993). The epidemiology of personality disorders: A 1990 update. *Journal of Personality Disorders, 7,* 44–62.

Weissman, M. M., & Myers, J. K. (1978). Affective disorders in a U.S. urban community. *Archives of General Psychiatry, 35,* 1304–1311.

Wells, K., Stewart, A., Hays, R., Burnam, M., Rogers, W., Daniels, M., Berry, S., Greenfield, S., & Ware, J. (1989). The functioning and well-being of depressed patients: Results from the Medical Outcomes Study. *JAMA, 262,* 914–919.

Wittchen, H-U. (1994). Reliability and validity studies of the WHO–Composite International Diagnostic Interview (CIDI): A critical review. *Journal of Psychiatric Research, 28,* 57–84.

Wohlfarth, T. D., van den Brink, W., Ormel, J., Koeter, M. W., & Oldehinkel, A. J. (1993). The relationship between social dysfunctioning and psychopathology among primary care attenders. *British Journal of Psychiatry, 163,* 37–44.

World Health Organization. (1977). *Manual of the international statistical classification of diseases, injuries, and causes of death* (9th rev.). Geneva: Author.

World Health Organization. (1990). *Composite International Diagnostic Interview (CIDI), Version 1.0.* Geneva: Author.

Zahner, G.E.P., Hsieh, C. C., & Fleming, J. A. (1995). Introduction to epidemiologic research methods. In M. T. Tsaung, M. Tohen, & G.E.P. Zahner (Eds.), *Textbook in psychiatric epidemiology* (pp. 23–54). New York: John Wiley & Sons.

Zimmerman, M. (1994). Diagnosing personality disorders: A review of issues and research methods. *Archives of General Psychiatry, 51,* 225–245.

---

*The authors appreciate the helpful comments of Evelyn Bromet, Sheldon Danziger, Phil Leaf, and Uli Wittchen. More detailed results of the National Comorbidity Survey can be obtained by consulting the NCS homepage, http://www.hcp.med.harvard.edu/ncs.*

# Classification and Diagnostic Assessment

Janet B. W. Williams

A 48-year-old married stockbroker is admitted to the medical service of a hospital by his internist after he appeared at her private office for the third time in a month insisting that he is having a heart attack. The cardiologist's workup is completely negative.

The patient states that his heart problem started six months ago when he had a sudden episode of terror, chest pain, palpitations, sweating, and shortness of breath while driving across a bridge on his way to work. His father and aunt had both had heart problems, and the patient was sure he was developing a similar illness. Not wanting to alarm his wife and children, he initially said nothing; but when the attacks began to recur, he consulted his internist. The internist found nothing wrong and told him he should try to relax, take more time off from work, and develop some leisure interests. In spite of his attempts to follow this advice, the attacks recurred with increasing intensity and frequency.

The patient claims that he believes the doctors who say there is nothing wrong with his heart, but during an attack he still becomes concerned that he is having a heart attack and will die (adapted from Spitzer, Skodol, Gibbon, & Williams, 1981).

What is the diagnosis? Heart attack? Depression? Anxiety neurosis? If this patient were seen in an emergency room, he would probably be given an EKG and perhaps other tests to rule out myocardial infarction or heart attack. Once this was ruled out, if the year were 1975, his condition would likely have been diagnosed as anxiety neurosis: either psychotherapy alone (some would even treat this with psychoanalytically oriented psychotherapy or psychoanalysis) or psychotherapy and an anxiolytic medication such as diazepam or another tranquilizer would have been prescribed. Over time, the anxiety symptoms might resolve, but in any case the patient would probably not have gotten immediate relief.

Since 1980, however, the diagnosis and treatment of such a case are different. According to the *Diagnostic and Statistical Manual of Mental Disorders*, fourth edition,

Portions of this chapter have previously appeared in *The American Psychiatric Press Textbook of Psychiatry* (3rd ed.; R. E. Hales, S. C. Yudofsky, & J. A. Talbott, eds.), Washington, DC: American Psychiatric Press, in press.

(DSM-IV) (APA, 1994), and its immediate predecessors, the third edition (DSM-III) (APA, 1980) and third edition, revised (DSM-III-R) (APA, 1987), the diagnosis of panic disorder would clearly account for this man's symptoms of sudden discrete periods of extreme fear, accompanied by physical symptoms such as chest pain, heart palpitations, sweating, shortness of breath, and a fear that he will die during the attack. Furthermore, these symptoms seem to occur at times other than during life-threatening circumstances and are not precipitated just by exposure to a phobic stimulus. The diagnosis of panic disorder indicates specific and often dramatically effective treatment: an antidepressant medication, combined with behavior therapy if there is anticipatory anxiety and avoidance. This treatment works in a high percentage of cases. This case illustrates, as well as any case can, the importance of accurate assessment and diagnosis and also the great strides that have been made in psychiatric classification in the past 20 years.

This chapter discusses the importance of diagnosis and assessment, the general principles guiding the DSM-IV and strategies useful to the clinician in making diagnoses. Features of the major categories themselves are reviewed within specific chapters in Part One of this book.

## Why Diagnose?

Why assign diagnoses at all? Why not just describe the cases that we see and treat them according to the symptoms that they have? Why is it necessary to label people?

First, we must be clear that it is not people we are labeling; it is disorders that people have. Health professionals should never refer to someone as "a schizophrenic" or "a depressive," but rather as "a person with schizophrenia," or as "someone who has depression," just as they have places to live, friends, families, and other possible disorders as well. This avoids the mistaken connotation that someone with a mental disorder has only that and lacks other attributes and roles in life. It also avoids implying that all people with a particular mental disorder are alike; on the contrary, they may differ in many important ways that can affect treatment and outcome. For these reasons, DSM-III and subsequent editions avoided using diagnostic terms as descriptive nouns (Spitzer & Williams, 1979). In addition, in DSM-IV the people evaluated are not referred to as patients. It was recognized during the development of DSM-III that the use of this word might limit the use of the manual by some mental health professionals, including many social workers, who do not traditionally refer to their clientele as patients. In a further attempt to facilitate the use of the DSM by the various mental health professions, the terms "physician" and "psychiatrist" are not used. Instead, users are referred to as "clinicians" and "mental health professionals."

It is important for health professionals to have a language with which to communicate; giving names to the groups of symptoms that we see over and over allows us a shorthand way of describing the entities with which we deal. It is much more efficient to be able to say that a client has major depressive disorder, rather than having to say that a client has "depressed mood and has lost interest in things; she also has trouble sleeping, has lost her appetite, has trouble concentrating and thinks about suicide." Certainly this fuller description conveys more specific information and may in some settings be a more useful description, but in most instances, the abbreviated diagnostic term is all that is required to make a particular point. A diagnostic classification, as a listing of these various diagnostic terms, allows us to keep track of them.

# What Is a Mental Disorder?

It is recognized that more precise boundaries for the concept *mental disorder* cannot be specified, just as they cannot be for *physical disorder* (Wakefield, 1992). However, the following definition guided the development of DSM-III, DSM-III-R, and DSM-IV and was helpful when deciding which syndromes should be included as mental disorders and determining how they should be defined. What follows is from DSM-IV (APA, 1994).

> Each of the mental disorders is conceptualized as a clinically significant be-havioral or psychological syndrome or pattern that occurs in an individual and that is associated with present distress (e.g., a painful symptom) or disabil-ity (e.g., impairment in one or more important areas of functioning) or with a significantly increased risk of suffering death, pain, disability, or an important loss of freedom. In addition, this syndrome or pattern must not be merely an expectable and culturally sanctioned response to a particular event, for exam-ple, the death of a loved one. Whatever its original cause, it must currently be considered a manifestation of a behavioral, psychological, or biological dys-function in the individual. Neither deviant behavior (e.g., political, religious, or sexual) nor conflicts that are primarily between the individual and society are mental disorders unless the deviance or conflict is a symptom of a dys-function in the individual, as described above. (pp. xxi–xxii)

A common misunderstanding about the disorders in DSM-IV is that each cate-gory represents a discrete entity with distinct boundaries between it and other men-tal disorders and between it and normality. Although the disorders by necessity have been defined as distinctly as possible, there are continuing controversies about the interrelationships among many of the categories. The current categorical and mul-tiaxial system does draw boundaries where in fact there may be a continuum. For example, although DSM-IV defines major depressive disorder and dysthymic disor-der as two specific depressive disorders, many people believe that these two disor-ders represent merely different points on a continuum of depressive symptoms rather than two distinct entities. Also, many believe that the personality disorders defined in DSM-IV are only points on a continuum of personality traits. Future re-search will have to answer the question of whether it would be more useful to adopt an approach in which scaled ratings of disturbance are made in certain areas of psychopathology rather than discrete diagnoses.

# Diagnostic Validity

The validity of a diagnosis is the extent to which it serves the multiple purposes for which it is intended. There are four major types of validity that are applied to psy-chiatric diagnoses: face, descriptive, predictive, and construct. *Face validity* is the ex-tent to which, on the face of it, the definition of a disorder seems reasonable as a description of a particular clinical entity and allows professionals to communicate about the disorder. For example, the list of symptoms that define the DSM-IV cate-gory of panic disorder has significant face validity because clinicians generally agree that these are the signs and symptoms they see in their patients who have panic at-tacks. *Descriptive validity* is the extent to which the defining features of a diagnostic category are unique to that category. For example, the DSM-IV definition of a manic episode has a lot of descriptive validity because its clinical features clearly distinguish it from other categories: euphoric mood and decreased need for sleep are rarely seen in other disorders. On the other hand, the category of generalized anxiety disorder has less descriptive validity because its essential features, excessive anxiety and worry, are often present in people with other mental disorders.

If a diagnosis has high *predictive validity*, it is useful for predicting the natural history and treatment response of a person with the disorder. For example, the category of panic disorder has high predictive validity because there is a high likelihood that a person with this disorder will develop agoraphobia as a complication, and, as described above, there is a high probability that there will be a good response to certain treatments. Finally, construct validity is the highest form of validity and the form for which most of the mental disorders have the least evidence. *Construct validity* is the extent to which we understand the etiology or pathophysiologic process of a disorder. Evidence for the construct validity of a disorder includes a genetic factor, a biologic mechanism, and social and environmental factors that cause the disorder.

## DSM-III

In 1952, the sixth edition of the World Health Organization's (WHO) International Classification of Diseases (ICD) expanded to include mental disorders. The ICD is a classification system used all over the world that lists all medical disorders and their codes, but without descriptions or diagnostic criteria. In that same year, the APA produced the first edition of its *Diagnostic and Statistical Manual of Mental Disorders* (APA, 1952). The DSM listed codes and names for all the mental disorders that were recognized in the ICD and contained a glossary of mental disorders with a brief description of their characteristics.

DSM-II (APA, 1968) also included brief descriptions of all the mental disorders (see Figure 2-1 for an example). DSM-II used two factors to determine the assignment of disorders: (1) whether a condition was considered to be psychotic or neurotic and (2) the nature of the presumed cause (*endogenous,* which meant reactive to a psychosocial stressor, or the result of an established personality pattern). DSM-III (APA, 1980) changed to a descriptive, atheoretical approach to classification and was based on the severity of specified symptoms and the course of the disorder (First, Donovan, & Frances, 1996). The various revisions of the DSM have paralleled editions of the ICD, so that the current DSM-IV is compatible with the clinical modification of ICD-9 (ICD-9-CM) that is currently in use in the United States as well as with the 10th revision of the ICD (ICD-10) now in use overseas.

The impact of DSM-III was remarkable. Soon after its publication, it became widely accepted in the United States as the common language of mental health clinicians and researchers for communicating about the disorders for which they have professional responsibility. All major textbooks of psychiatry and other textbooks that discuss psychopathology either made extensive reference to DSM-III or largely adopted its terminology and concepts, and it was used as a major teaching tool in medical student education and residency training classes (Williams, Spitzer, & Skodol, 1985).

DSM-III was a manual of "firsts": for the first time, definitions with specified diagnostic criteria were provided for each category of mental disorder (see Figure 2-1 for an example of diagnostic criteria from DSM-IV that are similar to those in DSM-III); for the first time, a system for multiaxial diagnosis was provided (see below); and for the first time, national field trials, in which more than 12,000 patients were evaluated, were conducted to test the manual before its final adoption (Spitzer

FIGURE **2-1**

## DSM-II and DSM-IV Diagnostic Criteria

### DSM-II Diagnostic Criteria for Drug Dependence

This category is for patients who are addicted to or dependent on drugs other than alcohol, tobacco, and ordinary caffeine-containing beverages. Dependence on medically prescribed drugs is also excluded so long as the drug is medically indicated and the intake is proportionate to the medical need. The diagnosis requires evidence of habitual use or a clear sense of need for the drug. Withdrawal symptoms are not the only evidence of dependence; while always present when opium derivatives are withdrawn, they may be entirely absent when cocaine or marijuana are withdrawn. The diagnosis may stand alone or be coupled with any other diagnosis.

### DSM-IV Diagnostic Criteria for Substance Dependence

A maladaptive pattern of substance use, leading to clinically significant impairment or distress, as manifested by three (or more) of the following, occurring at any time in the same 12-month period:

(1) tolerance, as defined by either of the following:
    (a) a need for markedly increased amounts of the substance to achieve intoxication or desired effect
    (b) markedly diminished effect with continued use of the same amount of the substance

(2) withdrawal, as manifested by either of the following:
    (a) the characteristic withdrawal syndrome for the substance (refer to Criteria A and B of the criteria sets for withdrawal from the specific substances)
    (b) the same (or a closely related) substance is taken to relieve or avoid withdrawal symptoms

(3) the substance is often taken in larger amounts or over a longer period than was intended

(4) there is a persistent desire or unsuccessful efforts to cut down or control substance use

(5) a great deal of time is spent in activities necessary to obtain the substance (e.g., visiting multiple doctors or driving long distances), use the substance (e.g., chain-smoking), or recover from its effects

(6) important social, occupational, or recreational activities are given up or reduced because of substance use

(7) the substance use is continued despite knowledge of having a persistent or recurrent physical or psychological problem that is likely to have been caused or exacerbated by the substance (e.g., current cocaine use despite recognition of cocaine-induced depression, or continued drinking despite recognition that an ulcer was made worse by alcohol consumption)

Sources: American Psychiatric Association. (1968). *Diagnostic and statistical manual of mental disorders* (2nd ed.). Washington, DC: Author. American Psychiatric Association. (1994). *Diagnostic and statistical manual of mental disorders* (4th ed.). Washington, DC: Author.

& Forman, 1979; Spitzer, Forman, & Nee, 1979). The publication of DSM-III in 1980 sparked an explosion of research into psychiatric diagnoses and their treatments that has continued to the present. In the years since the publication of DSM-III, several thousand articles that directly address some aspect of it have appeared in the scientific literature (Skodol & Spitzer, 1987; Widiger, Frances, Pincus, First, & Davis, 1994).

It is necessary to have a generally agreed-on definition of a disorder's defining characteristics and what differentiates it from other similar disorders. This allows clinicians and researchers to study the disorder and its treatment, to begin to understand its etiology, and when an effective treatment is developed, to identify people with the same disorder who might benefit from that treatment. Thus, for proper diagnosis, especially for those conditions for which an effective treatment exists, it is important to have a specified definition. The availability of the standard definitions in DSM-III has facilitated research with groups of patients and clients who are relatively homogeneous with respect to their psychiatric symptoms.

As our diagnostic classification system has become refined over time, relationships between some diagnoses and some treatments have become clearer. Unfortunately, even with DSM-IV, relatively few diagnoses are yet directly associated with specific effective treatments, although the most progress in this regard has been made for the major and common categories such as mood disorders and anxiety disorders. Although DSM-III and its diagnostic criteria represented a general consensus in the field at the time, they were by no means noncontroversial (Kirk & Kutchins, 1992). However, specified diagnostic criteria have enabled us to learn much more about these conditions, which in turn has facilitated the refinement of their definitions based on growing clinical experience and empirical evidence. Each subsequent edition of the classification (that is, DSM-III-R and now DSM-IV) has reflected interim results of this cycle of definition, study, and definition refinement. Although much more is known now about these disorders than in 1980, undoubtedly this cycle will continue for many years to come and over time will continue to lead to improved treatments for many of the mental disorders.

DSM-III also had considerable influence internationally, although it was intended primarily for use in the United States (Spitzer, Williams, & Skodol, 1983). A testimony to its success is that in addition to fairly widespread use abroad, many of its basic features, such as the inclusion of specified diagnostic criteria, were adopted for inclusion in an official research version of the mental disorders chapter of the ICD-10. DSM-III and its successors have been translated into many languages and are used routinely by teachers and researchers in other countries. Input from research with peoplefrom various social and cultural backgrounds has increased significantly with each revision of the DSM and will undoubtedly continue to provide information that will be useful for future revisions.

## DSM-IV

The development of DSM-IV involved several important efforts. First, comprehensive literature reviews were conducted in many areas of the classification, including controversial areas and areas in which recent scientific findings might suggest changes in the classification, text, or criteria. Second, analyses of sets of data from already completed studies or studies in progress were funded by the John D. and Catherine T. MacArthur Foundation to answer specific nosologic questions. Finally, 12 field trials were funded by the National Institute of Mental Health (NIMH), the National Institute on Drug Abuse (NIDA), and the National Institute on Alcohol Abuse and Alcoholism (NIAAA) to study the impact of changes that were being considered for inclusion in DSM-IV. Some features of DSM-IV are described below. These and other general features are further described in the introduction to DSM-IV.

### DIAGNOSTIC CRITERIA

As mentioned above, specified diagnostic criteria are included in DSM-IV for every specific category. They have been revised from those in previous editions based on continued clinical experience and new empirical findings.

### DESCRIPTIVE APPROACH

By and large, clinicians can agree on the defining features of most of the mental disorders despite disagreement about their causes. For this reason, the mental disorders in DSM-IV (as was also true in DSM-III and DSM-III-R) are defined by their descriptive features without reference to etiologic theories, except for those disorders whose etiology or pathophysiologic process is known. This generally descriptive, or atheoretical, approach has enabled clinicians of varying theoretical orientations to use this classification; in other words, clinicians can generally agree on the identification of these conditions but still preserve their own approaches to understanding and treating them.

## DIAGNOSTIC HIERARCHIES

For some disorders in DSM-IV, the diagnostic criteria follow hierarchic principles so that a diagnosis lower in the hierarchy is not given (even if its diagnostic criteria are met) if the criteria for a diagnosis higher in the hierarchy also are met for the same symptomatology. For example, both diagnoses of major depressive episode and adjustment disorder with depressed mood would not be given for the same disturbance, even if the symptomatic criteria for both disorders are met. This is operationalized in the wording of an exclusion criterion for adjustment disorder: "The stress-related disturbance does not meet the criteria for another specific Axis I disorder and is not merely an exacerbation of a pre-existing Axis I or Axis II disorder" (APA, 1994, p. 626).

In DSM-IV there are two main hierarchic principles:

1. Disorders due to a general medical condition and substance-induced disorders pre-empt the diagnosis of any other disorder that could produce the same symptoms, if a general medical condition or substance can be identified. For example, a patient with a major depressive syndrome may be diagnosed as having major depressive disorder, mood disorder due to hypothyroidism, or hallucinogen mood disorder. If the history or laboratory tests reveal that the depression began during the course of hypothyroidism or during hallucinogen intoxication, the clinician should consider one of the two latter diagnoses rather than major depressive disorder. However, if no general medical condition, specific substance intoxication, or withdrawal is identified as the cause of the mood disturbance and the criteria for a major depressive disorder are met, it is the mood disorder (that is, major depressive disorder) that should be diagnosed.

2. When a more pervasive disorder commonly has essential or associated symptoms that are the defining symptoms of a less pervasive disorder, only the more pervasive disorder is diagnosed if its diagnostic criteria are met. For example, if chronic mild depression is present only when the essential features of schizophrenia also are present, only schizophrenia is diagnosed rather than schizophrenia and dysthymic disorder (to account for the chronic mild depression), because depressive symptoms are commonly associated with schizophrenia.

The decisions of which diagnostic hierarchies to impose and which to abandon were made to balance competing goals of clinical validity (that is, not pre-empting the diagnosis of disorders with differential predictive validity) and parsimony (that is, not encouraging a diagnosis for every symptom present). If all the hierarchies were suspended, many people would receive many diagnoses. For example, in many cases of schizophrenia there also are depression, anxiety, and often somatoform symptoms. Without any diagnostic hierarchies, an approach advocated by some, such cases could receive diagnoses of major depressive disorder, dysthymic disorder, generalized anxiety disorder, social phobia, and undifferentiated somatoform disorder, as well as schizophrenia. Such a list might distract the clinician from concentrating on treatment of the schizophrenia, when many of the other symptoms might resolve on their own once the acute phase of schizophrenia resolves.

## MULTIAXIAL SYSTEM FOR EVALUATION

As mentioned above, DSM-III took a major step forward by incorporating, for the first time in an official diagnostic system in this country, a multiaxial system for evaluation (Williams, 1985a, 1985b). The basic concept of such a system is that the clinician is expected to evaluate each subject according to each of several areas of information that are assumed to be of high clinical value. Use of a multiaxial system ensures that attention is given to certain types of disorders, aspects of the environment, and areas of functioning that might be overlooked if the focus were on assessing a single presenting problem. Ideally, each domain, called an "axis," is assessed independently of the others, although in practice they often are related. Together, they represent a view of the person's condition that is more comprehensive than an evaluation limited to mental disorder diagnoses. Although not empirically demonstrated, it is assumed that a multiaxial evaluation is more useful for planning treatment and evaluating prognosis because it better reflects the interrelated complexities of the various biological, psychological, and social aspects of a person's condition. For social workers, a multiaxial system embodies and reaffirms the importance of a biopsychosocial approach.

The DSM-IV multiaxial system consists of five axes, the first three of which are diagnostic (see Figure 2-2; Williams, 1997). All the mental disorders are included in the first two axes: Axis I is for clinical disorders and other conditions that may be a focus of clinical attention, and Axis II is for personality disorders and mental retardation. The provision of a separate axis for personality disorders and mental retardation ensures that consideration is given to the possible presence of these disorders that might otherwise be overlooked when attention is directed to the usually more florid Axis I disorders. For example, in the case of a major depressive disorder with psychotic features and schizotypal personality disorder, the clinician might inadvertently overlook the personality disorder because its features are so overshadowed by the

FIGURE **2-2**

| **DSM-IV Multiaxial System** | |
| --- | --- |
| **AXIS** | **DESCRIPTION** |
| I | Clinical Disorders |
| | Other Conditions That May Be a Focus of Clinical Attention |
| II | Personality Disorders |
| | Mental Retardation |
| III | General Medical Conditions |
| IV | Psychosocial and Environmental Problems |
| V | Global Assessment of Functioning |

SOURCE: American Psychiatric Association. (1994). *Diagnostic and statistical manual of mental disorders* (4th ed.). Washington, DC: Author.

psychotic symptoms associated with the depression. In many instances, disorders will be present on both Axes I and II, and in such cases, all appropriate diagnoses should be recorded. This Axis I–Axis II convention has undoubtedly been at least partially responsible for the tremendous increase in research and clinical attention that has been directed to the personality disorders in the 1980s and 1990s.

Axis III is for listing current general medical conditions that the clinician believes are potentially relevant to the understanding or management of the case. General medical conditions can be related to mental disorders in a variety of ways. In some cases, it is clear that the general medical condition is etiologic to (or the cause of) the development or worsening of a mental disorder (for example, anxiety disorder from hyperthyroidism) and that the mechanism for this effect is physiologic. In other instances, the general medical disorder may not seem to be etiologic, but is important in the overall management of the case (for example, a person with diabetes mellitus admitted to the hospital for an exacerbation of schizophrenia, for whom insulin management must be monitored). Sometimes a general medical disorder has important prognostic or treatment implications for the mental disorder as in a case with both major depressive disorder and cardiac arrhythmia, in which the choice of pharmacotherapy is influenced by the general medical condition. When a social worker or other nonphysician conducts a multiaxial evaluation, this area of functioning should still be evaluated by asking the client a question such as "How has your health been?" The information provided by the client should be recorded on Axis III, along with a notation about the source of the information, for example, "diabetes [by report of the client]" or "No general medical condition [by report of the client and confirmed in the chart by Dr. X]." It is important not to omit this axis and also to indicate that a medical diagnosis has been made only by a medical professional.

The fourth axis in DSM-IV provides a checklist for recording psychosocial and environmental problems that may affect the diagnosis, treatment planning, and prognosis of the person's mental disorders (on Axes I and II). A psychosocial or environmental problem may be a negative life event, an environmental difficulty, an interpersonal stress, an inadequacy of social supports or personal resources, or another problem that describes the context in which a person's difficulties have developed. The list of problem categories to be considered on Axis IV includes problems with one's primary support group; problems related to the social environment; inadequate access to health care services; problems related to interaction with the legal system; and educational, occupational, housing, economic, and other psychosocial problems. In general, only those problems that have been present during the year before the evaluation should be noted; in many cases it is appropriate to record more than one problem. When a psychosocial or environmental problem is the primary focus of clinical attention, it also is recorded on Axis I with its corresponding code from the section listing other conditions that may be a focus of clinical attention.

The Global Assessment of Functioning (GAF) Scale on Axis V, as shown in Figure 2-3, summarizes psychological, social, and occupational functioning on a continuum of mental health and illness. Studies have shown that clinical ratings of overall severity of disturbance are reliable and related to treatment utilization (Curran, Miller, Zwick, Monti, & Stout, 1980; Fenichel & Murphy, 1985; Gordon, Jardiolin, & Gordon, 1985; Husby, 1985; Mezzich, Evanczuk, Mathias, & Coffman, 1984). GAF ratings are made for current functioning at the time of evaluation and generally reflect the current need for treatment or care. Ratings may be made for other time periods (for example, past year) for special purposes.

Although surely many other areas of functioning are important for clinicians to consider in planning for treatment, for a multiaxial system to have maximal clinical usefulness, a limited number of axes must exist. These five were selected to represent the minimal number of areas of clinical information that would be of maximal clinical utility regardless of treatment approach and treatment context (that is, what

FIGURE **2-3**

## DSM-IV Axis V: Global Assessment of Functioning Scale

*Consider psychological, social, and occupational functioning on a hypothetical continuum of mental health–illness. Do not include impairment in functioning due to physical (or environmental) limitations.*

**CODE** (*Note:* Use intermediate codes when appropriate, e.g., 45, 68, 72).

**100**
|
**91**
Superior functioning in a wide range of activities, life's problems never seem to get out of hand, is sought out by others because of his or her many positive qualities. No symptoms.

**90**
|
**81**
Absent or minimal symptoms (e.g., mild anxiety before an exam); good functioning in all areas, interested and involved in a wide range of activities, socially effective, generally satisfied with life, no more than everyday problems or concerns (e.g., an occasional argument with family members).

**80**
|
**71**
If symptoms are present, they are transient and expectable reactions to psychosocial stressors (e.g., difficulty concentrating after family argument); no more than slight impairment in social, occupational, or school functioning (e.g., temporarily falling behind in schoolwork).

**70**
|
**61**
Some mild symptoms (e.g., depressed mood and mild insomnia) OR some difficulty in social, occupational, or school functioning (e.g., occasional truancy or theft within the household), but generally functioning pretty well, has some meaningful interpersonal relationships.

**60**
|
**51**
Moderate symptoms (e.g., flat affect and circumstantial speech, occasional panic attacks) OR moderate difficulty in social, occupational, or school functioning (e.g., few friends or conflicts with peers or co-workers).

**50**
|
**41**
Serious symptoms (e.g., suicidal ideation, severe obsessional rituals, frequent shoplifting) OR any serious impairment in social, occupational, or school functioning (e.g., no friends, unable to keep a job).

**40**
|
**31**
Some impairment in reality testing or communication (e.g., speech is at times illogical, obscure, or irrelevant) OR major impairment in several areas, such as work or school, family relations, judgment, thinking, or mood (e.g., depressed man avoids friends, neglects family, and is unable to work; child frequently beats up younger children, is defiant at home, and is failing at school).

**30**
|
**21**
Behavior is considerably influenced by delusions or hallucinations OR serious impairment in communication or judgment (e.g., sometimes incoherent, acts grossly inappropriately, suicidal preoccupation) OR inability to function in almost all areas (e.g., stays in bed all day; no job, home, or friends).

**20**
|
**11**
Some danger of hurting self or others (e.g., suicide attempts without clear expectation of death; frequently violent; manic excitement) OR occasionally fails to maintain minimal personal hygiene (e.g., smears feces) OR gross impairment in communication (e.g., largely incoherent or mute).

**10**
|
**1**
Persistent danger of severely hurting self or others (e.g., recurrent violence) OR persistent inability to maintain minimal personal hygiene OR serious suicidal act with clear expectation of death.

**0**    Inadequate information.

SOURCE: American Psychiatric Association. (1994). *Diagnostic and statistical manual of mental disorders* (4th ed.). Washington, DC: Author.

basic information every clinician would want to consider about every case). A prototypic recording form (see Figure 2-4) is provided in DSM-IV to facilitate the use of all five axes.

A word of caution: As noted in the introduction to DSM-IV, it is necessary to obtain much more information beyond a DSM-IV multiaxial evaluation before an adequate treatment plan can be formulated for any person. A DSM-IV diagnosis represents only the initial step in a comprehensive evaluation leading to a treatment plan.

FIGURE **2-4**

## DSM-IV Multiaxial Evaluation Report Form

**AXIS I:  Clinical Disorders**
        **Other Conditions That May Be a Focus of Clinical Attention**

Diagnostic code        DSM-IV Name

— — —.— —        _____

— — —.— —        _____

— — —.— —        _____

— — —.— —        _____

**AXIS II:  Personality Disorders**
         **Mental Retardation**

Diagnostic code        DSM-IV Name

— — —.— —        _____

— — —.— —        _____

**AXIS III:  General Medical Conditions**

ICD-9-CM Code        ICD-9-CM Name

— — —.— —        _____

— — —.— —        _____

— — —.— —        _____

**AXIS IV:  Psychosocial and Environmental Problems**

*Check:*

☐  Problems with primary support group   *Specify:*_____

☐  Problems related to the social environment   *Specify:*_____

☐  Educational problems   *Specify:*_____

☐  Occupational problems   *Specify:*_____

☐  Housing problems   *Specify:*_____

☐  Economic problems   *Specify:*_____

☐  Problems with access to health care services   *Specify:*_____

☐  Problems related to interaction with the legal system/crime   *Specify:*_____

☐  Other psychosocial and environmental problems   *Specify:*_____

**AXIS V:  Global Assessment of Functioning Scale**        *Score:* _ _ _
                                            *Time frame:* _____

SOURCE: American Psychiatric Association. (1994). *Diagnostic and statistical manual of mental disorders* (4th ed.). Washington, DC: Author.

The additional necessary information will, of course, be determined in part by the theoretical orientation of the clinician and may emphasize psychological, biological, or social aspects of the functioning of the individual being evaluated.

## SYSTEMATIC DESCRIPTIONS

DSM-IV, as did its immediate predecessors, includes standard categories of information to offer a complete description of the features of the various disorders. The description of each category begins with its *diagnostic features*, the clinical signs and symptoms that are required to make the diagnosis. This is followed by a discussion of the disorder's *associated features and disorders*, which can include associated descriptive features and mental disorders that often are associated with the disorder but are not essential for making the diagnosis; associated laboratory findings that may be diagnostic (as in some sleep disorders), confirmatory of the construct of the disorder, or merely complications of the disorder; and associated physical examination signs, symptoms, and general medical conditions that may be of diagnostic significance but are not essential to the diagnosis (for example, dental erosion resulting from vomiting associated with bulimia nervosa) or that are merely associated conditions. A section addressing specific *culture, age, and gender features* describes variations in the presentation of the disorder that may be attributable to a person's cultural setting, age, or gender (including prevalence and sex ratio). Under *prevalence*, data are provided on point and lifetime prevalence and incidence of the disorder. These data are provided for different clinical settings (for example, inpatient or outpatient) when known. The section on *course* describes the typical lifetime patterns of presentation and evolution of the disorder. This may include information on the usual age at onset, mode of onset (for example, abrupt or insidious), chronicity, typical duration of episodes, and progression over time (for example, stationary, worsening, or improving). The *familial pattern* section provides data on the frequency of the disorder among first-degree biological relatives of those with the disorder compared with the general population. Each category also includes a discussion of *differential diagnosis*, describing how to distinguish this disorder from other disorders that have some similar presenting characteristics.

## CROSS-CULTURAL CONSIDERATIONS

DSM-IV has been translated into many languages and is widely used in other parts of the world. Somewhat surprisingly, its use in cultures vastly different from those of most of the people who were mainly responsible for developing it has generally been successful (Spitzer, 1983; Spitzer et al., 1983). In DSM-IV, cross-cultural considerations received even more attention than in previous editions, supported by a conference on culture held to address needed changes in the text and criteria to make them more useful and accurate across cultures (Mezzich, Kleinman, Fabrega, & Parron, 1996).

Three additional innovative features were added to DSM-IV. First, because of evidence suggesting that the symptoms and course of a number of DSM-IV disorders are influenced by local cultural factors, a new section that describes culturally related features was added to the text for many disorders. In the text for major depressive episode, for example, the DSM-IV states, "In some cultures, depression may be experienced largely in somatic terms, rather than with sadness or guilt. Complaints of 'nerves' and headaches (in Latino and Mediterranean cultures), of weakness, tiredness, or 'imbalance' (in Chinese and Asian cultures), of problems of the 'heart' (in Middle Eastern cultures), or of being 'heartbroken' (among Hopi) may express the depressive experience" (APA, 1994, p. 324). Second, descriptions of some culturally related syndromes were added as examples to not otherwise speci-fied categories (for example, possession added as an example to dissociative disorder not otherwise specified), and a glossary of 25 of the best studied "culture-bound syndromes" and idioms of distress that may be encountered in clinical practice in North America was added as an appendix to DSM-IV. Finally, an outline for cultur-al formulation also was added to the appendix. This outline is meant to supplement the DSM-IV multiaxial system and to address difficulties that may be encountered in applying DSM-IV criteria in a multicultural environment. The introduction to DSM-IV cautions clinicians to pay attention to their clients' ethnic and cultural contexts. This outline provides help to the clinician in conducting a systematic eval-uation of the ways in which the person's cultural context might be related to their clinical care.

## RELATIONAL DISTURBANCES

DSM-III and its successors often have been criticized for their exclusive focus on mental disorders that occur in people. This has restricted their usefulness in the diag-nosis and treatment of problems that occur in the family and other relational units, and family therapists have not embraced DSM-III and DSM-III-R mainly for that reason (Wynne, 1987). Early in the development of DSM-IV, a Coalition on Family Diagnosis was formed by professional groups dealing with these issues to consider possible changes that might be made in DSM-IV. This resulted in several new fea-tures, including the addition of a group of relational problems to the section of con-ditions that may be a focus of clinical attention. This new grouping includes relation-al problems related to a mental disorder or general medical condition, parent–child relational problems, partner relational problems, sibling relational problems, and re-lational problems not otherwise specified (NOS). In addition, an optional axis called the Global Assessment of Relational Functioning (GARF) Scale appears in an ap-pendix to DSM-IV.

## WOMEN'S ISSUES

People with expertise in various areas of women's issues were appointed to review the text and criteria for DSM-IV to ensure that women's issues received adequate attention.

## AS AN EDUCATIONAL TOOL

Certain features of DSM-IV contribute to its usefulness as an educational tool in teaching students about basic psychopathology (Skodol, Spitzer, & Williams, 1981). A beginning section in DSM-IV provides explanations of the diagnostic criteria, the organization of the text descriptions of the disorders, and the terms and conventions used throughout the manual. A separate chapter describes the multiaxial system in detail. The manual also contains several appendixes (some of which have been de-scribed above) that are useful in teaching. Most of these are designed to make the manual more user friendly, that is, to facilitate its use by clinicians and researchers. A small forest of decision trees is provided to make the differential diagnostic process easier by helping clinicians understand the organization and hierarchic structure of the classification. Using one of these trees, a clinician can follow a series of questions to rule in or out various disorders. The decision tree for anxiety disorders is presented in Figure 2-5.

A glossary of technical terms defines terms that are included in the diagnostic criteria of DSM-IV. An alphabetic listing of the diagnostic categories and a numeric listing of the codes are included as separate appendixes, as are listings of selected ICD codes for general medical conditions and corresponding ICD-10 codes for DSM-IV disorders. Published with DSM-IV is the Mini-D, a pocket-sized quick reference guide containing the diagnostic criteria. Another useful teaching tool is the *DSM-IV Case Book* (Spitzer, Gibbon, Skodol, Williams, & First, 1994), which presents many case vignettes, each with a discussion of the DSM-IV differential diagnosis.

## Diagnostic Assessment

Treatment selection, goal setting, and psychoeducation all depend on the accuracy of the diagnostic formulation; therefore, the determination of an accurate psychiatric diagnosis is the first step in clinical management. A thorough and accurate assessment is more likely to result in a feasible and helpful treatment plan. But how is such a comprehensive evaluation to be accomplished?

The development of diagnostic criteria for each mental disorder has made possible the development of diagnostic interview guides that provide some structure to the process of clinical assessment across a range of psychiatric diagnoses. In these instruments, questions are provided for the interviewers to help them elicit the information necessary to make the appropriate diagnostic decisions. By specifying the questions to be asked, these interview guides help reduce diagnostic errors that may occur when different clinicians base their diagnostic judgments on different information or when clinicians fail to cover an important area of information. Diagnostic interview guides have been shown to produce more accurate psychiatric diagnoses than unstructured clinical interviews (Kranzler et al., 1995).

Structured interviews offer major advantages to clinicians and researchers. First, they guide interviewers to make diagnoses using an agreed-on diagnostic nomenclature and definitions; this process generally enhances the reliability with which diagnoses are made. In addition, there is a tendency for clinicians to focus exclusively on a patient's chief complaint and to forget to inquire systematically about other potentially significant comorbid symptoms. Structured interviews help circumvent this problem by ensuring that a thorough differential diagnosis is made, one that considers all of the diagnostic possibilities, including comorbid conditions.

Accurate diagnostic assessment requires both clinical judgment and experience. More often than not, a psychiatric interview must be modified to meet the needs of a patient's background (cultural and educational), personality, or psychopathology. For example, a question may need to be rephrased in a more simplified way if English is not the patient's primary language or if it is evident that the patient is unsure about the meaning of the question. Furthermore, when interviewing patients who are psychotic, evidence for delusions and hallucinations comes from the patient's description of his or her presenting problem rather than from the answer to any specific yes–no question. Interview guides encourage the clinician to ask the patient to provide substantiating examples to ensure that when a patient provides a "yes" or "no" answer to a close-ended question, he or she has truly understood the intent of the question. Thus, diagnostic interview guides can help even relatively new clinicians make

FIGURE **2-5**

## DSM-IV Decision Tree for Differential Diagnosis: Anxiety Disorders

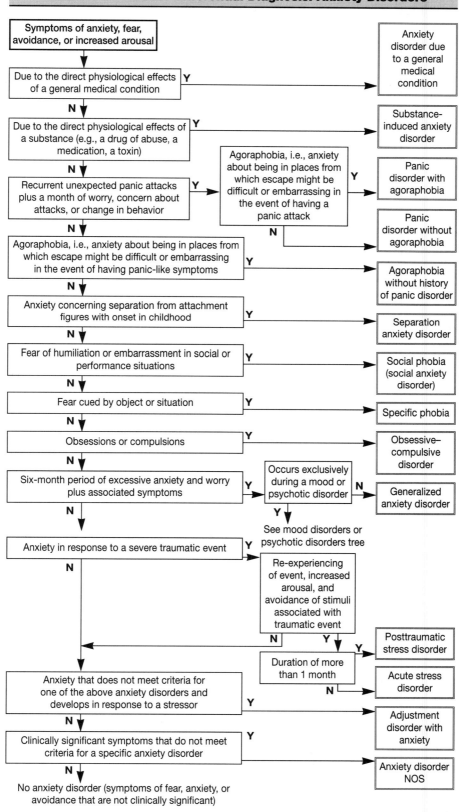

Source: American Psychiatric Association. (1994). *Diagnostic and statistical manual of mental disorders* (4th ed.). Washington, DC: Author.

psychiatric diagnoses as reliably as expert clinicians because they facilitate the evaluation and recording of which specific symptoms are present and which are absent.

Structured interview guides have been used mainly by researchers, who have a special interest in standardizing diagnostic assessments and ensuring that all the patients in a given study are homogeneous with respect to diagnosis. However, the need for accurate, reliable psychiatric diagnosis is not confined to study populations. Treatment selection, level-of-care determination, and goal setting critically depend on comprehensive and accurate diagnostic assessment. With managed care and the need for accountability in assessing and treating mental disorders, structured interviews may now have a place in the routine assessment of patients in clinical settings.

The diagnostic interview guides currently in most widespread use are described below. Additional interview guides not reviewed here are targeted to one diagnostic area, such as anxiety disorders (Di Nardo, Moras, Barlow, Rapee, & Brown, 1993) and personality disorders (First, Gibbon, Spitzer, Williams, & Benjamin, 1997; Loranger et al., 1994; Pfohl, Blum, & Zimmerman, 1997). Similar interview guides have been developed to cover diagnoses often found in children and adolescents (Gutterman, O'Brien, & Young, 1987; Hodges, 1993).

## FEATURES OF STRUCTURED INTERVIEWS

Structured diagnostic interviews differ in several important ways. For one, the degree of structure imposed on the interaction between the interviewer and the patient–subject may differ, from fully structured (in which all the interviewer's questions are exactly specified and no clinical judgment is used) or semistructured (in which many of the questions are spelled out, but the interviewer is required to exercise some judgment in choosing which questions to ask or in supplementing the specified questions) to very unstructured (in which few or no questions are specified for the interviewer). Structured diagnostic interviews also vary by some practical issues, such as the qualifications required for interviewers, training requirements, and how long the interview takes to administer. Finally, diagnostic interview guides differ in their psychometric characteristics such as reliability and validity.

The validity of an instrument is a thorny issue. It is meaningful only when compared with some kind of a gold standard. Unfortunately, for psychiatric diagnosis no obvious gold standard exists to use as a yardstick for measuring the validity of an interview. No blood test or imaging technique can provide the definitive diagnosis of a mental disorder. Clearly, psychiatric diagnoses derived from unstructured clinical interviews cannot by themselves form the basis for a gold standard because, as discussed above, structured interviews may be more valid than unstructured interviews. In the absence of gold, Spitzer (1983) has coined the term "LEAD standard" (Longitudinal observation by Experts using All available Data as sources of information) to describe the elements of the most valid psychiatric diagnostic judgments. Although criticized for itself being fallible, in the absence of valid biological indicators of mental illness, this LEAD standard remains the best standard available.

## DIAGNOSTIC INTERVIEW GUIDES

### DIS/CIDI

The Diagnostic Interview Schedule (DIS) was developed in 1981 in response to an NIMH request for a diagnostic procedure that could be administered by lay interviewers for use in a large-scale epidemiologic survey of the incidence of mental disorders in the general population (Robins, Helzer, Croughan, & Ratcliff, 1981). The plan to conduct more than 20,000 face-to-face interviews made it impractical to have clinicians making the psychiatric diagnoses. The DIS interview is fully structured so that no clinical judgment is required in making the ratings. Although it was developed as an epidemiologic tool, it also has been used in a number of clinical settings over the years. It has a relatively wide diagnostic coverage, including mood disorders, anxiety disorders, substance use disorders, schizophrenia, somatization disorder, antisocial personality disorder, and eating disorders. The Composite International Diagnostic Interview (CIDI) (Robins et al., 1988; Wittchen, 1994; Wittchen et al., 1991) is an international modification of the DIS that follows the same format of the DIS but makes ICD-10 diagnoses in addition to DSM-III-R and DSM-IV diagnoses. The administration time for the DIS and CIDI ranges from one hour (for a relatively straightforward subject) to three hours (for a talkative patient with a complicated lifetime history).

Although these instruments have been used in some studies by clinical interviewers, they are fully structured to minimize the amount of judgment required to administer them and thus do not make use of the skill of an experienced clinician interviewer, which many believe is essential to ensure the validity of the diagnostic assessments (Spitzer, 1983). The main advantage of the DIS and CIDI is that these interviews can be administered by interviewers without clinical training or by computer (Greist et al., 1987; Mathisen, Evans, & Meyers, 1987).

## SCID

The most widely used general clinical diagnostic interview guide is the Structured Clinical Interview for DSM-IV (SCID) (First, Gibbon, Spitzer, Williams, & Benjamin, 1997; First, Spitzer, Gibbon, & Williams, 1997a; Segal, Hersen, & Van Hasselt, 1994; Skre, Onstad, Torgersen, & Kringlen, 1991; Spitzer, Williams, Gibbon, & First, 1992; Williams et al., 1992). The SCID, a semistructured interview for making the major DSM-IV Axis I diagnoses, covers mood, anxiety, psychotic, substance use, somatoform, eating, and adjustment disorders. The SCID begins with an open-ended overview of the present illness and past episodes of psychopathology, followed by a systematic review of the presence or absence of particular items from the DSM-IV criteria. This overview provides an opportunity for the subject to describe the presenting problem in his or her own words, and allows the collection of certain types of information that may not be covered in the course of assessing specific diagnostic criteria later in the interview (for example, previous treatment, social and occupational functioning, and context of the development of the psychopathology). The sequence of questions in the SCID is designed to approximate the differential diagnostic process of an experienced clinician. Because the DSM-IV diagnostic criteria are embedded in the SCID and are assessed as the interview progresses, the interviewer is in effect continually testing diagnostic hypotheses. Figure 2-6 illustrates the SCID question for trouble concentrating, with the corresponding DSM-IV diagnostic criterion in the center column.

Ordinarily, the SCID is administered in a single sitting and takes from 60 to 90 minutes, although in some cases (for example, a particularly complex psychiatric history and inability of the subject to describe his or her psychopathology succinctly) it may take two hours or more. There are two versions of the SCID for Axis I disorders: (1) a clinician version, which covers only those diagnoses most commonly seen in clinical practice and excludes many subtypes and diagnostic specifiers, and

FIGURE **2-6**

**Structured Clinical Interview for DSM-IV (SCID): Item Example**

**Interview Questions**

Did you have trouble thinking or concentrating?
(What kinds of things did it interfere with?)
(Nearly every day?)

**IF NO:** Was it hard to make decisions about
everyday things?

**Diagnostic Criteria**

Diminished ability to think or concentrate, or
indecisiveness, nearly every day (either by
objective account or as observed by others)

SOURCE: First, M. B., Spitzer, R. L., Gibbon, M., & Williams, J.B.W. (1997). *Structured Clinical Interview for DSM-IV Axis I Disorders (SCID)*. New York: New York State Psychiatric Institute, Biometrics Research Department.

(2) a research version, which includes a number of subtypes, severity and course specifiers, and disorders that are diagnostically useful for researchers but that may not be of general interest to clinicians. A version of the SCID for assessing Axis II Personality Disorders also is available (First, Spitzer, Gibbon, & Williams, 1995; First, Spitzer, Gibbon, Williams, Davies, et al., 1995), as is a computer-administered screening version that would be given before the SCID interview to alert the interviewer to those diagnostic domains in which psychopathology is most likely present.[1]

## PRIME-MD

With the managed care movement in the 1990s, primary care clinicians are playing an increasingly prominent role in our health care system. More and more, they are becoming the gatekeepers to specialized care, so that now most initial evaluations for entry into the health care system are conducted by primary care clinicians. Years of research have indicated that mental disorders are present as a primary or associated condition in at least 20 percent of primary care outpatients, and in fact, most cases of mental disorders are treated by primary care physicians (PCPs) rather than mental health professionals. Further, studies also have consistently shown that PCPs in the office setting fail to diagnose and treat approximately 50 percent of mental disorders in their patients. Major obstacles to the recognition of mental disorders by PCPs include inadequate knowledge of the diagnostic criteria for these disorders, uncertainty about the best questions to ask to evaluate whether those criteria are met, and time limitations inherent in a busy office setting.

Because PCPs are increasingly becoming the treatment providers for most people with mental disorders, interview guides have recently been developed for use in primary care. The most widely used of these instruments is the PRIME-MD (Primary Care Evaluation of Mental Disorders) (Spitzer, Williams, et al., 1994). PRIME-MD, the first psychiatric diagnostic interview schedule designed for PCPs, is a standardized but brief and easy diagnostic assessment procedure that evaluates the four groups of mental disorders (mood, anxiety, alcohol, and somatoform disorders) most commonly encountered in the general population and primary care settings. It also evaluates eating disorders, which have more recently been shown to be common in the general population. In extensive field testing, the PRIME-MD proved to have sound psychometric characteristics, but PCPs complained about the eight and a half minutes (on average) it took to administer. Therefore, currently under development is

[1]The Internet address for the SCID Web page is http://cpmcnet.columbia.edu/dept/scid/

a self-report version that relies on the patient to provide more symptomatic information that the clinician can review to make a diagnosis more quickly.

### *DIAGNOSTIC RELIABILITY*

With structured interviews, the psychometric properties of greatest importance are reliability and validity. Reliability is an indicator of diagnostic agreement and is measured in one of two ways: (1) *joint interrater reliability* measures the extent to which different clinicians observing the same interview agree on the diagnosis, and (2) *test–retest interrater reliability* measures the agreement between two clinicians each independently administering the interview to the same client at different times. Reliability is typically calculated for each diagnosis (or diagnostic grouping) included in the structured interview using the kappa statistic, which corrects for chance agreement (Cohen, 1960).

Clinicians and researchers often are interested in knowing the reliability of a particular structured instrument. This is not a meaningful question, however, because measured reliability depends on the design of the particular reliability study. A study that measures joint reliability, for example, will always obtain higher reliability than a study using the test–retest method because the clinicians are, in fact, basing their ratings on exactly the same phenomena. The base rates of the diagnoses in the population studied and characteristics of the interviewers also affect the reliability obtained, because it is harder to achieve good reliability in a population with rare or very frequent diagnoses, and interviewers who have worked together for a long time will get higher reliability than interviewers who have never observed each other before. For these reasons, it is not meaningful to compare instruments with respect to reliability unless the instruments are observed head-to-head in the same study. Reliability statistics are most useful in ensuring that a certain degree of agreement is attainable with a particular instrument, although this does not necessarily predict the actual level of reliability that would be achieved in one's own application of the interview. Some critics of psychiatric diagnostic reliability fail to acknowledge that diagnostic unreliability is not a problem unique to psychiatry. In fact, some of the most trusted diagnostic tests in medicine have very low reliability (for example, the interpretation of X rays) (Elmore, Wells, Lee, Howard, & Feinstein, 1994; Etchells, Bell, & Robb, 1997).

The diagnostic reliability of an assessment procedure reflects the ability of clinicians to agree on a psychiatric diagnosis given a particular clinical presentation. Although good reliability does not assure good diagnostic validity, poor reliability places an upper limit on diagnostic validity. A number of factors (sources of error variance) may contribute to diagnostic unreliability, including differences in what the patient or client reports at different times, differences in how clinicians interview and interpret the clinical information, and differences in the rules by which clinicians make diagnostic judgments (Williams, in press). As noted above, the innovations of diagnostic criteria and structured interview guides have improved diagnostic reliability.

## Screening Scales for Assessment

Rating scales exist to measure nearly every aspect of psychopathology and functioning. Although too numerous to describe in this volume, the reader is referred to several compendia of psychiatric rating scales (Thompson, 1989; Van Riezen & Segal, 1988). In addition, the APA (in press) is preparing a *Handbook of Psychiatric Measures* that will evaluate some of the current measures available and describe how to choose, use, and interpret them in a clinical setting.

When evaluating the usefulness or accuracy (validity) of a particular diagnostic test or procedure, it is necessary to evaluate it against some standard procedure assumed to be valid. This is referred to as "procedural validity" and should not be confused with diagnostic validity discussed above (Spitzer & Williams, 1985).

The validity of a new test or procedure is generally evaluated by comparing its results to some standard test or procedure that serves as the criterion. The validity of the new test is measured against that criterion with three statistical indices: sensitivity, specificity, and predictive power. These concepts are fully described and illustrated in a classic article by Baldessarini, Finklestein, and Arana (1983).

These concepts may be easiest to understand in the case of a new test to screen for a particular diagnosis. The *sensitivity* of the new screening test is calculated as the percentage of true cases it correctly identifies as having the diagnosis (that is, its true-positive rate). The *specificity* is the percentage of noncases that it correctly identifies as not having the diagnosis (its true-negative rate). Finally, the *predictive power* of the new test is the percentage of total cases in which the test agrees with the criterion, that is, the total number of cases that both tests agree have the diagnosis, plus the total number of cases that both tests agree do not have the diagnosis, all divided by the total number of cases. The predictive power of a test can be broken down into positive predictive power and negative predictive power. A test's total predictive power is a summation of these two statistics.

When evaluating the usefulness or appropriateness of a screening scale for a particular task, one must consider its psychometric characteristics. Depending on the consequences of identifying a case, one must decide whether it is more important to identify true cases (high sensitivity) or minimize the identification of false cases (specificity). For example, if one is evaluating a diagnostic test for a serious illness for which the treatment is fairly innocuous, it may be more important to maximize the identification of cases, even if the trade-off is falsely identifying a certain percentage of cases. One could argue that this applies to depression. The consequences of not identifying a true case can be severe (suicide, job loss, and family disruption), whereas the consequences of giving psychotherapy or prescribing an antidepressant medication for someone who does not really need it are not so grave.

## Importance to Social Workers of Classification and Diagnostic Assessment

DSM-III, DSM-III-R, and DSM-IV have not been without their critics, including social workers (Kirk & Kutchins, 1992; Kutchins & Kirk, 1987). However, recognizing that DSM is still an imperfect system, one must balance the improvements in mental health practice that it has facilitated with possible drawbacks to the system, such as an implied reification of the diagnostic categories and a greater number of categories that could potentially become stigmatizing labels. Despite these potential negatives, the increasing precision of the classification of mental disorders has undoubtedly facilitated recent important clinical and research advances, such as more effective psychotherapeutic and pharmacologic treatments for panic disorder and major depressive disorder, as well as significant genetic findings such as those that are already paving the way to cures for some general medical disorders. The drawbacks to patients or clients and mental health professionals, on balance, seem few in comparison to the potential gains of using DSM-IV.

In most psychiatric treatment facilities, the language of DSM-IV is the standard terminology used in diagnostic case discussions. Familiarity with DSM-IV often becomes required for participation in such discussions. The specificity of the diagnostic criteria in DSM-IV and the consequent increase in diagnostic reliability have made it possible for researchers to select groups of subjects that are more homogeneous diagnostically. And it is important for researchers in the social sciences to pay attention to diagnostic variables because many social variables are influenced by and have influence on psychopathology.

Assessment goes hand in hand with classification: Assignment to the proper diagnosis within a classification requires a skilled assessment. Proper longitudinal assessment also is crucial because it allows us to evaluate the efficacy of our interventions. It is important for social workers to be familiar with the diagnostic criteria and multiaxial system of DSM-IV because of its universality as a tool for communication among mental health professionals, its contribution to effective evaluation and treatment planning, its usefulness for teaching psychopathology, and its potential as a basis for research. However, if we are to be as effective as possible in alleviating our clients' suffering, we must become knowledgeable about diagnosis and classification, as well as being adept at assessment.

# References

American Psychiatric Association. (1952). *Diagnostic and statistical manual of mental disorders.* Washington, DC: Author.

American Psychiatric Association. (1968). *Diagnostic and statistical manual of mental disorders* (2nd ed.). Washington, DC: Author.

American Psychiatric Association. (1980). *Diagnostic and statistical manual of mental disorders* (3rd ed.). Washington, DC: Author.

American Psychiatric Association. (1987). *Diagnostic and statistical manual of mental disorders* (3rd ed., rev.). Washington, DC: Author.

American Psychiatric Association. (1994). *Diagnostic and statistical manual of mental disorders* (4th ed.). Washington, DC: Author.

American Psychiatric Association, Task Force on the Handbook of Psychiatric Measures. (in press). *The handbook of psychiatric measures: A task force report of the American Psychiatric Association.* Washington, DC: Author.

Baldessarini, R. J., Finklestein, S., & Arana, G. W. (1983). The predictive power of diagnostic tests and the effect of prevalence of illness. *Archives of General Psychiatry, 40,* 569–573.

Cohen, J. (1960). A coefficient of agreement for nominal scales. *Educational and Psychological Measurement 20,* 37–46.

Curran, J. P., Miller, I. W., III, Zwick, W. R., Monti, P. M., & Stout, R. L. (1980). The socially inadequate patient: Incidence rate, demographic and clinical features, and hospital and posthospital functioning. *Journal of Consulting and Clinical Psychology, 48,* 375–382.

Di Nardo, P., Moras, K., Barlow, D. H., Rapee, R. M., & Brown, T. A. (1993). Reliability of DSM-III-R anxiety disorder categories. Using the Anxiety Disorders Interview Schedule–Revised (ADIS–R). *Archives of General Psychiatry, 50,* 251–256.

Elmore, J. G., Wells, C. K., Lee, C. H., Howard, D. H., & Feinstein, A. R. (1994). Variability in radiologists' interpretations of mammograms. *New England Journal of Medicine, 331,* 1493–1499.

Etchells, E., Bell, C., & Robb, K. (1997). Does this patient have an abnormal systolic murmur? *JAMA, 277,* 564–571.

Fenichel, G. S., & Murphy, J. G. (1985). Factors that predict psychiatric consultation in the emergency department. *Medical Care, 23,* 258–265.

First, M. B., Donovan, S., & Frances, A. (1996). Nosology of chronic mood disorders. *Psychiatric Clinics of North America, 19,* 29–39.

First, M. B., Gibbon, M., Spitzer, R. L., Williams, J.B.W., & Benjamin, L. S. (1997). *Structured Clinical Interview for DSM-IV Axis II Personality Disorders (SCID-II).* Washington, DC: American Psychiatric Press.

First, M. B., Spitzer, R. L., Gibbon, M., & Williams, J.B.W. (1995). The Structured Clinical Interview for DSM-III-R Personality Disorders (SCID-II). Part I: Description. *Journal of Personality Disorders, 9,* 83–91.

First, M. B., Spitzer, R. L., Gibbon, M., & Williams, J.B.W. (1997a). *Structured Clinical Interview for DSM-IV Axis I Disorders–Clinician Version (SCID–CV).* Washington, DC: American Psychiatric Press.

First, M. B., Spitzer, R. L., Gibbon, M., & Williams, J.B.W. (1997b). *Structured Clinical Interview for DSM-IV Axis I Disorders (SCID).* New York: New York State Psychiatric Institute, Biometrics Research Department.

First, M. B., Spitzer, R. L., Gibbon, M., Williams, J.B.W., Davies, M., Borus, J., Howes, M. J., Kane, J., Pope, H. G., Jr., & Rounsaville, B. (1995). The Structured Clinical Interview for DSM-III-R Personality Disorders (SCID-II). Part II: Multi-site test–retest reliability study. *Journal of Personality Disorders, 9,* 92–104.

Gordon, R. E., Jardiolin, P., & Gordon, K. K. (1985). Predicting length of hospital stay of psychiatric patients. *Journal of American Psychiatry, 142,* 235–237.

Greist, J. H., Klein, M. H., Erdman, H. P., Bires, J. K., Bass, S. M., Machtinger, P. E., & Kresge, D. G. (1987). Comparison of computer- and interviewer-administered versions of the Diagnostic Interview Schedule. *Hospital and Community Psychiatry, 38,* 1304–1311.

Gutterman, E. M., O'Brien, J. D., & Young, J. G. (1987). Structured diagnostic interviews for children and adolescents: Current status and future directions. *Journal of the American Academy of Child and Adolescent Psychiatry, 26,* 621–630.

Hodges, K. (1993). Structured interviews for assessing children. *Journal of Child Psychology and Psychiatry and Allied Disciplines, 34,* 49–68.

Husby, R. (1985). Short-term dynamic psychotherapy. V. Global assessment scale as an instrument for description and measurement of changes for 33 neurotic patients. *Psychotherapy and Psychosomatics, 43,* 28–31.

Kirk, S. A., & Kutchins, H. (1992). *The selling of DSM: The rhetoric of science in psychiatry.* New York: Aldine de Gruyter.

Kranzler, H. R., Kadden, R. M., Burleson, J. A., Babor, T. F., Apter, A., & Rounsaville, B. J. (1995). Validity of psychiatric diagnoses in patients with substance use disorders: Is the interview more important than the interviewer? *Comprehensive Psychiatry, 36,* 278–288.

Kutchins, H., & Kirk, S. A. (1987). DSM-III and social work malpractice. *Social Work, 32,* 205–211.

Loranger, A. W., Sartorius, N., Andreoli, A., Berger, P., Buchheim, P., Channabasavanna, S. M., Coid, B., Dahl, A., Diekstra, R. F., & Ferguson, B. (1994). The International Personality Disorder Examination. The World Health Organization/Alcohol, Drug Abuse, and Mental Health Administration International Pilot Study of Personality Disorders. *Archives of General Psychiatry, 51,* 215–224.

Mathisen, K. S., Evans, F. J., & Meyers, K. (1987). Evaluation of a computerized version of the Diagnostic Interview Schedule. *Hospital and Community Psychiatry, 38,* 1311–1315.

Mezzich, J. E., Evanczuk, K. J., Mathias, R. J., & Coffman, G. A. (1984). Admission decisions and multiaxial diagnosis. *Archives of General Psychiatry, 41,* 1001–1004.

Mezzich, J. E., Kleinman, A., Fabrega, H., & Parron, D. L. (1996). *Culture and psychiatric diagnosis: A DSM-IV perspective.* Washington, DC: American Psychiatric Press.

Pfohl, B., Blum, N., & Zimmerman, M. (1997). *Structured Interview for DSM-IV Personality (SIDP-IV).* Washington, DC: American Psychiatric Press.

Robins, L. N., Helzer, J. E., Croughan, J., & Ratcliff, K. S. (1981). National Institute of Mental Health Diagnostic Interview Schedule: Its history, characteristics, and validity. *Archives of General Psychiatry, 38,* 381–389.

Robins, L. N., Wing, J., Wittchen, H. U., Helzer, J. E., Babor, T. F., Burke, J., Farmer, A., Jablenski, A., Pickens, R., Regier, D. A., Sartorius, N., & Towle, L. H. (1988). The Composite International Diagnostic Interview. An epidemiologic instrument suitable for use in conjunction with different diagnostic systems and in different cultures. *Archives of General Psychiatry, 45,* 1069–1077.

Segal, D. L., Hersen, M., & Van Hasselt, V. B. (1994). Reliability of the Structured Clinical Interview for DSM-III-R: An evaluative review. *Comprehensive Psychiatry, 35,* 316–327.

Skodol, A. E., & Spitzer, R. L. (Eds.). (1987). *An annotated bibliography of DSM-III.* Washington, DC: American Psychiatric Press.

Skodol, A. E., Spitzer, R. L., & Williams, J.B.W. (1981). Teaching and learning DSM-III. *American Journal of Psychiatry, 32,* 243–244.

Skre, I., Onstad, S., Torgersen, S., & Kringlen, E. (1991). High interrater reliability for the Structured Clinical Interview for DSM-III-R Axis I (SCID-I). *Acta Psychiatrica Scandinavica, 84,* 167–173.

Spitzer, R. L. (1983). Psychiatric diagnosis: Are clinicians still necessary? *Comprehensive Psychiatry, 24,* 399–411.

Spitzer, R. L., & Forman, J.B.W. (1979). DSM-III field trials: II. Initial experience with the multiaxial system. *American Journal of Psychiatry, 136,* 818–820.

Spitzer, R. L., Forman, J.B.W., & Nee, J. (1979). DSM-III field trials: I. Initial interrater diagnostic reliability. *American Journal of Psychiatry, 136,* 815–817.

Spitzer, R. L., Gibbon, M., Skodol, A. E., Williams, J.B.W., & First, M. B. (1994). *DSM-IV case book.* Washington, DC: American Psychiatric Press.

Spitzer, R. L., Skodol, A. E., Gibbon, M., & Williams, J.B.W. (1981). *DSM-III case book.* Washington, DC: American Psychiatric Association.

Spitzer, R. L., & Williams, J.B.W. (1979). Dehumanizing descriptors? *American Journal of Psychiatry, 136,* 1481.

Spitzer, R. L., & Williams, J.B.W. (1985). Classification of mental disorders. In H. Kaplan & B. Sadock (Eds.), *Comprehensive textbook of psychiatry* (4th ed., pp. 591–613). Baltimore: Williams & Wilkins.

Spitzer, R. L., Williams, J.B.W., Gibbon, M., & First, M. B. (1992). The Structured Clinical Interview for DSM-III-R (SCID). I: History, rationale and description. *Archives of General Psychiatry, 49,* 624–629.

Spitzer, R. L., Williams, J.B.W., Kroenke, K., Linzer, M., deGruy, F. V., Hahn, S. R., Brody, D., & Johnson, J. G. (1994). Utility of a new procedure for diagnosing mental disorders in primary care: The PRIME-MD 1000 study. *JAMA, 272,* 1749–1756.

Spitzer, R. L., Williams, J.B.W., & Skodol, A. E. (Eds.) (1983). *International perspectives on DSM-III.* Washington, DC: American Psychiatric Press.

Thompson, C. (Ed.). (1989). *The instruments of psychiatric research.* Chichester, England: John Wiley & Sons.

Van Riezen, H., & Segal, M. (1988). *Comparative evaluation of rating scale for clinical psychopharmacology.* Amsterdam: Elsevier.

Wakefield, J. C. (1992). The concept of mental disorder: On the boundary between biological facts and social values. *American Psychologist, 47,* 373–388.

Widiger, T. A., Frances, A. J., Pincus, H. A., First, M. B., & Davis, W. W. (1994). *DSM-IV sourcebook* (Vol. 1). Washington, DC: American Psychiatric Press.

Williams, J.B.W. (1985a). The multiaxial system of DSM-III: Where did it come from and where should it go? I. Its origins and critiques. *Archives of General Psychiatry, 42,* 175–180.

Williams, J.B.W. (1985b). The multiaxial system of DSM-III: Where did it come from and where should it go? II. Empirical studies, innovations, recommendations. *Archives of General Psychiatry, 42,* 181–186.

Williams, J.B.W. (1997). The DSM-IV multiaxial system. In T. A. Widiger, A. J. Frances, H. A. Pincus, R. Ross, M. B. First, & W. Davis (Eds.), *DSM-IV sourcebook* (Vol. 3, pp. 393–400). Washington, DC: American Psychiatric Press.

Williams, J.B.W. (in press). Psychiatric classification. In R. E. Hales, S. C. Yudofsky, & J. A. Talbott (Eds.), *The American Psychiatric Press textbook of psychiatry* (3rd ed.). Washington, DC: American Psychiatric Press.

Williams, J.B.W., Gibbon, M., First, M. B., Spitzer, R. L., Davies, M., Borus, J., Howes, M. J., Kane, J., Pope, H. G., Jr., Rounsaville, B., & Wittchen, H-U. (1992). The Structured Clinical Interview for DSM-III-R (SCID). II: Multi-site test–retest reliability. *Archives of General Psychiatry, 49,* 630–636.

Williams, J.B.W., Spitzer, R. L., & Skodol, A. E. (1985). DSM-III in residency training: Results of a national survey. *American Journal of Psychiatry, 142,* 755–758.

Wittchen, H-U. (1994). Reliability and validity studies of the WHO–Composite International Diagnostic Interview (CIDI): A critical review. *Journal of Psychiatric Research, 28,* 57–84.

Wittchen, H-U., Robins, L. N., Cottler, L. B., Sartorius, N., Burke, J. D., & Regier, D. (1991). Cross-cultural feasibility, reliability and sources of variance of the Composite International Diagnostic Interview (CIDI). The Multicentre WHO/ADAMHA field trials. *British Journal of Psychiatry, 159,* 645–653.

Wynne, L. C. (1987). A preliminary proposal for strengthening the multiaxial approach of DSM-III: Possible family-oriented revisions. In G. L. Tischler (Ed.), *Diagnosis and classification in psychiatry: A critical appraisal of DSM-III* (pp. 477–488). Cambridge, England: Cambridge University Press.

# Mood Disorders

Lee W. Badger and Elizabeth H. Rand

**M**ood disorders exact a dreadful toll on families, on the nation's economy, and especially on the 11 million Americans who suffer from them (Greenberg, Stiglin, Finkelstein, & Berndt, 1993). Depressed people endure greater hardship and discomfort than those with most chronic physical illnesses. Among serious illnesses, only advanced coronary artery disease results in more days spent in bed, and only arthritis causes more chronic pain (Wells et al., 1989). In the long run, the social cost of depression is comparable to that of AIDS, cancer, or heart disease ("How Much," 1994).

A study conducted by a team of economists at Massachusetts Institute of Technology found that the cost of major depression, bipolar disorder, and dysthymia amounts to $43.7 billion a year, 55 percent of which ($24 billion) results from absenteeism and lowered productivity among the 72 percent of depressed people who are in the labor force. Twenty-eight percent ($12 billion) goes to the cost of treatment, and 17 percent results from the more than 18,000 associated suicides (at least half of those who commit suicide are severely depressed). These striking figures do not include the associated costs of addiction to tobacco and alcohol and of physical illness, which often co-occur with mood disorders. Nor do the estimates take into account the substantial financial (to say nothing of the emotional) cost to family members who lose time from work and must provide household services for a relative who is depressed (Greenberg et al., 1993).

Despite the significant costs of depression and other mood disorders, these illnesses are neither widely recognized nor adequately treated (Higgins, 1994). A case in point is the greater than one-third of bipolar patients in the recent National Depressive and Manic–Depressive Association (NDMDA) Survey who reported being ill for more than 10 years before receiving a correct diagnosis (Lish, Dime-Meenan, Whybrow, Price, & Hirschfeld, 1994). In the past decade, we also have learned that more than one-half of all people who suffer from mental disorders seek medical help in the primary care rather than in the mental health specialty sector (Regier, Narrow, et al., 1993) and that between 50 percent and 80 percent of these patients' illnesses go unrecognized or misdiagnosed (Higgins, 1994). This problem occurs despite the fact that depression is the most frequent disorder of any kind that primary care physicians are called on to treat (Katon & Sullivan, 1990). Recently, Schulberg et al. (1995) and Katon et al. (1995) demonstrated that integrating mental health professionals into primary care results in dramatic improvement in patient outcome. Future decades will witness increased research activity aimed at addressing a variety of collaborative models to improve the provision of mental health care. Which profession or professions are ultimately selected will be crucial. As deGruy (in press) concluded, "Mental health care cannot be divorced from primary medical care, and all attempts to do so are doomed to failure. Primary care cannot be practiced without addressing mental health concerns, and all attempts to do so will result in inferior care" (p. D-3).

This chapter summarizes the major research concerning mood disorders over the past two decades. The results of this body of research have led to considerable alterations in the manner in which mood disorders are now classified, in our understanding of their prevalence and distribution, in an awareness of their biological and psychosocial origins, and in the appreciation of the cost to patients and society. Perhaps of greatest importance, we have begun to understand better the ways in which mood disorders are experienced by those who suffer from them.

## Epidemiology and Risk Factors

*Epidemiology* is the branch of medicine that studies the distribution of disorders, the prevalence or number of active cases at a given time, and the incidence or number of new cases during a specified time period. Any epidemiologic investigation depends on the system of classification selected to define the disorder's inclusion and exclusion criteria. Because classification of mood disorders has occasionally undergone both rapid and revolutionary change, it is not surprising to find wide variability in current estimates of prevalence and incidence of mood disorders. Despite such variability, the findings from epidemiologic studies provide crucial information for understanding the etiology, treatment, and future prevention of these diseases.

Nine recent epidemiologic surveys conducted around the world, including the five-site Epidemiologic Catchment Area (ECA) studies conducted in the mid-1980s in the United States, have conclusively confirmed that mood disorders occur across nations and cultures. The point prevalence of mood disturbance, moreover, increases linearly as the focus moves from the community in general (2 percent to 4 percent) to primary care settings (5 percent to 10 percent) to inpatient medical settings (6 percent to 14 percent) (Burville, 1995; Jaffe, Froom, & Galambos, 1994; Williams, Kerber, Mulrow, Medina, & Aguilar, 1995).

The ECA studies of the 1980s represented the first large-scale community-based epidemiologic survey to measure the prevalence of mental disorders in the United States. From the ECA data, the phenomenon of substantial psychiatric comorbidity became apparent. More than 60 percent of respondents with one lifetime psychiatric disorder were found to have two or more disorders (Robins et al., 1984). The ECA studies reported a lifetime prevalence for affective disorders of 8 percent for people over age 18 (Regier, Narrow, et al., 1993; Robins & Regier, 1991). However, the more recent National Comorbidity Survey (NCS) reported much higher lifetime rates—between 17 percent and 19 percent (Kessler et al., 1994), an almost twofold increase. The latter rates are remarkably similar to the 16 percent to 20 percent reported in the earlier Zurich epidemiologic study (Angst & Dobler-Mikola, 1985) as well as in 11 other studies done worldwide (Wittchen, Knauper, & Kessler, 1994). The obvious discrepancy in rates is a concern to epidemiologists and continues to be under review (Table 3-1).

TABLE **3-1**

| Ranges in Lifetime Prevalence Rates of Mood Disorders | |
| --- | --- |
| DISORDER | RATES (%) |
| Major depression | 8–20 |
| Dysthymia | 3–8 |
| Bipolar I and Bipolar II disorders | 0.6–3 |
| Minor and subthreshold depression | 6–23 |

Rates for dysthymia ranged from 3 percent to 8 percent across all surveys, and the rates for Bipolar I and II disorders, which are considerably less common, ranged from 0.6 percent to 3.0 percent (Anthony & Petronis, 1991; Regier, Narrow, et al., 1993; Wittchen et al., 1994). In the only epidemiologic study to separate Bipolar I and Bipolar II disorders, Weissman and Myers (1978) found a prevalence of 0.6 percent for each and a lifetime prevalence of 0.4 percent for cyclothymic personality; other studies reviewed by Howland and Thase (1993) have shown considerably higher rates, suggesting that cyclothymia may be at least as prevalent as Bipolar I.

The lifetime prevalence of minor and subthreshold depressions has been reported at 23 percent (Johnson, Weissman, & Klerman, 1992), although the DSM-IV mood disorders field trial noted prevalences of 6 percent for minor depression and 2 percent for recurrent brief depression (Keller et al., 1995). In a re-analysis of the ECA data, Judd, Rapaport, Paulus, and Brown (1994) reported a lifetime prevalence of 11.8 percent for subsyndromal symptomatic depression (SSD), with women representing two-thirds of those impaired.

An epidemiologic and clinical risk factor is a specific characteristic or condition whose presence is associated with an increased prospect that a specific disorder is present or that it will develop. Risk factors and the etiology of a disorder are thus inexorably interrelated. Some recent research, described below, has helped clarify the contributions of various risk factors to mood disorders; however, some of it has simply added to our uncertainty.

## AGE

Substantial evidence indicates that the rates of both major depression and bipolar disorder are increasing and that onset is occurring at an earlier age with each generation (Dysthymia Working Group, 1992). Although these findings appear consistent worldwide, variations in the long- and short-term trends suggest that the rates are inclined, not surprisingly, to be affected by differing historical, economic, and social indices (Lavori et al., 1993).

The risk of major depression is low in childhood, increases substantially with adolescence, and appears to attain its highest prevalence in young adulthood (18–29 years). Studies of elderly populations have proved inconsistent so far. Some studies have reported high rates of depression among older men and women (Blazer & Williams, 1980; Weissman & Myers, 1978), especially those over age 84 (Burke, Burke, Regier, & Rae, 1990), whereas others have reported low rates (Ernst & Angst, 1992; Parker, 1987; Regier, Farmer, et al., 1993). Unfortunately, the recent NCS included only people under age 55.

Of the two forms of dysthymia (early and late onset), early onset is the most frequent. Its prevalence peaks among adults ages 45 to 64 and declines thereafter (Weissman, Leaf, Bruce, & Florio, 1988). There is emerging evidence that elderly dysthymic patients may differ from younger patients; in other words, they are not just "young dysthymic patients who simply grew older" (Devanand et al., 1994, p. 1592).

Bipolar disorder has an earlier age of onset (18 and 22 years, on average, for Bipolar I and Bipolar II disorders, respectively) than most of the nonbipolar mood disorders (Weissman, Leaf, Bruce, et al., 1988), although 59 percent of adults with bipolar disorder in the NDMDA survey claimed onset during childhood or adolescence (Lish et al., 1994). Minor depression also appears to be most prevalent in young adults (25–34 years; Judd et al., 1994). Goodwin and Jamison (1990) pooled data from 22 studies and found an average weighted mean of age 28 for onset of bipolar disorder, although the median is probably younger.

## GENDER

Gender does not seem to be an important factor in the distribution of mood disorder in young children; the sex ratio for major depression of prepubertal age is 1:1. However, by age 15, girls have twice as many depressive episodes as boys (Weissman & Klerman, 1977), and this appears to be true cross-culturally (Wolk & Weissman, 1995). The point prevalence for major depression is from 4.5 percent to 9.3 percent for women and 2.3 percent to 3.2 percent for men, with a lifetime risk of 20 percent to 25 percent for women and 7 percent to 12 percent for men (American Psychiatric Association [APA], 1993). Approximately the same sex ratio (1.5 to 3.0) applies to dysthymia as well (Weissman, Leaf, Bruce, et al., 1988), whereas for minor depression the ratio is somewhat more equivalent (Judd et al., 1994). The incidence of postpartum depression ranges broadly from 6.8 percent to 16.0 percent, depending on the diagnostic criteria used and the time of symptom onset, although one study found that 25 percent of adolescent mothers experience the disorder (Stowe & Nemeroff, 1995).

The sex ratio for bipolar disorder, by contrast, for both children and adults is close to unity (Boyd & Weissman, 1981). The National Institute of Mental Health (NIMH) collaborative study corroborated that women tend to have the depressive type of illness, whereas men more often have the manic form (Coryell et al., 1989). Although cyclothymia is found in some studies to be more prevalent among females than males, Weissman and Myers (1978) showed the same prevalence in males and females as is seen in bipolar disorder.

## RACE AND ETHNICITY

In the NCS and ECA studies, black Americans had a lower one-year prevalence (2.2 percent) of major depression than either whites (2.8 percent) or Hispanic Americans (3.3 percent), but this did not constitute a statistically significant difference by race or ethnicity (Anthony & Petronis, 1991; Kessler et al., 1994; Regier, Narrow, et al., 1993; Weissman, Bruce, Leaf, Florio, & Holzer, 1991). Unlike the NCS studies, the ECA studies did not find that Hispanics have significantly higher rates than non-Hispanics (Burville, 1995). The unevenness of these results reflects a diversity in methodologies, including sample selection and uncontrolled effects of marginality and social roles (Anthony & Petronis, 1991).

Although early studies reported higher rates of bipolar disorder in black than in white people, these studies were confounded by the same factors as were depression studies. Although there has been a historic tendency to misdiagnose manic–depressive illness as schizophrenia within the black population (Mukherjee, Shukla, Woodle, Rosen, & Olarte, 1983), recent studies, including the ECA data, have reported equal rates of bipolar disorder in black and white people (Blazer et al., 1985; Weissman & Myers, 1978).

The potential for variability of rates of disorder within the same ethnic or racial groups is rarely addressed. In other words, is there an intracultural diversity? Dressler and Badger (1985) compared rates of depressive symptoms across three regionally distinct, predominantly African American communities and found markedly different rates. The data indicated that different sociocultural processes involving stressors and support systems were the most likely explanation for the observed differences.

## SOCIOECONOMIC STATUS

As in so many other areas, researchers have reported either higher rates of major depression and dysthymia among lower income and less educated groups (Bruce, Takeuchi, & Leaf, 1991; Regier, Narrow, et al., 1993; Robins & Regier, 1991; Stansfeld & Marmot, 1992) or, counterintuitively, no relationship at all (Weissman et al., 1991; Weissman, Leaf, Bruce, et al., 1988). There is accumulating and persuasive evidence, however, that the prevalence and level of depression are lower among employed than among unemployed people, for both men and women, especially when unemployment lasts as long as six months (Anthony & Petronis, 1991; Weissman et al., 1991). People who are suffering from subsyndromal symptomatic depression also have been found to be more frequent recipients of disability and welfare benefits than are people who are free from depressive symptoms (Judd et al., 1994).

In a retrospective study, Alnaes and Torgersen (1993) found that bipolar patients reported economic and job-related problems even more often than patients with depressive disorders. Only one-third of the bipolar respondents in the NDMDA survey reported being employed full-time, despite the fact that more than 80 percent of the sample had at least some college education. In addition, nearly one-third reported receiving some public assistance (Lish et al., 1994).

Whether unemployment is a causal condition for either of these mood disorders remains unknown, although longitudinal, prospective evidence appears to contradict the argument that depression leads to unemployment (Anthony & Petronis, 1991). Clearly, however, the illness substantially undermines a person's ability to obtain or sustain occupational success.

## MARITAL STATUS

There is an increased risk for major depression and dysthymia among separated, divorced, and widowed adults, and this finding supports the etiological theories of depression that implicate the stress of marital disruption (Hirschfeld & Cross, 1981; Weissman et al., 1991). Living alone also is a significant risk factor; major depression is twice as likely to affect men and women living alone as those living with others. The NDMDA survey reported that 25 percent of the bipolar respondents had never been married, and more than half were not married at the time that they responded to the survey (Lish et al., 1994).

## RELIGION

Evidence is sketchy regarding the importance of religion or religious affiliation. One report from the Durham, North Carolina, site of the ECA survey asserted that the likelihood of major depression among people affiliated with the Pentecostal church was three times greater than among people with other religious affiliations. However, additional carefully designed studies are needed to understand the complex interactions between mental health and religion, as both a belief system and a social institution (Meador et al., 1992).

## RELATIONSHIP AMONG RISK FACTORS

As shown in Table 3-2, those at highest risk for major depression, dysthymia, and minor depression appear to be women, young adults, unmarried people, unemployed people, and those who have experienced a recent interpersonal loss. The risk factors for bipolar disorder differ substantially; gender, marital status, education, and socioeconomic status do not appear to influence risk. However, there is considerable difference of opinion as to whether any of these epidemiologic risk findings are valid or, conversely, whether they are artifacts of research design and sampling cohorts (Anthony & Petronis, 1991). The differences in rates reported across various epidemiologic surveys probably result from differences in the way depression was diagnosed, the often considerable cultural barriers to expression, and the age composition of the samples selected. Despite the variations, however, it is reasonable to conclude that mood disturbances affect at least as many as 16 percent of American adults and thereby represent a major public health problem.

TABLE **3-2**

### Probable Epidemiologic Risk Factors for Mood Disorder

| DISORDER | AGE | GENDER (RATIO) | RACE AND ETHNICITY[a] | MARITAL STATUS | SOCIOECONOMIC STATUS |
|---|---|---|---|---|---|
| Major depression | 18–29 | female (2:1) | Hispanic | unmarried | low, undereducated |
| Dysthymia | 45–64 | female (1.5:3) | — | unmarried | low, undereducated |
| Minor, subthreshold | 25–34 | equivalent | — | unmarried | low, undereducated |
| Bipolar I, Bipolar II, and cyclothymia | 18–29 | equivalent | equivalent | no association | professional |

**Summary:** Those at highest risk for major depression, dysthymia, and minor depression appear to be women, young adults, the unmarried, the unemployed, and those people who have experienced a recent interpersonal loss. The risk factors for bipolar disorder differ substantially; gender, marital status, education, or socioeconomic status do not appear to influence risk.

[a]There is no evidence that race alone is a primary etiologic factor. Socioeconomic status is likely to account for any race and ethnic differences.
NOTE: — = unknown.

Additional methodological variations impede full understanding of the relationships among risk factors and depressive episodes. Studies developed to investigate the association between race and depression, as an example, have often compared data from lower socioeconomic groups of African Americans with those generated from middle-class white groups. The current ambiguity concerning rates of depression among elderly men and women also raises questions about the methodology of cohort studies in which respondents are asked to recall previous psychopathology (Burville, 1995). Rates of depression in elderly populations have even been reported without controlling for gender and marital status, both of which are strongly associated with age and mood disorders (Comstock & Helsing, 1976). Whereas the introduction of structured psychiatric interview schedules and specific diagnostic criteria in the 1970s may have greatly advanced our understanding of the epidemiology of mood disorders, concerns remain that epidemiologic surveys, guided by these fixed criteria, impose a false homogeneity on conditions that are essentially heterogeneous (Jones, 1989).

Following a review of numerous community surveys and ECA findings, Simon and Von Korff (1992) suggested that effects of study methods also may contribute to the apparent temporal trends in the prevalence of depression and that cross-sectional surveys may underestimate lifetime psychiatric morbidity among older respondents. In other words, generational changes in the lifetime risk of depression or other psychiatric disorders may not be reliably assessed by cross-sectional survey data (Simon & Von Korff, 1992). Therefore, it is wise to be cautious about accepting the findings of any epidemiologic study in the absence of prospective longitudinal and developmental epidemiologic investigations (Angold & Worthman, 1993).

## Unipolar Mood Disorders

As described by Williams in chapter 2, both classification and diagnostic systems establish categories into which disorders are placed; the latter also specify criteria that can be used to operationalize the disorders. Both systems, especially the more explicit diagnostic systems, have profound implications for research and subsequent understanding of the epidemiology, etiology, and course of disorders as well as for developing effective treatment. The accumulated research results are used to adjust classification inclusion and exclusion criteria accordingly. Therefore, it is not surprising that classification is a slowly evolving process.

The World Health Organization (WHO) sponsored the development of a classification system beginning at the turn of this century—the *International Classification of Diseases* (ICD). However, it did not begin to include mental disorders until the sixth edition in 1952. The ICD is a classification system into which disorders are assigned without explanation and without diagnostic criteria. Also in 1952, the APA produced the first edition of its *Diagnostic and Statistical Manual of Mental Disorders* (DSM). This manual, containing a glossary of mental disorders with their characteristics, constituted the first official publication to focus on clinical and diagnostic rather than on statistical utility (APA, 1994). The second edition of the manual (DSM-II) (APA, 1968) used two factors to determine the assignment of disorders: (1) whether a condition was considered to be psychotic or neurotic and (2) the nature of the presumed cause (either endogenous or reactive to a psychosocial stressor, or the result of an established personality pattern) (First, Donovan, & Frances, 1996). DSM-III (APA, 1980), on the other hand, used a descriptive, atheoretical approach to classification based on the severity of specified symptoms and the course of the disorder (First et al., 1996). Unipolar and bipolar disorders were thus separated for the first time. Largely because of Akiskal's path-breaking work and despite considerable controversy, the category of dysthymia was introduced to reclassify long-term depression as a mood rather than a neurotic disorder. In the similarly atheoretical DSM-III-R (APA, 1987), mood disorders were characterized by the number of symptoms simultaneously present, their quality, and their duration. The possibility of chronicity of major depression was introduced by allowing a chronic specifier (First et al., 1996), the symptom requirement for dysthymia was adjusted, and it became possible for the first time to diagnose together major depression and dysthymia, informally called "double depression." The main problem with this admittedly superior DSM-III-R classification system, however, was that it failed to clarify how to distinguish between differences in the course and the severity of the latter two disorders (Keller, Hanks, & Klein, 1996; Keller et al., 1995).

The conceptualization and classification of chronic major depression and dysthymia continue to engage the attention of researchers and clinicians. In fact, APA initiated the DSM-IV mood disorders field trial, a multisite, collaborative, naturalistic study that was completed in 1992, in an attempt to assess the relationships among major depression, dysthymia, minor depression, and depressive personality (Keller et al., 1995). Simultaneously and in close collaboration with the DSM-IV work groups, the ICD-10 was developed by the WHO.[1] DSM-IV codes and terms are fully compatible with the mental and behavioral disorders chapter in ICD-10 so that when the latter does come into use as the official reporting system, no changes will be required (APA, 1994).

Since its introduction as a diagnostic rather than classification system, the DSM system has revolutionized the field of psychiatry and fostered an explosion in knowledge about mental illness (deGruy, in press). The DSM-IV is about 50 percent longer than DSM-III-R, which was published seven years earlier, but the space devoted to mood disorders has more than tripled. The DSM-IV classification retains the general outline of DSM-III-R, but there are many changes resulting from new discoveries. The significant research findings from the DSM-IV field trials, as well as other related noteworthy investigations, and the resulting DSM-IV modifications in the classification of mood disorders, are described below and shown in Table 3-3.

## TYPES OF DISORDERS

### Major Depressive Disorder

Two types of major depression have been postulated.[2] The first, which seems to have internal causation (probably biological), is referred to as "melancholic" or "endogenous depression." A second type, which probably results from characterologic,

---

[1] As established by international treaty, DSM-IV is linked to the ICD system for federal (Medicare and Veterans Administration hospitals) billing purposes (Liebowitz, 1993b).

[2] Not everyone agrees. Parker and colleagues (1991) argued that neurotic depression is a pseudo-entity that is clinically meaningless. They advise clinicians not to assume neurotic depression following exclusion of endogenous depression but rather to consider a heterogeneous group of options, including anxiety and personality disorders.

TABLE **3-3**

### Classification of Unipolar Mood Disorders According to DSM-IV

| DISORDER | CHARACTERISTICS |
| --- | --- |
| **Major depressive disorder** | |
| With melancholic features | Psychomotor retardation and agitation, late insomnia, weight and appetite loss, feelings of guilt |
| With psychotic features | Delusions or hallucinations, or both |
| Chronic depression | Clusters of episodes, or single episodes separated by years |
| With atypical features | Overeating, oversleeping, leaden paralysis, and hypersensitivity to rejection |
| With seasonal pattern | Sleep, appetite, and weight increase in winter depression and decrease in summer depression (or vice versa) |
| With postpartum onset | Mild dysphoria or irritability to psychosis or severe depression |
| **Dysthymic Disorder** | Long-standing, more or less chronic, lack of interest in one's usual pleasurable activities |
| **Depression Not Otherwise Specified**[a] | |
| Premenstrual dysphoric disorder | Depressive symptoms four to five days preceding menstruation; none after |
| Minor depressive disorder | Two or more depressive symptoms, for two or more weeks, with associated social or occupational dysfunction |
| Recurrent brief depressive disorder | Episodes last three days but otherwise fulfill the symptomatic criteria for major depression |
| Mixed anxiety–depressive disorder | Anxiety symptoms with symptoms of depression |
| Depressive personality disorder | Pervasive pattern of depressive cognitions and behaviors by early childhood |

[a]Also found in the Appendix to DSM-IV.

personal, or neurotic responses to precipitating events, in addition to biological causes, is generally referred to as "exogenous" or "reactive depression." Psychosocial factors are most frequently implicated in the latter type. Early versions of the DSM reflected the two types of depression, but despite their continued currency, later revisions dropped the distinction. The DSM-IV category of "Adjustment Disorder with Depressed Mood" is used in instances in which a mood disturbance is provoked by a psychosocial stressor, but symptoms are not sufficient in duration or number to meet criteria for major depressive disorder. If the symptoms are sufficient in number to meet criteria for major depression, regardless of whether there was an identifiable stressor, major depression is the correct diagnosis.

The mood disorder field trials investigated the reliability and utility of six course-based patterns of major depression derived from all possible configurations of single or recurrent episodes, with or without preceding dysthymia, and with or without full recovery between episodes (Keller et al., 1995). The vast majority (91 percent) of trial subjects could be classified within one of these patterns, and it thus was thought that sufficient support existed for a course-based classification system for major depression in DSM-IV (Keller et al., 1995; Keller et al., 1996). According to this system, major depression may include one or more of the patterns described below.

*Major Depressive Disorder with Melancholic Features*

As will be a theme throughout this chapter, despite extensive research in mood disorders, the results in almost all arenas remain uncertain. For example, whereas Maes, Schotte, and colleagues (1991) concluded from their research that melancholic features constitute a discrete biological class of major depression rather than occupy a place along a continuum from minor to major to melancholic depression, Rush and Weissenburger (1994) concluded from their comprehensive review that there was less than consistent validity for melancholic depression as a distinct subtype. The DSM-IV work group at one time considered deleting the melancholic modifier but elected to retain the designation because of its apparent clinical utility in determining treatment options and even broadened it by requiring either unreactive mood or pervasive anhedonia. Although the concept of melancholia has a long history, additional research is needed to empirically test the associated biological and psychological features.

*Major Depressive Disorder with Psychotic Features*

Collective research findings support the clinical significance of psychotic depression and, therefore, it is maintained as a distinct subtype in DSM-IV (Johnson, Horwath, & Weissman, 1991). Schatzberg and Rothschild (1992) found statistically significant differences between psychotic and nonpsychotic depression in many areas, such as the biology, familial transmission, course and outcome, and response to treatment. All of these, especially in combination, point to its clinical importance as a separate diagnosis. In the conclusion of their extensive review, Dubovsky and Thomas (1992) proposed that the "greatest theoretical challenge presented by psychotic depression is to understand how disturbances of thought and affect influence each other to produce a distinct syndrome that is more than the sum of its parts" (p. 1195).

*Chronic Depressive Disorder*

In the early 1900s, Kraepelin (1921) characterized chronic depression as a biologically derived depressive temperament. Some years later, psychoanalytic theory conceptualized chronic depression altogether differently and maintained that it was based on a person's particular (and perhaps peculiar) childhood development (Shea & Hirschfeld, 1996). In the early editions of the DSM, chronic depression was classified as a personality disorder and as a neurosis. In recent years, however, increasing attention has focused on the chronicity of several of the mood as well as personality disorders. In the 1980s, Akiskal and colleagues successfully identified and validated two subtypes of chronic depression (Akiskal, 1983; Akiskal, King, Rosenthal, Robinson, & Scott-Strauss, 1981; Akiskal et al., 1980): (1) major depression, with a chronic specifier, and (2) dysthymia, with fewer depressive symptoms. Both are now recognized by the APA and included in DSM-IV.

*Major Depressive Disorder with Atypical Features*

Using prospective data from the vast ECA studies, Horwath, Johnson, and Weissman (1992) found substantial validity for atypical features (defined as overeating, oversleeping, leaden paralysis, and hypersensitivity to rejection) as a distinct subtype of major depression. Major depression with atypical features has been added to the DSM-IV to reflect important treatment implications of this unusual subtype.

### Major Depressive Disorder with Seasonal Pattern

For as many as 15 percent of patients with recurrent major depression, depressive episodes regularly recur on an annual basis. They may occur in one of two seasonal risk periods: recurrent fall–winter depression or, less frequently, recurrent spring–summer depression. The term "seasonal affective disorder" (SAD) has been used to describe this phenomenon. The opposite seasonal types of depression tend to have opposite vegetative symptoms; for example, sleep, appetite, and weight increase in winter depression and decrease in summer depression (Wehr, 1992). DSM-IV includes seasonal pattern as a course specifier, as did DSM-III-R.

### Major Depressive Disorder with Postpartum Onset

Postpartum disorders can range from mild dysphoria or irritability to psychosis or severe depression. Following a recent and comprehensive review of the literature, Dobie and Walker (1992) concluded that major depression after childbirth is probably the same illness as major depression at other times. However, the debate about whether postpartum depression represents a distinct entity remains unresolved (Stowe & Nemeroff, 1995). DSM-IV does include this new subtype as a course specifier for major depressive disorder and bipolar I and II disorders.

## Dysthymic Disorder

The term "dysthymia" was first introduced in 1980 in the DSM-III affective disorder section, replacing the category of "depressive neurosis" in the neuroses section of the former DSM-II. Derived from the earlier constructs of neurotic depression, chronic depression, and depressive personality, dysthymia was defined as a condition characterized by mild depressive symptoms present most of the time for a period of at least two years (Dysthymia Working Group, 1995; Klein et al., 1996). Akiskal's (1994b) review of the evidence found strong support for dysthymia as a primary affective disorder and one that often precedes major affective episodes, perhaps even by more than a decade. In fact, more than 90 percent of people with dysthymia developed subsequent cases of major depression, and more than 80 percent of patients with dysthymia also had major depression (Keller, 1993).

Although there is no consensus on whether dysthymia is a distinct mood disorder or a personality disorder (Keller, 1994b), later findings suggest that dysthymia and major depression are independent. Subsequent to the DSM-IV mood disorders field trials, a proposal ("alternative criterion B"; APA, 1994) was entertained to alter the DSM-III-R diagnostic criteria to emphasize the more representative cognitive and affective symptoms and to de-emphasize the less characteristic vegetative symptoms.

## Depressive Disorder Not Otherwise Specified (NOS)

Numerous presentations known to clinicians and reported in the literature do not meet criteria for any of the diagnostic categories in the DSM. Several of these involve alterations in mood—depressive, manic, or hypomanic—and have been categorized as depressive disorder NOS or as bipolar disorder NOS. Several proposals were made to the Mood Disorders Work Group to separate selected new categories of disorder from the NOS group. Following the trials, the work group identified several categories as meriting closer attention, including premenstrual dysphoric disorder (premenstrual syndrome), minor depression, recurrent brief depression, mixed anxiety–depression, and depressive personality disorder. Currently, these disorders are distributed together in DSM-IV as depressive disorder NOS or mood disorder NOS. They also are found in the DSM-IV appendix. Research findings over the past two decades have clarified these disorders, the most salient of which are described below.

### Premenstrual Dysphoric Disorder

Premenstrual syndrome (PMS) has been the subject of heated popular discussion as well as professional debate. It also has been variously defined, no doubt adding further to the confusion and controversy over its legitimacy as a disorder. Most definitions refer to the presence of depressive symptoms during the four or five days preceding menstruation and an absence of symptoms postmenstruation. In an extensive and comprehensive review of the literature on PMS, Bancroft (1993) noted that the conceptualization of PMS has not only medical and psychiatric implications, but potential adverse political consequences as well. The review led the author to propose a paradigm shift in the thinking about PMS involving a three-factor model: (1) a "timing factor" to account for the hormonal change, (2) a menstruation factor to include the process of build-up and shedding of the endometrium, and (3) a vulnerability factor to cover a variety of characteristics (psychosocial as well as biological) that serve to determine how vulnerable a woman will be to the first two factors. A virtue of this model, in addition to diffusing the political issue, is that the existing literature can be reappraised in a way that has considerable potential relevance to our understanding of PMS and major depressive disorder (Bancroft, 1993). There is accumulating evidence, for example, that recurrent premenstrual mood changes may increase the likelihood of chronic depressive disorder among vulnerable women. Harrison, Endicott, Nee, Glick, and Rabkin (1989) found a lifetime prevalence of major depression in 70 percent of women with a confirmed diagnosis of premenstrual syndrome. Following a comprehensive analysis of the literature, Endicott (1993) noted shrewdly that changes in the severity and periods of depressive symptoms should be noted by researchers, both in epidemiology and clinical trial studies, as well as by clinicians serving women with depression.

### Minor Depressive Disorder

The DSM-IV field trial was conducted in part to examine the occurrence of and disability associated with minor depressive disorder. After extensive investigation, however, the data were still inconclusive (Keller et al., 1995), and minor depressive disorder was placed in the DSM-IV appendix. Despite consistent reports of significant disability associated with minor depressive disorder, there remains considerable controversy over whether it should be assigned a separate disorder classification (Broadhead, Blazer, George, & Tse, 1990; Johnson et al., 1992; Judd et al., 1994).

### Recurrent Brief Depressive Disorder (RBD)

Another mission of the field trials was to investigate the validity of recurrent brief depression as a distinct mood disorder subtype. RBD is identical to major depression in the number and severity of symptoms, but it lasts for periods of less than two weeks and recurs at least monthly for one year or longer. Since 91 percent of all field trial patients had current or lifetime major depressive disorder or dysthymic disorder, the work group concluded that the evidence was not persuasive enough, either for or against the proposed category, to include it as a unique entity. Therefore, RBD can be found alongside minor depressive disorder in the appendix to DSM-IV (Keller et al., 1995).

### Mixed Anxiety–Depressive Disorder

Diagnostic criteria for mixed anxiety–depressive disorder closely parallel the categories of depression NOS and anxiety NOS. It has become increasingly clear that as many as 60 percent of patients with major depressive disorder also have symptoms of anxiety or anxiety disorders (Keller & Hanks, 1995), which has led to speculation about whether mixed anxiety–depressive disorder might actually be a distinct subtype of either a unipolar depression or anxiety disorder. Coryell, Endicott, and Winokur (1992) concluded their extensive investigation by noting that anxiety syndromes appear to be prognostically significant but not indicators of an additional disorder. Because the ICD-10 includes a category of mixed anxiety and depression, the DSM-IV task force, amid considerable controversy, made the decision to include it in the DSM-IV appendix (Liebowitz, 1993b; Preskorn & Fast, 1993).

### Depressive Personality Disorder

Depressive personality was in the past subsumed categorically under a wide variety of mood and personality disorders (Hirschfeld & Holzer, 1994). Particularly in recent years, many researchers and clinicians have argued for the formal recognition of depressive personality as a distinct entity (Keller et al., 1996; Phillips, Gunderson, Hirschfeld, & Smith, 1990). Klein and Miller (1993) found significant (although modest in magnitude) relationships between depressive personality and lifetime DSM-III diagnoses of major depression and dysthymia, indicating that these are distinct although overlapping constructs. This conclusion also was supported by the DSM-IV mood disorder field trials (Keller et al., 1996). Keller and colleagues claimed, as did Klein and Miller (1993) and Hirschfeld and Holzer (1994), that these results provide significant evidence to justify the validity of depressive personality disorder. Depressive personality disorder is a clinically important condition with significant social and occupational morbidity and, although it is not subsumed by existing mood disorder or personality categories, it can be viewed as falling within the affective spectrum. Nevertheless, the decision was made to list depressive personality disorder in the DSM-IV appendix and await further study.

## Subthreshold Depression

The term "subthreshold" is loosely used in the literature to refer to a wide variety of depressive conditions that do not meet DSM criteria (including the NOS categories) for any mood disorder (Angst & Hochstrasser, 1994; Broadhead et al., 1990; Wells et al., 1989). Chiefly during the past decade, concern has been growing about the unexpected impairment that appears to be associated with subthreshold mood disorders. To explain by example, in just the past few years a new category, subsyndromal symptomatic depression (SSD), has been proposed as an unrecognized clinical condition of considerable health importance (Judd et al., 1994). SSD is divided into two types, with and without mood disturbance, and requires the simultaneous presence of two or more depressive symptoms for two weeks or longer with associated social dysfunction. The first type overlaps with the DSM-IV category of minor depressive disorder, whereas the latter, with prevalent symptoms of hypersomnia and weight gain, is similar but not identical to the DSM-IV category of atypical depressive disorder. Because there is still a lack of information on what subthreshold depressive symptoms represent (that is, whether they are secondary to other psychiatric or physical disorders or whether they characterize a primary affective illness), no current standard exists for measuring them (Sherbourne et al., 1994). It is expected that this disorder will receive considerable research and clinical attention in the near future.

## Summary

Many questions remain about the conceptualization and classification of mood disorders, especially chronic depression, dysthymic disorder, and the subthreshold conditions. The line dividing chronic mood disturbance from personality disorder remains difficult to define (Hiller et al., 1994), particularly because comorbidity is commonly reported (Hirschfeld et al., 1989). Despite the inclusion of dysthymic disorder as a mood disorder in both the DSM-IV and the ICD-10, it has been argued that it would be better conceptualized as a personality disorder. Even the validity of the diagnostic requirement for major depressive disorder of a two-week duration of depressed mood or anhedonia has been questioned (Judd et al., 1994). One of the major challenges for the ongoing process of classification of mood disorders is the development of a system that reflects the wide variation in the severity and course seen in clinical practice (Keller et al., 1995). Greater clarification of the uncertainties described above will continue to be the center of research attention over the next decades so that diagnosis may become more accurate and treatment more effective.

## *PATHOGENESIS*

The unipolar mood disorders represent heterogeneous, multifactorial disorders. Genetic and early environmental factors appear to influence temperament and response to adverse life events and together are likely to regulate a person's vulnerability to depression (Kendler, Kessler, Neale, Heath, & Eaves, 1993). Therefore, understanding the etiology of mood disorders necessitates considering genetic and other biological factors, personality and temperament, and psychosocial risk factors (Kendler et al., 1993). There has been extensive research activity in the past two decades and (especially regarding the biology of mood disorders) much exploration of new territory. Recent discoveries are described below.

## Genetics

A genetic marker should be more prevalent in people with a disorder, in this case significant mood disturbances, than in those without and should be a trait rather than a state-dependent marker. In other words, it should be present even after recovery from the illness (Nathan & Schatzberg, 1994). A consistent finding for at least two decades has been that the incidence of depression and the other mood disorders is one and one-half to three times higher among people with relatives who have mood disorders than among people without such relatives (Regier, Farmer, et al., 1993; Weissman, Leckman, Merikangas, Gammon, & Prusoff, 1984). Children of parents suffering from depression have consistently been found to be at significant risk for developing depressive disorders (Hammen, 1991; Keller et al., 1986; Weissman et al., 1987). Keller et al. (1986) reported that an astonishing 40 percent of daughters of parents with affective disorder developed a depressive disorder by age 17. As striking as these findings are, they do not explain whether the association results from a genetic loading or from upbringing and life experience. After all, families in which a parent suffers from depression may be more likely to have chronic parental dysfunction, which may be the primary factor contributing to any subsequent negative outcomes for the children (Marton & Maharaj, 1993).

Twin and adoption studies have attempted to elucidate the nature-versus-nurture debate. If there is a genetic factor, then a twin with a depressed identical (monozygotic) twin should be more likely to have the disorder than a twin with a depressed fraternal (dizygotic) twin, even if the twins are reared in separate environments. However to date, results of numerous twin studies have been inconclusive. For example, Andrews, Stewart, Allen, and Henderson (1990) found no etiologic role for genetic factors, but more recent results have typically shown a genetic component (Kendler et al., 1993; Kendler et al., 1995; Kendler, Neale, Kessler, Heath, & Eaves, 1992a, 1992b, 1994; Kendler, Walters, et al., 1994; McGuffin & Katz, 1989; Moldin, Reich, & Rice, 1991). In fact, Kendler and colleagues concluded that genetic factors play a substantial causal role in depression, although whether they are necessary or sufficient is not yet known. The authors based their conclusion on the consistency of data, which showed a two to three times greater concordance rate among monozygotic than among dizygotic twins (Kendler et al., 1993; Kendler et al., 1992a, 1992b; Kendler, Neale, et al., 1994; Kendler, Walters, et al., 1994). Kendler, Walters, and colleagues also concluded that environmental factors probably cause twin resemblance for the age at which they have their first episode, and genetic factors probably cause the degree of impairment and experience of changes in appetite, weight, and sleep.

Of the three major adoption studies of depression, two found significant evidence for genetic effects (Cadoret, O'Gorman, Heywood, & Troughton, 1985; Wender et al., 1986), whereas the other found greater support for the importance of environmental factors (von Knorring, Cloninger, Bohman, & Sigvardsson, 1983).

The extent of genetic influence appears to be the same for both broadly and narrowly defined forms of major depression. Both neurotic and endogenous depressions have been found to aggregate in families, although there is some indication that genetic factors have a more pronounced effect in the former (Torgersen, 1986). In cases beginning in childhood or adolescence, dysthymia is associated with high familial rates of mood disorders and a recurrent pattern of superimposed major depression.

All in all, then, heredity is extremely likely to be among the important predisposing factors for the mood disorders (Akiskal, 1992; Akiskal & Weise, 1992; Kendler, Walters, et al., 1994; McGuffin & Katz, 1989), accounting for as much as one-half of the variance among people with depressive symptoms (Kendler, Walters, et al., 1994). Kendler, Walters, and colleagues concluded that depressive symptoms in adulthood reflect enduring characteristics of temperament that are substantially influenced by hereditary factors but only mildly influenced by shared experiences in the family of origin.

### Neurobiology and Biological Risk Factors

The study of biological processes is an important way to establish the validity of psychiatric diagnoses and to promote the development of effective treatments (Howland & Thase, 1991). Especially in recent years, a considerable amount of research has identified potential neurophysiological processes that provide information essential to effective clinical decision making (Nathan & Schatzberg, 1994).

It is now accepted beyond reasonable doubt that depression is accompanied by neurochemical changes in the brain. Current theories remain unspecific as to the exact nature of these changes, although neurotransmitters are central to most hypotheses. These chemical messengers transmit electrical signals from one nerve cell to another, setting into motion the neural interactions that affect behavior, feeling, and thought processes. The major neurotransmitters believed to be involved are serotonin, norepinephrine, dopamine, and (a more recent addition) acetylcholine.[3] Based on an improved understanding of the biology of depression and the major role apparently played by the neurotransmitter serotonin (Owens & Nemeroff, 1994), the selective serotonin reuptake inhibitors (SSRIs) were introduced in 1987. They represent the first class of drugs that were developed to target a specific site. Current research also has focused attention on other central neurotransmitters, such as gamma-aminobutyric acid (GABA) and glutamic acid, and neuropeptides, such as corticotropin-releasing factor. Finally, heterocyclic amines, derived from fried and broiled meats, food dyes, soft drinks, and particularly cigarette and petroleum fumes, are increasingly implicated in the etiology of unipolar depression in susceptible people (Newman & Holden, 1993). It has even been suggested that these neurotoxins might account for the rising rates of depression reported in more highly developed nations.

Despite the difficulty of demonstrating a true genetic trait marker, there is evidence that low plasma GABA (an inhibitory neurotransmitter) may represent a biological marker of vulnerability for development of various mood disorders (Petty, 1994). Changes in plasma concentrations of GABA reflect brain GABA activity, and concentrations are significantly lower in about one-third of patients with major depressive disorder; concentrations also are low in patients with mania and in patients with bipolar disorder who are depressed. These low concentrations of GABA appear to persist after recovery from depression and are not increased by treatments that improve depressive symptoms (Petty, 1994).

Located deep within the brain, the hypothalamus is responsible for the regulation of the endocrine and autonomic nervous systems and controls food intake, sexual drive, sleep rhythms, and the synthesis and release of certain hormones. Abnormal functioning of this region is associated with depression and its corresponding symptoms of anorexia, decreased sexual interest, early morning wakening, and abnormal production of certain hormones. With respect to the latter, one of the surest findings in biological psychiatry is that patients with major depression have elevated plasma cortisol, a steroid hormone (Pariante, Nemeroff, & Miller, 1995). This understanding

---

[3]The etiological importance of these chemicals was discovered, ironically, when the drug reserpine (a hypertension medication used to treat schizophrenia during the 1960s) unexpectedly led to depression. Among its neurochemical effects, reserpine indirectly reduces the amount of serotonin and norepinephrine, and thus these neurotransmitters were implicated in the etiology of depression.

first emerged from the observation that patients with Cushing's disease, which is associated with an excess of cortisol, often suffer from extremely depressed moods. Using the knowledge that injected dexamethasone normally suppresses production of endogenous cortisol but does not do so in patients with Cushing's disease, mental health investigators tried the dexamethasone suppression test in patients with depression. They found that a significant proportion of bipolar and unipolar depressed patients, especially psychotically depressed patients (Coryell, Pfohl, & Zimmerman, 1984), also failed to suppress cortisol in response to exogenous dexamethasone. Unfortunately, although highly sensitive, this test has proved to be too nonspecific—many nonsuppressors have other disorders—to be a useful diagnostic tool for depression.

There are reports that growth hormone secretion is often blunted in depressed patients, compared with nondepressed people, when given an alpha-2 receptor antagonist such as clonidine. In fact, clonidine has recently been proposed as a possible diagnostic test, although it might be more useful for ruling out depression than confirming it (Schittecatte et al., 1994). However, other reports find no significant differences between patients with depressive disorder and healthy controls (Gann, Riemann, Stoll, Berger, & Muller, 1995).

An important recent finding is that patients who have attempted violent suicide also show evidence of dysregulation of the hypothalamic-pituitary-adrenal (HPA) axis (Roy, 1994). In a study reported by Ohmori, Arora, and Meltzer (1992), suicide and homicide victims had significantly higher cortical concentrations of HVA (homovanillic acid, a dopamine metabolite) than did those who died of physical disease, but not higher than those who died of accidents. In a review of his own studies, Roy (1994) concluded that depressed patients who had attempted suicide had significantly reduced cerebrospinal fluid (CSF) concentrations of HVA and significantly lower urinary outputs of HVA than patients who had not attempted suicide. Similarly, patients who repeatedly attempted suicide over a five-year follow-up period had significantly reduced concentrations compared with patients who made no further suicide attempts. These data suggest a role for diminished central dopaminergic neurotransmission in suicidal behavior among depressed people. In a finding directly implicating the HPA axis, Szigethy, Conwell, Forbes, Cox, and Caine (1994) found that the average postmortem weight of the adrenal glands in people who committed suicide was significantly higher than in a group of nonpsychiatric control subjects.

Thyroid function or dysfunction also has been implicated in mood disorders. Several studies indicate that subclinical hypothyroidism is more prevalent in chronic depression than in milder forms, implying that evaluation of thyroid function should always be included in the assessment of depression (Howland & Thase, 1991). Recently, Custro and colleagues (1994) added a new twist to the relationship between thyroid function and depression by reporting that thyroid disease may be secondary to endogenous depression. In other words, depression also may play a precipitating role in the development of thyroid disease.

Biological (especially endocrine) explanations for major depressive disorder seem among the most likely to elucidate the two-to-one female-to-male ratio that exists af) ter puberty (Wolk & Weissman, 1995). For example, there is some evidence that suicide attempts are more likely during the premenstrual phase of the menstrual cycle, and autopsy evidence points to a greater occurrence of completed suicides during the late luteal phase (Endicott, 1993). Although Abramowitz, Baker, and Fleischer (1982) found that a sizable number of women admitted to psychiatric hospitals for depression were admitted on the first day of menstruation or on the day before, they did not propose that hormonal changes directly cause depression. Instead, their conclusion was that hormones may aggravate a pre-existing condition.

Postpartum depression also seems to exhibit a hormonal component, although the specific biological mechanism has yet to be discovered. Recent research has shown that depressive illnesses at menopause do not differ from those experienced at other ages.[4] Women who are most vulnerable typically have a history of past depressive episodes (Pariser, 1993).

Depression has long been believed to be a psychological consequence of stress, and animal research has clearly demonstrated a profound effect of stress on the immune system. Recent developments suggest that both major depressive disorder and stressful life events may modify immune functions, affecting susceptibility to physical illness (Maes, 1995). Reports suggest that severe depression is characterized by immune dysfunction insofar as depressed people show abnormalities in certain cell types involved in the immune system when compared with healthy people (Marazziti et al., 1992). Once again, however, the exact nature of the involvement remains unclear. Some authors have described an immune suppression (Asnis & Miller, 1989), whereas others have described an immune activation (Maes et al., 1992). There is some inconclusive additional evidence that immunity may be differentially affected in men and women (Maes, DeMeester, et al., 1991).

Another interesting investigative area is the contribution of circadian rhythms, which control certain daily biological cycles, to the etiology of depression. In fact, the abnormal sleep pattern of depressed people was one of the earliest findings in biological psychiatry. The normal pattern of sleep begins with 90 minutes of non-REM sleep, which is followed by a first REM period; several more REM periods occur later in the sleep period. Many recent studies have shown that people with major depressive disorder usually have a prolonged period before falling asleep followed by a shortened period of sleep before entering the first REM period. These people experience increased wakefulness, have more REM periods (dream more) earlier in the night, tend to awaken earlier in the morning, and tend to have difficulty falling back to sleep. Upon recovery from depression, sleep patterns tend to return to normal (Beersma & van den Hoofdakker, 1992; Mendlewicz & Kerkhofs, 1991).[5] Recent sleep research also has revealed important evidence that strongly suggests a common pathophysiologic pathway for major depressive disorder and dysthymic disorder (Akiskal, 1994a).

A broader rhythm is the seasonal pattern seen in certain disorders. A relatively new area of research has begun to link some types of depression to the seasonal changes: depression in the fall and winter and normal (or mania) in the spring and summer. Occasionally the opposite occurs (Wehr, Sack, Rosenthal, & Cowdry, 1988). One etiologic theory relating depression to reduced light environments is supported by evidence that people with depression who are exposed to bright light have a positive therapeutic outcome (Wehr, 1992). Although no single biological system has been conclusively shown to be responsible for seasonal depression, the hormone

---

[4]Mental health experts once believed that women who experienced depression during menopause were suffering from involutional melancholia (a depressive illness), but this diagnosis is no longer in use.

[5]As many as 60 percent of depressed patients experience remission after a night of total or partial sleep deprivation (Leibenluft, 1996).

melatonin, the neurotransmitter serotonin, and the neuropeptide corticotropin-releasing hormone all have been implicated (Wehr, 1992).

## Neuroanatomy

No certainty exists about the pathophysiology of mood disorders and their underlying functional neuroanatomy. However, recent studies have benefited from the availability of computed tomography (CT scanning), magnetic resonance imaging (MRI), positron emission tomography (PET scanning), and single photon emission computed tomography (SPECT). These technologies provide an opportunity to study the neuroanatomical structure and the functioning of the brain at different stages of illness. For example, there is now evidence that patients with unipolar major depression may show a lower whole brain cerebral blood flow (CBF) and reduced regional CBF in the frontal, temporal, and parietal lobes (Sackeim et al., 1993; Thomas et al., 1993). There has been some disagreement with these findings, however. Maes and colleagues (1993) concluded that cortical CBF was relatively intact in their sample of 43 unipolar depressed subjects and 12 normal control subjects. Furthermore, these studies have been conducted only on hospitalized patients, and there is concern about the variability among the control groups (Goodwin & Jamison, 1990).

## Premorbid Personality Structure and Temperament

Some investigators have proposed that individual temperament, or personality, may provide the best explanation for the heterogeneity of mental disorders and their prognosis (Joyce & Paykel, 1989).[6] Winokur and Coryell (1991) proposed that temperament predisposes a person to abnormal affect and that the major underlying problem in the mood disorders is a lifelong personality disturbance that occasionally surfaces as major depressive disorder. Depressed patients with comorbid Axis II disorders appear to be temperamentally different from those who do not suffer from such comorbidity, suggesting that continued study of underlying temperament dimensions may increase our understanding of the patterns of comorbidity between major depressive disorder, other Axis I disorders, and personality disorders (Mulder, Joyce, & Cloninger, 1994).

One particular personality type, neuroticism, consistently has been found to be a dependable predictor of unipolar depression by a large number of investigators (Akiskal, 1992; Angst & Clayton, 1986; Hirschfeld et al., 1989; Keller et al., 1996; Maier, Lichtermann, Minges, & Huen, 1992; Scott, Eccleston, & Boys, 1992). Neuroticism characterizes a person who is emotionally unstable, vulnerable to stress, and prone to anxiety. It has been hypothesized that women are more likely to exhibit this personality, suggesting another possible clue to the mystery of the greater instance of depression among women than among men (Mulder et al., 1994). Many researchers and clinicians claim that the neurotic personality is long-standing and, therefore, the primary problem. Any mood disorder is a secondary problem (Maier

---

[6]Researchers in Europe have focused their attention on the etiological importance of personality features (also called "character"), whereas American researchers have tended to investigate temperament (genetic and constitutional factors of personality), with its closer link to biology (Akiskal, 1991). Many researchers use the terms interchangeably.

et al., 1992). Related sociological theories suggests that socialization differences predispose women to be depressed when under stress (Seligman, 1975), whereas men are more likely to become alcoholic (Weissman & Klerman, 1977).

Cloninger and his colleagues have proposed an expanded biosocial theory of personality, including both temperament and character, that may further understanding of the effects of early environment on psychopathology (Cloninger, Svrakic, & Pryzbeck, 1993). They have postulated three genetically independent traits, which have been labeled "harm avoidance" (for example, pessimistic worry), "reward dependence" (for example, social attachment and dependence) and "impulsive decision making." Their theory has recently been put to empirical test, and a number of interesting associations among patterns of depression and temperament will likely begin to emerge (Mulder et al., 1994).

Dysthymic disorder is thought to have underlying personality disturbance even more than major depressive disorder. For instance, in a study by Pepper and colleagues (1995), a significantly greater proportion of patients with dysthymic disorder (60 percent) than patients with episodic major depressive disorder (18 percent) met criteria for a personality disorder. The most common of these were borderline, histrionic, and avoidant personality disorders. Other studies have found less dramatic differences, however. In a study by Sanderson and colleagues, 50 percent of patients with major depressive disorder, 52 percent of patients with dysthymic disorder, and 69 percent of patients with double depression were diagnosed as having at least one personality disorder. Most commonly reported were avoidant and dependent personality disorders (Sanderson, Wetzler, Beck, & Betz, 1992). Whatever the true percentages, it appears indisputable that comorbidity is a common occurrence.

## Psychosocial Precipitants

Psychosocial factors are most frequently implicated in exogenous or reactive depression, as opposed to endogenous or melancholic depression, as described above under "Types of Disorders." Psychosocial factors include stressful life events as well as cultural and social factors.

### Stressful Life Events

Some studies have found almost no relationship between stressful life events and the onset of mood disorders (McGuffin, Katz, & Bebbington, 1988; Perris, von Knorring, & Perris, 1982), but an impressive number of others have reported the emergence of major depressive disorder following a substantial adverse life event, such as the sudden termination of a close relationship (Brown & Harris, 1978; Dohrenwend & Dohrenwend, 1974; Hammen et al., 1987; Kendler et al., 1995; Kessler, House, & Turner, 1987; Phelan et al., 1991; Warner, Mufson, & Weissman, 1995). Most notably, early childhood trauma, especially that caused by physical and sexual abuse, is identified as a significant risk factor for later development of psychotic depression (Livingston, 1987). More recent research suggests, however, that people who develop major depressive disorder may have abnormally acute reactions to the stresses of life events rather than more than their share of such events and, therefore, that life events may represent the prodromal manifestation of a mood disorder rather than its primary cause (Richardson, 1991). For example, Hammen (1991) found that although depressed women reported a greater rate of stressful life events than those who were not depressed, the women themselves were partially responsible for the difference. This possibility was supported by McNaughton, Patterson, Irwin, and Grant (1992), who suggested that the increased number of events reported by depressed patients might be partly attributable to dysfunctional behavior that produces depression-related events and that these events might in turn exacerbate depression. These findings suggest the necessity of psychosocial and psychotherapeutic intervention with depressed people.

An important new finding is that psychosocial stressors may play a greater role in the first episode of major depression and then a decreasing role in subsequent episodes. In his important 1992 article, based on solid empirical research, Post, the chief of the biological psychiatry branch of NIMH, proposed a neurophysiologic kindling-sensitization hypothesis to explain the longitudinal course of major depression. Post concluded, "Early clinical observations and recent systematic studies overwhelmingly document a greater role for psychosocial stressors in association with the first episode of major affective disorder than with subsequent episodes" (p. 999). Both stressors and episodes, he continued, "may leave residual traces and vulnerabilities to further occurrences," and the data suggest that "the biochemical and anatomical substrates underlying the affective disorders evolve over time as a function of recurrences, as does pharmacological responsivity" (p. 999). Each episode of major depression may further sensitize and permanently alter limbic and neurotransmitter systems, which may explain the gradual worsening of episodes over time. One implication of these findings is that aggressive treatment and maintenance therapy may be crucial for individuals experiencing their initial depressive episode.

## Cultural Factors

The DSM-IV marks a dramatically new level in the acknowledgment of the role of culture in shaping the presentation of symptoms and the course of each mood disorder, including major depression (Manson, 1995). Many disorder categories now include a systematic discussion of cultural variations in the presentation of symptoms, although there remain concerns that more cultural influence has been empirically discovered and should, therefore, have been included (Manson, 1995).

The experience and expression of dysphoria vary considerably across cultures, making the affective symptoms of the mood disorders particularly difficult to ascertain. Even the word "depressed" is absent from the lexicon of some cultures (Manson, 1995). As Manson concluded in a comprehensive review article, future revisions of the DSM must continue to emphasize clinical description, but it "needs to be extended beyond the middle and upper classes of American and European society," and a better understanding "must take into account the social contexts and cultural forces that shape one's everyday world" (p. 497).

## Social Factors

The family is typically the primary setting and context in which risk factors combine to increase vulnerability and precipitate actual depressive episodes (Schwab, Stephenson, & Bell, 1988). Family factors recently posited as contributory to the etiology of depression include, among others, violence (Bryer, Nelson, Miller, & Krol, 1987; Holmes & Robins, 1988), alcoholism (West & Prinz, 1987; Winokur & Coryell,

1991), parental mental illness (Kessler & Magee, 1993; Weissman et al., 1987), and the absence of maternal care in childhood (Parker & Hadzi-Pavlovic, 1984; Perris, 1983). A variable commonly found to be associated with mood disorder is the lack of intimate, confiding relationships (Price, Ketterer, & Bader, 1980). The supporting presence of close and sympathetic people during times of stress has been identified as a key buffer against the unhealthy consequences of stress (Brown & Harris, 1986). Research with monkeys and other primates has shown that animals, when socially isolated during infancy, develop behavior patterns similar to depressed humans (for example, despair, crying, withdrawal, appetite loss, disturbed sleep, and agitation). In an interesting recent study by McNaughton and colleagues (1992), it was found that depressed people reported significantly fewer social supports and less satisfaction with the emotional component of the support that was available. However, these studies have been correlational, and there is as yet no evidence in humans of a causal relationship between the quality of social life and clinical depression (Marton & Maharaj, 1993).

In a related vein, evidence concerning the association between death of a significant person and the development of depression remains inconclusive. Brown and Harris (1978) reported that the loss by death or separation of a parent or sibling before age 11 was a risk factor for depression; more recent investigations, however, have not been able to support the hypothesis that death of a parent in childhood is a direct cause of depression, or even significantly associated with the disorder (Crook & Eliot, 1980; Kendler et al., 1993; Perris, Homgren, von Knorring, & Perris, 1986; Ragan & McGlashan, 1986; Tennant, 1988). Evidence is equally equivocal regarding the relationship between loss of a spouse and the development of depression; Mor, McHorney, and Sherwood (1986) found no connection between death of a spouse and depression, whereas Zisook and Schuchter (1991) reported that almost one-quarter of bereaved spouses had major depression after two, seven, and 13 months. Karam (1994) found that the risk of recurrence of depressive episodes was unrelated to whether the depressive episodes were connected with grief.

## Summary

The impressive quantity and quality of the research conducted over the past few decades have contributed exponentially to knowledge about the etiology of mood disorders. However, there remains much to discover. Aggregated results of twin and adoption studies have been equivocal, and the precise nature of inheritance of any of the mood disorders is still far from certain (Akiskal, 1992). Little substantive progress has been made toward answering the question of how biological vulnerability and psychosocial adversity interact, despite a growing body of literature comparing both biological and genetic theories with psychosocial theories (Kendler et al., 1995). No research documents the relationship between adverse life events and the first onset of depression (Council on Scientific Affairs, 1993). Several factors also limit the usefulness of many of the research findings: a lack of diagnostic consistency across research populations, the overlap of symptom boundaries, the apparent frequency of comorbidity between the disorders, and the fact that most studies have been cross-sectional rather than longitudinal. It is still unclear, for example, whether major depression and dysthymia are each a heterogeneous group of conditions or, alternatively, different aspects of the same disorder (Howland & Thase, 1991; Muller, Hofschuster, Ackenheil, Mempel, & Eckstein, 1993). Notwithstanding

FIGURE **3-1**

## Mechanisms Implicated in the Etiology of Unipolar Mood Disorders

**Genetics**
1.5–3 times more common in family members
Three times more common in monozygotic than dizygotic twins

**Other Biological Factors**
Neurotransmitters: "too little or too much?"
Biological rhythms: sleep cycles and seasons
Hormones: cortisol
Immune system: suppression or activation?

**Personality and Temperament**
Neuroticism in major depression
Borderline, histrionic, and avoidant in dysthymia

**Psychosocial Factors**
Stressful life events
Social forces
Cultural forces

**Summary:** Biology and heredity may "set us up" for certain disorders, but psychosocial input is necessary for the mood disorder to materialize. It is equally plausible, however, that psychosocial factors set us up and our biology provides the mechanism that produces the disorder. Cause and effect have not been clarified (McNeal & Cimbolic, 1986).

some promising developments, there are as yet no definitive hormonal or blood tests for the diagnosis of depression or prediction of response to a given treatment. One of the eagerly anticipated outcomes of further identification of biological markers is the specification of meaningful categories and subtypes (Weissman et al., 1984). Such problems notwithstanding, it can be stated with considerable confidence that biology and heredity predispose certain people to both major depressive disorder and to dysthymic disorder (and perhaps to the subthreshold disorders as well) but that psychosocial factors are commonly required for their expression (Figure 3-1).

## PSYCHIATRIC COMORBIDITY

*Comorbidity* refers to the simultaneous occurrence of a second disorder, which may be either a psychiatric or a physical disorder, that may or may not influence the outcome, severity, and duration of a first disorder. Comorbid disorders may share certain etiological factors, such as negative life events or a common genetic predisposition (Monroe, 1990). Research interest in the comorbidity of psychiatric disorders is fairly recent, beginning only in the 1970s (Feinstein, 1970). However, it has been understood for some time that many drugs and neurologic and other medical disorders can cause symptoms of depression that complicate not only diagnosis and treatment but also an understanding of the etiology and course of depressive disorders. As many as four out of 10 people with major depression have histories of one or more nonmood psychiatric disorders (Sargeant, Bruce, Florio, & Weissman,

1990). The most frequent comorbid conditions are described below, beginning with other Axis I and II psychiatric disorders.

## Double Depression

A factor that strongly influences the course of depression is the presence of double depression, which occurs when major depressive disorder is superimposed on an underlying chronic dysthymic disorder (Keller, 1994a; Keller & Shapiro, 1982). Double depression typically begins insidiously in childhood or adolescence, pursues a low-grade intermittent course and is complicated by superimposed, highly recurrent major depressive episodes. Levitt and colleagues found that patients with double depression had an earlier age of onset of mood disturbance, more episodes of major depressive disorder, and more frequent concurrent anxiety disorders than patients with major depressive disorder alone (Levitt, Joffe, & MacDonald, 1991). The recovery rate of patients with double depression is understandably lower than that of patients with a single disorder (Keitner, Ryan, Miller, Kohn, & Epstein, 1991; Levitt et al., 1991; Wells, Burnam, Rogers, Hays, & Camp, 1992). In both the NIMH Collaborative Study on the Psychobiology of Depression (Keller & Shapiro, 1982) and the Medical Outcomes Study (Wells et al., 1992), patients with double depressive disorder had more severe episodes of major depression, were more likely to relapse, and experienced a greater number of depressive symptoms at each follow-up than did patients with major depressive disorder alone. In the collaborative study, 58 percent of patients recovered from an acute episode of major depressive disorder but did not recover from their underlying, chronic minor depressive state (Keller, 1993). Recovery rates appear to be equivalent for men and women (Keitner et al., 1991).

## Alcoholism

Coexisting depression and alcoholism are among the most frequent comorbid conditions in all psychiatry (Salloum et al., 1995). According to the ECA report, people with an alcohol abuse problem have almost twice the likelihood of having major depressive disorder as well (Helzer & Pryzbeck, 1988), and in women the likelihood may triple (Gorman, 1992). Alcoholism has been associated with an increased risk of suicide in adolescents and adults (Asnis et al., 1993; Pfeffer, Newcorn, Kaplan, Mizruchi, & Plutchik, 1988). The alcohol disorder appears likely to precede rather than follow the major depressive disorder (Gorman, 1992), although Petty (1992) concluded in a review that about 20 percent of people who were recently detoxified from alcohol subsequently develop depression. In several studies, alcoholism also has been associated with dysthymic disorder (Keller, 1994b).

## Anxiety

Research has shown that three out of five patients with depression display some anxiety symptoms (Keller & Hanks, 1995). Panic disorder is especially common among women who have major depressive disorder (Mulder et al., 1994). Symptoms of anxiety carry with them implications for the differential diagnosis of either disorder and expected adverse affects on the severity, course, and responsiveness to treatment (Liebowitz, 1993a; Van Valkenburg, Akiskal, Puzantian, & Rosenthal, 1984).

## Somatization Disorders

Smith (1992) reviewed the literature on the relationship between somatoform disorders and depression and, despite a disturbing lack of empirically based data, he discovered convincing evidence of a high prevalence of depression in patients with simultaneous somatoform disorder and chronic pain. Only one study in the past 15 years, however, reported the effect of treatment, and then on only two patients (both responded positively to antidepressant therapy). Smith concluded, fairly, that there is pressing need for empirical exploration of the epidemiology, course, and treatment of, and the prognosis of patients with coexisting somatoform and mood disorders.

## Dementia, Including Alzheimer's Disease

Perhaps more than half of all patients with Alzheimer's disease, especially women, also have dysthymic or major depressive disorders. However, these comorbid disorders appear to have different origins. Migliorelli and colleagues (1995) suggested that dysthymic disorders in elderly people may be an emotional reaction to progressive cognitive decline, whereas major depressive disorder may result from biological factors.

The differentiation between dementia and depression is complex. In some cases, both depression and dementia coexist as primary conditions. In others, depressive symptoms may be the first sign of dementia. In still other cases, an elderly person who has depression may exhibit signs of dementia (such as memory loss, confusion, and disorientation) and have what is currently called "pseudodementia."[7] There is substantial evidence that depression in elderly men and women is as treatable as depression in younger people, especially when a combination of psychotherapy and antidepressants is offered (Reynolds, Frank, Perel, Mazumdar, & Kupfer, 1995).

A primary purpose of a review by Emery and Oxman (1992) was to examine the validity of the common distinction made between depressive dementia as functional and reversible, and degenerative dementia as organic and irreversible. The authors concluded that depressive dementia may not be as reversible as previously thought.

## Personality (Axis II) Disorders

In a study reported by Nordstrom and colleagues, patients who had attempted suicide scored higher than age- and gender-matched control subjects on neuroticism, psychoticism, interpersonal aversiveness, indirect aggression, and a host of other negative personality features (Nordstrom, Schalling, & Asberg, 1995). Depressed people with borderline personality disorder, as reported in a study by Sullivan, Joyce, and Mulder (1994), had significantly earlier onset of depression and also demonstrated a higher prevalence of conduct disorder. Depression that coexists with the borderline personality spectrum of disorders (histrionic, narcissistic, and antisocial), expectedly, has a difficult course and poor outcome (Reich & Vasille, 1993).

---

[7]Differential diagnosis can be assisted by MRI readings of temporal lobe atrophy that provide good discrimination between Alzheimer's disease and major depressive disorder (O'Brien et al., 1994).

## *MEDICAL COMORBIDITY*

Whereas some depressive symptoms may be expected with medical illness, major depressive disorder is a serious and disabling disorder and is never an "appropriate" complication of or "normal response" to medical illness (Cassem, 1995). People with chronic medical illness have a good chance of developing a psychiatric disorder. They have a 28 percent higher rate of experiencing any disorder (for example, delusions) and a 13 percent higher rate of mood disorder (Wells, Golding, & Burnam, 1988). All health professionals must be vigilant in acknowledging depression, especially among hospitalized medical patients (Wool, 1990).

### Depressive Disorder Resulting from a General Medical Condition

DSM-III and DSM-III-R made no provisions among the affective or mood disorders for the category of depression secondary to medical illness and, in fact, organic mental disorder was a major depressive disorder exclusion criterion. Thus, a diagnosis of major depression in a medically ill person was permitted only as an organic mood disorder in both editions of the manual (Cassem, 1995). DSM-IV, however, includes mood disorders "due to a general medical condition," a designation for researchers and clinicians to use when a mood disorder is thought to be the direct physiological consequence of a medical condition.

The rates of depression among patients with central nervous system disorders such as Parkinson's, Huntington's, and Alzheimer's diseases, as well as stroke and epilepsy, are sufficiently high to suggest that basic neuronal changes have occurred (Cassem, 1995). Depression occurs in roughly half of all patients with Parkinson's disease and is associated with significant cognitive decline (Cummings, 1992). Estimated rates have ranged relatively narrowly, from 20 percent to 45 percent, in spinal cord injury patients (Kishi, Robinson, & Forrester, 1994), although in post-stroke patients the range is from 18 percent to 61 percent (Burville et al., 1995). The same uncertainty of scope surrounds other medical disorders, such as HIV and AIDS, in which the prevalence of comorbid depression ranges from 0 to 18.4 percent (Cassem, 1995). When psychiatric sequelae occur in any of these disorders, their etiological bases may be biological, genetic, or psychological. The influence of depression on recovery remains unclear, although compelling new evidence suggests that recovery is related in part to the presence of adequate social support (Kishi et al., 1994; Parikh et al., 1990).

At least one-half of all patients with chronic pain report high levels of depression (Romano & Turner, 1985). It is not always easy to discern whether the depression is a response to living with chronic pain or whether the chronic pain is a symptom of a primary depression, or if the two are even related. Although studies attempting to link depression in patients with chronic pain to the life stages have been equivocal, it appears that as pain intensity increases, older patients feel less control, and depressive symptoms increase accordingly. Dworkin and Gitlin (1991) provided an excellent review of the research literature regarding the relationships between chronic pain and depression.

Many if not most patients recovering from myocardial infarctions experience major depression. Frasure-Smith, Lesperance, and Talajic (1993) reported a research finding of considerable importance: It appears that major depression in recovering patients is an independent risk factor for mortality, equivalent to a prior heart attack.

Variable yet high rates of major depression also have been reported in patients with many less traumatic, although chronic and progressive, medical conditions.[8] Forty-two percent of all patients with chronic obstructive pulmonary disease (Gift & McCrone, 1993), 21 percent to 34 percent of patients with rheumatoid arthritis (Morrow, Parker, & Russell, 1994), and 18 percent of patients with diabetes (Lustman, Griffith, Gavard, & Clouse, 1992) experience depression. Virtually all patients with severe hypothyroidism are found to have serious concurrent depression (Haggerty & Prange, 1995). In recent studies, 20 percent to 71 percent of people suffering from chronic fatigue syndrome also were found to have either major depressive disorder or dysthymic disorder (Bombardier & Buchwald, 1995; Kruesi, Dale, & Straus, 1989). McDaniel and colleagues reviewed the literature on the diagnosis, biology, and treatment of depression in cancer patients and reported a huge variation in rates—from a low of 1.5 percent to a high of 50.0 percent—when prevalence was categorized by the cancer site (McDaniel, Musselman, Porter, Reed, & Nemeroff, 1995). Such a wide range of response surely lends support to the position that depression is not a normal response of someone who has a diagnosis of cancer.

### Drug-Induced Depression

DSM-III-R classified drug-induced depression under "organic mood disorder," but DSM-IV includes a new category called "substance-induced mood disorder" to be used in cases in which the mood disorder is judged to be the direct physiological consequence of a medication or a "street" drug. The number of drugs that have been identified as occasionally causing depression is nearly endless. Antihypertensive medications are most likely to cause depressive symptoms because they decrease norepinephrine (Dworkin & Gitlin, 1991). An informative review of the literature by Patten and Lamarre (1992) found no empirical evidence of unique or characteristic clinical features in patients with drug-induced depression, although they conceded that the existing research was largely anecdotal and often poorly designed.

### Summary

Although interest in comorbidity is relatively new, the literature is already voluminous. Mood disorders are highly prevalent in patients with chronic medical and other psychiatric conditions and are associated with high medical care utilization (Katon & Sullivan, 1990). It will be vital to learn the extent to which depression is comorbid with specific psychiatric disorders in order to better understand common etiological factors and the development of treatment interventions (Lewinsohn, Rohde, Seeley, & Hops, 1991).

## COURSE AND PROGNOSIS

An understanding of the course of mood disorders validates diagnostic criteria and assists in the identification of new subtypes, in the estimation of treatment needs,

---

[8]In 1980, Hall published a list of 25 disorders that often produce depression. Katon and Sullivan (1990) and Cassem (1995) have published comprehensive reviews of the literature on the association between depression and chronic medical illness.

TABLE **3-4**

**Terminology for the Course of Major Depressive Disorder**

| TERM | DEFINITION |
| --- | --- |
| Episode | A period of two weeks or longer |
| Remission | Few or no symptoms are present |
| Relapse | Incomplete resolution of an episode |
| Full recovery | A minimum of eight weeks with few or no symptoms |
| Recurrence(s) | Instance(s) of a completely new episode |

SOURCE: Frank, E., Prien, R. F., Jarrett, R. B., Keller, M. B., Kupfer, D. J., Lavori, P. W., Rush, A. J., & Weissman, M. M. (1991). Conceptualization and rationalization for consensus definitions of terms in major depressive disorder: Remission, recovery, relapse and recurrence. *Archives of General Psychiatry, 48,* 851–855.

and in the prediction of outcome. For the past 20 years at least, it has been generally acknowledged that mood disorders encompass wide variability in onset, course, and range of severity (Akiskal, 1983; Coryell & Winokur, 1992; Karam, 1994; Keller, 1994a; Keller et al., 1992; Keller & Shapiro, 1982; Scott et al., 1992; Wells et al., 1992). Although the terminology used to describe the course of mood disorders is basic to its understanding, dissimilarity in definitions has thwarted the clear interpretation of research findings. To remedy this critical problem, Frank and colleagues (1991) proposed the following consensus definitions (Table 3-4): People who suffer from mood disorder *episodes* (a period of two weeks or longer) may have periods of *remission* (in which few or no symptoms are present) or *relapse* (incomplete resolution of an episode), or if the person is fortunate, he or she may have *full recovery* (a minimum of eight weeks with few or no symptoms). They may have one or more *recurrences* (instances of a completely new episode) or a single episode (Frank et al., 1991). These or another set of definitions may one day prevail, but to date the profession is dependent on research in which there is considerable ambiguity. Despite this problem, research over the past two decades has uncovered a great deal about the course of depressive disorders.

## Major Depressive Disorder

Symptoms of major depressive disorder usually develop over days or weeks. More than one-half of all patients exhibit low-grade depressive conditions before experiencing a major depressive episode (Keller & Shapiro, 1982). A prodromal period, with mild symptoms of anxiety and depression, may be experienced for several weeks or months. The duration of episodes also varies, although the average untreated episode lasts six months or longer (APA, 1994). The average age of onset is 20 years, and one-half of all people with depression will have had their first episode before they reach age 40; however, major depressive disorder may begin at any age (APA, 1993).

According to *Practice Guidelines for Major Depressive Disorder in Adults* (APA, 1993), one-half of those suffering from major depression will experience just one episode. Several other investigations, however, submit that this may be an overestimate (Goodwin & Jamison, 1990; Post, Rubinow, & Ballenger, 1984). A study by Cassano and colleagues (1993) reported that a mere one-third of 687 consecutive inpatients and outpatients with primary major depressive disorder experienced a single episode. Systematic evaluation of familial, sociodemographic, temperamental, and symptomatic factors led the authors to divide patients into two nearly equivalent categories. The first group, as composed of patients whose first episode occurred after age 45, were more likely to experience both isolated episodes and a greater frequency of antecedent life stressors. The second group included patients who experienced their first episode, superimposed on either depressive or hyperthymic temperaments, before age 45. These patients suffered greater severity of illness, higher rates of attempted suicide, greater anxiety and somatization, and more frequent psychotic tendencies. They also had a greater potential for recurrence (Cassano et al., 1993).

A group of patients who represent a challenge to current classification are those patients with unipolar depression who share certain characteristics with patients who have bipolar disorder. They have been described as "pseudounipolar" and are characterized by early age of onset, high frequency of recurrence, and a family history of bipolar illness (Akiskal et al., 1985). There is also a considerable interest in characteristics that predict switching from unipolar to bipolar disorder, although in a study reported by Coryell and colleagues (1995), fewer than 6 percent of people who initially had unipolar disorder switched to Bipolar I disorder in a 10-year follow-up period, and another 5 percent had a hypomanic episode. The researchers found that psychosis and a family history of mania predicted shifts to Bipolar I disorder and that an initial chronic depressive episode with an early age of onset predicted later development of Bipolar II disorder.

### Chronic Depressive Disorder

Widespread acceptance of the fact of both episodic and chronic forms of depression now exists (Howland, 1993a), thanks to Akiskal's studies of the phenomenology and course of chronic depression in the early 1970s and to the reports of the longitudinal NIMH Collaborative Study of the Psychobiology of Depression in the 1980s. A patient may experience chronic depression in a variety of ways. Some people may have clusters of episodes, whereas others may have single episodes separated by years (APA, 1993; Keller, 1993). A significant number of patients experience multiple or long episodes and never return to their predepression state (Akiskal et al., 1980; Angst, 1988). The Collaborative Study examined the course of illness at six-month intervals for five years and at annual intervals thereafter for a minimum of 10 years and estimated recovery within one year to be only 70 percent. Just 18 percent to 25 percent of those still depressed after one year recovered within the next five years (Keller et al., 1992; Maj, Veltro, Pirozzi, Lobrace, & Magliano, 1992). Of the original number, a sizable 12 percent were still depressed at the end of the five years, and 7 percent were still depressed at the end of 10 years (Keller et al., 1992; Keller et al., 1996). These people with chronic depression experienced subcriteria symptoms of depression, resembling chronic minor depressive disorder or dysthymic disorder, most of the time. These findings are similar to those reported by Angst (1988) from the Zurich Study as well. Clinically, it is important to determine whether a patient has had previous episodes because those are the strongest predictors of future episodes: Two previous episodes predict a 50 percent to 90 percent probability of recurrence, and three or more previous episodes predict a greater than 90 percent probability (Keller et al., 1992). It is noteworthy that in both the Zurich

(Angst, 1988) and the Rand Medical Outcomes studies (Wells et al., 1992), there was no conspicuous association between any sociodemographic factors and the recurrence of depressive episodes.

It comes as no surprise that the type and amount of treatment provided patients with depression has an effect on the duration and severity of the disorder. Nevertheless, there remains much controversy about the ideal combination and duration of treatment and its effect on the recurrence or chronicity of episodes. Increasingly, professionals argue that treatment should be continued even for those patients who have fully recovered (Keller, 1994a). In fact, there is some evidence that if treatment is continued for at least three years following the acute episode, subsequent episodes can be prevented (Frank et al., 1990; Post et al., 1984). Before a clinician commits a patient to such long-term treatment, however, it is important to be reasonably sure that the patient will suffer recurrence without treatment.

## Melancholic Depression

The principal features of melancholic depression are psychomotor retardation and agitation, late insomnia, weight and appetite loss, feelings of guilt, and delusions. These symptoms occur in nearly all psychotic depressions as well as in many depressions without psychosis. People who experience an episode of major depression with melancholic features will not necessarily experience the next episode of major depression in the same form, although nonmelancholic episodes are more likely to become melancholic with increasing age. Otherwise, melancholia is not associated with a unique course (Rush & Weissenburger, 1994). However, melancholic features are generally thought to predict a good response to ECT and to antidepressants (Peselow, Sanfilipo, Difiglia, & Fieve, 1992).

## Psychotic Depression

If a major depressive episode is accompanied by delusions or hallucinations, or both, it is described as "psychotic" or "delusional." Delusions without hallucinations occur in about one-half to two-thirds of all patients with psychotic depression; people experience hallucinations without delusions in fewer than 25 percent of instances (Dubovsky & Thomas, 1992). Approximately 20 percent of patients with psychotic depression have bipolar disorder, compared with 10 percent of depressed patients without psychotic features (Aronson, Shukla, Hoff, & Cook, 1988). Patients with psychotic depression are generally more severely depressed than patients who are depressed but without psychosis, and unfortunately, once a person has experienced a psychotic episode, subsequent episodes are likely to be psychotic (Helms & Smith, 1983).

In a study of the functional status of patients with psychotic depression, schizoaffective disorder, and schizophrenia, Tsuang and Coryell (1993) found that baseline diagnosis was a powerful predictor of long-term outcome; patients with psychotic depression had much better outcomes than patients with schizoaffective disorder or schizophrenia. All in all, however, psychotic depressions have a low rate of spontaneous recovery (Coryell et al., 1984) and a rare response in clinical trials to placebo medication (Dubovsky & Thomas, 1992).

## Atypical Depression

Horwath and colleagues (1992) described major depressive disorder with atypical features as associated with a younger age of onset; more psychomotor slowing; and more comorbid panic disorder, drug abuse or dependence, and somatization disorder, compared with major depressive disorder without these features. These associated features are not predictive of rapid recovery.

## Postpartum Depression

Conclusions about postpartum depression are as equivocal as in most other areas of depression research. The same inconsistency in definitions of depression and in distinctions among subtypes (for example, between postpartum psychosis and postpartum depression) hamper interpretation of the research findings. Studies suggest that psychosocial stressors, such as a poor marital relationship, may be particularly important etiologic factors in postpartum depression (Wolk & Weissman, 1995). Some studies indicate that women with postpartum depression experience shorter duration of symptoms and better outcomes than do women who are otherwise depressed, whereas others have found serious morbidity, up to four years, following delivery (Dobie & Walker, 1992). The onset, severity, and duration of postpartum depression are variable. Greater than 60 percent of patients have symptom onset within six weeks of delivery. Once a woman has experienced a postpartum depression, she is at increased risk (the reported range is 30 percent to 50 percent) with subsequent pregnancies (Garvey, Tuason, Lumry, & Hofman, 1983). Many women with postpartum depression do not exhibit the classic symptoms of depression; instead they manifest a mood lability that some have labeled a depressed form of puerperal bipolar disorder (Brockington, Margison, Schofield, & Knight, 1988).

## Dysthymic Disorder

Dysthymic disorder is a chronic form of mood disorder, although it is symptomatically less severe than major depressive disorder. Nonetheless, it can affect every aspect of a person's life, with devastating results. Compelling evidence exists that patients with dysthymic disorder are at increased risk for deteriorating general health and social dysfunction and that they are heavy users of medical services (Howland, 1993b). Dysthymic disorder typically has an insidious onset at early age. The person's experience of depressed mood has a tendency to be more subjective than objective. In other words, the mood does not feel clearly differentiated from the patient's usual sense of himself or herself (Dysthymia Working Group, 1995). The depression is experienced as a long-standing, more or less chronic anhedonia or lack of interest in one's usual pleasurable activities. Marked disturbances in appetite or psychomotor function are unusual (Dysthymia Working Group, 1995).

A high prevalence of comorbidity is associated with dysthymic disorder. More than three-quarters of patients have additional psychiatric disorders (Weissman, Leaf, Bruce, et al., 1988), including major depressive disorder, alcoholism, anxiety, and personality disorders (Howland, 1993a). Keller and Shapiro (1982) demonstrated that more than 90 percent of people with dysthymic disorder developed subsequent cases of major depressive disorder after a median duration of five years. Little wonder that the result was a longer recovery time and consequentially high rates of recurrence and chronicity (Keller et al., 1992).

## Recurrent Brief Depression

The longitudinal epidemiologic Zurich study identified brief but recurrent episodes of depression with severity of symptoms, impairment, and distress equivalent to major depressive disorder. Average episodes last three days, but they otherwise fulfill the symptomatic criteria for major depressive disorder. RBD is characterized by frequent episodes lasting less than two weeks and is reported to be a common, disabling illness with a chronic, relapsing course (Angst & Hochstrasser, 1994; Montgomery & Montgomery, 1992). RBD also is associated with considerable suicidality and treatment-seeking and has high comorbidity with anxiety disorders. In addition, there is persuasive evidence that as many as 31 percent of patients with SAD also can be characterized as having RBD (Kasper, Ruhmann, Hasse, & Mollerr, 1992). As might be expected, patients with combined major depressive disorder and RBD have been reported to be more severely affected and have a higher attempted suicide rate than patients with only one of these conditions (Angst & Hochstrasser, 1994).

## Minor Depressive Disorder and Subsyndromal Symptomatic Depression

Interest in the subsyndromal forms of depression, particularly minor depression and subsyndromal symptomatic depression, has grown substantially over the past 10 years. Unfortunately, it is difficult to sort out the research findings because of the variety of definitions and diagnoses used. Nevertheless, three analyses of the ECA data have confirmed that minor depressive disorder, the essential feature of which is the experience of at least two but less than five depressive symptoms for a minimum of two weeks, is real and that it accounts for substantial days lost from work and poor social and role functioning (Broadhead et al., 1990; Johnson et al., 1992; Judd et al., 1994). The Medical Outcomes Study also reported that depressive symptoms alone in people who did not have major depressive or dysthymic disorders were associated with significant social dysfunction and disability. In fact, these patients were less well off than patients suffering from several major medical conditions, including diabetes and hypertension (Wells et al., 1989). Minor depressive disorder is thus neither a normal nor a benign condition (Judd et al., 1994). The proposed category of subsyndromal symptomatic depression is likewise associated with substantial social dysfunction and disability (Judd et al., 1994).

## Functional Impairment

The extremely important Medical Outcomes Study, with its sample of over 20,000 patients, vividly described the terrible impairment in most domains of physical and social functioning among people with major depression as well as people exhibiting only the subthreshold depressive symptoms described above (Wells et al., 1989). Both groups functioned less well than people with such major medical conditions as hypertension, diabetes, and arthritis (Klerman, 1989; Wells et al., 1989; Wells et al., 1992). In addition, patients with subthreshold depression experienced limitations in daily functioning, including more days in bed, just as severely as patients with major depression (Broadhead et al., 1990; Johnson et al., 1992).

## Prognosis

Depression clearly guarantees significant morbidity and mortality compared with other mental disorders and other medical conditions. Nonetheless, depression is thought to have a favorable prognosis (Manschreck & Leighton, 1992). Such optimism is warranted in part because of the long-standing (since the late 1800s) observation that in some cases depression spontaneously remits and that untreated patients may enjoy periods of complete freedom from symptoms (Keller, 1993; Kraepelin, 1921). Developments in the effectiveness of antidepressants and various psychotherapies have provided substantial reasons for optimism. It seems that 80 percent to 90 percent of people with a major depressive disorder can be treated successfully (Regier et al., 1988).

It also is evident that just one person in three who suffers from a mood disorder ever seeks treatment (Regier, Narrow, et al., 1993) despite the accumulating evidence of the severity of illness. In part because of a lack of treatment, as many as 15 percent to 20 percent of patients with depression develop chronicity, and up to 20 percent commit suicide. The remainder spend as much as one-fifth of their lives suffering from the disorder (Angst, 1992). In the face of a growing appreciation for the chronicity of depressive illness, the traditional optimism may be fading.

Some studies have reported that people whose depression is clearly related to a significant psychosocial precursor with rapid onset of symptoms seem to have a greater likelihood of quick and complete recovery than those whose depression is of the melancholic type. In the NIMH Collaborative Study, recovery was slowed when there was a longer initial episode before treatment was initiated (Coryell, Endicott, & Keller, 1990; Keller, 1993; Keller et al., 1992). It was especially interesting, because it is counterintuitive, that the severity of depressive symptoms did not emerge as a predictor until study groups had been followed for five years or more (Keller, 1993). The Medical Outcomes Study researchers reported the poorest clinical outcomes for patients with double depression, especially for those patients with high initial symptom severity. More important, however, they discovered that patients with dysthymia, even in the absence of major depression, had similarly poor outcomes relative to patients with major depression alone. They also reported a fascinating finding that has special implications for psychosocial treatment: The combined significance of the severity of depressive symptoms, functional status, and general well-being had greater prognostic weight even than the particular type of depressive disorder (Wells et al., 1989; Wells et al., 1992). They concluded that patients with several depressive symptoms should be carefully monitored for at least one year for possible emerging major depression (Wells et al., 1992).

With respect to the subthreshold depressive disorders, numerous studies have indicated that the strongest correlates of outcome are psychosocial factors such as employment, domestic conditions, and life events (Miranda & Munoz, 1994). Of course, this strongly suggests the likely benefit of psychosocial treatments. In fact, in a comprehensive review of treatment studies for minor depression, Conte and Karasu (1992) encountered strong preliminary evidence that psychological and psychosocial treatment is indeed effective. They argued for the funding of well-controlled investigations with clearly defined interventions.

## *SUMMARY*

This review of the research has explored the ways in which a person experiences a course of depression. Some of the conclusions have been based on the findings of the recent and extensive research efforts of the NIMH Collaborative, the Zurich, and the Medical Outcomes studies. To place these findings in clinical perspective, however, it is essential to recognize that, unfortunately, most of the patients studied have received inadequate treatment for their mood disorder (Angst, 1988; Keller, 1993; Wells et al., 1992). Therefore, what has been reported is largely untreated or undertreated depression. There is irrefutable evidence that vigorous pharmacologic intervention is beneficial for patients with most forms of mood disorders, including dysthymic disorder, and that aggressive and responsible treatment predicts a more swift and positive outcome (Akiskal, 1991; Howland, 1991; Howland, 1993a). No comparable volumes of research exist that describe information about the course of depression when it is adequately treated. There is a great opportunity to better understand the natural course and treated course of all types of depression when greater standardization in research methods has been achieved.

# Bipolar Disorders

States of melancholia and mania have been described for the past 2,000 years (Goodwin & Jamison, 1990), but not until this century has a standard model of manic–depressive illness been available. German psychiatrist Emil Kraepelin (1921) clearly distinguished between the two major psychoses: (1) dementia praecox, which later became known as schizophrenia, and (2) manic–depressive insanity. Thirty years later, Leonhard (1979), also a German psychiatrist, further distinguished between patients who experienced both manic and depressed episodes, whom he called "bipolar," and those who experienced only depressed episodes. Subsequently, Dunner and colleagues proposed a distinction between the patients whose manic episodes were severe enough to require hospitalization—the Bipolar I patients— and those whose manic episodes were less severe—the Bipolar II patients (Dunner, Gershon, & Goodwin, 1976). Angst (1978) identified a subgroup of bipolar patients whose manic and depressed moods were both less severe; the disorder was eventually classified as cyclothymia.

The unipolar–bipolar distinction was first incorporated into American nosology in 1980 with the publication of the DSM-III.[9] Cyclothymic disorder was included, as was Bipolar I, but Bipolar II disorder was recognized only in the residual category akin to the one created for residual unipolar disorders, called bipolar disorder NOS. DSM-IV has continued to refine the subtypes within the bipolar spectrum, also known as manic–depressive illness, such that they now include four syndromes: (1) Bipolar I, characterized by one or more manic or mixed (that is, both depressed and manic) episodes; (2) Bipolar II, characterized by at least one hypomanic episode in addition to one or more major depressive episodes; (3) cyclothymic disorder, which is identified by numerous periods of hypomanic symptoms and subthreshold depressive symptoms; and (4) the residual category described above.

---

[9]The First International Conference on Bipolar Disorder was held in 1994 at the University of Pittsburgh.

## TYPES OF DISORDERS

### Bipolar I

In DSM-IV, six separate subtypes are listed for Bipolar I disorder. One of these may designate a single manic episode, whereas the remaining five are used to describe the quality of the most recent episode (that is, whether it was manic, hypomanic, mixed, depressed, or unspecified). As with the diagnosis of unipolar major depressive disorder, additional specifiers are available to describe the pattern of episode recurrence. These include rapid cycling, which indicates at least four episodes in a year; the presence or absence of interepisode recovery; and the emergence of a seasonal pattern in the depressed episodes. DSM-IV also provides additional specifiers for the severity of the episode, the presence of psychotic or catatonic features, postpartum onset, and further characterization of the mood (that is, if it is depressed, chronic, or has melancholic or atypical features).

Five areas of classification in which researchers and nosologists have recently been particularly interested include (1) the long-term stability and prediction of switching or shifting between mania and depression; (2) the validity of the mixed-state modifier; (3) the validity of the rapid cycling specification; (4) the overlap with nonbipolar disorders; and (5) the greater efficacy and utility of proposed alternative classification systems. Recent research findings in these areas are described below.

### Long-Term Stability

The long-term stability of original diagnoses is especially important to both clinicians and researchers involved with bipolar disorders because patients may exhibit one pathological state, such as mania, and only later reveal (or retrospectively recognize) the presence of other states, such as depression. Nonetheless, there is evidence of significant diagnostic stability. In 1995, Coryell and colleagues published the results of a 10-year prospective study of people who switched from one mood disorder to another. They found that only one in 10 people with a unipolar depressive disorder later experienced either a manic or hypomanic episode, and even fewer (8 percent) with Bipolar II disorder converted to Bipolar I. Fewer still, just 7 percent, who had been previously diagnosed with Bipolar I disorder had subsequent hypomania (that is, a Bipolar II–type subthreshold manic episode) during a 10-year follow-up.

Akiskal et al. (1995) reported similar results from their 11-year prospective study. Thirteen percent of patients with unipolar depression switched to one of the bipolar disorders. Those few (less than 4 percent) who switched to Bipolar I, however, were otherwise similar to their depressed counterparts who had never experienced a manic episode. People who switched to Bipolar II disorder (9 percent) differed from the others in that they had experienced onset of depression at a considerably younger age.[10] The combined findings from these two longitudinal, prospective studies provide considerable evidence for the diagnostic stability among the bipolar disorders.

---

[10]The temperamental profile, which was apparent during the depressive episodes and included mood lability, social anxiety, and daydreaming, also was a good predictor of switching (Akiskal et al., 1995).

## Validity of the Mixed State

The mixed state (also called "dysphoric mania") was described early in this century by Kraepelin (1921) to specify people who have mania and depression at the same time. In a 1995 review, Swann estimated the prevalence of the mixed state to be between 30 percent and 40 percent of all patients with bipolar disorders and more common among women and in families with a history of major depressive disorder or depressive personality.

McElroy and colleagues reviewed 17 studies of mixed state and found substantial evidence of a distinct entity (McElroy et al., 1992). Although they were unable to identify any characteristic demographic features, they did conclude that mixed episodes predict a more difficult course than either manic or depressed episodes alone. Swann (1995) reported that the risk for a mixed state is increased by the presence of substance abuse, neurologic disorder, or developmental disorders.

Although the mixed state is consistently recognized as a common occurrence, debate persists about precise classification and diagnostic criteria. In contrast to the DSM-III-R, which allowed for ultra-rapid cycling between the two states, DSM-IV requires a simultaneous full manic episode and full major depressive episode (a shorter duration allowed) for diagnosis.

## Rapid Cycling

Rapid cycling refers to the experience of at least four manic, hypomanic, mixed, or major depressive episodes during a single year. In the early 1970s, the literature suggested that these patients did not respond well to lithium. Rapid cycling was therefore recognized as a lithium-resistant subtype of bipolar disorder, and alternative modes of treatment were explored.[11]

About 15 percent of patients with bipolar disorder experience rapid cycling (Wehr et al., 1988). Bauer and his colleagues (1994) conducted a DSM-IV workgroup study to determine the validity of certain bipolar disorder specifiers and subtypes and to decide whether rapid cycling should be included as a course modifier. The work group compiled an excellent review of rapid-cycling research, although it was compelled to conclude that all previous studies, taken together, were equivocal. The group found that patients with rapid cycling included more patients of higher socioeconomic levels and more women than men. Maj, Magliano, Pirozzi, Marasco, and Guarneri (1994) also determined that patients with rapid cycling tended to be older, had been ill longer, had more hospitalizations, and had been prescribed more neuroleptic treatments than had patients without rapid cycling. Wehr et al. (1988) had shown earlier that rapid cycling can be induced by antidepressants in patients with bipolar disorder, and because patients suffering from it tend to respond differently to medication than do patients without rapid cycling,[12] it seemed likely that rapid cycling represented a unique subtype. Cumulative findings have thus supported the validity of rapid cycling as a course modifier for both Bipolar I disorder

---

[11]Patients with rapid cycling respond less well to lithium and better to valproate than do patients without it, although use of valproate frequently results in depression (Calabrese, Rapport, Kimmel, Reece, & Woyshville, 1993). Evidence such as this suggests that rapid cycling may represent a truly unique subtype rather than an extreme condition.

[12]Patients with rapid cycling tend to respond to medication differently from patients without rapid cycling; specifically, they respond less well to lithium and better to anticonvulsants (Wehr et al., 1988).

and Bipolar II disorder diagnoses. Therefore, it has been included as such in the DSM-IV.

### Overlap with Nonbipolar Disorders

There are several problematic classification areas apart from the current DSM-IV bipolar spectrum (Blacker & Tsuang, 1992; McElroy, Keck, & Strakowski, 1996). One of these is the overlap across diagnostic criteria for schizophrenia and for bipolar disorder, especially schizoaffective disorder, for which DSM-IV requires specific symptoms of schizophrenia concurrent with a major depressive, mixed, or manic episode (APA, 1994). The illness may be further subtyped as bipolar or depressive. Although the mood symptoms must constitute much of the episode, there also must be a two-week period of delusions or hallucinations without a mood disturbance. It remains to be learned whether schizoaffective disorder is a mood disorder, a non-schizophrenic psychotic disorder, or a mixture of schizophrenia and mood disorder. Some investigators have argued that people with manic symptoms are more like the mood disorder group, whereas those with depressed symptoms are more like the psychotic group (Goodwin & Jamison, 1990).

A further classification challenge is presented by those patients with bipolar depression who share certain characteristics with patients with bipolar disorder. Cassano and colleagues defined a temperament type—namely, hyperthymic—that when seen among patients with unipolar depression may indicate an underlying bipolar disorder (Cassano, Akiskal, Savino, Musetti, & Perugi, 1992). These patients have been described as "pseudounipolar" (Akiskal et al., 1985) and are identified by early age of onset, high frequency of recurrence, and a family history of bipolar disorder. When patients with pseudounipolar disorder are treated with antidepressants, they may switch and begin to exhibit a bipolar course (Akiskal & Akiskal, 1988; Cassano et al., 1992), further suggesting a possible classification overlap worthy of continued investigation.

### Alternative Classification Systems

Beginning in the early 1980s, Blacker and Tsuang suggested considering an alternative classification system for bipolar disorders (Blacker & Tsuang, 1992). Their argument, which remains pertinent despite the publication of the DSM-IV, was that the current categorical and multiaxial system draws boundaries where, in fact, there may be a continuum (for example, mania and hypomania), resulting in criteria of questionable validity and reliability. Although they acknowledged the appeal and utility of the current system, they proposed that consideration be given to scaled or probabilistic classification systems. They further proposed greater reliance on practice guidelines for clinical use and suggested using different systems altogether for research purposes, thereby not trying to build one system of nosology to serve all possible needs. Swann (1995) proposed another classification system for mood disorders that is based on behavioral rather than mood disturbances.[13] He argued that such a classification system might be more useful for treatment than the current system.

---

[13]Swann's (1995) proposal includes affective arousal, which would be high in both agitated depression and mixed mania and correlates with norepinephrine turnover; increased motor and goal-oriented activity that is high only in the manic states; and psychic pain, which is high in all states except mania.

## Bipolar II

Bipolar II was first described by Dunner, Fleiss, and Fieve in 1976 and earned a place as a distinct diagnostic entity in 1994 by its separation from the DSM-III-R NOS category. Like Bipolar I, Bipolar II is a rare disorder with a similarly low prevalence of only 0.6 percent (Goodwin & Jamison, 1990; Weissman, 1978). The diagnosis requires at least one major depressive episode and one hypomanic, or sub-threshold manic, episode.[14] In addition, there must be neither a full manic nor a mixed episode. If either have ever been present, the diagnosis is Bipolar I disorder. In summarizing data comparing patients with Bipolar I and Bipolar II disorder, Cassano and colleagues (1992) noted that although they were similar in age of on-set, number of total episodes, and number of episodes of major depressive disorder, patients with Bipolar II disorder had fewer hospitalizations, a more chronic course, more suicidal behavior, and greater comorbidity. Coryell and colleagues (1995) have shown that these combined features support the classification of Bipolar II as a distinct entity.

Bipolar II, like Bipolar I, is a rare disorder with a similarly low prevalence of only 0.6 percent (Goodwin & Jamison, 1990; Weissman, 1978). Patients with Bipolar II disorder, moreover, are more likely than patients with Bipolar I disorder to develop a depressive episode, which suggests that they are not intermediate between Bipolar I and major depression (Weissman, 1978). Coryell and colleagues demonstrated further support for the stability of the diagnostics by demonstrating that during a two-year study period, just 4 percent of patients originally diagnosed as having Bipolar II disorder were subsequently given a Bipolar I diagnosis (Coryell, Andreasen, Endicott, & Keller, 1987). The higher prevalence of a hyperthymic temperament among Bipolar II than among Bipolar I patients also provides support for the classification and diagnostic separation of the two disorders (Cassano et al., 1992).

## Cyclothymic Disorder

Cyclothymia has been recognized as one of the manic–depressive illnesses since early in this century. Kraepelin (1921) believed it was a condition that predisposed people to more severe mood disorders. Although cyclothymia was first included in DSM-III in 1980, research on all aspects of this disorder has lagged behind that of the major mood disorders. One difficulty has been that people with chronic low-grade conditions are less likely to seek treatment and are thus not as likely to come to the attention of investigators. Another problem that applies to cyclothymia, as well as to Bipolar II, is that the conditions with minor symptomatology tend to have less diagnostic reliability and result in a more heterogeneous grouping of patients (Andreasen et al., 1981). There is some question whether cyclothymic disorder is a distinct disorder or whether it represents an early stage of Bipolar I or II. According to Goodwin and Jamison's (1990) summary of existent studies, it appears that approximately one-third of patients with cyclothymic disorder will eventually develop the full syndrome of bipolar illness. In their 1993 review, Howland and Thase arrived at the indeterminate conclusion that although cyclothymic disorder is neither

---

[14]These subthreshold manic episodes are sometimes extremely difficult to discern (Andreasen et al., 1981).

a necessary nor a sufficient condition for the later development of Bipolar disorder, there is certainly a subgroup of cyclothymic patients who will develop Bipolar I or II disorders. An alternative position, therefore, is that cyclothymic disorder, or even cyclothymic temperament, may be a useful marker for what will later become a more severe disorder (Akiskal, 1994b).

Cyclothymic disorder appears to be more closely related to Bipolar II than to Bipolar I. Both cyclothymic disorder and Bipolar II disorder require hypomanic episodes and the absence of true mania. Like the rapid-cycling course for patients with both Bipolar I and II, cyclothymic disorder requires numerous episodes over a two-year period, yet patients with rapid cycling and cyclothymic disorder are less responsive to lithium treatment than are patients with Bipolar I disorder.[15] The clinical characteristics, longitudinal course, and family histories among cyclothymic patients suggest that many have a form of bipolar disorder, although as it is currently defined, cyclothymia has proved to be so variable that this is not true of all patients.

Patients with early-onset rapid cycling are more likely to have had a cyclothymic temperament than patients with late-onset rapid cycling (Kukopoulos et al., 1983). The high prevalence in rapid cycling among women is not found in cyclothymic disorder, and a higher rate of cyclothymic disorder in families of people with rapid cycling, as opposed to nonrapid cycling, has not been confirmed (Nurnberger et al., 1988). On these bases, Howland and Thase (1993) concluded that cyclothymic disorder and rapid cycling generally are not overlapping.

### Summary

Although it is clear from this review of current research that the diagnostic criteria for the bipolar disorders have improved greatly with the publication of DSM-IV, many classification issues remain unsettled. Blacker and Tsuang (1992) suggested that current disputes concerning the boundaries of bipolar disorder result, at least in part, from the nosologic process itself. The current uncertainties about bipolar disorders and their relationships to personality and other psychiatric disorders will continue to provide fertile ground for discussion of both the specific diagnostic guidelines and the nature of classification itself.

## *PATHOGENESIS*

A full understanding of the pathophysiology of bipolar disorder remains elusive. Nonetheless, it is clear that the bipolar spectrum of illness represents significant brain disease that is the end product of a mixture of biological and environmental factors. Hypothesized associations are described below.

### Genetics

Family, twin, and adoption studies all have contributed to a genetic hypothesis for the etiology of bipolar disorder. There is now little doubt that bipolar disorder involves, at least in part, a genetically transmitted vulnerability. In their summary of

---

[15]People with cyclothymic disorder tend to develop hypomania when administered antidepressants, and only 50 percent respond to lithium, again making them more like patients with Bipolar II disorder than like those with Bipolar I disorder (Akiskal, 1994b).

family studies since the early 1980s, Gershon and Nurnberger (1995a) concluded that more patients who had bipolar disorder than patients who had unipolar illness had relatives with bipolar disorder. In fact, first-degree relatives of probands with bipolar disorder, compared with people who are unaffected, have an estimated tenfold risk of bipolar disorder (Mendlewicz, 1994). Gershon and Nurnberger calculated that a child with one parent with bipolar disorder has a 30 percent chance of having a mood disorder and a 50 percent to 75 percent risk if the second parent also has bipolar disorder. Regardless of how impressive these family studies are, they cannot differentiate environmental from genetic influences.

Twin and adoption studies have attempted to elucidate this distinction. As described above, if a genetic factor exists, then a twin with an identical twin (who theoretically shares 100 percent of genetic material) with bipolar disorder should be more likely to have bipolar disorder than a twin with a fraternal twin (who shares only 50 percent of genetic material) who has bipolar disorder, even if the twins are reared in separate environments. Twin studies provide compelling evidence for the heritability of bipolar disorder. Concordance rates for bipolar disorder tabulated by Berrettini (1995) across seven twin studies found an impressive 65 percent rate for identical twins and only a 14 percent rate for fraternal twins. These cumulative rates confirm those that had been reported in the earlier, landmark Danish twin studies in the 1970s which showed 67 percent and 20 percent concordance rates (Gershon, 1990). It also has been found that concordance rates are positively correlated with disorder severity (Berrettini, 1995).

Although they are powerful and persuasive, twin studies do not eliminate the confounding factor of environment as well as adoption studies do. Berretini (1995) reviewed studies that had compared biological relatives of patients with bipolar disorder who had been adopted, with biological relatives of patients with bipolar disorder who had not been adopted. He found that the risk was similar in both groups. In other words, environment played little or no role in the etiology of bipolar disorder.[16] Nevertheless, because of the limited number of studies and small number of probands in the adoption literature, these studies do not yet provide the level of support for the genetic transmission hypothesis that has been provided by twin studies (Gershon, 1990).

One of the most exciting areas of recent psychiatric research has been the use of molecular genetic techniques to help locate and identify genes related to specific psychiatric illnesses. "Linkage analysis," as this is called, is a method that can be used to localize disease vulnerability genes to a specific region on the human genome. Through such studies, several chromosomes have emerged as promising candidates for transmitting susceptibility to bipolar disorder. The excitement over linkage studies began with the report of a genetic linkage between chromosome 11 and bipolar disorder in an Old Order Amish pedigree (Egeland et al., 1987). Although replications were not successful,[17] continuing analysis of that same pedigree,

---

[16]Berretini (1995) cited a major 1977 study in which Mendlewicz had compared biological relatives of affected adoptees and biological relatives of nonaffected adoptees and had estimated a 31 percent risk in biological relatives of adoptees with bipolar disorder and a 26 percent risk in biological relatives of nonadopted patients with bipolar disorder. In other words, the rates were remarkably similar.

[17]The connection between chromosome 11 and bipolar disorder in an Old Order Amish pedigree (Egeland et al., 1987) has been contradicted by numerous subsequent studies (Mendlewicz et al., 1991; Mitchell et al., 1991).

in which bipolar disorder and other mood disorders occurred at an unusually high rate, has demonstrated evidence for linkage to other genes, namely on chromosomes 6, 13, and 15 (National Institutes of Health [NIH], 1996). Additional recent reports suggest that the X chromosome and chromosomes 4, 15, and 18 also may transmit susceptibility to bipolar disorder (Berrettini, 1995; Craddock & McGuffin, 1993; Gershon, 1995; NIH, 1996). Conversely, there is evidence that chromosome 21 may confer protection from bipolar disorder in some patients with trisomy 21. Replication of these findings will be crucial, especially because the methods used in the studies to date have been strongly criticized.[18]

The biological research on Bipolar II disorder is not extensive, although there is evidence that genetics might play a substantial role in its etiology. By way of illustration, when Endicott and colleagues (1985) compared probands with Bipolar I and II disorders, they found that each group had more relatives who had experienced the same rather than the other type of disorder. Goodwin and Jamison (1990) reviewed four studies from the 1980s and drew a similar conclusion, strongly suggesting that the disorders are distinct from one another, but are genetically linked. More recently, Simpson and colleagues (1993) conducted a study of first-degree relatives of probands with Bipolar I and Bipolar II disorders and concluded that Bipolar II disorder is genetically related but less complex than Bipolar I disorder. In their opinion, accurate diagnosis of Bipolar II disorder will be crucial in finding any genetic loci underlying bipolar disorders generally.

In the 1970s, Bertelsen and colleagues found that if one identical twin had manic–depressive illness, the other twin, if not manic–depressive, often had a cyclothymic syndrome (Bertelsen, Harvald, & Hauge, 1977). This evidence provided early support for the positive relationship of cyclothymic disorder to the bipolar spectrum. According to nearly all family studies, patients with cyclothymia have an increased familial risk for both bipolar and unipolar disorders. This finding is in interesting contrast to the evidence reported above that patients with unipolar depression have increased familial risk for that same disorder but have no increased risk for either cyclothymic or other bipolar disorders (Heun & Maier, 1993). Akiskal and colleagues (1985) reported that a substantial percentage of high-risk children (children of patients with bipolar disorder) have cyclothymic disorder, which tends to occur early in adolescence and, for the overwhelming majority, subsequently develops into Bipolar I or II disorder.

## Neurobiology and Biological Risk Factors

Researchers have been interested in biochemical models of the pathophysiology of bipolar disorder for several decades.[19] The relevant literature includes studies of neurotransmitters and their interactions, neuroendocrine abnormalities, the more recently identified neuropeptides, and the membrane transport systems and their related electrolytes. Additional investigations have focused on potential sites of neuroanatomical lesions, electrophysiological functions, and possible immunologic and

---

[18]Linkage studies have used diagnoses made by clinicians who were not blind to the status of the probands. Further reliability studies are needed given the serious impact of diagnostic misclassifications on genetic linkage results (Maziade et al., 1992).

[19]See Goodwin and Jamison's (1990) excellent comprehensive review of the primary research literature on the biochemistry and pathophysiology of bipolar disorders.

viral etiologies. Most recently, considerable attention has been directed at sleep, sea-sonality, and other rhythmic phenomena that are commonly dysregulated in mood disorders.

Some of the earliest biological investigations probed the monoaminergic neuro-transmitter systems, including norepinephrine, dopamine and serotonin. Initially, each of these neurotransmitters was considered in isolation; subsequently, relation-ships among them were explored. One recent theory, the more complex, so-called permissive hypothesis, has postulated that a single neurotransmitter might serve to keep the others in balance (Goodwin & Jamison, 1990). From the simplest notion that depression represents a deficiency and mania in excess of a single neurotrans-mitter, models have become increasingly more complex, now involving interactions among the monoamines, other neurotransmitters (such as acetylcholine and GABA), and enzyme modulators.[20] Because plasma GABA (an inhibitory neurotransmitter) concentrations are low both in patients with mania and in those with bipolar disor-der who are depressed, there may be evidence of a biological marker for the devel-opment of various mood disorders (Petty, 1994). Potter, Rudorfer, and Linnoila (1988) and Goodwin and Jamison (1990) concluded that norepinephrine remains the neurotransmitter most consistently implicated in bipolar disorder and that the pharmacologic probes used to study other neurotransmitters, including the GABA system, can be shown to interact with the norepinephrine system at one level or an-other.

The neuroendocrine system has been among the most intensely studied for its potential contribution to the etiology of mood disorders, stemming in part from clinical observations that both depression and mania are associated with changes in thyroid hormone and cortisol levels. Nevertheless, research results to date are com-plex and inconclusive. Whereas most research has approached hormone activity as secondary to neurotransmitter activity (hormones and neurotransmitters cannot be viewed independently[21]), there is increasing interest in the primary effect of hor-mones on the brain itself (Goodwin & Jamison, 1990). For example, the patients who have rapid cycling are more likely to be female and to have a high incidence of thyroid hormone abnormality. Wehr and colleagues at NIMH have postulated that these abnormalities act directly on the brain and, therefore, are not simply a conse-quence of the bipolar disorder (Wehr, 1991).

Perhaps the most exciting area of research in the pathophysiology of bipolar disorder derives from its clinically observed rhythmic patterns on the one hand and the apparent dysregulation of normal rhythms, such as sleep, on the other hand. There are a variety of circadian rhythm disturbances in bipolar disorder, most no-tably the decreased need for sleep while in the manic state and the tendency for people in the depressed state to sleep too much. In fact, sleep loss not only precedes mania, it may trigger it (Wehr, 1991). Research findings on alterations in sleep archi-tecture of patients with unipolar disorder are fairly consistent, but the same is not

---

[20]Probes for exploring neurotransmitter activity have included the chemicals themselves and their receptors as well as their metabolites, which can be found variously in cerebrospinal flu-id, plasma, and urine. In addition, the effects of pharmacologic compounds, both clinically and on neurotransmitter activity, can be observed.

[21]Neurotransmitters influence the synthesis and release of hormones, and hormones influ-ence the effects of the neurotransmitters. Therefore, they undoubtedly influence each other (Gold, Goodwin, & Chrousos, 1988).

true for patients with bipolar disorder in either phase (Goodwin & Jamison, 1990). However, sleep research has the potential to identify a trait marker for bipolar disorder because studies have shown patients with bipolar disorder to be sensitive to cholinergic induction of REM sleep, even when in an euthymic, untreated state (Gershon & Nurnberger, 1995b; Goodwin & Jamison, 1990).

In addition to the daily rhythmic pattern, there also is a long-recognized and common seasonal pattern in the mood disorders. Of the 10 percent of patients who have a seasonal mood disorder syndrome, almost one-half have bipolar disorder (Faedda et al., 1993). The syndrome tends to be expressed either at extremes of light and temperature (winter and summer) or at extremes of the rate of change of light and temperature (fall and spring). Melatonin, a hormone that is synthesized by the pineal gland at night and inhibited by light, has received a great deal of recent attention because it is intricately related to both daily and seasonal rhythms. This finding may explain why the incidence of mania peaks in the summer.[22] Furthermore, Nurnberger and colleagues (1988) showed that even adults at risk (those with relatives who have bipolar disorder) but without the disorder showed a greater sensitivity to the suppression of melatonin secretion. Thus, two possible biological markers for bipolar disorder are sensitivity to bright-light suppression of nighttime melatonin release and cholinergic induction of REM sleep.

Like the hormones, the neuropeptides have been increasingly implicated in the etiology of the bipolar disorders. They include somatostatin, corticotropin-releasing factor, and vasopressin as well as several others that have slow but persistent effects consistent with both the clinical course of bipolar disorder and the benefit of medication (Berrettini et al., 1987). As a result, in part, of the knowledge that neuropeptides may regulate the flow of fluid and electrolytes, electrolyte and cell membrane abnormalities also have been identified as related to the pathophysiology of bipolar disorders.[23] Recent research has focused particularly on the enzymes regulating sodium and potassium ion fluxes across membranes and on any secondary messengers activated by signals at the membrane itself (Dubovsky, Murphy, Christiano, & Lee, 1992; el-Mallakh & Wyatt, 1995). Abnormalities at this level may be central to the pathophysiology of bipolar disorder, but the precise elaboration remains unknown.

In the mid-1980s, Post and colleagues (1986) proposed a behavioral kindling–sensitization hypothesis of the pathophysiology of bipolar disorder. This model holds particular promise because it allows for the integration of both genetic vulnerability and environmental factors. It was developed from observations that bipolar disorder is generally recurrent, that recurrence increases with both age and the number of previous episodes, and that episodes are similar for a given patient. The evidence assembled by Post and colleagues suggests that some patients with manic–depressive illness have early episodes triggered by stress followed by more serious episodes that are not necessarily so triggered. Their explanation is that these patients experience behavioral sensitization in which repeated stimulations produce increasingly severe

---

[22]However, seasonal mood disorder also may take the form of summer depression and winter hypomania (Wehr & Rosenthal, 1989).

[23]Observations of changes in the volume of body water of patients, the importance of cations in nerve transmissions, and the fact that lithium has a stabilizing effect on patients' clinical condition also point to an etiologic role for electrolytes and cell membranes (Goodwin & Jamison, 1990).

reactions and electrophysiological kindling, such that after repeat episodes a stimulus is no longer required.[24]

Limited literature suggests other possible biological pathways for bipolar disorders. For example, the possibility of a viral or immunologic basis for the bipolar disorders, as for unipolar disorders, has been proposed. After their comprehensive review, however, Yolken and Torrey (1995) concluded that the data point toward an infectious etiology. A definite link has not been established. There also has been the suggestion that pathophysiological differences may exist between Bipolar I and II and that brain high-energy phosphate metabolism may be impaired in patients with Bipolar II disorder (Kato et al., 1994).

There are few biological studies of patients with cyclothymic disorder. Howland and Thase (1993) concluded from those they were able to find that there is a likelihood that future findings will be similar to those for other mood disorders. By way of example, Depue and colleagues found an abnormal function of the hypothalamic–pituitary–adrenal axis in patients with cyclothymic disorder similar to the abnormalities found in patients with major depressive disorder (Depue, Kleiman, Davis, Hutchinson, & Kraus, 1985).

## Neuroanatomy

It is unlikely that there exists a simple, discrete neuroanatomical lesion underlying bipolar disorder. However, clinical observations of complete remission in some patients and pharmacologic response even in patients whose disorder is known to be due to a brain lesion highlight the promise of neuroanatomical findings for increased understanding of the pathophysiology of bipolar disorders (Goodwin & Jamison, 1990). Structural imaging techniques, such as CT scans and MRIs, have greatly facilitated the investigation of neuroanatomy. So have more recently developed techniques for imaging functional activities of the live brain, such as glucose uptake and metabolism through PET scanning and blood flow through regional CBF and SPECT. Despite many advances, including the reports of a preponderance of left-sided abnormalities in depressed states and right-sided abnormalities in manic states, many internal inconsistencies and unanswered questions remain.

## Premorbid Personality Structure and Temperament

There is considerable research interest in the observed overlap of personality types and the symptoms of bipolar disorder. Akiskal and collaborators (1995) identified four affective dispositions—dysthymia, irritability, hyperthymia, and cyclothymia—that exist as a continuum with the major mood states. They proposed that the latter three be recognized as temperamental markers for bipolar disorder. The Bipolar II disorder subtype, they reported, can best be understood by a stable lability of mood across the life span (that is, a trait), which intrudes into and possibly accentuates depressive episodes (that is, depressive states), thereby creating an intimate interweaving

---

[24]This important etiologic model has the following components: both genetic factors and stress may be predisposing; there are threshold effects; repeat episodes are often similar; later episodes may not require a trigger; youth increases vulnerability; and repeated episodes of one phase may lead to a form of compensation manifested in a switch to another phase (Goodwin & Jamison, 1990).

of trait and state. They suggested, and Deltito (1993) provided corroboration, that this temperamental profile is valid and, they added, may be more fundamental in defining the affective dysregulation of Bipolar II disorder than the hypomanic episodes that are emphasized in DSM-IV (Akiskal et al., 1995).

## Psychosocial Precipitants

Because there is strong evidence of genetic susceptibility to bipolar disorder, the role of environmental stressors may have more to do with the precipitation of episodes than with the etiology of the disorder per se (Goodwin & Jamison, 1990). However, numerous studies have shown that stressful events precede earlier episodes rather than later ones, and thus, at least early on, stressors may activate a pre-existing vulnerability (Post et al., 1986).

Pregnancy, which may be considered a stressor for some women under certain conditions, can precipitate either a manic or a depressive episode. Packer (1992) reported that 20 percent of women with bipolar disorder have manic episodes during or after pregnancy. It is not clear, however, whether this may result from a discontinuation of prophylactic medication, from physiological changes during pregnancy, or from psychological stress.

## Summary

In a recent publication, Carroll (1994) summarized the evidence that supports a primary role for biological factors in the etiology of the bipolar disorders. Carroll concluded that the data from twin and adoption studies suggest transmission does not segregate in families as a single dominant or recessive gene, but that there is a complex interaction among more than one gene and environmental factors. The author cited the persistent evidence of circadian patterns of physiological change, especially those of appetite and sleep, and the apparent deterioration in the course of illness over time as providing further potency for biological hypotheses.

It was initially hypothesized that an environmental effect interacting with biological vulnerability could explain the apparent trend toward an increasingly earlier age of onset of bipolar disorder (Dysthymia Working Group, 1992). The discovery of a phenomenon known as "DNA repeat expansions," however, has generated an alternative hypothesis that proposes the trend may be a reflection of a new form of rapid genetic change (Gershon, 1995).

Additional compelling support for the biological foundation of the bipolar disorders comes from evidence of an association of right-sided lesions in secondary episodes of mania and of left-sided lesions in depression, as well as the substantial benefit that can be derived from pharmacologic treatments in both the manic and depressive phases. Cyclothymic disorder also appears to have some genetic basis. The few biological studies that exist point to the likelihood of eventual findings similar to the other mood disorders (Howland & Thase, 1993).

## *COMORBIDITY*

The study of comorbidity may help us understand the pathophysiology of mental disorders and is crucial to treatment planning because co-occurrence of two or more disorders is often associated with poor response and poor outcome (Strakowski, McElroy, Keck, & West, 1994).

FIGURE **3-2**

**Psychiatric Comorbidity with Bipolar Disorders**

**Bipolar I**
50–90 percent have two or more comorbid disorders
Nearly half have a comorbid alcohol abuse or dependence problem
Most prevalent Axis II diagnoses are borderline personality and histrionic personality
disorders

**Bipolar II**
Comorbidity may be a hallmark of Bipolar II disorder
Chronic depressive disorder, premenstrual dysphoria, and alcoholism
As high as 59 percent comorbidity with persistent eating disorders

**Cyclothymic Disorder**
Strongly associated with borderline personality disorder

## Psychiatric Comorbidity

The NCS of the early 1990s was intended specifically to measure comorbidity among psychiatric disorders (see also chapter 1). Kessler et al. (1994) reported that more than one-half of affected people had two or more disorders. Brady and Sonne (1995) reported that nearly 90 percent of those with the more severe diagnoses had three or more disorders. Although the co-occurrence of mania with other psychiatric disorders has yet to be studied as extensively as its co-occurrence with depression, there appears to be an equally high frequency (Figure 3-2). Strakowski et al. (1994) reviewed the literature up to 1994 and identified high rates of comorbidity with obsessive–compulsive disorder, bulimia nervosa, panic disorder, impulse control disorders, some personality disorders, and substance abuse. Unfortunately, the number of studies upon which these conclusions have been based is small, and few of the studies were either prospective or controlled.[25]

Comorbidity with other psychiatric disorders may be a hallmark of Bipolar II disorder. Endicott and colleagues (1985) found that more women with Bipolar II than Bipolar I disorder had a tendency to suffer from chronic depressive disorder, premenstrual dysphoria, and alcoholism. Bipolar II also appears to be a common (as high as 59 percent) comorbid finding in hospitalized patients with severe persistent eating disorders (Simpson, al-Mufti, Andersen, & DePaulo, 1992). Because comorbidity is known to increase rates of chronicity and contribute to complications in Bipolar II disorder, these observations underscore the seriousness of the condition. It is clear as well that many patients who initially have cyclothymic disorder later develop other bipolar disorders, and according to DSM-IV criteria, these patients would have psychiatric comorbidity among at least two of the bipolar disorders.

---

[25]Strakowski et al. (1994) concluded their review with questions for further research: Does a comorbid psychiatric disorder whose onset occurred first represent a prodromal symptom, a risk factor, or an actual cause of bipolar disorder? When the comorbid disorder occurs simultaneously, is it distinct or a variable presentation of the same disorder?

*Alcohol and Drug Abuse*

Substance abuse is the most frequently studied comorbid psychiatric disorder (Akiskal et al., 1995) and certainly one of the most common. Regier et al. (1990) reported from the ECA data that 46 percent of people with bipolar disorder had a comorbid alcohol abuse or dependence problem, and 61 percent had an alcohol or other drug abuse diagnosis.[26] In a 10-year follow-up of 70 patients with both bipolar disorder and alcoholism, Winokur and colleagues (1994) did not find a greater rate of independent alcoholism in the families, thus suggesting that alcoholism is typically a secondary disorder. Brady and Sonne (1995) discovered that substance use negatively affects the course and prognosis of bipolar disorder and is associated with more irritable and dysphoric mood states, increased treatment resistance, and a greater need for hospitalization. In a rare study of cyclothymia, alcoholism, and drug abuse, Akiskal and colleagues found high rates of alcoholism and drug abuse among patients with cyclothymic disorder who were experiencing an extended course (Akiskal, Djenderedijian, Rosenthal, & Khani, 1977).

*Personality (Axis II) Disorders*

The reported prevalence of personality disorders in patients with bipolar disorder varies widely (O'Connell, Mayo, & Sciutto, 1991). The most prevalent Axis II diagnosis appears to be borderline personality disorder, followed by histrionic personality disorder (Jackson et al., 1991). Baxter and associates and Levitt and colleagues looked at co-occurrence in another way. Both groups of researchers found that, among patients hospitalized for borderline personality disorder, few also received bipolar disorder diagnoses (Baxter, Edell, Gerner, Fairbanks, & Gwirtsman, 1984; Levitt, Joffe, Ennis, MacDonald, & Kutcher, 1990).

It appears that patients with borderline personality disorder are likely to have mood symptoms similar to those seen in cyclothymic disorder (Howland & Thase, 1993). Howland & Thase (1993) summarized current investigations of the relationship among cyclothymic disorder, Bipolar II disorder, rapid cycling, dysthymic disorder, and the personality disorders. Their review included the conceptual history of cyclothymia, clinical phenomenology, family history, biological studies, and treatment. The cumulative results suggested that some forms of cyclothymia are strongly associated with borderline personality disorder (Levitt et al., 1990) but that the condition is clinically heterogeneous (Howland & Thase, 1993).

## Medical Comorbidity

In 1978, Krauthammer and Klerman first proposed that mania believed to be a direct physiological consequence of a medical condition or the result of an ingested substance be considered a distinct bipolar disorder subtype. In DSM-IV, however, these secondary mood disorders are classified as mood disorders resulting from a general medical condition or substance-induced mood disorders. Goodwin and Jamison (1990) have provided a comprehensive review of the known organic causes of secondary bipolar disorder, but specific studies of medical comorbidity with cyclothymic disorder appear not to exist.

---

[26]Strakowski et al. (1994) likewise found the rate of comorbid alcohol abuse or dependence to be in the 20 percent to 60 percent range.

*Bipolar Disorder Resulting from a General Medical Condition*

In the absence of positive proof of a causative relationship between two disorders, their chronological relationship, course, and any unusual aspects of presentation can shed light on the nature of their association. For example, one area of considerable research interest is the possibility of locating a neuroanatomical lesion that is originally produced by a medical disorder and then, in turn, causes secondary mania. Strakowski et al. (1994) concluded from their review of the literature that "mania in the setting of significant neurologic disorders seems to result from lesions involving right-sided subcortical structures . . . cortical areas closely linked to the limbic system" (p. 307). They noted that other pathophysiological data regarding bipolar disorder (for example, neuroendocrine, neuroimaging, and circadian rhythm studies) also suggest hypothalamic abnormalities and, therefore, both primary and secondary mania may share at least a pathophysiological step.

Some researchers have claimed that the higher rate of thyroid dysfunction among women than among men accounts for their numbers among patients with rapid cycling. In 1988, however, Wehr and colleagues (1988) found that their rate of thyroid disease among female patients with rapid cycling, who accounted for 92 percent of all patients, was no greater than the rate among patients without rapid cycling and that there was no relationship between menstrual cycles and manic–depressive cycles.

Evans, Byerly, and Greer (1995) reviewed the research on several conditions associated with secondary mania, including late-onset mania, closed-head injury, and HIV infection. They found conflicting reports with regard to late-onset mania. Most studies, however, reported few family members with bipolar disorder, a disproportionate amount of neurologic impairment among patients with late onset, a tendency toward treatment resistance, and a higher rate of mortality. It is notable that all of these patterns support a nongenetic etiology for late-onset mania. Patients with closed-head injury and patients with AIDS showed a high prevalence of secondary mania (Evans et al., 1995). Patients who have AIDS and bipolar disorder seemed less likely to have a personal or family history of mood disorders, and patients with closed-head injury had atypical symptoms. Both of these features support an organic rather than genetic etiology.

The comorbidy of bipolar disorder with numerous disorders other than these four, including multiple sclerosis and migraine (Jaffe et al., 1994), has been observed, but causality has not been established (Strakowski et al., 1994). Another form of comorbidity may exist, such as when a medical condition and a bipolar disorder co-occur but are not causally related. Nevertheless, the one disorder may represent a risk factor or may affect the course or outcome of the other. Some disorders, such as migraine, may represent an alternative expression of the bipolar disorder. Strakowski and colleagues (1994) cited two studies that reported that roughly one in five patients with mania had some kind of medical comorbidity, but they refrained from drawing any further conclusions because of inadequate sample sizes and an absence of longitudinal or prospective designs.

## Drug-Induced Bipolar Disorder

Recreational drug use and alcohol abuse are relatively common among patients with bipolar disorder, which adds to the difficulty of diagnosis. Goodwin and Jamison (1990) described both the street drugs and the therapeutic drugs that are likely to precipitate manic episodes. Among the former are hallucinogens, amphetamines, cocaine, and marijuana. Among the therapeutic drugs are steroids, L-dopa, and the antidepressants, the latter precipitating a manic episode or rapid cycling in an estimated 15 percent to 20 percent of patients treated in general psychiatric practice and 50 percent of patients treated in specialist research units and in clinics for patients with refractory depression (Fawcett, 1994).

## Summary

The question of the role of comorbid disorders in the etiology of bipolar disorder remains unanswered, although it is clear that comorbidity adversely affects the course of bipolar disorder (Kessler et al., 1994). Existing studies are limited in number, they often have inadequate sample size to establish causality, and they rarely have prospective designs. Several issues regarding the co-occurrence of bipolar and other disorders, therefore, are unsettled, such as which demographic factors predict comorbidity, why and when patients with bipolar disorder are most likely to engage in substance abuse, and whether substance abuse precipitates manic episodes or is, alternatively, a prodromal syndrome. Because most people who are available for study are themselves psychiatric patients, little is known about either the natural course or the psychiatric and medical comorbidity of people who are not patients.

## COURSE AND PROGNOSIS

Bipolar disorder is a devastating brain disease that involves episodes of mania and depression. Mania characteristically begins with hypomania, which then progresses to the point at which social and occupational functioning is disrupted. Speech is generally rapid, and behavior is hyperactive. Manic episodes are characterized by elated or irritable mood, increased energy, decreased need for sleep, poor judgment and lack of insight, and often reckless or irresponsible behavior. Manic episodes may alternate with profound depressions characterized by pervasive sadness, hopelessness, and an inability to eat, sleep, concentrate, or even move.

A substantial number, about one in five, of patients with bipolar disorder take their own lives (Goodwin & Jamison, 1990). Contrary to earlier belief, patients suffering from a mixed state, characterized by simultaneous manic and depressive symptoms, have even higher rates of suicide than do depressed patients (Dilsaver, Chen, Swann, Shoaib, & Krajewski, 1994). Strakowski et al.'s recent study further suggests that it is not the mixed state itself but the severity of the depressive symptoms that is associated with suicidality (Strakowski, McElroy, Keck, & West, 1996).

Typically, a patient with bipolar disorder will experience approximately eight to 10 episodes of mania or depression in his or her lifetime. As has been described above, some patients have rapid-cycling disorder and experience many more episodes. Just over one-half of patients with bipolar disorder present first with a manic episode and almost one-half present with a depressive episode. The variation across studies is considerable. During manic–depressive cycles, patients show variable clinical presentations including dramatic fluctuations of mood, energy, activity, information processing, and behavior (Carroll, 1994).

Age at onset is a key factor in the differential diagnosis of bipolar disorder and also may affect the course of illness. Early age at onset reflects higher familial loading (Strober, 1992), and numerous studies have reported associated psychotic features (Angst, 1986). Coryell and colleagues (1995) reported that young age at onset and chronicity, taken together, predicted a shift from a nonbipolar disorder to Bipolar II disorder, whereas a family history of mania or psychosis predicts a shift to Bipolar I disorder.

The rate of late-onset bipolar disorder has not been firmly established (Young, 1992), but these patients appear less likely to have relatives with bipolar disorder, and their mania is more likely to be secondary to medical, especially neurologic, problems or drug treatments (Strakowski et al., 1994).

Kraepelin's (1921) distinction between manic–depressive illness and dementia praecox was based on his observations that the former was episodic rather than chronic and, furthermore, had a more benign impact. Goodwin and Jamison (1990), however, examined the early studies that had demonstrated a high rate of single-episode manic–depressive illness and concluded that the methodologies used were faulty and the study populations included many patients with unipolar syndromes. Today, it is clear that bipolar disorder is a lifelong illness, often with recurrent episodes.

It is clinically important to ascertain how long an episode is likely to last and whether the course of illness will remain chronic. Kessler and colleagues (1994) studied these factors among patients grouped according to whether they had a purely manic, purely depressed, or mixed or cycling pattern. They found that patients with pure mania recovered the most quickly, usually in five weeks; the patients with pure depression recovered in about nine weeks; and those patients with features of both disorders, either simultaneously or in cycles, generally recovered at about 14 weeks. Rates of chronicity, defined as remaining ill for more than a year, were 7 percent, 22 percent, and 32 percent in these groups, respectively.

It also is clinically important to determine the cycle length, that is, the length of time from the beginning of one episode to the beginning of the next. Because it tends to be constant in a given person, cycle length reflects the duration of a symptom-free interval. Rapid cycling also worsens the course of bipolar disorder, and cycling within an episode markedly increases the probability of a chronic condition. Rapid cycling tends to occur more often in women than in men and to occur later in the illness (Wehr et al., 1988). Although early studies found increasingly short cycle length over the course of an illness, more recent data indicate that cycle length remains constant over time (Winokur et al., 1994).

In a 1985 study, Endicott and colleagues found no significant differences in age at onset, cycling within episodes, number of psychotic episodes, or rate of suicide between patients with Bipolar I and Bipolar II disorders. Using data from a five-year prospective follow-up study comparing patients with Bipolar I, Bipolar II, and major depression, Coryell and colleagues (1989) reported that both bipolar groups had higher relapse rates than did patients with unipolar depression and had higher rates of manic, hypomanic, and depressive episodes. Not surprisingly, the patients with Bipolar II disorder were less likely to be hospitalized or to develop full-blown mania than were the patients with Bipolar I disorder. Overall, the need for hospitalization and medication during depressive episodes was equivalent among the three groups.

Cyclothymic disorder, like dysthymic disorder, is a chronic disorder that lasts at least two years and includes numerous periods with hypomanic symptoms and numerous periods with depressive symptoms (APA, 1994). It will be important in future research to distinguish those patients who have a chronic mood disorder that is stable and will not progress to Bipolar I or II from those patients for whom the syndrome is prodromal and from those who have another condition altogether.

## Functional Impairment

Coryell and colleagues (1993) found that patients with unipolar or bipolar disorder suffered significant impairment at nearly every level of psychosocial functioning, including work, family, marital status, nonmarital interpersonal relationships, and recreational enjoyment. A naturalistic study by Goldberg, Harrow, and Grossman (1995) found that 60 percent of patients with bipolar disorder had severe difficulty in at least one area of functioning at both two-year and four-and-one-half-year follow-up. Compared with a group of patients with unipolar disorder, those with bipolar disorders had more rehospitalizations, worse work function, and worse overall outcomes. Romans and McPherson (1992) examined social interactions of patients with bipolar disorder with their marital partners and with others and, when compared to a community sample, found that both kinds of relationships were impoverished.

## Prognosis

Harrow and colleagues studied the outcomes for patients with mania about 18 months after hospital discharge and found that only 26 percent of those patients were doing well; 34 percent were doing poorly, and 40 percent still had some impairment (Harrow, Goldberg, Grossman, & Meltzer, 1990). Forty-two percent had been rehospitalized at least once during the study period. Those findings support earlier work by Winokur, Clayton, and Reich (1969). Since the Harrow et al. study, Winokur and collaborators (1994) have published the results of a 10-year follow-up of 131 patients in the NIMH Collaborative Study of the Psychobiology of Depression. They found that almost 90 percent of the patients had at least one additional hospitalization, but 96 percent experienced at least one period of eight or more weeks without an episode. In other words, only 4 percent of patients remained chronic throughout. Patients with a family history of mania had a greater-than-average number of episodes.

## Summary

These studies taken together explain the changing view of bipolar disorder. Earlier thought to have a remitting course with an overall favorable outcome, bipolar disorder is now recognized as having a difficult and often deteriorating course. Patients with bipolar disorder, especially of the mixed-state variety, are at even greater risk of suicide than are patients with major depression. The longer the illness, the older the patient, and the greater the predominance of manic rather than depressed episodes, the worse the outcome for patients with bipolar disorder. Patients with rapid-cycling disorder and with concurrent medical or psychiatric disorders have particularly severe impairment and an especially difficult course.

Bipolar II disorder is a new entry to DSM-IV. It is similar in many ways to Bipolar I disorder but is characterized by greater chronicity, higher suicide rates and, especially, greater comorbidity than Bipolar I disorder. Research into the etiology and course of Bipolar II is limited, although there is developing evidence to support a biological and temperamental basis. An important avenue for future research will be to distinguish those patients who have a chronic and stable mood disorder that will not progress to Bipolar I or Bipolar II disorder both from those patients whose syndrome is prodromal and from those patients who may have another condition altogether, such as a personality disorder (Howland & Thase, 1993).

# References

Abramowitz, E. S., Baker, A. H., & Fleischer, S. F. (1982). Onset of depressive psychiatric crises and the menstrual cycle. *American Journal of Psychiatry, 139,* 475–478.

Akiskal, H. S. (1983). Dysthymic disorder: Psychopathology of proposed chronic depressive subtypes. *American Journal of Psychiatry, 140,* 11–20.

Akiskal, H. S. (1991). Chronic depression. *Bulletin of the Menninger Clinic, 55,* 156–171.

Akiskal, H. S. (1992). Mood disorders. In R. Berkow & A. Fletcher (Eds.), *Merck manual* (16th ed., pp. 1592–1614). Rahway, NJ: Merck Research Laboratories.

Akiskal, H. S. (1994a). Dysthymia: Clinical and external validity. *Acta Psychiatrica Scandinavica, 383*(Suppl.), 19–23.

Akiskal, H. S. (1994b). Dysthymic and cyclothymic depressions: Therapeutic considerations. *Journal of Clinical Psychiatry, 55*(Suppl.), 46–52.

Akiskal, H. S., & Akiskal, K. (1988). Re-assessing the prevalence of bipolar disorders: Clinical significance and artistic creativity. *Psychiatrie et Psychobiologie [Psychiatry and Psychobiology]* 3, 295–365.

Akiskal, H., Djenderedijian, A., Rosenthal, R., & Khani, M. (1977). Cyclothymic disorder: Validating criteria for inclusion in the bipolar affective group. *American Journal of Psychiatry, 134,* 1227–1233.

Akiskal, H. S., Downs, J., Jordan, P., Watson, S., Daugherty, D., & Pruitt, D. B. (1985). Affective disorders in referred children and younger siblings of manic–depressives: Mode of onset and prospective course. *Archives of General Psychiatry, 42,* 996–1003.

Akiskal, H. S., King, D., Rosenthal, T. L., Robinson, D., & Scott-Strauss, A. (1981). Chronic depression: Part I. Clinical and familial characteristics in 137 probands. *Journal of Affective Disorders, 3,* 297–315.

Akiskal, H. S., Maser, J. D., Zeller, P. J., Endicott, J., Coryell, W., Keller, M., Warshaw, M., Clayton, P., & Goodwin, F. (1995). Switching from "unipolar" to Bipolar II: An 11-year prospective study of clinical and temperamental predictors in 559 patients. *Archives of General Psychiatry, 52,* 114–123.

Akiskal, H. S., Rosenthal, T. L., Haykal, R. F., Lemmi, H., Rosenthal, R. H., & Scott-Strauss, A. (1980). Characterologic depressions: Clinical and sleep EEG findings separating "subaffective dysthymias" from "character spectrum disorders." *Archives of General Psychiatry, 37,* 777–783.

Akiskal, H. S., & Weise, R. E. (1992). The clinical spectrum of so-called "minor" depressions. *American Journal of Psychotherapy, 46,* 9–22.

Alnaes, R., & Torgersen, S. (1993). Mood disorders: Developmental and precipitating events. *Canadian Journal of Psychiatry, 38,* 217–224.

American Psychiatric Association. (1952). *Diagnostic and statistical manual of mental disorders.* Washington, DC: Author.

American Psychiatric Association. (1968). *Diagnostic and statistical manual of mental disorders* (2nd ed.). Washington, DC: Author.

American Psychiatric Association. (1980). *Diagnostic and statistical manual of mental disorders* (3rd ed.). Washington, DC: Author.

American Psychiatric Association. (1987). *Diagnostic and statistical manual of mental disorders* (3rd ed., rev.). Washington, DC: Author.

American Psychiatric Association. (1993). Practice guideline for major depressive disorder in adults. *American Journal of Psychiatry, 150*(Suppl.), 1–26.

American Psychiatric Association. (1994). *Diagnostic and statistical manual of mental disorders* (4th ed.). Washington, DC: Author.

Andreasen, N. C., Grove, W. M., Shapiro, R. W., Keller, M. B., Hirschfeld, M. A., & McDonald-Scott, P. (1981). Reliability of lifetime diagnosis. *Archives of General Psychiatry, 38*, 400–405.

Andrews, G., Stewart, G., Allen, R., & Henderson, A. S. (1990). The genetics of six neurotic disorders: A twin study. *Psychological Medicine, 21*, 329–335.

Angold, A., & Worthman, C. W. (1993). Puberty onset of gender differences in rates of depression: A developmental, epidemiologic and neuroendocrine perspective. *Journal of Affective Disorders, 29*, 145–158.

Angst, J. (1978). The course of affective disorders: II. Typology of bipolar manic–depressive illness. *Archives of Psychiatry Nervenkrankheiten, 226*, 65–73.

Angst, J. (1986). The course of major depression, atypical bipolar disorder, and bipolar disorder. In G. Klerman & N. Matussek (Eds.), *New results in depression research* (pp. 26–35). Berlin: Springer-Verlag.

Angst, J. (1988). Clinical course of affective disorders. In T. Helgason & R. J. Daly (Eds.), *Depressive illness: Prediction of course and outcome* (pp. 23–46). Berlin: Springer-Verlag.

Angst, J. (1992). How recurrent and predictable is depressive illness? In S. Montgomery & F. Rouillon (Eds.), *Long-term treatment of depression* (pp. 1–13). New York: John Wiley & Sons.

Angst, J., & Clayton, P. (1986). Premorbid personality of depressive, bipolar, and schizophrenic patients with special reference to suicidal issues. *Comprehensive Psychiatry, 27*, 511–532.

Angst, J., & Dobler-Mikola, A. (1985). The Zurich Study: VI. A continuum from depression to anxiety disorders. *European Archives of Psychiatry and Neurological Sciences, 23*, 179–186.

Angst, J., & Hochstrasser, B. (1994). Recurrent brief depression: The Zurich Study. *Journal of Clinical Psychiatry, 55*(Suppl.), 3–9.

Anthony, J., & Petronis, K. R. (1991). Suspected risk factors for depression among adults 18–44 years old. *Epidemiology, 2*, 123–132.

Aronson, T. A., Shukla, S., Hoff, A., & Cook, B. (1988). Proposed delusional depression subtypes: Preliminary evidence from a retrospective study of phenomenology and treatment course. *Journal of Affective Disorders, 14*, 69–74.

Asnis, G. M., Friedman, T. A., Sanderson, W. C., Kaplan, M. L., Van Praag, H. M., & Harkavy-Friedman, J. M. (1993). Suicidal behaviors in adult psychiatric outpatients. I. Description and prevalence. *American Journal of Psychiatry, 150*, 108–112.

Asnis, G. M., & Miller, A. H. (1989). Phenomenology and biology of depression: Potential mechanisms for neuromodulation of immunity. In I. H. Miller (Ed.), *Depressive disorders and immunity* (pp. 51–63). Washington, DC: American Psychiatric Press.

Bancroft, J. (1993). The premenstrual syndrome: A reappraisal of the concept and evidence. *Psychological Medicine, 24*(Monograph Suppl.), 1–47.

Bauer, M. S., Calabrese, J., Dunner, D. L., Post, R., Whybrow, P. C., Gyulai, L., Tay, L. K., Younkin, S. R., Byrnum, D., Lavori, P., & Price, R. A. (1994). Multisite data reanalysis of the validity of rapid cycling as a course modifier for bipolar disorder in DSM-IV. *American Journal of Psychiatry, 151,* 506–515.

Baxter, L., Edell, W., Gerner, R., Fairbanks, L., & Gwirtsman, H. (1984). Dexamethasone suppression test and Axis I diagnoses of inpatients with DSM-III borderline personality disorder. *Journal of Clinical Psychiatry, 45,* 150–153.

Beersma, D. G., & van den Hoofdakker, R. H. (1992). Can non-REM sleep be depressogenic? *Journal of Affective Disorders, 24,* 101–108.

Berrettini, W. (1995). Diagnostic and genetic issues of depression and bipolar illness. *Pharmacotherapy, 15*(Suppl.), 69S–75S.

Berrettini, W. H., Nurnberger, J.I.J., Zerbe, R. L., Gold, P. W., Chrousos, G. P., & Tomai, T. (1987). CSF neuropeptides in euthymic bipolar patients and controls. *British Journal of Psychiatry, 150,* 208–212.

Bertelsen, A., Harvald, B., & Hauge, M. (1977). A Danish twin study of manic–depressive disorders. *British Journal of Psychiatry, 130,* 330–351.

Blacker, D., & Tsuang, M. T. (1992). Contested boundaries of bipolar disorder and the limits of categorical diagnosis in psychiatry. *American Journal of Psychiatry, 149,* 1473–1483.

Blazer, D., George, L. K., Landerman, R., Pennybacker, M., Melville, M. L., Woodbury, M., Manton, K., Jordan, K., & Locke, B. (1985). Psychiatric disorders: A rural/urban comparison. *Archives of General Psychiatry, 42,* 651–656.

Blazer, D., & Williams, C. D. (1980). Epidemiology of dysphoria and depression in an elderly population. *American Journal of Psychiatry, 137,* 439–444.

Bombardier, C. H., & Buchwald, D. (1995). Outcome and prognosis of patients with chronic fatigue vs. chronic fatigue syndrome. *Archives of Internal Medicine, 155,* 2105–2110.

Boyd, J. H., & Weissman, M. M. (1981). Epidemiology of affective disorders: A re-examination and future directions. *Archives of General Psychiatry, 38,* 1039–1046.

Brady, K., & Sonne, S. C. (1995). The relationship between substance abuse and bipolar disorder. *Journal of Clinical Psychiatry, 56*(Suppl. 3), 19–24.

Broadhead, W. E., Blazer, D. G., George, L. K., & Tse, C. K. (1990). Depression, disability, and days lost from work in a prospective epidemiological survey. *JAMA, 264,* 2524–2528.

Brockington, I. F., Margison, F. R., Schofield, E. M., & Knight, R.J.E. (1988). The clinical picture of the depressed form of puerperal psychosis. *Journal of Affective Disorders, 15,* 29–37.

Brown, G. W., & Harris, T. O. (1978). *Social origins of depression: A study of psychiatric disorder in women.* London: Tavistock.

Brown, G. W., & Harris, T. O. (1986). Establishing causal links: The Bedford College studies of depression. In H. Katshnig (Ed.), *Life events and psychiatric disorders* (pp. 107–187). Cambridge, England: Cambridge University Press.

Bruce, M. L., Takeuchi, D. T., & Leaf, P. J. (1991). Poverty and psychiatric status: Longitudinal evidence from the New Haven Epidemiological Catchment Area Study. *Archives of General Psychiatry, 48,* 470–474.

Bryer, J. B., Nelson, B. A., Miller, J. B., & Krol, P. A. (1987). Childhood sexual and physical abuse as factors in adult psychiatric illness. *American Journal of Psychiatry, 144,* 1426–1430.

Burke, K. C., Burke, J. D., Jr., Regier, D. A., & Rae, D. S. (1990). Age at onset of selected mental disorders in five community populations. *Archives of General Psychiatry, 47,* 511–518.

Burville, P. W. (1995). Recent progress in the epidemiology of major depression. *Epidemiologic Reviews, 17,* 21–31.

Burville, P. W., Johnson, G. A., Jamrozik, K. D., Anderson, C. S., Stewart-Wynne, E. G., & Chakera, T.M.H. (1995). Prevalence of depression after stroke: The Perth Community Stroke Study. *British Journal of Psychiatry, 166,* 320–327.

Cadoret, R. J., O'Gorman, T. W., Heywood, E., & Troughton, E. (1985). Genetic and environmental factors in major depression. *Journal of Affective Disorders, 9,* 155–164.

Calabrese, J. R., Rapport, D. J., Kimmel, S. E., Reece, B., & Woyshville, M. J. (1993). Rapid cycling bipolar disorder and its treatment with valproate. *Canadian Journal of Psychiatry, 38*(Suppl. 2), S57–S61.

Carroll, B. J. (1994). Brain mechanisms in manic depression. *Clinical Chemistry, 40,* 303–308.

Cassano, G. B., Akiskal, H. S., Savino, M., Musetti, L., & Perugi, G. (1992). Proposed subtypes of Bipolar II and related disorders: With hypomanic episodes (or cyclothymia) and with hyperthymic temperament. *Journal of Affective Disorders, 26,* 127–140.

Cassano, G. B., Akiskal, H. S., Savino, M., Soriani, A., Musetti, L., & Perugi, G. (1993). Single episode of major depressive disorder. First episode of recurrent mood disorder or distinct subtype of late-onset depression? *European Archives of Psychiatry and Clinical Neuroscience, 242,* 373–380.

Cassem, E. H. (1995). Depressive disorders in the medically ill: An overview. *Psychosomatics, 36,* S2–S10.

Cloninger, C. R., Svrakic, D. M., & Pryzbeck, T. R. (1993). A psychobiological model of temperament and character. *Archives of General Psychiatry, 50,* 975–990.

Comstock, G. W., & Helsing, K. J. (1976). Symptoms of depression in two communities. *Psychological Medicine, 6,* 551–563.

Conte, H. C., & Karasu, T. B. (1992). A review of treatment studies of minor depression: 1980–1991. *American Journal of Psychotherapy, 46,* 59–74.

Coryell, W., Andreasen, N. C., Endicott, J., & Keller, M. (1987). The significance of past mania or hypomania in the course and outcome of major depression. *American Journal of Psychiatry, 144,* 309–315.

Coryell, W., Endicott, J., & Keller, M. (1990). Outcome of patients with chronic affective disorders: A five-year follow-up. *American Journal of Psychiatry, 147,* 1627–1633.

Coryell, W., Endicott, J., Maser, J. D., Keller, M. B., Leon, A. C., & Akiskal, H. S. (1995). Long-term stability of polarity distinctions in the affective disorders. *American Journal of Psychiatry, 152,* 385–390.

Coryell, W., Endicott, J., & Winokur, G. (1992). Anxiety syndromes as epiphenomena of primary major depression: Outcome and familial psychopathology. *American Journal of Psychiatry, 149,* 100–107.

Coryell, W., Keller, M., Endicott, J., Andreasen, N., Clayton, P., & Hirschfeld, R. (1989). Bipolar II illness: Course and outcome over a five-year period. *Psychological Medicine, 19,* 129–142.

Coryell, W., Pfohl, B., & Zimmerman, M. (1984). The clinical and neuroendocrine features of psychotic depression. *Journal of Nervous and Mental Disease, 172,* 521–528.

Coryell, W., Scheftner, W., Keller, M., Endicott, J., Maser, J., & Klerman, G. L. (1993). The enduring psychosocial consequences of mania and depression. *American Journal of Psychiatry, 150,* 720–727.

Coryell, W., & Winokur, G. (1992). Course and outcome. In E. S. Paykel (Ed.), *Handbook of affective disorders* (pp. 89–108). New York: Guilford Press.

Council on Scientific Affairs. (1993). The etiological features of depression in adults. *Archives of Family Medicine, 2,* 76–84.

Craddock, N., & McGuffin, P. (1993). Approaches to the genetics of affective disorders. *Annals of Medicine, 25,* 317–322.

Crook, T., & Eliot, J. (1980). Parental death during childhood and adult depression: A critical review of the literature. *Psychological Bulletin, 87,* 289–299.

Cummings, J. L. (1992). Depression and Parkinson's disease: A review. *American Journal of Psychiatry, 149,* 443–454.

Custro, N., Scafidi, V., LoBaido, R., Nastri, L., Abbate, G., Cuffaro, M. P., Gallo, S., Vienna, G., & Notarbartolo, A. (1994). Subclinical hypothyroidism resulting from autoimmune thyroiditis in female patients with endogenous depression. *Journal of Endocrinological Investigation, 17,* 641–646.

deGruy, F. V. (in press). Mental health care in the primary care setting. In Committee on the Future of Primary Care, Institute of Medicine (Eds.), *Primary care: America's health in a new era.* Washington, DC: National Academy Press.

Deltito, J. A. (1993). The effect of valproate on bipolar spectrum temperamental disorders. *Journal of Clinical Psychiatry, 54,* 300–304.

Depue, R. A., Kleiman, R. M., Davis, P., Hutchinson, M., & Kraus, S. P. (1985). The behavioral high-risk paradigm and bipolar affective disorder, VIII: Serum free control in nonpatient cyclothymic subjects selected by the General Behavior Inventory. *American Journal of Psychiatry, 142,* 175–181.

Devanand, D. P., Nobler, M. S., Singer, T., Kiersky, J. E., Turret, N., Roose, S. P., & Sackheim, H. A. (1994). Is dysthymia a different disorder in the elderly? *American Journal of Psychiatry, 151,* 1592–1599.

Dilsaver, S. C., Chen, Y-W., Swann, A. C., Shoaib, A. M., & Krajewski, K. J. (1994). Suicidality in patients with pure and depressive mania. *American Journal of Psychiatry, 151,* 1312–1315.

Dobie, S. A., & Walker, E. A. (1992). Depression after childbirth. *Journal of the American Board of Family Practice, 5,* 303–311.

Dohrenwend, B. S., & Dohrenwend, B. P. (1974). *Stressful life events: Their nature and effects.* New York: John Wiley & Sons.

Dressler, W. W., & Badger, L. W. (1985). Epidemiology of depressive symptoms in black communities: A comparative analysis. *Journal of Nervous and Mental Disease, 173,* 212–220.

Dubovsky, S. L., Murphy, J., Christiano, J., & Lee, C. (1992). The calcium second messenger system in bipolar disorders: Data supporting new research directions. *Journal of Neuropsychiatry, 4,* 3–14.

Dubovsky, S. L., & Thomas, M. (1992). Psychotic depression: Advances in conceptualization and treatment. *Hospital and Community Psychiatry, 43,* 1189–1198.

Dunner, D., Fleiss, J., & Fieve, R. (1976). Lithium carbonate prophylaxis failure. *British Journal of Psychiatry, 129,* 40–44.

Dunner, D. L., Gershon, E., & Goodwin, F. (1976). Heritable factors in the severity of affective illness. *Biological Psychiatry, 11,* 31–42.

Dworkin, R. H., & Gitlin, M. J. (1991). Clinical aspects of depression in chronic pain patients. *Clinical Journal of Pain, 7,* 79–94.

Dysthymia Working Group. (1992). The changing rate of major depression: Cross-national comparisons. *JAMA, 268,* 3098–3105.

Dysthymia Working Group. (1995). Dysthymia in clinical practice. *British Journal of Psychiatry, 166,* 174–183.

Egeland, J. A., Gerhard, D. S., Pauls, D. L., Sussex, J. N., Kidd, K. K., Allen, C. R., Hostetter, A. M., & Housman, D. E. (1987). Bipolar affective disorders linked to DNA markers on chromosome 11. *Nature, 325*, 783–787.

el-Mallakh, R. S., & Wyatt, R. J. (1995). The Na,K-ATPase hypothesis for bipolar illness. *Biological Psychiatry, 37*, 235–244.

Emery, V. O., & Oxman, T. E. (1992). Update on the dementia spectrum of depression. *American Journal of Psychiatry, 149*, 305–317.

Endicott, J. (1993). The menstrual cycle and mood disorders. *Journal of Affective Disorders, 29*, 193–200.

Endicott, J., Nee, J., Andreasen, J., Clayton, P., Keller, M., & Coryell, W. (1985). Bipolar II: Combine or keep separate? *Journal of Affective Disorders, 8*, 17–28.

Ernst, C., & Angst, J. (1992). The Zurich Study: XII. Sex differences in depression: Evidence from longitudinal epidemiological data. *European Archives of Psychiatry and Clinical Neuroscience, 241*, 222–230.

Evans, D. L., Byerly, M. J., & Greer, R. A. (1995). Secondary mania: Diagnosis and treatment. *Journal of Clinical Psychiatry, 56*(Suppl. 3), 31–37.

Faedda, G. L., Tondo, L., Teicher, M. H., Baldessarini, R. J., Gelbard, H. A., & Floris, G. F. (1993). Seasonal mood disorders. Patterns of seasonal recurrence in mania and depression. *Archives of General Psychiatry, 50*, 17–23.

Fawcett, J. (1994). *Treatment of refractory and rapid-cycling bipolar disorder.* Available June 1996 from www.wpic.pitt.edu/research/bipolr2.htm.

Feinstein, A. R. (1970). The pre-therapeutic classification of co-morbidity in chronic disease. *Journal of Chronic Diseases, 23*, 455–468.

First, M. B., Donovan, S., & Frances, A. (1996). Nosology of chronic mood disorders. *Psychiatric Clinics of North America, 19*(1), 29–39.

Frank, E., Perel, J. M., Cornes, C., Jarrett, D. B., Mallinger, A. G., Thase, M. E., McEachran, A. B., & Grochocinski, V. J. (1990). Three-year outcomes for maintenance therapy in recurrent depression. *Archives of General Psychiatry, 47*, 1093–1099.

Frank, E., Prien, R. F., Jarrett, R. B., Keller, M. B., Kupfer, D. J., Lavori, P. W., Rush, A. J., & Weissman, M. M. (1991). Conceptualization and rationalization for consensus definitions of terms in major depressive disorder: Remission, recovery, relapse and recurrence. *Archives of General Psychiatry, 48*, 851–855.

Frasure-Smith, N., Lesperance, F., & Talajic, M. (1993). Depression following myocardial infarction. *JAMA, 270*, 1819–1825.

Gann, H., Riemann, D., Stoll, S., Berger, M., & Muller, W. E. (1995). Growth-hormone response to clonidine in panic disorder patients in comparison to patients with major depression and healthy controls. *Psychopharmacology, 28*, 80–83.

Garvey, M. J., Tuason, V. B., Lumry, A. E., & Hofman, N. G. (1983). Occurrence of depression in the postpartum state. *Journal of Affective Disorders, 5*, 97–101.

Gershon, E. S. (1990). Genetics. In F. K. Goodwin & K. R. Jamison (Eds.), *Manic–depressive illness* (pp. 373–401). New York: Oxford University Press.

Gershon, E. S. (1995). Recent developments in genetics of bipolar illness. In G. Gessa, W. Fratta, L. Pani, & G. Serra (Eds.), *Depression and mania: From neurobiology to treatment* (pp. 85–98). New York: Raven Press.

Gershon, E., & Nurnberger, J. I. (1995a). Bipolar illness. In J. M. Oldham & M. B. Riba (Eds.), *Psychiatric genetics* (pp. 405–424). Washington, DC: American Psychiatric Press.

Gershon, E. S., & Nurnberger, J. I., Jr. (1995b). Review of psychiatry. In J. M. Oldham & M. B. Riba (Eds.), *Review of psychiatry* (Vol. 14, pp. 405–460). Washington, DC: American Psychiatric Press.

Gift, A. G., & McCrone, S. H. (1993). Depression in patients with COPD. *Heart and Lung, 22*, 289–297.

Gold, P. W., Goodwin, F. K., & Chrousos, G. P. (1988). Clinical and biochemical manifestations of depression. Relation to the neurobiology of stress. *New England Journal of Medicine, 319*, 413–420.

Goldberg, J. F., Harrow, M., & Grossman, L. (1995). Course and outcome in bipolar affective disorder: A longitudinal follow-up study. *American Journal of Psychiatry, 152*, 379–384.

Goodwin, F. K., & Jamison, K. R. (1990). *Manic–depressive illness.* New York: Oxford University Press.

Gorman, D. M. (1992). Distinguishing primary and secondary disorders in studies of alcohol dependence and depression. *Drug and Alcohol Review, 11*, 23–29.

Greenberg, P. E., Stiglin, L. E., Finkelstein, S. N., & Berndt, E. R. (1993). The economic burden of depression. *Journal of Clinical Psychiatry, 54*, 405–418.

Haggerty, J. J., & Prange, A. J. (1995). Borderline hypothyroidism and depression. *Annual Review of Medicine, 46*, 37–46.

Hall, R.C.W. (1980). *Psychiatric presentations of medical illness: Somatopsychic disorders.* New York: SP Medical and Scientific Books.

Hammen, C. (1991). Generation of stress in the course of unipolar depression. *Journal of Abnormal Psychology, 100*, 555–561.

Hammen, C., Gordon, D., Burge, D., Adrian, C., Jaenicke, C., & Hiroto, D. (1987). Maternal affective disorders, illness and stress: Risk for children's psychopathology. *American Journal of Psychiatry, 144*, 736–741.

Harrison, W. M., Endicott, J., Nee, J., Glick, H., & Rabkin, J. G. (1989). Characteristics of women seeking treatment for premenstrual syndrome. *Psychosomatics, 30*, 405–411.

Harrow, M., Goldberg, J. F., Grossman, L. S., & Meltzer, H. Y. (1990). Outcome in manic disorders. *Archives of General Psychiatry, 47*, 665–671.

Helms, P. M., & Smith, R. E. (1983). Recurrent psychotic depression: Evidence of diagnostic stability. *Journal of Affective Disorders, 5*, 51–54.

Helzer, J. E., & Pryzbeck, T. R. (1988). The co-occurrence of alcoholism with other psychiatric disorders in the general population and its impact on treatment. *Journal of the Study of Alcohol, 49*, 219–224.

Heun, R., & Maier, W. (1993). The distinction of Bipolar II disorder from Bipolar I and recurrent unipolar depression: Results of a controlled family study. *Acta Psychiatrica Scandinavica, 87*, 279–284.

Higgins, E. (1994). A review of unrecognized mental illness in primary care: Prevalence, natural history, and efforts to change the course. *Archives of Family Medicine, 3*, 899–907.

Hiller, W., Dichtl, G., Hecht, H., Hundt, W., Mombour, W., & von Zerssen, D. (1994). Evaluating the new ICD-10 categories of depressive episode and recurrent depressive disorder. *Journal of Affective Disorders, 31*, 49–60.

Hirschfeld, R.M.A., & Cross, C. K. (1981). Psychosocial risk factors for depression. In D. A. Regier & G. Allen (Eds.), *Risk factor research in the major mental disorders* (pp. 55–67). Rockville, MD: National Institute of Mental Health.

Hirschfeld, R. M., & Holzer, C.E.R. (1994). Depressive personality disorder: Clinical implications. *Journal of Clinical Psychiatry, 55*(Suppl.), 10–17.

Hirschfeld, R.M.A., Klerman, G. L., Lavori, P. W., Keller, M. B., Griffith, P., & Coryell, W. (1989). Premorbid personality assessments of first onset of major depression. *Archives of General Psychiatry, 46*, 345–350.

Holmes, S. J., & Robins, L. N. (1988). The role of parental disciplinary practices in the development of depression and alcoholism. *Psychiatry, 51,* 24–36.

Horwath, E., Johnson, J., & Weissman, M. M. (1992). The validity of major depression with atypical features based on a community study. *Journal of Affective Disorders, 26,* 117–125.

How much does depression cost society? (1994, October). *Harvard Mental Health Newsletter,* pp. 1–2.

Howland, R. H. (1991). Pharmacotherapy of dysthymia: A review. *Journal of Clinical Psychopharmacology, 11,* 83–92.

Howland, R. H. (1993a). Chronic depression. *Hospital and Community Psychiatry, 44,* 633–639.

Howland, R. H. (1993b). General health, health care utilization, and medical comorbidity in dysthymia. *International Journal of Psychiatry in Medicine, 23,* 211–238.

Howland, R. H., & Thase, M. E. (1991). Biological studies of dysthymia. *Biological Psychiatry, 30,* 283–304.

Howland, R. H., & Thase, M. E. (1993). A comprehensive review of cyclothymic disorder. *Journal of Nervous and Mental Disease, 181,* 485–493.

Jackson, H. J., Whiteside, H. L., Bates, G. W., Bell, R., Rudd, R. P., & Edwards, J. (1991). Diagnosing personality disorders in psychiatric inpatients. *Acta Psychiatrica Scandinavica, 83,* 206–213.

Jaffe, A., Froom, J., & Galambos, N. (1994). Minor depression and functional impairment. *Archives of Family Medicine, 3,* 1081–1086.

Johnson, J., Horwath, E., & Weissman, M. M. (1991). The validity of major depression with psychotic features based on a community sample. *Archives of General Psychiatry, 48,* 1075–1081.

Johnson, J., Weissman, M. M., & Klerman, G. L. (1992). Service utilization and social morbidity associated with depressive symptoms in the community. *JAMA, 267,* 1478–1483.

Jones, B. D. (1989). Epidemiology of depression (discussion of the paper by McCormick). *Psychiatric Journal of the University of Ottawa, 14,* 349–351.

Joyce, P. R., & Paykel, E. S. (1989). Predictors of drug response in depression. *Archives of General Psychiatry, 46,* 89–99.

Judd, L. L., Rapaport, M. H., Paulus, M. P., & Brown, J. L. (1994). Subsyndromal symptomatic depression: A new mood disorder? *Journal of Clinical Psychiatry, 55*(Suppl.), 18–28.

Karam, E. G. (1994). The nosological status of bereavement-related depressions. *British Journal of Psychiatry, 165,* 48–52.

Kasper, S., Ruhmann, S., Hasse, T., & Mollerr, H. J. (1992). Recurrent brief depression and its relationship to seasonal affective disorder. *European Archives of Psychiatry and Clinical Neuroscience, 242,* 20–26.

Kato, T., Takahashi, S., Shioiri, T., Murashita, J., Hamakawa, H., & Inubushi, T. (1994). Reduction of brain phosphocreatine in bipolar II disorder detected by phosphorus-31 magnetic resonance spectroscopy. *Journal of Affective Disorders, 31,* 125–133.

Katon, W., & Sullivan, M. (1990). Depression and chronic medical illness. *Journal of Clinical Psychiatry, 51*(Suppl.), 3–11.

Katon, W., Von Korff, M., Lin, E., Simon, G., Walker, E., Bush, T., & Ludman, E. (1995). Collaborative management to achieve treatment guidelines: Impact on depression in primary care. *JAMA, 273,* 1026–1031.

Keitner, G. I., Ryan, C. E., Miller, I. W., Kohn, R., & Epstein, N. B. (1991). 12-month outcome of patients with major depression and co-morbid psychiatric or medical illness (compound depression). *American Journal of Psychiatry, 148,* 345–350.

Keller, M. B. (1993). Overview of depression: Chronicity, recurrence, morbidity and the need for maintenance treatment. *Rhode Island Medicine, 76,* 381–386.

Keller, M. B. (1994a). Depression: A long-term illness. *British Journal of Psychiatry, 165* (Suppl.), 9–15.

Keller, M. B. (1994b). Dysthymia in clinical practice: Course, outcome and impact on the community. *Acta Psychiatrica Scandinavica, 383*(Suppl.), 24–34.

Keller, M., Beardslee, W., Dorer, D., Lavori, P. W., Samuelson, H., & Klerman, G. R. (1986). Impact of severity and chronicity of parental affective illness on adaptive functioning and psychopathology in children. *Archives of General Psychiatry, 43,* 930–937.

Keller, M. B., & Hanks, D. L. (1995). Anxiety symptom relief in depression treatment outcomes. *Journal of Clinical Psychiatry, 56*(Suppl. 6), 22–29.

Keller, M. B., Hanks, D. L., & Klein, D. N. (1996). Summary of the DSM-IV mood disorders field trial and issue overview. *Psychiatric Clinics of North American, 19*(1), 1–28.

Keller, M. B., Klein, D., Hirschfeld, R.M.A., Kocsis, J. H., McCullough, J. P., Miller, I., First, M. B., Holzer, C. P., III, Keitner, G. I., Marin, D. B., & Shea, T. (1995). Results of the DSM-IV mood disorders field trial. *American Journal of Psychiatry, 152,* 843–849.

Keller, M. B., Lavori, P. W., Endicott, J., Coryell, W., Hirschfeld, R. M., & Shea, T. (1992). Time to recovery, chronicity, and levels of psychopathology in major depression: A 5-year prospective follow-up. *Archives of General Psychiatry, 49,* 788–792.

Keller, M. B., & Shapiro, R. W. (1982). "Double depression": Superimposition of acute depressive episodes on chronic depressive disorders. *American Journal of Psychiatry, 139,* 438–442.

Kendler, K. S., Kessler, R. C., Neale, M. C., Heath, A. C., & Eaves, L. J. (1993). The prediction of major depression in women: Toward an integrated etiological model. *American Journal of Psychiatry, 150,* 1139–1148.

Kendler, K. S., Kessler, R. C., Walters, E. E., MacLean, C., Neale, M. C., Heath, A. C., & Eaves, L. J. (1995). Stressful life events, genetic liability, and the onset of an episode of major depression in women. *American Journal of Psychiatry, 152,* 833–842.

Kendler, K. S., Neale, M. C., Kessler, R. C., Heath, A. C., & Eaves, L. J. (1992a). A population-based twin study of major depression in women: The impact of varying definitions of illness. *Archives of General Psychiatry, 49,* 257–256.

Kendler, K. S., Neale, M. C., Kessler, R. C., Heath, A. C., & Eaves, L. J. (1992b). Major depression and generalized anxiety disorder. Same genes, (partly) different environments? *Archives of General Psychiatry, 49,* 716–722.

Kendler, K. S., Neale, M. C., Kessler, R. C., Heath, A. C., & Eaves, L. J. (1994). The clinical characteristics of major depression as indices of the familial risk to illness. *British Journal of Psychiatry, 165,* 66–72.

Kendler, K. S., Walters, E. E., Truett, R., Heath, A. C., Neale, M. C., Martin, N. G., & Eaves, L. J. (1994). Sources of individual differences in depressive symptoms: Analysis of two samples of twins and their families. *American Journal of Psychiatry, 51,* 1605–1614.

Kessler, R. C., House, J. S., & Turner, J. B. (1987). Unemployment and health in a community sample. *Journal of Health and Social Behavior, 28,* 51–59.

Kessler, R. C., & Magee, W. J. (1993). Childhood adversities and adult depression: Basic patterns of association in a US survey. *Psychological Medicine, 23,* 679–690.

Kessler, R. C., McCanagle, K. A., Zhao, S., Nelson, C. B., Hughes, M., Eshleman, S., Wittchen, H. U., & Kendler, K. S. (1994). Lifetime and 12-month prevalence of DSM-III-R psychiatric disorders in the United States. *Archives of General Psychiatry, 51,* 8–19.

Kishi, Y., Robinson, R. G., & Forrester, A. W. (1994). Prospective longitudinal study of depression following spinal cord injury. *Journal of Neuropsychiatry, 6,* 237–244.

Klein, D. N., Kocsis, J. H., McCullough, J. P., Holzer, C. E., Hirschfeld, R.M.A., & Keller, M. B. (1996). Symptomatology in dysthymic and major depressive disorder. *Psychiatric Clinics of North America, 19(1),* 41–53.

Klein, D. N., & Miller, G. A. (1993). Depressive personality in nonclinical subjects. *American Journal of Psychiatry, 150,* 1718–1724.

Klerman, G. L. (1989). Depressive disorders. *Archives of General Psychiatry, 46,* 856–858.

Kraepelin, E. (1921). *Manic–depressive insanity and paranoia.* Edinburgh: E and S Livingstone.

Krauthammer, C., & Klerman, G. L. (1978). Secondary mania: Manic syndromes associated with antecedent physical illness or drugs. *Archives of General Psychiatry, 35,* 1333–1339.

Kruesi, M. J., Dale, J., & Straus, S. E. (1989). Psychiatric diagnoses in patients who have chronic fatigue syndrome. *Journal of Clinical Psychiatry, 50,* 53–56.

Kukopoulos, A., Caliari, B., Tundo, A., Minnai, G., Floris, G., Regindali, D., & Tondo, L. (1983). Rapid cyclers, temperament, and antidepressants. *Comprehensive Psychiatry, 24,* 249–258.

Lavori, P. W., Warshaw, M., Klerman, G., Mueller, T. I., Leon, A., Rice, J., & Akiskal, H. (1993). Secular trends in lifetime onset of MDD stratified by selected sociodemographic risk factors. *Journal of Psychiatric Research, 27,* 95–109.

Leibenluft, E. (1996). *Circadian rhythms factor in rapid-cycling bipolar disorder.* Available Summer 1996 from www.mhsource.com/edu/psytimes/p960533.html.

Leonhard, K. (1979). *The classification of endogeneous psychosis* (Russell Berman, Trans.). New York: Irvington. Originally published in 1957.

Levitt, A. J., Joffe, R. T., Ennis, J., MacDonald, C., & Kutcher, S. P. (1990). The prevalence of cyclothymia in borderline personality disorder. *Journal of Clinical Psychiatry, 51,* 335–339.

Levitt, A. J., Joffe, R. T., & MacDonald, C. (1991). Life course of depressive illness and characteristics of current episode in patients with double depression. *Journal of Nervous and Mental Disease, 179,* 678–682.

Lewinsohn, P. M., Rohde, P., Seeley, J. R., & Hops, H. (1991). Co-morbidity of unipolar disorder I. Major depression with dysthymia. *Journal of Abnormal Psychology, 100,* 205–213.

Liebowitz, M. R. (1993a). Depression with anxiety and atypical depression. *Journal of Clinical Psychiatry, 54*(Suppl.) 10–14.

Liebowitz, M. R. (1993b). Mixed anxiety and depression: Should it be included in DSM-IV? *Journal of Clinical Psychiatry, 54*(Suppl.), 4–7.

Lish, J. D., Dime-Meenan, S., Whybrow, P. C., Price, R. A., & Hirschfeld, R.M.A. (1994). The National Depressive and Manic–Depressive Association (DMDA) survey of bipolar members. *Journal of Affective Disorders, 31,* 281–294.

Livingston, R. (1987). Sexually and physically abused children. *Journal of the American Academy of Child and Adolescent Psychiatry, 26,* 413–415.

Lustman, P. J., Griffith, L. S., Gavard, J. A., & Clouse, R. E. (1992). Depression in adults with diabetes. *Diabetes Care, 15,* 1631–1639.

Maes, M. (1995). Evidence for an immune response in major depression: A review and hypothesis. *Progress in Neuropharmacological and Biological Psychiatry, 19,* 11–38.

Maes, M., DeMeester, I., Vanhoof, G., Scharpe, S., Bosmans, E., Vandervorst, C., Verkerk, R., Minner, B., Suy, E., & Raus, J. (1991). Decreased serum dipeptidyl peptidase IV activity in major depression. *Biological Psychiatry, 30,* 577–586.

Maes, M., Dierck, R., Meltzer, H. Y., Ingels, M., Schotte, C., Vandewoude, M., Calabrese, J., & Cosyns, P. (1993). Regional cerebral blood flow in unipolar depression measured with TC-99M-HMPAO single proton photoemission computed tomography: Negative findings. *Psychiatry Research, 50,* 77–88.

Maes, M., Lambrechts, J., Bosmans, E., Jacobs, J., Suy, E., Vandervorst, C., Dejonckheere, C., Minner, B., & Raus, J. (1992). Evidence for a systemic immune activation during depression: Results of leukocyte enumeration by flow cytometry in conjunction with monoclonal antibody staining. *Psychological Medicine, 22,* 45–53.

Maes, M., Schotte, C., D'Hondt, P., Vanderwoude, M., Scharpe, S., & Cosyns, P. (1991). Biological heterogeneity of melancholia: Results of pattern recognition methods. *Journal of Psychiatric Research, 25*(3), 95–108.

Maier, W., Lichtermann, D., Minges, J., & Huen, R. (1992). Personality traits in subjects at risk for unipolar depression: A family study perspective. *Journal of Affective Disorders, 24,* 153–163.

Maj, M., Magliano, L., Pirozzi, R., Marasco, C., & Guarneri, M. (1994). Validity of rapid cycling as a course specifier for bipolar disorder. *American Journal of Psychiatry, 151,* 1015–1019.

Maj, M., Veltro, F., Pirozzi, R., Lobrace, S., & Magliano, L. (1992). Pattern of recurrence of illness after recovery from an episode of major depression: A prospective study. *American Journal of Psychiatry, 149,* 795–800.

Manschreck, T. C., & Leighton, A. H. (1992). Reducing disability in mood disorders and schizophrenia. *Hospital and Community Psychiatry, 43,* 179–180.

Manson, S. M. (1995). Culture and depression. *Psychiatric Clinics of North America, 18,* 487–501.

Marazziti, D., Ambrogi, F., Vanacore, R., Mignani, V., Savino, M., Palego, L., Cassano, G. B., & Akiskal, H. S. (1992). Immune cell imbalance in major depressive and panic disorders. *Neuropsychobiology, 26,* 23–26.

Marton, P., & Maharaj, M. A. (1993). Family factors in adolescent unipolar depression. *Canadian Journal of Psychiatry, 38,* 373–382.

Maziade, M., Roy, M. A., Fournier, J. P., Cliche, D., Merette, C., Caron, C., Garneau, Y., Montgrain, N., Shriqui, C., & Dion, C. (1992). Reliability of best-estimated diagnosis in genetic linkage studies of major psychoses: Results from the Quebec pedigree studies. *American Journal of Psychiatry, 149,* 1674–1686.

McDaniel, S. J., Musselman, D. L., Porter, M. R., Reed, D. A., & Nemeroff, C. B. (1995). Depression in patients with cancer. *Archives of General Psychiatry, 52,* 89–99.

McElroy, S. L., Keck, P. E., Pope, H. G., Hudson, J. I., Faedda, G. L., & Swann, A. C. (1992). Clinical and research implications of the diagnosis of dysphoric or mixed mania or hypomania. *American Journal of Psychiatry, 149,* 1633–1644.

McElroy, S. L., Keck, P. E., & Strakowski, S. M. (1996). Mania, psychosis, and antipsychotics. *Journal of Clinical Psychiatry, 57*(Suppl. 3), 14–26.

McGuffin, P., & Katz, R. (1989). The genetics of depression and manic–depressive illness. *British Journal of Psychiatry, 155,* 294–304.

McGuffin, P., Katz, R., & Bebbington, P. (1988). The Camberwell Collaborative Depression Study, III: Depression and adversity in the relatives of depressed probands. *British Journal of Psychiatry, 152,* 775–782.

McNaughton, M. E., Patterson, T. L., Irwin, M. R., & Grant, I. (1992). The relationship of life adversity, social support, and coping to hospitalization with major depression. *Journal of Nervous and Mental Disease, 180,* 491–497.

McNeal, E. T., & Cimbolic, P. (1986). Antidepressants and biochemical theories of depression. *Psychological Bulletin, 99,* 361–374.

Meador, K. G., Koenig, H. G., Hughes, D. C., Blazer, D. G., Turnbull, J., & George, L. K. (1992). Religious affiliation and major depression. *Hospital and Community Psychiatry, 43,* 1204–1208.

Mendlewicz, J. (1994). The search for a manic depressive gene: From classical to molecular genetics. In F. Bloom (Ed.), *Progress in brain research* (Vol. 100, pp. 255–259). New York: Elsevier Science.

Mendlewicz, J., & Kerkhofs, M. (1991). Sleep electroencephalography in depressive illness. A collaborative study by the World Health Organization. *British Journal of Psychiatry, 159,* 505–509.

Mendlewicz, J., Leboyer, M., deBruyn, A., Malafosse, A., Sevy, S., Hirsch, D., Van Broeckhover, C., & Mallet, J. (1991). Absence of linkage between chromosome 11P15 markers and manic–depressive illness in a Belgian pedigree. *American Journal of Psychiatry, 148,* 1683–1687.

Migliorelli, R., Teson, A., Sabe, L., Petracchi, M., Leiguarda, R., & Starkstein, S. E. (1995). Prevalence and correlates of dysthymia and major depression among patients with Alzheimer's disease. *American Journal of Psychiatry, 151,* 37–44.

Miranda, J., & Munoz, R. (1994). Intervention for minor depression in primary care. *Psychosomatic Medicine, 56,* 36–142.

Mitchell, P., Waters, B., Morrison, N., Sine, J., Donald, J., & Eisman, J. (1991). Close linkage of bipolar disorder to chromosome 11 markers is excluded in two large Australian pedigrees. *Journal of Affective Disorders, 21,* 23–32.

Moldin, S., Reich, T., & Rice, J. (1991). Current perspectives on the genetics of unipolar depression. *Behavioral Genetics, 21,* 211–242.

Monroe, S. (1990). Psychosocial factors in anxiety and depression. In J. D. Maser & C. R. Cloninger (Eds.), *Co-morbidity in anxiety and mood disorders* (pp. 463–498). Washington, DC: American Psychiatric Press.

Montgomery, S. A., & Montgomery, D. (1992). Features of recurrent brief depression. *Encephale, 18*(Special Issue 4), 521–523.

Mor, V., McHorney, C., & Sherwood, S. (1986). Secondary morbidity among the recently bereaved. *American Journal of Psychiatry, 143,* 158–163.

Morrow, K. A., Parker, J. C., & Russell, J. L. (1994). Clinical implications of depression in rheumatoid arthritis. *Arthritis Care and Research, 7,* 58–63.

Mukherjee, S., Shukla, S., Woodle, J., Rosen, A. M., & Olarte, S. (1983). Misdiagnosis of schizophrenia in bipolar patients: A multi-ethnic comparison. *American Journal of Psychiatry, 140,* 1571–1574.

Mulder, R. T., Joyce, P. R., & Cloninger, C. R. (1994). Temperament and early environment influence co-morbidity and personality disorders in major depression. *Comprehensive Psychiatry, 35,* 225–233.

Muller, N., Hofschuster, E., Ackenheil, M., Mempel, W., & Eckstein, R. (1993). Investigations of the cellular immunity during depression and the free interval: Evidence for an immune activation in affective psychosis. *Progress in Neuro-Psychopharmacology and Biological Psychiatry, 17,* 713–730.

Nathan, K. I., & Schatzberg, A. F. (Eds.). (1994). *Mood disorders* (Vol. 13). Washington, DC: American Psychiatric Press.

National Institutes of Health. (1996). *Scientists close in on multiple gene sites for manic depressive illness.* Available from *Science Daily,* http://www.sciencedaily.com/1996/April/03/story1. htm.

Newman, J. C., & Holden, R. J. (1993). The "cerebral diabetes" paradigm for unipolar depression. *Medical Hypotheses, 41,* 391–408.

Nordstrom, P., Schalling, D., & Asberg, M. (1995). Temperamental vulnerability in attempted suicide. *Acta Psychiatrica Scandinavica, 92,* 155–160.

Nurnberger, J. I., Berrettini, W., Tamarkin, L., Hamovit, J., Norton, J., & Gershon, E. S. (1988). Supersensitivity to melatonin suppression by bright light in young people at risk for affective disorder. *Neuropsychopharmacology, 1,* 217–223.

O'Brien, J. T., Desmond, P., Ames, D., Schweitzer, I., Tuckwell, V., & Tress, B. (1994). The differentiation of depression from dementia by temporal lobe magnetic resonance imaging. *Psychological Medicine, 24,* 633–640.

O'Connell, R. A., Mayo, J. A., & Sciutto, M. S. (1991). PDQ-R personality disorders in bipolar patients. *Journal of Affective Disorders, 23,* 217–221.

Ohmori, T., Arora, R. C., & Meltzer, H. Y. (1992). Serotonergic measures in suicide brain: The concentration of 5-HIAA, HVA, and tryptophan in frontal cortex of suicide victims. *Biological Psychiatry, 32,* 57–71.

Owens, M. J., & Nemeroff, C. B. (1994). Role of serotonin in the pathophysiology of depression: Focus on the serotonin transporter. *Clinical Chemistry, 40,* 288–295.

Packer, S. (1992). Family planning for women with bipolar disorder. *Hospital and Community Psychiatry, 43,* 479–482.

Pariante, C. M., Nemeroff, C. B., & Miller, A. H. (1995). Glucocorticoid receptors in depression. *Israeli Journal of Medicine, 31,* 705–712.

Parikh, R. M., Robinson, R. G., Lipsey, J. R., Starstein, S. E., Federoff, J. P., & Price, T. R. (1990). Impact of poststroke depression on recovery in activities of daily living over a 2-year follow-up. *Archives of Neurology, 47,* 785–789.

Pariser, S. F. (1993). Women and mood disorders. Menarche to menopause. *Annals of Clinical Psychiatry, 5,* 249–254.

Parker, G. (1987). Are the lifetime prevalence estimates in the ECA study accurate? *Psychological Medicine, 17,* 275–282.

Parker, G., & Hadzi-Pavlovic, D. (1984). Modification of levels of depression in mother-bereaved women by parental and marital relationships. *Psychological Medicine, 14,* 125–135.

Parker, G., Hall, W., Boyce, P., Hadzi-Pavlovic, D., Mitchell, P., Wilhelm, K., Brodaty, H., Hickie, I., & Eyers, K. (1991). Depression subtyping: Unitary, binary or arbitrary. *Australian and New Zealand Journal of Psychiatry, 2,* 63–76.

Patten, S. B., & Lamarre, C. J. (1992). Can drug-induced depressions be identified by their clinical features? *Canadian Journal of Psychiatry, 37,* 213–215.

Pepper, C. M., Klein, D. N., Anderson, R. L., Riso, R. L., Ouimette, P. C., & Lizardi, C. (1995). DSM-III-R Axis II co-morbidity in dysthymia and major depression. *American Journal of Psychiatry, 152,* 239–247.

Perris, C., Homgren, S., von Knorring, L., & Perris, H. (1986). Parental loss by death in early childhood of depressed parents and of their healthy siblings. *British Journal of Psychiatry, 148,* 165–169.

Perris, H. (1983). Deprivation in childhood and life events in depression. *Archives of Psychiatry and Neurological Sciences, 233,* 489–498.

Perris, H., von Knorring, L., & Perris, C. (1982). Genetic vulnerability for depression and life events. *Neuropsychobiology, 8,* 241–247.

Peselow, E. D., Sanfilipo, M. P., Difiglia, C., & Fieve, R. R. (1992). Melancholic/endogenous depression and response to somatic treatment and placebo. *American Journal of Psychiatry, 149,* 1324–1334.

Petty, F. (1992). The depressed alcoholic: Clinical features and medical management. *General Hospital Psychiatry, 14,* 258–264.

Petty, F. (1994). Plasma concentrations of gamma-aminobutyric acid (GABA) and mood disorders: A blood test for manic depressive disease? *Clinical Chemistry, 40,* 296–302.

Pfeffer, C. R., Newcorn, J., Kaplan, G., Mizruchi, M. S., & Plutchik, R. (1988). Suicidal behavior in adolescent psychiatric inpatients. *Journal of the American Academy of Child and Adolescent Psychiatry, 27,* 357–361.

Phelan, J., Schwartz, J. E., Bromet, E. J., Dew, M. A., Parkinson, D. K., Schulberg, H. C., Dunn, L. O., Blane, H., & Curtis, E. C. (1991). Work stress, family stress, and depression in professional and managerial employees. *Psychological Medicine, 21,* 999–1021.

Phillips, K., Gunderson, J., Hirschfeld, R., & Smith, L. E. (1990). A review of the depressive personality. *American Journal of Psychiatry, 147,* 830–837.

Post, R. M. (1992). Transduction of psychosocial stress into the neurobiology of recurrent affective disorder. *American Journal of Psychiatry, 149,* 999–1010.

Post, R. M., Rubinow, D. R., & Ballenger, J. C. (1984). Conditioning, sensitizing, and kindling: Implications for the course of affective illness. In R. M. Post & J. C. Ballenger (Eds.), *Neurobiology of mood disorders* (pp. 432–466). Baltimore: Williams & Wilkins.

Post, R. M., Rubinow, D. R., & Ballenger, J. C. (1986). Conditioning and sensitization in the longitudinal course of affective illness. *British Journal of Psychiatry, 149,* 191–201.

Potter, W. Z., Rudorfer, M. V., & Linnoila, M. (Eds.). (1988). *New clinical studies support a role of norepinephrine antidepressant action.* New York: Alan R. Liss.

Preskorn, S. H., & Fast, G. A. (1993). Beyond signs and symptoms: The case against a mixed anxiety and depression category. *Journal of Clinical Psychiatry, 54*(Suppl.), 24–32.

Price, R. H., Ketterer, R. F., & Bader, B. C. (Eds.). (1980). *Prevention in community mental health: Research, policy and practice.* Beverly Hills, CA: Sage Publications.

Ragan, P. V., & McGlashan, T. H. (1986). Childhood parental death and adult psychopathology. *American Journal of Psychiatry, 143,* 153–157.

Regier, D. A., Farmer, M. E., Rae, D. S., Locke, B. Z., Keith, S., Judd, L., & Goodwin, K. (1990). Co-morbidity of mental disorders with alcohol and other drug abuse. *JAMA, 264,* 2511–2518.

Regier, D. A., Farmer, M. E., Rae, D. S., Myers, J. K., Kramer, J. K., Robins, L. N., George, L. K., Karno, M., & Locke, B. Z. (1993). One-month prevalence of mental disorders in the United States and sociodemographic characteristics: The Epidemiologic Catchment Area Study. *Acta Psychiatrica Scandinavica, 88,* 35–47.

Regier, D. A., Hirschfeld, R.M.A., Goodwin, F. K., Burke, J. D., Lazar, J. B., & Judd, L. L. (1988). The NIMH depression, awareness, recognition, and treatment program: Structure, aims, and scientific basis. *American Journal of Psychiatry, 145,* 1351–1357.

Regier, D. A., Narrow, W. E., Rae, D. S., Manderscheid, R. W., Locke, B. Z., & Goodwin, F. K. (1993). The de facto U.S. mental and addictive disorders service system:

Epidemiologic Catchment Area prospective 1-year prevalence rates of disorders and services. *Archives of General Psychiatry, 50,* 85–94.

Reich, J., & Vasille, R. (1993). The effect of personality disorders on the treatment outcome of Axis I conditions: An update. *Journal of Nervous and Mental Disease, 181,* 475–484.

Reynolds, C. F., Frank, E., Perel, J. M., Mazumdar, S., & Kupfer, D. J. (1995). Maintenance therapies for late-life recurrent major depression: Research and review circa 1995. *International Psychogeriatrics, 7*(Suppl.), 27–39.

Richardson, J. S. (1991). Animal models of depression reflect changing views on the essence and etiology of depressive disorders in humans. *Progress in Neuro-Psychopharmacology and Biological Psychiatry, 15,* 199–204.

Robins, L. N., Helzer, J. E., Weissman, M. M., Orvaschel, H., Gruenberg, E., Burke, J. D., Jr., & Regier, D. A. (1984). Lifetime prevalence of specific psychiatric disorders in three sites. *Archives of General Psychiatry, 41,* 949–958.

Robins, L. N., & Regier, D. A. (1991). *Psychiatric disorders in America: The Epidemiological Catchment Area Study.* New York: Free Press.

Romano, J. M., & Turner, J. A. (1985). Chronic pain and depression: Does the evidence support a relationship? *Psychological Bulletin, 97,* 18–34.

Romans, S. E., & McPherson, H. M. (1992). The social networks of bipolar affective disorder patients. *Journal of Affective Disorders, 25,* 221–228.

Roy, A. (1994). Recent biological studies of suicide. *Suicide and Life-Threatening Behavior, 24,* 10–14.

Rush, A. J., & Weissenburger, J. E. (1994). Melancholic symptom features and DSM-IV. *American Journal of Psychiatry, 151,* 489–498.

Sackeim, H. A., Prohovnik, I., Moeller, J. R., Mayeux, R., Stern, Y., & Devanand, D. P. (1993). Regional cerebral blood flow in mood disorders. II. Comparison of major depression and Alzheimer's disease. *Journal of Nuclear Medicine, 34,* 1090–1101.

Salloum, I. M., Mezzich, J. E., Cornelius, J., Day, N. L., Delay, D., & Kirisci, L. (1995). Clinical profile of co-morbid major depression and alcohol use disorders in an initial psychiatric evaluation. *Comprehensive Psychiatry, 36,* 260–266.

Sanderson, W. C., Wetzler, S., Beck, A. T., & Betz, F. (1992). Prevalence of personality disorders in patients with major depression and dysthymia. *Psychiatric Research, 42,* 93–99.

Sargeant, J. K., Bruce, M. L., Florio, L. P., & Weissman, M. M. (1990). Factors associated with 1-year outcome of major depression in the community. *Archives of General Psychiatry, 47,* 519–526.

Schatzberg, A. F., & Rothschild, A. J. (1992). Psychotic (delusional) major depression: Should it be included as a distinct syndrome in DSM-IV? *American Journal of Psychiatry, 149,* 733–745.

Schittecatte, M., Charles, G., Machowski, R., Dumont, F., Garcia-Valentin, J., Wilmotte, J., Papart, P., Pitchot, W., Wauthy, J., Ansseau, M., Hoffmann, G., & Pelc, I. (1994). Effects of gender and diagnosis on growth hormone response to clonidine for major depression: A large-scale multicenter study. *American Journal of Psychiatry, 151,* 216–220.

Schulberg, H. C., Madonia, M. J., Block, M. R., Coulehan, J. L., Scott, C. P., Rodriguez, E., & Black, A. (1995). Major depression in primary care practice: Clinical characteristics and treatment implications. *Psychosomatics, 36,* 129–137.

Schwab, J., Stephenson, J. J., & Bell, R. A. (1988). Risk for depression in families over time: A pilot epidemiologic study. *Hospital and Community Psychiatry, 39,* 58–62.

Scott, J., Eccleston, D., & Boys, R. (1992). Can we predict the persistence of depression? *British Journal of Psychiatry, 161,* 633–637.

Seligman, M.E.P. (1975). *Helplessness: On depression, development and death.* New York: Freeman.

Shea, M. T., & Hirschfeld, R.M.A. (1996). Chronic mood disorder and depressive personality. *Psychiatric Clinics of North America, 19*(1), 103–120.

Sherbourne, C. D., Wells, K. B., Hays, R. D., Rogers, W., Burnam, M. A., & Judd, L. L. (1994). Subthreshold depression and depressive disorder: Clinical characteristics of general medical and mental health specialty outpatients. *American Journal of Psychiatry, 151,* 1777–1784.

Simon, G. E., & Von Korff, M. (1992). Reevaluation of secular trends in depression rates. *American Journal of Epidemiology, 135,* 1411–1422.

Simpson, S. G., al-Mufti, R., Andersen, A. E., & DePaulo, J.R.J. (1992). Bipolar II affective disorder in eating disorder inpatients. *Journal of Nervous and Mental Disease, 180,* 719–722.

Simpson, S. G., Folstein, S. E., Meyers, D. A., McMahon, F. J., Brusco, D. M., & DePaulo, J.R.J. (1993). Bipolar II: The most common bipolar phenotype? *American Journal of Psychiatry, 150,* 901–903.

Smith, G. R. (1992). The epidemiology and treatment of depression when it coexists with somatoform disorders, somatization, or pain. *General Hospital Psychiatry, 14,* 265–272.

Stansfeld, S. A., & Marmot, M. G. (1992). Social class and minor psychiatric disorder in British civil servants: A validated screening survey using the General Health Questionnaire. *Psychological Medicine, 22,* 739–749.

Stowe, Z. N., & Nemeroff, C. B. (1995). Women at risk for postpartum-onset major depression. *American Journal of Obstetrics and Gynecology, 173,* 639–645.

Strakowski, S. M., McElroy, S. L., Keck, P. E., & West, S. A. (1994). The co-occurrence of mania with medical and other psychiatric disorders. *International Journal of Psychiatry in Medicine, 24,* 305–328.

Strakowski, S. M., McElroy, S. L., Keck, P. E., & West, S. A. (1996). Suicidality among patients with mixed and manic bipolar disorder. *American Journal of Psychiatry, 153,* 674–676.

Strober, M. (1992). Relevance of early age-of-onset in genetic studies of bipolar affective disorder. *Journal of the American Academy of Child and Adolescent Psychiatry, 31,* 606–610.

Sullivan, P. F., Joyce, P. R., & Mulder, R. T. (1994). Borderline personality disorder in major depression. *Journal of Nervous and Mental Disease, 182,* 508–516.

Swann, A. C. (1995). Mixed or dysphoric manic states: Psychopathology and treatment. *Journal of Clinical Psychiatry, 56*(Suppl. 3), 6–10.

Szigethy, E., Conwell, Y., Forbes, N. T., Cox, C., & Caine, E. D. (1994). Adrenal weight and morphology in victims of completed suicide. *Biological Psychiatry, 36,* 374–380.

Tennant, C. (1988). Parental loss in childhood. *Archives of General Psychiatry, 45,* 1045–1050.

Thomas, P., Vaiva, G., Samaille, E., Maron, M., Alaix, C., Steinling, M., & Goudemand, M. (1993). Cerebral blood flow in major depression and dysthymia. *Journal of Affective Disorders, 29,* 235–242.

Torgersen, S. (1986). Genetic factors in moderately severe and mild affective disorders. *Archives of General Psychiatry, 43,* 222–236.

Tsuang, D., & Coryell, W. (1993). An 8-year follow-up of patients with DSM-III-R psychotic depression, schizoaffective disorder, and schizophrenia. *American Journal of Psychiatry, 150,* 1182–1188.

Van Valkenburg, C., Akiskal, H. S., Puzantian, V., & Rosenthal, T. (1984). Anxious depression: Clinical, family history, and naturalistic outcome comparisons with panic and major depressive disorder. *Journal of Affective Disorders, 6,* 677–682.

von Knorring, A. L., Cloninger, C. R., Bohman, M., & Sigvardsson, S. (1983). An adoption study of depressive disorders and substance abuse. *Archives of General Psychiatry, 40,* 943–950.

Warner, V., Mufson, L., & Weissman, M. M. (1995). Offspring at high and low risk for depression and anxiety: Mechanisms of psychiatric disorder. *Journal of the American Academy of Child and Adolescent Psychiatry, 34,* 786–797.

Wehr, T. A. (1991). Sleep-loss as a possible mediator of diverse causes of mania. *British Journal of Psychiatry, 159,* 576–578.

Wehr, T. A. (1992). Seasonal vulnerability to depression. Implications for etiology and treatment. *Encephale, 18*(Special Issue 4), 479–483.

Wehr, T. A., & Rosenthal, N. E. (1989). Seasonality and affective illness. *American Journal of Psychiatry, 146,* 829–839.

Wehr, T. A., Sack, D. A., Rosenthal, N. E., & Cowdry, R. W. (1988). Rapid cycling affective disorder: Contributing factors and treatment responses in 51 patients. *American Journal of Psychiatry, 145,* 179–184.

Weissman, M. M. (1978). Affective disorders in a U.S. urban community: The use of research diagnostic criteria in an epidemiological survey. *Archives of General Psychiatry, 35,* 1304–1311.

Weissman, M. M., Bruce, M. L., Leaf, P. J., Florio, L. P., & Holzer, C. E. (1991). Affective disorders. In L. N. Robins & D. E. Regier (Eds.), *Psychiatric disorders in America* (pp. 53–80). New York: Free Press.

Weissman, M. M., Gammon, G. D., John, K., Merikangas, K. R., Warner, V., Prusoff, B. A., & Scholomskas, D. (1987). Children of depressed parents: Increased psychopathology and early onset of major depression. *Archives of General Psychiatry, 44,* 847–853.

Weissman, M. M., & Klerman, G. L. (1977). Sex differences and the epidemiology of depression. *Archives of General Psychiatry, 34,* 98–111.

Weissman, M. M., Leaf, P. J., Bruce, M. L., & Florio, L. (1988). The epidemiology of dysthymia in five communities: Rates, risks, co-morbidity and treatment. *American Journal of Psychiatry, 145,* 815–819.

Weissman, M. M., Leaf, P. J., Tischler, G. L., Blazer, D. G., Kanno, M., Bruce, M. L., & Florio, L. P. (1988). Affective disorders in five United States communities. *Psychological Medicine, 18,* 141–153.

Weissman, M. M., Leckman, J. F., Merikangas, K. R., Gammon, G. D., & Prusoff, B. A. (1984). Depression and anxiety disorders in parents and children: Results from the Yale Family Study. *Archives of General Psychiatry, 41,* 845–852.

Weissman, M. M., & Myers, J. (1978). Affective disorders in a U.S. urban community: The use of RDC criteria in an epidemiological survey. *Archives of General Psychiatry, 35,* 1304–1311.

Wells, K. B., Burnam, M. A., Rogers, W., Hays, R., & Camp, P. (1992). The course of depression in adult outpatients: Results from the Medical Outcomes Study. *Archives of General Psychiatry, 49,* 788–794.

Wells, K. B., Golding, J. M., & Burnam, M. A. (1988). Psychiatric disorder in a sample of the general population with and without chronic medical conditions. *American Journal of Psychiatry, 145,* 976–981.

Wells, K. B., Stewart, A., Hays, R. D., Burnam, M. A., Rogers, W., Daniel, M., Berry, S., Greenfield, S., & Ware, J. (1989). The functioning and well-being of depressed patients. Results from the Medical Outcomes Study. *JAMA, 262,* 914–919.

Wender, P. H., Kety, S. S., Rosenthal, D., Schulsinger, F., Ortmann, J., & Lunde, I. (1986). Psychiatric disorders in the biological and adoptive families of adopted individuals with affective disorder. *Archives of General Psychiatry, 43,* 923–929.

West, M. O., & Prinz, R. J. (1987). Parental alcoholism and childhood pathology. *Psychological Bulletin, 102,* 204–218.

Williams, J. W., Kerber, C. A., Mulrow, C. D., Medina, A., & Aguilar, C. (1995). Depressive disorders in primary care: Prevalence, functional disability, and identification. *Journal of General Internal Medicine, 10,* 7–12.

Winokur, G., Clayton, P. J., & Reich, T. (Eds.). (1969). *Manic–depressive illness.* St. Louis: C. V. Mosby.

Winokur, G., & Coryell, W. (1991). Familial alcoholism in primary unipolar depressive disease. *American Journal of Psychiatry, 148,* 184–188.

Winokur, G., Coryell, W., Akiskal, H. S., Endicott, J., Keller, M., & Mueller, T. (1994). Manic–depressive (bipolar) disorder: The course in light of a prospective ten-year follow-up of 131 patients. *Acta Psychiatrica Scandinavica, 89,* 102–110.

Wittchen, H., Knauper, B., & Kessler, R. C. (1994). Lifetime risk of depression. *British Journal of Psychiatry, 26*(Suppl.), 16–22.

Wolk, S. I., & Weissman, M. M. (1995). *Women and depression: An update* (Vol. 14). Washington, DC: American Psychiatric Press.

Wool, M. S. (1990). Understanding depression in medical patients. Part I: Diagnostic considerations. *Social Work in Health Care, 14*(4), 25–38.

World Health Organization. (1952). *International classification of disease* (6th ed.). Geneva: Author.

Yolken, R. H., & Torrey, E. F. (1995, January). Viruses, schizophrenia, and bipolar disorder. *Clinical Microbiology Review,* pp. 131–145.

Young, R. C. (1992). Geriatric mania. *Clinical Geriatric Medicine, 8,* 387–399.

Zisook, S., & Schuchter, S. R. (1991). Depression through the first year after the death of a spouse. *American Journal of Psychiatry, 148,* 1346–1352.

# Anxiety Disorders

Gail Steketee, Barbara L. Van Noppen, Iris Cohen, and Laura Clary

In this chapter, we review findings regarding multiple aspects of the psychopathology of four of the major anxiety disorders, including panic disorder and agoraphobia, social phobia, generalized anxiety disorder (GAD), and obsessive–compulsive
disorder (OCD). (A discussion of psychopathological aspects of posttraumatic stress
disorder [PTSD] is included in chapter 8). We have omitted discussion of specific
phobias because these rarely lead to sufficient distress by themselves to bring clients
into a clinic, although they are often present as co-occurring conditions alongside
other disorders.

Within the sections describing each anxiety condition below, we present the diagnostic criteria for the disorder, noting changes in recent years. We then address
disorder prevalence and clinical characteristics as well as common settings in which
each presents. Effects on functioning, psychosocial and familial aspects, and issues of
diversity are discussed, followed by common comorbid conditions and the clinical
challenge these generate. Finally, we comment on research and clinical priorities regarding important missing information about these disorders as well as the implications for treatment from the psychopathological findings presented.

## Panic Disorder and Agoraphobia

### DIAGNOSTIC CRITERIA

Panic or anxiety attacks and agoraphobic avoidance have been described in the literature for more than 100 years (see, for example, Westphal, 1871). More recently,
although greater clarity has been evident in descriptions of these symptoms and
their interrelationship, considerable debate has focused on the classification of the
various forms of panic and agoraphobia. According to the fourth edition of the *Diagnostic and Statistical Manual of Mental Disorders* (DSM-IV) from the American Psychiatric Association (APA, 1994), three disorders can be diagnosed: (1) panic disorder;
(2) panic disorder with agoraphobia (PDA); and (3) agoraphobia without history of
panic disorder (AWOPD). The current criteria for panic disorder require both recurrent unexpected panic attacks and a persistent concern about having additional
attacks, or worry about consequences of the attack, such as losing control, having a
heart attack, or going crazy. To prevent confusion with other conditions, DSM-IV

states that panic attacks must occur independently of possible medication causes and should not be better explained by other conditions such as social phobia, specific phobias, OCD, or PTSD. For children, panic disorder is distinguished from separation anxiety.

A *panic attack*, often called an anxiety attack by those who have them, is defined as a discrete period of intense fear or discomfort, in which at least four of the following physical and psychological symptoms develop abruptly and reach a peak within 10 minutes: palpitations or pounding heart, chest pain or pressure, sweating, trembling or shaking, feeling short of breath, feeling of choking, abdominal distress, feeling dizzy or faint, feeling unreal or depersonalized (detached from oneself), numbness or tingling, chills or hot flushes, fear of losing control or going crazy, and fear of dying (APA, 1994). Usually, panic attacks are short-lived, occurring within a 10-20 minute period, although the physical and emotional aftereffects can persist for an hour or more. Having one or more of these attacks does not necessarily signal panic disorder because the latter also is defined by how frequently attacks occur as well as how concerned the person is about them and whether his or her behavior reflects this fear.

*Agoraphobia* is characterized by anxiety about being in places or situations where a panic attack might occur and from which escape might be difficult or embarrassing. Such fears typically involve a characteristic cluster of situations, such as being some distance from home alone, being in a crowd, standing in line, or being on a bridge, and traveling in a bus, train, or automobile. Some people with agoraphobia require the presence of a "safe" companion, and under such circumstances they may be able to travel anywhere freely. Like panic attacks, agoraphobia is not diagnosed as a separate disorder but as part of either PDA or AWOPD. This latter diagnosis occurs relatively rarely, and it appears that like their counterparts with panic disorders, these people typically are avoiding places where they fear that anxiety symptoms will become unmanageable (Goisman, Warshaw, et al., 1995). Thus, what appears to be a continuum of panic and agoraphobia has been somewhat arbitrarily assigned to three diagnostic categories.

## EPIDEMIOLOGY

In the early 1980s, the Epidemiologic Catchment Area (ECA) study was conducted in five communities in the United States, surveying more than 18,000 adults across several sites (Weissman, 1994; see also chapter 1). The ECA study provided extensive information about a variety of psychiatric disorders, although findings are somewhat controversial because of its diagnostic instrument, which may have led to underestimates of disorder prevalence. ECA estimates indicate that panic disorders afflict between 1.6 percent and 2.9 percent of women and between 0.4 percent and 1.7 percent of men in the general population (Katon, 1994), or approximately twice as many women as men. A Canadian study reported similar rates for women (1.7 percent) and men (0.8 percent) (Dick, Bland, & Newman, 1994), with comparable lifetime prevalence of 2.0 percent and six-month prevalence of 1.2 percent reported by Wittchen and Essau (1993).

Panic disorder tends to run a chronic course, with episodes of intermittent panic attacks lasting an average of six to eight years; complete remission is rare (Noyes, Garvey, Cook, & Samuelson, 1989; Wittchen & Essau, 1993). Among patients seeking treatment, Keller et al. (1994) reported that a naturalistic follow-up at one year showed a 39 percent probability of full remission for patients with panic disorder only and a 17 percent probability of remission for those with PDA, suggesting that the natural course may be somewhat better for those with panic alone and that even with treatment, most patients retain some, if not most, of their symptoms.

Although panic disorders have variable onset, the usual age is between 18 and 35, with slightly earlier onset in women than in men (Dick et al., 1994; Liebowitz & Fyer, 1994; Wittchen & Essau, 1993). Panic disorders are most commonly found between ages 25 and 44, and they rarely begin among those over age 65 (Weissman, 1994). However, recent data indicated a surprisingly high prevalence rate in patients ages 60 and over: 9.4 percent of 540 subjects reported panic disorder (Raj, Corvea, & Dagon, 1993). In this group, onset at age 60 or above had occurred in 5.7 percent. Such a discrepancy in prevalence rates among elderly people could be a result of methodological and diagnostic criteria differences, but further research is needed to clarify this point. Onset is often preceded by a significant life stressor. Early speculations that a history of childhood separation anxiety can herald later panic disorder and agoraphobia have been supported by Battaglia and colleagues (1995), although overall, the findings have not strongly supported this supposition (for a review, see McNally, 1994).

The distribution of the various panic disorders within the population is unclear. Goisman and colleagues' (1994) study of clinic patients showed that PDA was the most common of the three diagnosable conditions. In contrast, studies of nonclinical subjects showed that panic disorder was more frequent: 50 percent of those with panic disorder reported no symptoms of agoraphobia (Eaton, Kessler, Wittchen, & Magee, 1994). These discrepancies probably result from differences in sampling of clinic patients and nonclinical participants. Nonetheless, a lack of diagnostic consistency throughout research studies and controversial models of panic disorder course (see Barlow, 1988) have contributed to limited clarity on the proportions of the various panic disorders in the community.

The limited data on racial and ethnic group differences in the prevalence of panic disorders suggests that African American and white populations have similar frequencies (Horwath, Johnson, & Hornig, 1993). A study of two Northwest coast Indian villages in the United States found that a high proportion of residents (14 percent) met criteria for panic disorder (Neligh, Baron, Braun, & Czarnecki, 1990). Rates consistent with U.S. data are provided by Japanese researchers, who observed a 1 percent prevalence rate of panic disorder and agoraphobia (Aoki, Fujihara, & Kitamura, 1994). In examining prevalence across cultures, it is important to note that panic disorders, as defined by DSM criteria, may manifest as somewhat different syndromes with various presenting symptomologies. For example, Bell and colleagues observed an association of panic disorder and isolated sleep paralysis that had symptoms of tachycardia, hyperventilation, and fear on awakening or falling asleep (Bell, Dixie-Bell, & Thompson, 1986). Likewise, Liebowitz et al. (1994) investigated an illness in Hispanic culture called *ataque de nervios* (attack of nerves), which overlaps with panic disorder but is a more inclusive categorization. In their sample, such attacks were present in 70 percent of people seeking treatment at an anxiety disorders clinic. A large percentage appeared to have labeled panic disorder as *ataque de nervios*. This finding signals the importance of linguistic clarity in identifying panic disorder and related symptoms.

## CLINICAL CHARACTERISTICS

It is not surprising that people with panic disorder often seek assistance in medical settings, particularly emergency rooms, complaining of anxiety, tension, and health concerns (such as heart attacks). Patients with panic disorder show high use of general medical services and report more medical problems (Katon, 1994). Panic disorder symptoms are often misinterpreted by medical staff as medical disorders (Weissman, 1990); therefore, the diagnosis of panic disorder may go unrecognized. Indeed, health-related concerns are common clinical characteristics of panic disorders. Research participants with panic disorder have been found to interpret body sensations but not external events as more threatening than do nonclinical research participants (Westling & Ost, 1995). In a similar vein, Ehlers (1993) found that compared with control patients, panic patients tended to shift their attention toward physically threatening cues and rated bodily symptoms associated with anxiety or panic as more dangerous. Greater attention to and negative interpretations of bodily sensations or misinterpretations appear to be prominent clinical characteristics of panic disorder patients, as suggested by early researchers (Goldstein & Chambless, 1978).

The ability to function and a person's quality of life are often adversely affected by their panic disorder, with impairment evident in poor physical and emotional health, alcohol and drug abuse, suicide attempts, decreased time on hobbies, poorer marital functioning, increased financial dependency, increased use of general medical and psychiatric professionals, use of minor tranquilizers and antidepressants, and use of hospital emergency rooms (Markowitz, Weissman, Ouellette, Lishe, & Klerman, 1989; Telch, Schmidt, Jaimez, Jacquin, & Harrington, 1995). Interestingly, among clinical patients, AWOPD and PDA were associated with worse functioning than panic alone (Gelernter, Stein, Tancer, & Uhde, 1992; Goisman et al., 1994). In a study of patients with panic and agoraphobia, Cox, Swinson, Shulman, Kuch, and Reichman (1993) found that women showed more phobic avoidance than men, but men reported more alcohol use than women and perceived alcohol to be a more effective strategy in coping with anxiety. It is unclear whether the increased avoidance among women or alcohol use among men led to more problematic outcomes. Interestingly, one study indicated that those who developed avoidance behavior before onset of the full panic syndrome less often reported fullblown agoraphobia (Buller, Maier, Goldenberg, Lavori, & Benkert, 1991). Perhaps behavior that inhibits the experience of frequent or severe panic attacks lessens the likelihood of developing a more severe agoraphobic syndrome.

Extensive controversy exists over whether panic disorder increases the likelihood of attempting suicide. From the ECA study data, Weissman (1990) concluded that panic disorder and panic attacks were more strongly related to suicide attempts than other mental disorders. In contrast, Cox and colleagues found that only 1 percent of clinic patients with panic disorder had attempted suicide in the preceding year (Cox, Direnfeld, Swinson, & Norton, 1994). Both epidemiologic and clinic studies agreed that the presence of depression in panic patients substantially increased the likelihood of suicide attempts (Johnson, Weissman, & Klerman, 1990; Warshaw, Massion, Peterson, Pratt, & Keller, 1995), suggesting that depressive disorders provide the impetus to suicide rather than panic disorder itself. Interestingly, a Japanese study reported low to nonexistent rates of suicidal behavior among panic patients (Shioiri, Murashita, Kato, Fujii, & Takahashi, 1996). Suicidality in panic patients, at least in part, may be culturally based.

With regard to clinical differences in patients with panic disorder in African American and white communities, although both groups had similar symptoms, African American patients had a more severe syndrome, with more phobic symptoms, unnecessary psychiatric hospitalizations, medical emergency room visits, isolated sleep paralysis, childhood trauma, and life stressors (Chambless & Williams, 1995; Friedman, Paradis, & Hatch, 1994). They also sought help from a mental health professional at one-fifth the rate of white people (Horwath et al., 1993). At the end of exposure treatment, African Americans remained more severe on measures of phobic avoidance (Chambless & Williams, 1995), suggesting that these patients may suffer more severe symptoms and respond somewhat less well to conventional treatments.

## COMORBIDITY

Researchers have repeatedly shown that panic disorder is often comorbid with a variety of other mental health diagnoses. Approximately 70 percent of patients with panic disorder have Axis I comorbidity and 50 percent have Axis II personality comorbidity (Dick et al., 1994; Shear, Leon, & Spielman, 1994). Most common among the Axis I comorbid conditions are mood disorders, with as many as two-thirds reporting past or present depression. Rates of secondary comorbid depressive disorders occurring after the onset of panic appear to be lower than primary depressions, but concomitant symptoms are found in approximately 25 percent (see Reich et al., 1993). Other common accompanying conditions include alcohol dependence (19 percent for women and 32 percent for men) and social phobia (up to 46 percent) (see McNally, 1994). Recent findings suggest that alcohol use may be a form of self-medication, particularly in panic patients comorbid for both depression and social phobia (see Rosenbaum, Pollock, Otto, & Pollack, 1995).

Consistent with findings regarding greater impairment among those with agoraphobia, a recent study also indicated that compared with those with panic disorder, PDA patients showed a higher prevalence of comorbid diagnoses, including major depression, dysthymia, social phobia, GAD, and OCD (Starcevic, Uhlenhuth, Kellner, & Pathak, 1992). Among comorbid personality disorders in panic and agoraphobic patients, anxious cluster personality disorders predominate, including avoidant, dependent, and histrionic personality (see, for example, Chambless, Renneberg, Goldstein, & Gracely, 1992), with dependent disorders not surprisingly more common among those with agoraphobic avoidance (Hoffart, Thornes, Hedley, & Strand, 1994; Reich, Noyes, & Troughton, 1987). Because some comorbid conditions, particularly anxious cluster personality disorders, tend to remit with improvement in the panic condition (Mavissakalian & Hamann, 1987), it is not clear whether they play an etiologic role in panic, are secondary developments, or derive from some common underlying pathogenetic factor. Research addressing this question must necessarily be highly sophisticated to control for myriad factors.

## BIOLOGICAL ASPECTS

Several studies have focused on possible cardiac abnormalities associated with panic. In most cases, panic disorder occurs in patients with normal coronary arteries (Beitman, Mukerji, Flaker, & Basha, 1988). However, mitral valve prolapse is found more often in people with panic disorder than in other members of the population, although there is some controversy about this conclusion (Margraf, Ehlers, & Roth, 1988; McNally, 1994). Thus, cardiac-related anomalies may exist in some patients with panic disorder, but their role in development of the disorder is unclear.

People who panic are known to respond with significantly higher respiratory and lower tidal volume to carbon dioxide than controls, suggesting an abnormal respiratory control mechanism (Papp, Martinez, Klein, Coplan, & Gorman, 1995). It is unclear whether such respiratory problems predate panic attacks and are instrumental in their development or are merely symptoms induced by the panic state. Whatever its role, Margraf (1993) and others have argued that although hyperventilation is not unique to panic disorder, it plays a prominent role as a trigger for ongoing panic attacks. That treatment combining hyperventilation provocation and respiratory training markedly diminished the frequency of panic attacks (de Beurs, Lange, van Dyck, & Koele, 1995) attests to the benefits of adopting this model.

Of considerable interest to researchers investigating biological processes related to panic disorders is the effective use of pharmacologic treatments. Panic attacks have responded to a range of agents, including monoamine oxidase inhibitors (MAOIs), tricyclic antidepressants, and high-potency benzodiazepines (see Hollister, 1992; Klerman, 1992). Extensive literature on the differential efficacy of various pharmacologic treatments for panic and agoraphobia is reviewed in chapter 11 (see also McNally, 1994; Wolfe & Maser, 1994).

## ETIOLOGIC THEORIES

Disagreements among researchers supporting biological models and those supporting cognitive–behavioral models have been strident in recent years but have sparked many studies in an effort to explain the onset of panic disorders. A sufficient amount of research accumulated has enabled the National Institute of Mental Health (NIMH) to sponsor a consensus conference focused mainly on treatment studies but also indirectly on etiologic models on which treatments were based (see Wolfe & Maser, 1994).

Psychophysiological models include possible biochemical mechanisms (Heninger, 1994), hyperventilation or suffocation alarm responses (Klein & Gorman, 1987; Ley, 1985), and genetically linked neurochemical dysfunctions (Woodman, 1993). Evidence for biochemical mechanisms derives mainly from challenge or provocation studies using sodium lactate, carbon dioxide, and adrenaline, among other substances, to produce panic in the laboratory. This research has identified several chemical mechanisms for panic induction, but underlying dysregulation in a single system that would explain the various findings has not been evident (for a review, see McNally, 1994). Furthermoer, despite research linking hyperventilation to panic, findings have not strongly supported hyperventilation as an etiologic factor, except in a limited number of cases. Recent theoretical proposals by Klein (1993) regarding suffocation alarm have not been fully tested.

Woodman (1993) reviewed genetic research and found strong evidence for a genetic predisposition for panic disorder. First-degree relatives of people with panic disorders have a significantly higher prevalence of panic disorder than relatives of patients without panic disorder (Kushner, Thomas, Bartels, & Beitman, 1992). Furthermore, the former group had a greater risk of having an anxiety disorder, including panic; their risk was greater than that of relatives of patients with GAD, major depression, or controls (Mendlewicz, Papdimitriou, & Wilmotte, 1993).

Consistent with these findings, Horwath et al. (1995) found that agoraphobia and social phobia were concentrated in relatives of patients with panic disorder. Thus, some genetic linkage is apparent, but other factors are certainly involved.

Perhaps the most strongly supported etiologic model is a cognitive–behavioral theory of panic and agoraphobia that centers on the idea that patients learn to fear the physical symptoms of anxiety and panic in a vicious repeating cycle of perceived threat, apprehension, body sensations, and catastrophic misinterpretation of symptoms (see, for example, Clark, 1986; Goldstein & Chambless, 1978). They then attempt to avoid situations that might increase these sensations. Recent research in a biological challenge study of PDA patients supported a cognitive model of panic and safety signal theory of panic but did not support a biological model (Carter, Hollon, Carson, & Shelton, 1995). From a treatment standpoint, Westling and Ost (1995) observed that panic disorder patients who had completed cognitive–behavior therapy or applied relaxation training modeled on cognitive and behavioral theories had reduced levels of threat perception from bodily sensations comparable to controls. Overall, numerous studies support aspects of a cognitive model of panic. Cognitive techniques alone and in conjunction with behavioral methods, including relaxation and in vivo exposure, have led to improvement in patients' symptoms and functioning. (For thorough reviews, see McNally, 1994; Wolfe & Maser, 1994.)

## IMPLICATIONS FOR TREATMENT

The clinical course and presentation of panic disorders suggests that people presenting with unexplained or atypical medical conditions on a repeated basis should be considered for possible panic disorder diagnoses and referred to a mental health professional. This approach is particularly appropriate for people with relatives who report a history of panic. Both cognitive–behavioral and psychopharmacologic methods of treatment have shown good success independently and in combination. However, the treatment methods are likely to demonstrate even better results if further refinement of the models of panic and agoraphobic avoidance can be accomplished to clarify more precisely the biological mechanisms as well as their interaction with cognitive and behavioral processes.

# Social Phobia

## DIAGNOSTIC CRITERIA

Shyness and bashfulness in social situations are inextricably human experiences. Marks (1969) recounted the description that Hippocrates gave of a man with a social phobia who avoided social situations because he feared being disgraced and observed. Janet (1903) described similar patients who feared observation while speaking, writing, or playing the piano. First introduced into psychiatric diagnostic nomenclature in 1980 with the publication of DSM-III, social phobia was defined as an irrational fear and wish to avoid situations of scrutiny by others (APA, 1980). DSM-IV added clarity about the types of feared contexts (performance fears, humiliation, embarrassment, showing anxiety symptoms) and noted that the anxiety may take the form of a panic attack. Social and performance situations are either avoided or "endured with intense anxiety." Fears may be generalized broadly across many situations (generalized subtype) or may be more situation specific. Social phobia is common in childhood (Strauss & Last, 1993) and is evident in peer as well as adult interactions. Such fears are expressed through crying, tantrums, freezing, and avoiding situations with unfamiliar people.

It is important to distinguish social phobia in children and adults from alternative diagnoses such as avoidant disorder. In adults, a diagnosis of avoidant personality disorder should be given if fears and avoidance are widely generalized beyond ordinary social situations. The social phobia diagnosis is excluded if anxiety could be attributed to drug use or medication or is better accounted for by other conditions such as panic disorder, separation anxiety disorder, body dysmorphic disorder, a pervasive developmental disorder, or schizoid personality disorder. In addition, social phobia is not diagnosed when embarrassing psychiatric or medical symptoms (for example, stuttering, Parkinson's disease, and severe disfigurement) are responsible for social fears and avoidance. Nevertheless, some treatments for social anxiety remain relevant for some physically based conditions that cause embarrassment.

According to research findings, most people who seek treatment for social phobia fear and avoid two or more situations (Holt, Heimberg, Hope, & Liebowitz, 1992; Turner, Beidel, Dancu, & Keys, 1986) and show significant interruption in social or occupational functioning. Those with generalized social anxiety have shown few qualitative differences but are more distressed than people with circumscribed social fears (Heimberg, Hope, Dodge, & Becker, 1990; Turner, Beidel, & Townsley, 1992). People with specific social phobias also tend to respond better to pharmacotherapy and behavioral therapy than their generalized counterparts. Thus, generalized social phobia appears to be the more problematic condition.

Pollard and Henderson (1988) noted that many people fear embarrassment but their symptoms do not meet diagnostic criteria because their fear or avoidance is limited to one situation and they do not develop functional impairment (Schneier, Johnson, Hornig, Liebowitz, & Weissman, 1992). Shy people fear negative evaluation in social situations (Ludwig & Lazarus, 1983) and show similar somatic arousal including blushing, palpitations, trembling, and sweating (Amies, Gelder, & Shaw, 1983; Turner, Beidel, & Townsley, 1990) but have an earlier onset and are less functionally impaired than those with full social phobia (Turner et al., 1990). Given the resemblance in physiological responses and reported fears, test anxiety may be considered a discrete form of social phobia (Schneier et al., 1994). Oberlander, Schneier, and Liebowitz (1994) reported that social anxiety secondary to comorbid medical or psychiatric conditions can be responsive to the same treatment as that used for social phobias.

## EPIDEMIOLOGY

According to ECA studies, social phobia occurs more often among women, although differences by gender are not so striking as for panic disorders. Six-month prevalence rates ranged from 0.9 percent to 1.7 percent for men and 1.5 percent to 2.6 percent for women (Myers et al., 1984), with 2.4 percent (six million adults) experiencing social phobia at some point in their lives (Schneier et al., 1992). This prevalence rate may be considerably higher when diagnostic criteria include people with more generalized fears (Hope & Heimberg, 1993). In fact, the National Comorbidity Survey, using DSM-III-R criteria that allowed inclusion of avoidant personality disorder and the generalized subtype, revealed a much higher lifetime prevalence rate of 13.3 percent (Kessler et al., 1994). Prevalence rates of social phobia have varied somewhat across countries, with East Asian studies reporting the lowest prevalence: South Korea, 0.5 percent (Lee et al., 1990); Taiwan, 0.6 percent

(Hwu, Yeh, & Chang, 1989); and Italy, 1.0 percent (Faravelli, Innocenti, & Girdinelli, 1989). Three English-speaking sites reported the highest rates: Canada, 1.7 percent; four U.S. sites, 2.4 percent; and New Zealand, 3.0 percent. These differences may be explained in part by variation in cultural contexts in which social fears are expressed or by lack of sensitivity in the assessment instruments to detect culturally relevant symptoms. Particularly in multicultural societies, diagnostic procedures must take into consideration the differing presentations of social anxiety across cultures as well as the possible tendency to underreport because of embarrassment.

## CLINICAL CHARACTERISTICS

Symptoms of social phobia are diverse and include distress and avoidance of various types of social contexts. In a clinical sample of 88 patients, Turner and colleagues (1990) found that an average of 5.6 social situations created at least moderate distress. Turner et al. (1992) suggested that subgroups of people with social phobia may be characterized by the different types of situations feared. Some people with social phobia fear social performance situations, such as eating or speaking in front of others, whereas others experience fear in more general social interactions such as talking on the telephone and meeting new people. Racial concerns regarding devaluation by the dominant culture may play a role for some nonwhite people (see Fink, Turner, & Beidel, 1996). Those with performance concerns might differ from those with social interaction concerns, although as yet no empirical data support this clinical impression (Liebowitz, 1987; Turner et al., 1992). Similarly, in the literature on shyness, Buss (1980) distinguished two subgroups based on the presence or absence of scrutiny from others.

Situations that are typically feared or avoided by those with social phobias include speaking, eating and drinking in public, writing in the presence of others, taking tests, initiating and maintaining conversations, attending social gatherings or parties, and using public restrooms. Of these, public speaking is the most commonly feared situation, with meetings, parties, and conversations with authority figures also frequently avoided (Holt et al., 1992; Schneier et al., 1992). The size, gender, and social status of the audience, as well as the formality of the situation, may mediate the degree of distress experienced, with formal speaking situations (Turner et al., 1986) and opposite-sex interactions (Dodge, Heimberg, Nyman, & O'Brien, 1987) producing more distress and avoidance.

The course of social anxiety appears to be relatively chronic (Campbell & Rapee, 1994; Lovibond & Rapee, 1993). Social phobia has been associated with a pervasive pattern of interference in social, occupational, and academic functioning (Turner, Beidel, Borden, Stanley, & Jacob, 1991), but no studies have yet measured quality of life specifically. Examples of interference include entertainers with stage fright who have had to cancel performances or take a hiatus in their careers. Those with fear of using public toilets, a problem traditionally called "bashful bladder," may avoid going out in public or schedule their travels carefully around the availability of private restrooms. Other fears, however, such as excessive concern about writing or blushing in front of others, may be endured with dread, the suffering unnoticed by others and interference with functioning less evident.

Onset of social phobia typically occurs in the mid to late teenage years (Mannuzza, Fyer, Liebowitz, & Klein, 1990; Turner et al., 1986), although most seek treatment much later, at an average age of 30 (Butler, Cullington, Munby, Amies, & Gelder, 1984). Schneier et al. (1992) found that 47 percent of people reported onset before age 10, and it appears that in children social phobia can be readily diagnosed before this age (Beidel, 1991). Fears of social situations can occur from early infancy, although the fear of negative evaluation by others, a core feature of the diagnosis, may not develop until later in life (Crozier & Burnham, 1990; Garcia-Coll, Kagan, & Reznick, 1984).

Interestingly, although nearly twice as many women as men in the general population have social phobia, in clinical settings the gender distribution is nearly equal (Solyom, Ledwidge, & Solyom, 1986). Thus, men with social phobia seem more likely to seek treatment than women, perhaps because of the interference in functioning that may pose a greater problem for men than for women in traditional Western societies.

Studies of familial patterns of social phobia have found a higher incidence of social phobia in the first-degree relatives of those with social phobias compared with other disorders (Fyer, Mannuzza, Chapman, Liebowitz, & Klein, 1993; Reich & Yates, 1988). Most of the reports on parental characteristics are retrospective, revealing that people with social phobias rate their parents as more overprotective and rejecting and less emotionally warm than their nonclinical counterparts (Arrindell, Emmelkamp, Monsma, & Brilman, 1983). Not surprisingly, people with social phobias are less likely to be married (Schneier et al., 1992). Chapman (1993) observed that when they do marry, they tend to chose others with similar histories. The highest rates of social phobia are found among the lowest socioeconomic groups (Schneier et al., 1992).

## COMORBIDITY

Approximately 50 percent of patients with social phobia have comorbid disorders (Sanderson, Di Nardo, Rapee, & Barlow, 1990; Turner et al., 1991). Higher rates (69 percent) were reported in community studies, and 77 percent of this group reported that social phobia occurred first (Schneier et al., 1992). As for panic disorders, the most common comorbid diagnoses are other anxiety disorders, mood disorders, and substance abuse, with ECA study estimates of comorbid simple phobia at 59 percent, agoraphobia at 45 percent, alcohol abuse at 19 percent, major depression at 17 percent, and drug abuse at 13 percent. Turner and colleagues (1992) also reported that 33 percent had concurrent GAD. Comorbid dysthymia also was evident, with small percentages reporting concurrent panic disorder and OCD.

It is important for clinicians to distinguish social phobia from other psychiatric disorders that present with similar symptoms. As noted above, panic attacks can occur in social phobia but must be distinguished from panic disorder with or without agoraphobia, in which social fear occurs secondary to the fear of spontaneous panic attack. Likewise, people with depression tend to withdraw and avoid social situations, but this is due to lethargy or anhedonia rather than a fear of being judged by others. When substance abuse is present, the clinician may find investigating the order of onset helpful because alcohol and drugs are often used for self-medication beginning after the social phobia (Kushner, Sher, & Beitman, 1990; Smail, Stockwell, Canter, & Hodgson, 1984; Turner et al., 1986). If abuse is of long duration, it may require intervention before the causal social phobia is addressed.

With regard to Axis II comorbidity, Turner et al. (1991) found that 43 percent of their sample had coexisting personality disorders, in contrast to an earlier report of 17 percent by Klass, Di Nardo, and Barlow (1989). Consistent with findings for agoraphobia, the most common Axis II condition was avoidant personality disorder, and the differentiation between these two disorders can be difficult (Brown, Heimberg, & Juster, 1995; Widiger, 1992). Other concurrent Axis II disorders include OCD (13.2 percent) and histrionic personality (4.4 percent) with antisocial, dependent, paranoid, narcissistic, and borderline personality disorders rarely present (Turner et al., 1991).

## *ETIOLOGIC THEORIES*

Multiple factors are involved in the development of social phobia. In addition to the aggregation of social phobia in families, a genetic component has been supported by a single twin study, indicating higher concordance in monozygotic than dizygotic twins (Kendler, Neale, Kessler, Heath, & Eaves, 1992). However, the heritability of social phobia is only moderate, indicating that social phobia results from combined effects of genetic and other factors (Stemberger, Turner, Beidel, & Calhoun, 1995).

Little is known about neurobiological roots of social phobia. Various pharmacologic agents from different classes have proven to be efficacious in treating social phobia, arguing that this disorder represents a heterogenous group of neurobiological conditions or that the ultimate common pathway has not been determined (Nickell & Uhde, 1995). Liebowitz, Campeas, and Hollander (1987) elaborated on a dopaminergic neurotransmitter–receptor system hypothesis in the pathophysiology of social phobia. This hypothesis has been partly supported by the unusually high rate of social phobia in Parkinson's disease patients (Stein, Heuser, Juncos, & Uhde, 1990) and the responsivity of patients to MAOIs (Levin, Schneier, & Liebowitz, 1989). In a review of the biological studies, Nickell and Uhde (1995) concluded that the neurobiology of social phobia differed from that of panic and was more similar to controls. Few studies have examined neuroendocrine functioning in social phobia. Further investigation in these areas may lead to greater understanding of pathophysiology and perhaps of pharmacotherapy treatment mechanisms in social phobia.

Using an ethological model, Ohman (1986) viewed social fears as a by-product of dominance hierarchies that are characteristic of the social organization of some animal groups, particularly primates. A significant body of animal literature has studied the temperamental construct of behavioral inhibition thought to be a possible developmental precursor in social phobia (Stemberger et al., 1995). Behaviorally inhibited animals display characteristics seen in some people with social phobia: social anxiety, submissiveness, acquiescence, and timidity in social interactions (for a review, see Mineka & Zinbarg, 1995). Other studies found empirical support for a relationship among shyness, neuroticism, introversion, and inhibition (Higley & Suomi, 1989; Kagan, Reznick, Snidman, Gibbons, & Johnson, 1988). Many children identified as behaviorally inhibited have anxiety disorders characterized by social anxiety and fears that begin early and persist at least until age seven (Biederman et al., 1990; Kagan, Snidman, & Arcus, 1992). The onset of shyness also is early (Turner et al., 1990), and the symptoms of the two are similar. Stemberger et al. (1995) noted that shyness could be a predispositional temperamental factor toward social phobia, influenced by other variables, like traumatic conditioning and family history to determine the expression of the disorder.

Support for the relevance of conditioning experiences comes from Townsley (1992), who determined that 40 percent of those with generalized social phobia recalled traumatic conditioning experiences, as did 56 percent of those with specific social fears. Ohman et al. (Ohman, 1986; Ohman, Dimberg, & Ost, 1985) expanded on conditioning models with the concept of preparedness, an evolutionary-based predisposition to acquire fears of angry, critical, or rejecting faces. It may be that social phobia results from biological or psychological vulnerability to anxious apprehension of future social situations that could evoke anxiety.

Significant research has focused on cognitive models of social phobia. Clark and Wells (1995) offered a synthesis of several existing models, proposing that the interaction of previous experience and behavioral predisposition leads to assumptions about danger in one or more social situations. According to a cognitive model, fears of inappropriate or inept behavior that results in rejection or devaluation lead to automatic anxiety responses and negative social–evaluative thoughts. These interfere with the ability to accurately process social cues. The behavioral response to these phenomena is social withdrawal, evoking unfriendly responses from others, thus confirming the worst fears of someone with a social phobia.

## IMPLICATIONS FOR TREATMENT

It is clear from the etiologic models proposed above that treatment for social phobia spans the range of pharmacologic, behavioral, and cognitive treatments. Pharmacotherapy for social phobia spans a wide range of medications because research has demonstrated that several drug classes are effective. However, despite the growing literature on efficacy of medication, there is a high rate of relapse when benzodiazapines and MAOIs are discontinued within four months of treatment (for a review, see Potts & Davidson, 1995). Unfortunately, few studies have combined pharmacotherapy and psychosocial treatments (Clark & Agras, 1991; Falloon, Lloyd, & Harpin, 1981), although multiple causality models might support such combined methods.

Cognitive–behavioral treatments of social phobia have included social skills training, exposure therapy, relaxation techniques, rational emotive therapy, self-instructional training, systematic rational restructuring, and anxiety management training (see Butler & Wells, 1995; Heimberg & Juster, 1995). Hope and Heimberg (1993) described a promising group of cognitive–behavioral treatments for social phobia. Heimberg and Juster (1995) commented that new treatment interventions are needed to address subtypes of social phobia, comorbidity issues, and possible potentiating effects of treatment and pharmacotherapy combined. Further exploration of etiologic factors in social phobia subtypes might provide direction in the search for effective therapies.

# Generalized Anxiety Disorder

## DIAGNOSTIC CRITERIA

The precursor to GAD first appeared as an anxiety neurosis category in DSM-II to classify the symptoms of patients who were generally anxious over a prolonged period of time but did not demonstrate agoraphobic avoidance (Barlow, 1988; Borkovec & Whisman, 1996). Many clinicians found this vague definition inadequate, and DSM-III criteria were devised with greater specificity in mind. To this purpose, DSM-III excluded patients who had another mental disorder, moving GAD from anxiety neurosis to a residual category. Unfortunately, this decision introduced additional confusion, partly due to the high comorbidity rate of GAD with other anxiety disorders, leading to disagreement on the diagnosis of GAD across studies (Breslau & Davis, 1985). DSM-III-R then defined people with GAD as displaying excessive anxiety and uncontrollable worry about a number of events or activities not confined to other Axis I disorders (APA, 1987). Thus, this diagnosis could be made in addition to another disorder, provided that GAD symptoms could be clearly distinguished. Still, however, low diagnostic reliability has remained a problem (Brown, Barlow, & Liebowitz, 1994).

The current revision of GAD criteria in DSM-IV (APA, 1994) reflects an increased emphasis on the excessive-worry component and the elimination of autonomic hyperactivity symptoms from earlier versions. People must experience worry and excessive anxiety frequently for at least six months, with evidence of clinically significant distress or impaired functioning; symptoms cannot be due to a substance or medical condition (Brown et al., 1994). Several recent studies have found DSM-IV criteria to be reliable (Abel & Borkovec, 1995; Brown, Marten, & Barlow, 1995; Freeston & Dugas, 1994). However, in spite of the gains made in diagnostic criteria, questions continue to surround the diagnosis. Brown, Heimberg, and Juster (1995) observed that although 99 percent of the 390 subjects were diagnosed with GAD by both DSM-III-R and DSM-IV standards, a large percentage of patients with other diagnoses also had symptoms that met the criteria (35 percent to 92 percent), leading to questions about the specificity of symptoms defined for GAD. The authors suggested increasing the somatic criteria from three to four (out of six) symptoms to exclude some less distinct cases but worried that this change may prove to be overly restrictive. Barlow (1988) suggested that requiring more than one focus for apprehensive worry would ensure that anxiety was generalized and perhaps better distinguish it from other disorders.

People with GAD experience general chronic anxiety and describe themselves as always nervous and on edge, displaying both autonomic and motoric evidence of fear (Marten & Brown, 1993). These feelings do not climax in a panic attack but instead persist over long periods. GAD differs from other anxiety disorders in that anxious feelings are not precipitated by any single event or source and the clear avoidance behaviors of phobias are absent (Deffenbacher & Suinn, 1987). The defining feature of GAD appears to be worry, mainly about family, money, and work as well as health and other issues (Barlow, 1988; Craske, Rapee, Jackel, & Barlow, 1989). Compared with control patients (Craske et al., 1989), patients with this disorder showed less control over worrying, less awareness of the extent to which worrying was realistic, and less perceived success in alleviating worry. Thus, worry is characteristic of GAD but also may be a component in other anxiety disorders.

## EPIDEMIOLOGY

Because of confusion surrounding the clinical criteria for GAD, the prevalence rate in the general population remains unclear. The original DSM-III criteria yielded a prevalence rate of 2.0 percent to 5.2 percent of the general population across several studies (for reviews, see Barlow, 1988; Beck, Emery, & Greenberg, 1985; Coleman & Gantman, 1989). Using more specific DSM-III-R criteria, Kessler and associates (1994) found a similar rate of 1.6 percent for current prevalence and 5.1 percent for lifetime prevalence. However, the prevalence of GAD occurring without concurrent diagnosis of comorbid major depression or panic disorder is much reduced: 0.8 percent current and 1.6 percent lifetime. GAD appears to be more common among older adults, with the lowest rate found for ages 15 to 24 (2.0 percent lifetime) and the highest for ages 45 and older (10.3 percent lifetime) (Wittchen, Zhao, Kessler, & Eaton, 1994).

## CLINICAL CHARACTERISTICS

Like panic disorders, GAD patients are overwhelmingly female (Raskin, Peeke, Dickman, & Pinsker, 1982; Yonkers, Warshaw, Massion, & Keller, 1996), outnumbering male patients by at least two to one (Kessler et al., 1994). The onset of GAD often occurs between the late teenage years and early 20s, developing somewhat earlier and more gradually than some other anxiety disorders (Anderson, Noyes, & Crowe, 1984; Barlow, Blanchard, Vermilyea, Vermilyea, & Di Nardo, 1986; Coleman & Gantman, 1989). However, GAD can develop relatively late in adulthood, and it appears that patients with an early onset differ from those with a late onset. For example, early-onset patients were more likely to be female with a history of psychiatric conditions and other problems. Late-onset patients, however, were more likely to develop GAD following a stressful life event (Borkovec & Whisman, 1996). Typically, patients with GAD sought treatment in their 30s and 40s (Barlow, 1988; Raskin et al., 1982).

GAD tends to run a chronic, lifelong course (Anderson et al., 1984; Kessler et al., 1994), with earlier onset and longer duration than panic disorder (Anderson et al., 1984). Barlow, Blanchard, et al. (1986) reported that patients with GAD had severe generalized anxiety for 56 percent of their lives, whereas those with panic disorder reported such anxiety for 16 percent of their lives. The mean duration of illness was 20 years, and people with GAD rarely reported feeling well for prolonged periods of time (Yonkers et al., 1996), although they experienced some variation in their levels of anxiety (Mancuso, Townsend, & Mercante, 1993). Remission was rare, with rates of 15 percent at one year, increasing only to 25 percent by two years (Yonkers et al., 1996). For those who did remit, risk of relapse was encouragingly low: 7 percent after six months and 15 percent after one year. However, Brown et al. (1994) noted that even when patients did remit from GAD, about half continued to have anxiety symptoms associated with a comorbid anxiety disorder (Brown et al., 1994; Yonkers et al., 1996).

GAD appears to have an adverse impact on quality of life (Mancuso et al., 1993; Massion, Warshaw, & Keller, 1993). Although comorbidity with other disorders was associated with significantly higher rates of interference with daily life, help seeking, and taking medication, it is noteworthy that 59 percent of those diagnosed with GAD alone also reported problems in at least one of these areas (Wittchen et al., 1994).

Little research is available concerning racial, cultural, and socioeconomic aspects of GAD. White people did not differ from black people or Hispanics in prevalence of anxiety disorders (Kessler et al., 1994). Guarnaccia (1993) demonstrated GAD to be associated in Puerto Rico with *ataques de nervios*, described earlier in relation to panic disorder. Clearly, more research needs to be conducted in this area. In the general population, the prevalence rate of GAD appears to decline with an increase in income and education, indicating that worry is more common among lower socioeconomic groups (Kessler et al., 1994). Interestingly, the resources associated with higher socioeconomic status appeared to protect better against the onset or exacerbation of worries and fears than they did for sadness and associated mood disorders. However, in contrast to the general population, treatment-seeking patients with GAD tended to be well educated and middle class, holding high-level jobs.

With regard to other demographic variables, higher lifetime prevalence rates of GAD were found for previously married people than with currently married or never-married people (Kessler et al., 1994). Homemakers and unemployed respondents, who consisted primarily of those with long-term disabilities and early retirees, had significantly more GAD diagnoses than others. A higher lifetime prevalence of GAD was observed among those in the Northeast than in other parts of the country (Wittchen et al., 1994), suggesting that GAD more often afflicts those under stress.

## COMORBIDITY

As noted earlier, comorbidity rates among GAD and other anxiety disorders contribute to diagnostic confusion because the symptoms of GAD are often apparent in other anxiety disorders (Brown, Marten, et al., 1995). Respondents with lifetime GAD reported 90 percent lifetime comorbidity and 65 percent current comorbidity with another Axis I disorder (Wittchen et al., 1994). The majority of patient samples have lifetime histories of additional anxiety disorders (Goisman, Goldenberg, Vasile, & Keller, 1995; Yonkers et al., 1996). Comorbidity with panic disorder, social phobia, and simple phobias occurs most often (Borkovec, Abel, & Newman, 1995; Noyes, Woodman, Garvey, & Cook, 1992; Yonkers et al., 1996). Such a high rate of comorbidity brings into question whether GAD is an independent disorder, a residual disorder, the basis for other disorders, or the result of an underlying condition that generates apprehension and fear. Although high comorbidity could be due to inadequately specified criteria, it seems likely that common etiologic pathways are involved (Goisman, Goldenberg, et al., 1995).

GAD patients appear to share some ruminative processes displayed by OCD patients, but the role of compulsions among GAD is unclear. Whereas past evidence has demonstrated a lack of compulsive behavior (Deffenbacher & Suinn, 1987), recent evidence is less clear and suggests that compulsive checking may be related to some worry. Depression frequently co-occurs with GAD (Goisman, Goldenberg, et al., 1995; Weiller, Boyer, Lepine, & Lecrubier, 1994; Wittchen et al., 1994) but is not as commonly associated with GAD as with other anxiety disorders. Like panic, social phobia, and PTSD, GAD has a high rate of comorbidity with substance abuse, especially alcohol abuse (Brown & Barlow, 1992). GAD also is a relatively common accompaniment to eating disorders (Kendler, MacLean, Neale, & Kessler, 1991), Tourette's syndrome (Chee & Sachdev, 1994), attention deficit disorder (Shekim, Asarnow, Hess, & Zaucha, 1990), and PTSD (Hubbard, Realmuto, Northwood, & Masten, 1995).

Many studies have demonstrated a possible link between GAD and some types of Axis II personality disorders. Avoidant personality disorder co-occurs with GAD in 30 percent to 50 percent of cases (Brooks, Baltazar, & Munjack, 1989; Sanderson et al., 1990; Shadick & Borkovec, 1991). Among personality traits, interpersonal sensitivity appeared to be the most strongly associated with GAD (Mavissakalian, Hamann, Haidar, & de Groot, 1995). Borkovec (1994) has suggested that interpersonal developmental experiences might provide some etiologic basis for GAD, because GAD patients appear to be particularly concerned about interpersonal situations, and social phobia is the most common accompaniment.

## BIOLOGICAL ASPECTS

Limited genetic information exists about the heritability of GAD, although the disorder appears to be found fairly frequently among first-degree relatives (Noyes et al., 1992). However, GAD and major depressive disorder also share genetic factors according to family studies. The relatively low degree of heritability may argue for interpersonal or developmental factors, or both, in the etiology of GAD.

Recent research suggests that GAD is characterized by autonomic inflexibility. Lyonfields, Borkovec, and Thayer (1995) observed that GAD patients exhibited little vagal tone at baseline and little variation in heart rate and vagal tone during a worry task. Thayer, Friedman, and Borkovec (1996) proposed that this tonal deficiency was caused by the effects of worrisome thinking. Subjects also demonstrated classically conditioned responses to verbal threats, implying that GAD patients show increased attention and reactivity after repeated exposures to threat words. Attentional processes related to worry thus appear to be related to the neural regulation of the cardiovascular system, highlighting the important relationship of physiological mechanisms and cognitive processes in GAD. An etiologic model of biological components is further articulated below.

## ETIOLOGIC THEORIES

Recently, the cognitive role of worry has been explored by Borkovec (1994), who postulated that GAD-related worry involves abstract thought rather than (and perhaps to the exclusion of) imaginative thought processes. Typically, imagining a feared stimulus causes a cardiovascular response. The use of verbal thought instead of imagery in GAD patients may explain their lack of cardiovascular response in relation to controls (Lyonfields et al., 1995); worrying may actually block physiological sensations associated with anxiety. One of the primary roles of worry then may be to avoid aversive images and emotional anxiety. In this process, worry inhibits the emotional processing that is necessary for extinction of fears, thereby leading to a chronic anxiety.

Problem solving and tolerance for uncertainty or the need for safety signals also appear to play a role in GAD. Blais, Freeston, and Ladouceur (1994) reported that people with GAD had poorer problem evaluation and were less assured of their solutions than controls. They also spent more time in defining problems and produced fewer solutions. Dugas, Letarte, Rheaume, Freeston, and Ladouceur (1995) replicated this finding, and they further observed that worriers do not actually lack knowledge of problem solving; rather, they could not use it effectively. These researchers suggest that GAD subjects may have demonstrated these symptoms because of an intolerance of uncertainty rather than a tendency to worry, which is a matter for further investigation. Woody and Rachman (1994) argued that those with GAD have insufficient or ineffective safety signals and therefore rarely feel safe. Their generalized anxiety symptoms constitute a search for safety.

It also is possible that patients with GAD develop their worries to avoid traumatic memories. Such patients reported more traumatic experiences than controls, 65 percent of which were interpersonal in nature. Interestingly, despite the high frequency of traumas, these were not the focus of worries, suggesting again that worry serves an avoidance function. These traumas and possible ensuing interpretations of them may thus contribute to the origin or maintenance of GAD symptoms. In a related vein, Abel (1994) observed that patients with GAD had more difficulty identifying emotions on the Toronto Alexithymia Scale, implying that worrying may serve to avoid not only unpleasant imagery but also other emotions. Worrying then appears to constitute a process that maintains GAD and perhaps some other emotional disorders. Worrying may increase cognitive rigidity in ways that preclude emotional processing of traumas and the retrieval of realistic information and that further strengthen negative views of oneself and the world (Borkovec, 1994).

## IMPLICATIONS FOR TREATMENT

It is clear that further research is needed to test theories regarding worrying as an avoidance strategy and cognitive and physiological accompaniments to this process. Certainly the findings to date have significant implications for treatment. Such restriction in affective involvement suggests the potential usefulness of psychotherapies that increase access to pleasurable experiences and assist in emotional processing in general and of interpersonal contexts in particular.

The pervasive presence of apprehension and general anxiety in GAD, not surprisingly, has spawned several studies of the effects of anxiolytic medications, particularly benzodiazepines. Although there is significant evidence for their efficacy (Hoehn-Saric, McLeod, & Zimmerli, 1989; Roy-Byrne, Wingerson, Cowley, & Dager, 1993), it appears that as for other anxiety disorders, continued use of such medications is needed, or relapse is likely. Theoretical models suggesting that worry inhibits physiological, imagery, and emotional processes argue, however, that further reducing anxious feelings through medications may not be the best treatment option. Rather, psychological interventions that facilitate emotional processing and reduce worrying, perhaps in conjunction with anxiety-reducing medications, may be the most appropriate. Indeed, several studies support the benefits of cognitive–behavioral treatments and of interpersonal therapies (Borkovec & Costello, 1993; Butler, Fennell, Robson, & Gelder, 1991; Power, Simpson, Swanson, & Wallace, 1990).

# Obsessive–Compulsive Disorder

## DIAGNOSTIC CRITERIA

Throughout history, obsessive–compulsive symptoms have been described in literature (for example, William Shakespeare's Lady Macbeth) and in religious writings (Bainton, 1950). The beginning of the 20th century marked the start of clinical and scientific inquiry into OCD (Freud, 1925; Janet, 1903). OCD is characterized by recurrent obsessions or compulsions that provoke distress and interfere significantly with personal, social, or occupational functioning. The diagnostic criteria have undergone changes through the years, and DSM-IV (1994) reflects considerable improvement in their clarity.

Obsessions are intrusive thoughts, images, or impulses that are perceived as inappropriate and cause marked distress. Compulsions or rituals are purposeful behaviors or mental acts performed in response to an obsession to reduce discomfort and prevent a dreaded consequence. Thus, compulsions may be overt actions, such as washing, cleaning, checking, repeating actions, ordering objects, or hoarding objects, or they may be covert mental efforts such as praying, reviewing events, counting, and repeating words or phrases in one's head that neutralize anxiety or prevent a feared outcome. DSM-IV now includes a poor insight type of OCD, referring to people who fail to recognize the unreasonableness or excessiveness of their fears and actions.

To distinguish OCD from GAD, DSM defines obsessions as mental experiences that are not merely excessive worries about real-life problems. The content of the obsessions or compulsions must not reflect depression or another Axis I disorder. For example, a person with depression may have guilty ruminations, and a person with substance use disorder may be preoccupied with drugs, but these are not considered obsessions.

An emerging area of interest and controversy is the relationship between OCD and obsessive–compulsive spectrum disorders, which have typically included eating disorders, trichotillomania, hypochondriasis, body dysmorphic disorder, Tourette's syndrome, sexual addictions and paraphilias, pathological gambling, and impulsive personality disorders. Instead of categorical classification, Hollander (1993) proposed that these disorders may be viewed along a continuum of compulsivity and impulsivity, with a common inability to resist urges to perform repetitive behaviors. On one end of the spectrum are the compulsive risk-aversive disorders and at the other end are the impulsive risk-seeking disorders. Although many of these disorders share features with OCD, including some clinical symptoms, age of onset, course, comorbidity, etiology, familial transmission, and pharmacologic treatment response (Simeon, Hollander, & Cohen, 1994), there are several distinguishing features that raise caution against an assumption of similar underlying pathology. For example, the ruminations in body dysmorphic disorder and anorexia are egosyntonic (Steketee, 1993). Trichotillomania and other impulse control disorders (for example, gambling and kleptomania) rarely involve obsessive thoughts, a hallmark of OCD, and the "compulsive" behavior in these disorders is usually experienced as pleasurable rather than anxiety reducing.

## EPIDEMIOLOGY

OCD was once thought to be a rare illness with a poor prognosis, but is now recognized as the fourth most common psychiatric disorder in the United States. ECA reports suggest a six-month prevalence of 1.6 percent and lifetime prevalence of 2.5 percent (about 1 in 40 people) (Karno & Golding, 1991). These findings are supported by other studies in the United States (Henderson & Pollard, 1988) and abroad (Weissman et al., 1994).

## CLINICAL CHARACTERISTICS

Despite the variety of presentations of OCD, the phenomenologic features can be categorized into several main groupings. The most common obsessions, in descending order, are contamination, pathological doubt, somatic complaints, need for symmetry, aggressive impulses, and sexual impulses (Rasmussen & Eisen, 1990). The most common compulsions, in descending order, are checking, washing, counting, needing to ask or confess, ordering, and hoarding. It should be noted that these data were collected before the growing recognition of the prevalence of cognitive or mental rituals; thus, the frequency with which these occur is unclear. In addition to the above features, avoidance behaviors are very prominent in OCD; they account for interference in daily functioning and are a target of treatment in behavioral therapy.

Obsessive fears often focus on catastrophic consequences, such as developing AIDS, contaminating others, forgetting to do important things, and causing harm to others. People with washing and cleaning compulsions may report hour-long showers, carrying "handiwipes," and using disinfectants or excessive amounts of soap to wash. Checking rituals are usually intended to prevent harm, burglary, fire, mistakes, social embarrassment, or illness. Examples include retracing a route just driven to ensure no pedestrian was hit; repeatedly examining electrical outlets, plugs, and appliances; making sure checkbooks balance; making sure mailing envelopes are sealed; and excessively seeking reassurance from others. This final ritual can frustrate family members, who often bear the brunt of unremitting questioning to ease obsessive fears. Ordering and arranging objects usually reduces general discomfort or produces a sense of symmetry and satisfaction rather than preventing a perceived consequence. Hoarding involves the fear that an unimportant item might be needed in the future. Repeating rituals (such as walking back and forth through a doorway, putting clothes on and taking them off, opening and closing a door) are performed to magically undo an unwanted catastrophe. Mental or cognitive compulsions include counting to a "good number," reviewing actions to recall if a contaminated object was touched, and saying prayers to be absolved of sin or error.

In adulthood, unlike panic disorder and agoraphobia, OCD occurs nearly equally in men and women (Black, 1974; Rasmussen & Tsuang, 1986). However, during childhood, boys with OCD outnumber girls by two to one (Flament, 1994; Swedo, Rapoport, Leonard, Lenane, & Cheslow, 1989), probably because boys have earlier onset (ages 14 to 17) and more severe symptoms than girls, whose symptoms begin around age 19 (Rasmussen & Eisen, 1990). Rapoport (1986) indicated that about 50 percent of adults with OCD had symptoms that were manifest by age 15. Late-onset development of OCD is uncommon, with less than 15 percent of cases experiencing a first presentation of symptoms after age 35 (Rasmussen & Tsuang, 1986). The earlier onset in boys often occurs at a critical time period for development of social and especially heterosocial skills, making it difficult to fit in with peers and develop dating skills in later adolescence. Given this typical onset, it is not surprising that men with OCD have a much lower marriage rate than women and are more often found to be living in their parental home (Black, 1974).

The course of OCD is typically chronic or fluctuating. Most early studies were retrospective and emphasized chronicity (Karno & Golding, 1991). A review by Eisen and Steketee (1997) indicated that courses for most of adult clinical samples are chronic with some deterioration, although some patients experience occasional periods of partial remission. Most of these studies are on clinical populations, and little is known about the course of OCD in the general public.

Obsessions and compulsions span the full range of symptom severity, from minimal interference in daily functioning to extreme disability (Myers et al., 1984). Interestingly, although marital dysfunction has been observed, overall it appears that marital satisfaction in clinic patients with OCD is approximately similar to that of the normal population (Riggs, Hiss, & Foa, 1992). The family literature in OCD in the 1970s and early 1980s was limited to case reports or descriptive papers with a generally dynamic interpretation of the role of the symptom in the context of family issues, drawing largely from the field of systems theory. Family members are typically involved in the performance of rituals (Calvocoressi et al., 1995; Shafran, Ralph, & Tallis, 1995) and may offer invaluable information that carries both diagnostic and treatment implications (Van Noppen, Steketee, McCorkle, & Pato, 1997). The Family Accommodation Scale (Calvocoressi et al., 1995) appears to be a promising avenue for assessing the extent of family participation in rituals. Livingston-Van Noppen, Rasmussen, Eisen, and McCartney (1990) proposed that family responses to

OCD range along a continuum from accommodating to antagonistic. They suggested that extreme or inconsistent family reactions to symptoms (for example, reassurance giving, participation in washing or checking rituals, facilitation of avoidance, hostile reactions) could actually help maintain the disorder. Steketee (1993) reported that clients with OCD whose relatives believed they were malingering and could just stop their compulsions had poor outcome after behavioral therapy. Thus, there is a growing interest in the role of family responses to obsessive–compulsive symptoms and the implications for family behavioral treatment.

Flament and colleagues (1988) reported no relationship with race, socioeconomic status, or religion to OCD in a child and adolescent population. There have been similar findings in adult populations (Burnam et al., 1987; Karno & Golding, 1991). Despite their approximately equivalent prevalence rates, clients from communities of color have rarely presented at OCD clinics for treatment. Interestingly, a review of research on anxiety disorders in African Americans by Neal and Turner (1991) did not identify any such studies for OCD. More recently, a report suggested that some black Americans may present more often in medical settings such as dermatology clinics (Friedman, Hatch, Paradis, Popkin, & Shalita, 1995) and may have more severe symptoms (Chambless & Williams, 1995). OCD symptoms have been found to be similar across cultures (Khanna & Channabasavanna, 1987), although they may vary in content depending on culture or religion. For example, fears of developing tuberculosis or leprosy occurred in northern Sudan (Elsarrag, 1968), and *koro*, a fear of penile shrinkage, was reported in Chinese cultures (Lo, 1967). Such fears are rare in Western cultures.

## COMORBIDITY

Rasmussen and Eisen (1990) reported that 57 percent of patients with OCD seen at their clinic had a concurrent Axis I or Axis II diagnosis. Studies examining OCD and other co-occurring psychiatric disorders revealed that depression was the most common complication, with a high lifetime prevalence of 76 percent and current prevalence of up to 31 percent of cases (Barlow, Di Nardo, & Vermilyea, 1986; Rasmussen & Eisen, 1991). Depression accompanying OCD can be either primary or secondary to the OC symptoms. The next most common comorbid conditions are other anxiety disorders, including simple phobia (50 percent to 77 percent), panic disorder (11 percent to 27 percent), social phobia (18 percent), and agoraphobia (8 percent) (Karno, Golding, Sorenson, & Burnam, 1988; Mellman & Uhde, 1987; Rasmussen & Tsuang, 1986). Overall, the frequency of concurrent other anxiety disorders in OCD ranged from 25 percent to 70 percent across international studies (Weissman et al., 1994).

As noted above, a small percentage of OCD patients who otherwise are not psychotic display delusional or "overvalued" thinking (Insel & Akiskal, 1986; Kozak & Foa, 1994). These patients have little insight into the unreasonable or senseless nature of their symptoms. However, only a small percentage (less than 10 percent) actually go on to develop schizophrenia (Boyd et al., 1984; Fenton & McGlashan, 1986). Current psychosis was identified by Eisen and Rasmussen (1993) in only 14 percent of their OCD patients, and in a significant number of these cases, the only psychotic symptom was a delusional conviction about the reasonableness of the obsession rather than a broader psychotic disorder. Although psychosis appears to be a predictor of poor outcome of behavioral and pharmacological treatment, it is not clear whether this also is true of OCD with poor insight (Kozak & Foa, 1994).

Reports of alcohol abuse in an OCD population are contradictory. Some studies suggest lower than expected rates of alcohol dependence (Barlow, Di Nardo, et al., 1986; Reimann, McNally, & Cox, 1992), whereas others do not (Eisen & Rasmussen, 1989; Mellman & Uhde, 1987). Many patients report the onset of alcohol abuse after the OCD, suggesting that as for other anxiety disorders, alcohol may be used to self-medicate. Studies of OCD in alcohol-dependent patients reveal a 6 percent to 12 percent prevalence rate (Eisen & Rasmussen, 1989; Reimann et al., 1992).

There is a higher rate of Tourette's syndrome in OCD (7 percent) than is usually seen in the general population (Rasmussen & Eisen, 1991), and patients with it have very high rates of comorbid OCD and obsessive–compulsive symptoms (30 percent to 40 percent) (Robertson, Trimble, & Lees, 1988), suggesting some link between these disorders (see also Pauls, Towbin, Leckman, Zahner, & Cohen, 1986). Clinical researchers have drawn parallels between OCD and eating disorders. Rasmussen and Eisen (1991) reported that 17 percent of OCD clients had a lifetime history of an eating disorder. Conversely, Hudson, Pope, Yurgelun-Todd, Jonas, and Frankenburg (1987) found a 33 percent lifetime prevalence of OCD in subjects with bulimia and a 13 percent current incidence of OCD in a population with anorexia and bulimia. The frequent comorbidity of OCD with both Tourette's syndrome and eating disorders indicates a need for clinicians to attend to such possibilities during diagnostic interviewing and treatment planning.

With regard to personality disorders, Baer et al. (1990) found that 36 percent of a large sample with OCD met criteria for one or more DSM-III personality disorders. The most common of these were avoidant, dependent, and histrionic personality disorders (see also Steketee, 1990). These match closely the personality disorders associated with panic and agoraphobia (Mavissakalian, Hamann, & Jones, 1990). Interestingly, although less than one-quarter of those with OCD also meet criteria for obsessive–compulsive personality disorder (OCPD), these conditions are frequently confused, probably because a number of OCPD traits, such as rigidity and perfectionism, are frequently found in patients with OCD (Steketee, 1990). Nonetheless, significant differences between these conditions are evident: Repetitive acts of clients with OCD are typically ego-alien and usually resisted, whereas they are usually ego-syntonic in OCPD. Further, clients with OCPD often seek treatment because of others' complaints about their behavior, unlike most OCD clients, who recognize their behavior as excessive and inappropriate.

## ETIOLOGIC THEORIES

Several models have been proposed to account for the development and expression of OCD, which is generally presumed to arise from a complex interplay of biological, behavioral, and cognitive elements. Most clinicians draw from a blending of these models, and therefore a multimodal treatment approach has become common practice. Animal models of OCD have serious limitations because of obvious difficulty in studying cognitive aspects (such as obsessions) that are so fundamental to the disorder. Nonetheless, ethologists have observed similarities between displacement behaviors (for example, hoarding, grooming, pecking), stereotyped behaviors (for instance, scratching, masturbating, hair pulling), and compulsions (Insel & Winslow, 1990).

Biological models have concentrated on genetic factors and neurobiological (i.e., neuroanatomical, neurochemical, and neuroendocrine) factors. Most twin and family studies support the hypothesis that OCD is heritable, with higher concordance rates in monozygotic (65 percent) than dizygotic twins (15 percent) (Carey & Gottes-man, 1981; Rasmussen & Tsuang, 1986). Family studies also confirm a higher inci-dence of OCD in parents and siblings than in relatives of psychiatric controls (Black, Noyes, Goldstein, & Blum, 1992; Pauls, Alsobrook, Goodman, Rasmussen, & Leckman, 1995; Riddle et al., 1990). Perhaps even more prevalent than the diag-nosis of OCD are obsessive and compulsive traits in parents (for a review, see Steke-tee, 1993). A genetic vulnerability in conjunction with life stress and environment is suggested as causal by Turner, Beidel, and Nathan (1985).

High rates of head trauma or disease (for example, encephalitis, epilepsy, menin-gitis, and Sydenham's chorea) in OCD clients suggest an etiologic role of physiologi-cal processes related to these problems. Research exploring neuroanatomical abnor-malities in OCD has been based on newly available technology for brain imaging studies. Multiple areas of the brain have been implicated in this research, with dif-ferences reported mainly in the orbitofrontal cortex and limbic structures (Baxter et al., 1988; Insel & Winslow, 1990). Insel (1992) suggested a pathway that mediates obsessions and compulsions, connecting the striatum to the limbic structures and the orbitofrontal region of the cortex. Studies to date indicate that multiple path-ways are involved, and further investigation is required to illuminate specific mecha-nisms of action. Interesting findings were reported by Baxter, Schwartz, and Guze (1991), who compared metabolic rate changes in clients who improved from either pharmacotherapy or behavioral therapy and found a comparable treatment response in the activity of the caudate nucleus for both groups. This finding supports the in-fluence of effective psychological treatment on physiological processes.

Dysfunction in neurochemical processes, particularly in abnormalities in the neurotransmitter serotonin, also has been well studied. This research derives mainly from pharmacotherapy studies showing that the most efficacious medications for OCD are serotonin reuptake inhibitors, such as clomipramine (Anafranil), fluoxe-tine (Prozac), fluvoxamine (Luvox), sertraline (Zoloft), and paroxetine (Paxil) (for a review, see Greist, Jefferson, Kobak, Katzelnick, & Serlin, 1995). However, pharma-cologic challenges, platelet studies, and cerebrospinal studies of the role of sero-tonin in OCD have provided conflicting findings, indicating that serotonin irregu-larities alone cannot account for OCD symptoms (for example, Hollander et al., 1991; Zohar et al., 1989). The frequent emergence of OCD symptoms in adoles-cence, during pregnancy, after childbirth, and at menopause suggests that endocrine responses may play some role in the development of this disorder.

With regard to behavioral models of OCD, as Foa and Tillmanns (1980) noted and is now clearly articulated in DSM diagnostic criteria, obsessions generate anxi-ety and compulsions reduce this fear. In this two-stage theory of the acquisition and maintenance of fear and avoidance behavior, ordinary objects such as toilet seats or knives become associated with fear and anxiety by being paired with an aversive physical or mental experience (Rachman, 1977). This provokes immediate discom-fort and leads to avoidance, which is reinforced because it reduces anxiety. When passive avoidance is ineffective in decreasing anxiety, active escape strategies or compulsions such as cleaning or checking are used to restore feelings of safety or prevent harm (Rachman, 1976). That obsessions increase subjective and physiologi-cal discomfort and compulsions reduce discomfort is well documented in research studies (Boulougouris, Rabavilas, & Stefanis, 1977; Hornsveld, Kraaimaat, & van Dam-Baggen, 1979).

In addition to this conditioning model, informational learning or modeling ap-pear to play important roles (Foa & Kozak, 1986; Rachman & Wilson, 1980). For example, clients who flush toilets with their feet often say they are modeling the behavior after their parents' actions. However, although parental modeling may increase the likelihood of developing OCD, children with OCD often have rituals that differ substantially from those of their parents (Swedo et al., 1989). Furthermore, as noted above, the content of obsessions is influenced by the cultural and religious climate and the unique psychosocial history of the person. Behavioral treatment has evolved from this model and requires both exposure to external and mental obsessive cues and resistance to compulsions.

Cognitive models complement behavioral models by addressing the faulty cognitive processing inherent in OCD that may serve as a missing etiologic link. It is important to note that 80 percent to 99 percent of the general population report cognitive intrusions. This is therefore a "normal" phenomenon (Rachman & de Silva, 1978). However, those who go on to develop OCD react with more anxiety and have difficulty dismissing these intrusive experiences. Researchers in this area have studied various cognitive phenomena, including beliefs, memory, information processing, attitudes, and perceptions, to distinguish obsessive–compulsive thought processes from normative modes of thinking.

Foa and Kozak (1986) conceptualized OCD as an impairment in affective memory networks, characterized by an expectation of danger and an inability to generalize from experiences in which no harm occurred. Rituals are repeated frequently because they do not guarantee safety. Salkovskis (1989) proposed that obsessions develop from normal thoughts, images, and impulses that are associated with strong feelings of responsibility for harm to others, leading to self-criticism and efforts to remove or prevent blame and shame. Among others, Ladouceur and colleagues (1995) argued that a critical component of OCD is a flawed perception of the probability and severity of danger. Warren and Zgourides (1991) proposed a rational–emotive model in which a general biological vulnerability is influenced by developmental and learning factors that determine what are unacceptable thoughts and that form beliefs about the self, others, and the world. Recent studies using rational emotive therapy have yielded good outcomes (Emmelkamp & Beens, 1991), although evidence supporting the theoretical underpinnings of this model has not yet accrued.

The literature on cognitive features in OCD highlights a number of recurring themes that include the overestimation of risk or harm (Foa & Kozak, 1986), doubt about perceptions and memory, need for certainty, difficulty making decisions (Beech & Liddell, 1974; Guidano & Liotti, 1983; Reed, 1985), perfectionistic attitudes (McFall & Wollersheim, 1979; Pitman, 1987), excessive feelings of guilt and responsibility (Freeston, Ladouceur, Thibodeau, & Gagnon, 1992), and moralistic attitudes and rigid rules (Fitz, 1990; Steketee, Quay, & White, 1991). Considerable research is ongoing at present regarding the cognitive aspects of OCD to determine their potential role in development, maintenance, and treatment of this disorder.

## IMPLICATIONS FOR TREATMENT

In reviewing the above findings regarding the psychopathology of OCD, it is clear that this is a well-researched disorder about which much is now understood. It is evident that the wide variation in OC symptom manifestations has led to earlier diagnostic confusion and that more recent efforts at diagnosis using the functional relationship of obsessions and compulsions has improved both recognition of this condition and effective behavioral treatment. However, more clarity regarding the relationship or lack thereof to obsessive–compulsive spectrum disorders is needed. Some confusion remains regarding the importance of poor insight into obsessions and its relationship to insight in psychotic conditions. Treatments for OCD patients with very poor insight and schizotypal traits have generally included neuroleptics in combination with serotonergic medications and behavior therapy.

Further research on family responses relative to the maintenance of OC symptoms is likely to improve treatment efficacy. Information about cultural aspects is quite limited and may provide important insights for improving treatment access and effectiveness. The co-occurrence of OCD with other disorders has been extensively documented, but synergism among disorders is unclear, as are treatment implications of various comorbid conditions.

Among etiologic theories, those receiving the most recent attention are biological and cognitive mechanisms, with behavioral models generally well accepted. Although both pharmacologic and behavioral treatments have been well studied, the mechanism by which the former has its positive effects remains only partly specified. The usefulness of combining these methods has not been demonstrated despite the general belief that both biological and behavioral theories account for symptoms of OCD. Although exposure-based therapies appear to modify some beliefs, it is not clear that important cognitive defects are actually corrected. Cognitive therapies have been examined mainly in one center (Emmelkamp & Beens, 1991; Van Oppen et al., 1995), and more evidence that change in cognitive factors influences successful outcome is needed. Furthermore, much remains to be done to determine the role of beliefs and attitudes as well as perception, memory, and cognitive processing in the development and maintenance of OCD symptoms.

## Conclusion

Early classification systems lumped all phobias together, reflecting the then-prominent psychoanalytic conceptualization of phobias as symptomatic of unacceptable instinctual urges leading to anxious defense mechanisms. At the present time, several anxiety disorders are readily distinguishable, although questions remain about GAD and its potential importance in the development of all anxiety states.

It is clear from epidemiologic studies that anxiety disorders are common in the population. Costello (1982) estimated the prevalence among women to be as high as 19 percent. Women generally are afflicted and seek treatment more often than men for panic disorder and agoraphobia and GAD, but OCD and social phobia are found among men and women equally in treatment settings. Onsets for nearly all conditions occur by early adulthood, if not by midadolescence. Chronic conditions with accumulated functioning difficulties, comorbid anxiety, and depression are all too common. Surprisingly little information has accumulated regarding racial and cultural factors, although symptom patterns appear to differ only a little across cultures. However, treatment-seeking efforts may be quite different, and the relative absence of nonwhite patients applying to clinics, even when mental health treatment is available nearby, is noteworthy. Culturally accepted alternative patterns of help seeking (for example, medical clinics and the clergy) may explain this. In any case, some findings suggest that people of color, especially those of lower socioeconomic status, may suffer more severe symptoms with greater impairment.

Depression frequently co-occurs with anxiety disorders, and it appears that it is often a secondary consequence of the impairment. More information about anxiety disorders occurring secondary to depression and to other conditions would be helpful and might point to differential treatment strategies. The relatively high co-morbidity among anxiety disorders suggests some general vulnerability and an underlying pathway. Rosenbaum and colleagues (1995) suggest that the temperamental characteristic of behavioral inhibition (often evident in histories of patients with social phobia) may set the stage for psychosocial and biological factors to produce anxiety disorders. Accompanying anxious cluster personality disorders do not appear problematic and often remit with effective treatment (Mavissakalian & Hamann, 1987). More troublesome appear to be the odd and dramatic cluster comorbid diagnoses that may lead to a worse course and treatment outcome.

Biological components are clearly important in all of these disorders, especially in panic disorder, GAD, and OCD. Their role in etiology and the value of biological research studies to identify effective treatments remains unclear. In the future, we can expect to see considerably more research in this area and in cognitive models. It is hoped that this research will lead to better understanding of the development of anxiety and to more effective therapies.

# References

Abel, J. L. (1994, November). *Alexithymia in an analogue sample of generalized anxiety disorder and non-anxious matched controls.* Paper presented at the Annual Meeting of the Association for the Advancement of Behavior Therapy, San Diego.

Abel, J. L., & Borkovec, T. D. (1995). Generalizability of DSM-III-R generalized anxiety disorder to proposed DSM-IV criteria and cross-validation of proposed changes. *Journal of Anxiety Disorders, 9,* 103–115.

American Psychiatric Association. (1980). *Diagnostic and statistical manual of mental disorders* (3rd ed.). Washington, DC: Author.

American Psychiatric Association. (1987). *Diagnostic and statistical manual of mental disorders* (3rd ed., rev.). Washington, DC: Author.

American Psychiatric Association. (1994). *Diagnostic and statistical manual of mental disorders* (4th ed.). Washington, DC: Author.

Amies, P. L., Gelder, M. G., & Shaw, P. M. (1983). Social phobia: A comparative clinical study. *British Journal of Psychiatry, 142,* 174–179.

Anderson, D. T., Noyes, R., & Crowe, R. R. (1984). A comparison of panic disorder and generalized anxiety disorder. *American Journal of Psychiatry, 141,* 572–575.

Aoki, Y., Fujihara, S., & Kitamura, T. (1994). Panic attacks and panic disorder in a Japanese non-patient population: Epidemiology and psychosocial correlates. *Journal of Affective Disorders, 32,* 51–59.

Arrindell, W. A., Emmelkamp, P. M., Monsma, A., & Brilman, E. (1983). The role of perceived parental rearing practices in the aetiology of phobic disorders: A controlled study. *British Journal of Psychiatry, 143,* 183–187.

Baer, L., Jenike, M. A., Ricciardi, J. N., Holland, A. D., Seymour, R. J., Minichiello, W. E., & Buttolph, M. L. (1990). Standardized assessment of personality disorders in obsessive–compulsive disorder. *Archives of General Psychiatry, 47,* 826–830.

Bainton, R. H. (1950). *Here I stand: A life of Martin Luther.* New York: New American Library.

Barlow, D. H. (1988). *Anxiety and its disorders: The nature and treatment of anxiety and panic.* New York: Guilford Press.

Barlow, D. H., Blanchard, E. B., Vermilyea, J. A., Vermilyea, B. B., & Di Nardo, P. A. (1986). Generalized anxiety and generalized anxiety disorder: Description and reconceptualization. *American Journal of Psychiatry, 143,* 40–44.

Barlow, D. H., Di Nardo, P. A., & Vermilyea, B. B. (1986). Comorbidity and depression among the anxiety disorders. *Journal of Nervous and Mental Disease, 174,* 63–72.

Battaglia, M., Bertella, S., Politi, E., Bernardeschi, L., Perna, G., Gabriele, A., & Bellodi, L. (1995). Age at onset of panic disorder: Influence of familiar lability to the disease and of childhood separation anxiety disorder. *American Journal of Psychiatry, 152,* 1362–1364.

Baxter, L. R., Schwartz, J. M., & Guze, B. H. (1991). Brain imaging: Toward a neuroanatomy of OCD. In J. Zohar, T. Insel, & S. Rasmussen (Eds.), *The psychobiology of obsessive–compulsive disorder* (pp. 101–125). New York: Springer.

Baxter, L. R., Schwartz, J. M., Mazziotta, J. C., Phelps, M. E., Pahl, J. J., Guze, B. H., & Fairbanks, L. (1988). Cerebral glucose metabolism in nondepressed patients with obsessive–compulsive disorder. *American Journal of Psychiatry, 145,* 1560–1563.

Beck, A. T., Emery, G., & Greenburg, R. L. (1985). *Anxiety disorders and phobias: A cognitive perspective.* New York: Basic Books.

Beech, H. R., & Liddell, A. (1974). Decision making, mood states, and ritualistic behavior among obsessional patients. In H. R. Beech (Ed.), *Obsessional states* (pp. 143–160). London: Methuen.

Beidel, D. C. (1991). Social phobia and overanxious disorder in school-age children. *Journal of the American Academy of Child and Adolescent Psychiatry, 30,* 545–552.

Beitman, B. D., Mukerji, V., Flaker, G., & Basha, I. M. (1988). Panic disorder, cardiology patients, and atypical chest pain. *Psychiatric Clinics of North America, 11,* 387–397.

Bell, C. C., Dixie-Bell, D. D., & Thompson, B. (1986). Further studies on the prevalence of isolated sleep paralysis on black subjects. *Journal of the National Medical Association, 75,* 649–659.

Biederman, J., Rosenbaum, J. F., Hirshfeld, D. R., Faraone, S. V., Bolduc, E. A., Gersten, M., Meminger, S. R., Kagan, J., Snidman, N., & Reznick, J. S. (1990). Psychiatric correlates of behavioral inhibition in young children of parents with and without psychiatric disorders. *Archives of General Psychiatry, 47,* 21–26.

Black, D. (1974). The natural history of obsessional neurosis. In H. R. Beech (Ed.), *Obsessional states* (pp. 19–54). London: Methuen.

Black, D. W., Noyes, R., Goldstein, R. B., & Blum, N. (1992). A family study of obsessive–compulsive disorder. *Archives of General Psychiatry, 49,* 362–368.

Blais, F., Freeston, M. H., & Ladouceur, R. (1994, November). *How do clinical and nonclinical worriers solve problems?* Paper presented at the Annual Meeting of the Association of the Advancement of Behavior Therapy, San Diego.

Borkovec, T. D. (1994). The nature, functions, and origins of worry. In G.C.L. Davey & F. Tallis (Eds.), *Worrying: Perspectives in theory, assessment, and treatment* (pp. 5–34). New York: John Wiley & Sons.

Borkovec, T. D., Abel, J. L., & Newman, H. (1995). Effects of psychotherapy on comorbid conditions in generalized anxiety disorder. *Journal of Consulting and Clinical Psychology, 63,* 479–483.

Borkovec, T. D., & Costello, E. (1993). Efficacy of applied relaxation and cognitive–behavioral therapy in the treatment of generalized anxiety disorder. *Journal of Consulting and Clinical Psychology, 61,* 611–619.

Borkovec, T. D., & Whisman, M. A. (1996). Psychosocial treatment for generalized anxiety disorder. In M. Mavissakalian & R. Prien (Eds.), *Long-term treatments of anxiety disorders*. Washington, DC: American Psychiatric Press.

Boulougouris, J. C., Rabavilas, A. D., & Stefanis, C. (1977). Psychophysiological responses in obsessive–compulsive patients. *Behaviour Research and Therapy, 15*, 221–230.

Boyd, J. H., Burke, J. D. Gruenberg, E., Holzer, C. E., III, Rae, D. S., George, L. K., Karno, M., Stoltzman, R., McEvoy, L., & Nestadt, G. (1984). Exclusion criteria of DSM-III. *Archives of General Psychiatry, 41*, 983–989.

Breslau, N., & Davis, G. C. (1985). Generalized anxiety disorder: An empirical investigation of more stringent criteria. *Psychiatry Research, 15*, 231–238.

Brooks, R. B., Baltazar, P. L., & Munjack, D. J. (1989). Co-occurrence of personality disorders with panic disorder, social phobia, and generalized anxiety disorder: A review of the literature. *Journal of Anxiety Disorders, 3*, 259–285.

Brown, T. A., & Barlow, D. H. (1992). Comorbidity among anxiety disorders: Implications for treatment and DSM-IV. *Journal of Consulting and Clinical Psychology, 60*, 835–844.

Brown, T. A., Barlow, D. H., & Liebowitz, M. R. (1994). The empirical basis of generalized anxiety disorder. *American Journal of Psychiatry, 151*, 1272–1280.

Brown, E. J., Heimberg, R. G., & Juster, H. R. (1995). Social phobia subtype and avoidant personality disorder: Effect on severity of social phobia, impairment, and outcome of cognitive–behavioral treatment. *Behavior Therapy, 26*, 467–486.

Brown, T. A., Marten, P. A., & Barlow, D. H. (1995). Discriminant validity of the symptoms constituting the DSM-III-R and DSM-IV associated symptom criterion of generalized anxiety disorder. *Journal of Anxiety Disorders, 9*, 317–328.

Buller, R., Maier, W., Goldenberg, I. M., Lavori, P. W., & Benkert, O. (1991). Chronology of panic and avoidance, age of onset in panic disorder, and prediction of treatment response: A report from the Cross-National Collaborative Panic Study. *European Archives of Psychiatry and Clinical Neuroscience, 240*, 163–168.

Burnam, M. A., Hough, R. L., Escobar, J. I., Karno, M., Timbers, D. M., Telles, C. A., & Locke, B. Z. (1987). Six-month prevalence of specific disorders among Mexican Americans and non-Hispanic whites in Los Angeles. *Archives of General Psychiatry, 44*, 687–694.

Buss, A. H. (1980). *Self-consciousness and social anxiety*. San Francisco: Freeman.

Butler, G., Cullington, A., Munby, M., Amies, P., & Gelder, M. (1984). Exposure and anxiety management in the treatment of social phobia. *Journal of Consulting and Clinical Psychology, 52*, 642–650.

Butler, G., Fennel, M., Robson, P., & Gelder, M. (1991). Comparison of behavior therapy and cognitive behavior therapy in the treatment of generalized anxiety disorder. *Journal of Consulting and Clinical Psychology, 59*, 167–175.

Butler, G., & Wells, A. (1995). Cognitive–behavioral treatments: Clinical applications. In R. G. Heimberg, M. R. Liebowitz, D. A. Hope, & F. R. Schneier (Eds.), *Social phobia: Diagnosis, assessment, and treatment* (pp. 310–333). New York: Guilford Press.

Calvocoressi, L., Lewis, B., Harris, M., Trufan, S., Goodman, W., McDougle, C., & Price, L. (1995). Family accommodation in obsessive–compulsive disorder. *American Journal of Psychiatry, 152*, 441–443.

Campbell, M. A., & Rapee, R. M. (1994). The nature of feared outcome representations in children. *Journal of Abnormal Child Psychology, 22*, 99–111.

Carey, G., & Gottesman, I. I. (1981). Twin and family studies of anxiety, phobic and obsessive disorders. In D. Klien & J. Rabin (Eds.), *Anxiety: New research and changing concepts* (pp. 117–136). New York: Raven Press.

Carter, M. M., Hollon, S. D., Carson, R., & Shelton, R. C. (1995). Effects of a safe person on induced distress following a biological challenge in panic disorder with agoraphobia. *Journal of Abnormal Psychology, 104,* 156–163.

Chambless, D. L., Renneberg, B., Goldstein, A., & Gracely, E. J. (1992). MCMI-diagnosed personality disorders among agoraphobic outpatients: Prevalence and relationship to severity and treatment outcome. *Journal of Anxiety Disorders, 6,* 193–211.

Chambless, D. L., & Williams, K. E. (1995). A preliminary study of African Americans with agoraphobia: Symptom severity and outcome of treatment with in vivo exposure. *Behavior Therapy, 26,* 501–515.

Chapman, T. F. (1993). *Assortive mating and mental illness.* Unpublished doctoral dissertation, Yale University, New Haven, CT.

Chee, K-Y., & Sachdev, P. (1994). The clinical features of Tourette's disorder: An Australian study using a structured interview schedule. *Australian and New Zealand Journal of Psychiatry, 28,* 313–318.

Clark, D. B., & Agras, W. S. (1991). The assessment and treatment of performance anxiety in musicians. *American Journal of Psychiatry, 148,* 598–605.

Clark, D. M. (1986). A cognitive approach to panic. *Behaviour Research and Therapy, 24,* 461–470.

Clark, D. M., & Wells, A. (1995). A cognitive model of social phobia. In R. Heimberg, M. Liebowitz, D. Hope, & F. Schneier (Eds.), *Social phobia: Diagnosis, assessment and treatment* (pp. 69–93). New York: Guilford Press.

Coleman, R. E., & Gantman, C. A. (1989). Generalized anxiety disorder. In C. Lindemann (Ed.), *Handbook of phobia therapy: Rapid symptom relief in anxiety disorders* (pp. 113–143). Northvale, NJ: Jason Aronson.

Costello, C. G. (1982). Fears and phobias in women: A community study. *Journal of Abnormal Psychology, 91,* 280–286.

Cox, B. J., Direnfeld, D. M., Swinson, R. P., & Norton, G. R. (1994). Suicidal ideation and suicide attempts in panic disorder and social phobia. *American Journal of Psychiatry, 151,* 882–887.

Cox, B. J., Swinson, R. P., Shulman, I. D., Kuch, K., & Reichman, J. T. (1993). Gender effects and alcohol use in panic disorder with agoraphobia. *Behaviour Research and Therapy, 31,* 413–416.

Craske, M. G., Rapee, R. M., Jackel, L., & Barlow, D. H. (1989). Qualitative dimensions of worry in DSM-III-R generalized anxiety subjects and nonanxious controls. *Behaviour Research and Therapy, 27,* 397–402.

Crozier, W. R., & Burnham, M. (1990). Age-related differences in children's understanding of shyness. *British Journal of Developmental Psychology, 8,* 179–185.

de Beurs, E., Lange, A., van Dyck, R., & Koele, P. (1995). Respiratory training prior to exposure in vivo in the treatment of panic disorder with agoraphobia: Efficacy and predictors of outcome. *Australian and New Zealand Journal of Psychiatry, 29,* 104–113.

Deffenbacher, J. L., & Suinn, R. M. (1987). Generalized anxiety syndrome. In L. Michelson & L. M. Ascher (Eds.), *Anxiety and stress disorders* (pp. 332–360). New York: Guilford Press.

Dick, C. L., Bland, R. C., & Newman, S. C. (1994). Panic disorder. *Acta Psychiatrica Scandinavica, 89*(Suppl.), 45–53.

Dodge, C. S., Heimberg, R. G., Nyman, D., & O'Brien, G. T. (1987). Daily heterosocial interactions of high and low socially anxious college students: A diary study. *Behavior Therapy, 18,* 90–96.

Dugas, M., Letarte, H., Rheaume, J., Freeston, M. H., & Ladouceur, R. (1995). Worry and problem solving: Evidence of a specific relationship. *Cognitive Therapy and Research, 19,* 109–120.

Eaton, W. W., Kessler, R. C., Wittchen, H-U., & Magee, W. J. (1994). Panic and panic disorder in the United States. *American Journal of Psychiatry, 151,* 413–420.

Ehlers, A. (1993). Interoception and panic disorder. *Advances in Behaviour Research and Therapy, 15,* 3–21.

Eisen, J. L., & Rasmussen, S. A. (1989). Coexisting obsessive compulsive disorder and alcoholism. *Journal of Clinical Psychiatry, 50,* 96–98.

Eisen, J. L., & Rasmussen, S. A. (1993). Obsessive–compulsive disorder with psychotic features. *Journal of Clinical Psychiatry, 54,* 373–379.

Eisen, J. L., & Steketee, G. (1997). Course of illness in obsessive compulsive disorder. In L. Dickstein (Ed.), *Annual review of psychiatry: Volume 16: OCD across the lifecycle* (pp. III-73–III-95). Washington, DC: American Psychiatric Press.

Elsarrag, M. E. (1968). Psychiatry in the northern Sudan: A study in comparative psychiatry. *British Journal of Psychiatry, 114,* 945–948.

Emmelkamp, P.M.G., & Beens, H. (1991). Cognitive therapy with obsessive–compulsive disorder: A comparative evaluation. *Behaviour Research and Therapy, 29,* 293–300.

Falloon, I.R.H., Lloyd, G. G., & Harpin, R. E. (1981). The treatment of social phobia: Real-life rehearsal with nonprofessional therapists. *Journal of Nervous and Mental Disease, 169,* 180–184.

Faravelli, C. B., Innocenti, G. D., & Girdinelli, L. (1989). Epidemiology of anxiety disorders in Florence. *Acta Psychiatrica Scandinavica, 79,* 308–312.

Fenton, W. S., & McGlashan, T. H. (1986). The prognostic significance of obsessive–compulsive symptoms in schizophrenia (1985, Dallas, Texas). *American Journal of Psychiatry, 143,* 437–441.

Fink, C. M., Turner, S. M., & Beidel, D. C. (1996). Culturally relevant factors in the behavioral treatment of social phobia: A case study. *Journal of Anxiety Disorders, 10,* 201–210.

Fitz, A. (1990). Religious and familial factors in the etiology of OCD: A review. *Journal of Psychology and Theology, 18,* 141–147.

Flament, M. F. (1994). Recent findings in childhood onset obsessive–compulsive disorder. In E. Hollander, J. Zohar, D. Marazziti, & B. Olivier (Eds.), *Current insights in obsessive–compulsive disorder* (pp. 23–40). New York: John Wiley & Sons.

Flament, M. F., Whitaker, A., Rapoport, J. L., Davies, M., Berg, C. Z., Kalikow, K., Sceery, W., & Shaffer, D. (1988). Obsessive–compulsive disorder in adolescence: An epidemiological study. *Journal of the American Academy of Child and Adolescent Psychiatry, 27,* 764–771.

Foa, E. B., & Kozak, M. J. (1986). Emotional processing of fear: Exposure to corrective information. *Psychological Bulletin, 44,* 20–35.

Foa, E. B., & Tillmanns, A. (1980). The treatment of obsessive–compulsive neurosis. In A. Goldstein & E. B. Foa (Eds.), *Handbook of behavioral interventions: A clinical guide* (pp. 416–500). New York: John Wiley & Sons.

Freeston, M. H., & Dugas, M. (1994, November). *GAD: Support for DSM-IV modifications.* Paper presented at the Annual Meeting of the Association for the Advancement of Behavior Therapy, San Diego.

Freeston, M. H., Ladouceur, R., Thibodeau, N., & Gagnon, F. (1992). Cognitive intrusions in a non-clinical population: II. Associations with depressive, anxious, and compulsive symptoms. *Behaviour Research and Therapy, 30,* 263–272.

Freud, S. (1925). Notes upon a case of obsessional neurosis. In *Collected papers* (Vol. 3, pp. 293–383). London: Hogarth Press. Originally published in 1909.

Friedman, S., Hatch, M., Paradis, C. M., Popkin, M., & Shalita, A. R. (1995). Obsessive–compulsive disorders in two black ethnic groups: Incidence in an urban dermatology clinic. *Journal of Anxiety Disorders, 7,* 343–348.

Friedman, S., Paradis, C. M., & Hatch, M. (1994). Characteristics of African American and white patients with panic disorder and agoraphobia. *Hospital and Community Psychiatry, 45,* 798–803.

Fyer, A. J., Mannuzza, S., Chapman, T. F., Liebowitz, M. R., & Klein, D. F. (1993). A direct interview family study of socia phobia. *Archives of General Psychiatry, 50,* 286–293.

Garcia-Coll, C., Kagan, J., & Reznick, J. S. (1984). Behavioral inhibition in young children. *Child Development, 55,* 1005–1019.

Gelernter, C. S., Stein, M. B., Tancer, M. E., & Uhde, T. W. (1992). An examination of syndromal validity and diagnostic subtypes in social phobia and panic disorder. *Journal of Clinical Psychiatry, 52,* 23–27.

Goisman, R. M., Goldenberg, I., Vasile, R. G., & Keller, M. B. (1995). Comorbidity of anxiety disorders in a multicultural anxiety study. *Comprehensive Psychiatry, 36,* 303–311.

Goisman, R. M., Warshaw, M. G., Peterson, L. G., Rogers, M., Cuneo, P., Hunt, M., Tomlin-Albanese, J., Kazin, A., Gollan, J., Epstein-Kaye, T., Reich, J., & Keller, M. (1994). Panic, agoraphobia, and panic disorder with agoraphobia: Data from a multicenter anxiety disorders study. *Journal of Nervous and Mental Disease, 182,* 72–79.

Goisman, R. M., Warshaw, M. G., Steketee, G. S., Fierman, E. J., Rogers, M. P., Goldenberg, I., Weinshenker, N. J., Vasile, R. G., & Keller, M. B. (1995). DSM-IV and the disappearance of agoraphobia without a history of panic disorder: New data on a controversial diagnosis. *American Journal of Psychiatry, 152,* 1430–1443.

Goldstein, A. J., & Chambless, D. L. (1978). A reanalysis of agoraphobia. *Behavior Therapy, 9,* 47–59.

Greist, J. H., Jefferson, J. W., Kobak, K. A., Katzelnick, D. J., & Serlin, R. C. (1995). Efficacy and tolerability of serotonin transport inhibitors in obsessive–compulsive disorder. *Archives of General Psychiatry, 52,* 605–612.

Guarnaccia, P. J. (1993). *Ataques de nervios* in Puerto Rico: Culture-bound syndrome or popular illness? *Medical Anthropology, 15,* 157–170.

Guidano, V. L., & Liotti, G. (1983). *Cognitive processes and emotional disorders.* New York: Guilford Press.

Heimberg, R. G., Hope, D. A., Dodge, C. S., & Becker, R. E. (1990). DSM-III-R subtypes of social phobia: Comparison of generalized social phobics and public speaking phobics. *Journal of Nervous and Mental Disease, 178,* 172–179.

Heimberg, R. G., & Juster, H. R. (1995). Cognitive–behavioral treatments: Literature review. In R. G. Heimberg, M. R. Liebowitz, D. A. Hope, & F. R. Schneier (Eds.), *Social phobia: Diagnosis, assessment, and treatment* (pp. 261–309). New York: Guilford Press.

Henderson, J. G., & Pollard, C. A. (1988). Three types of obsessive compulsive disorder in a community sample. *Journal of Clinical Psychology, 44,* 747–752.

Heninger, G. R. (1994). Mechanism of action of drugs used in the pharmocotherapy of panic disorder. In B. E. Wolfe & J. D. Maser (Eds.), *Treatment of panic disorder* (pp. 91–102). Washington, DC: American Psychiatric Press.

Higley, J. D., & Suomi, S. J. (1989). Temperamental reactivity in nonhuman primates. In G. A. Kohnstamm, J. E. Bates, & M. K. Rothbart (Eds.), *Temperament in childhood* (pp. 153–167). New York: John Wiley & Sons.

Hoffart, A., Thornes, K., Hedley, L. M., & Strand, J. (1994). DSM-III-R Axis I and II disorders in agoraphobic patients with and without panic disorder. *Acta Psychiatrica Scandinavica, 89,* 186–191.

Hoehn-Saric, R., McLeod, D. R., & Zimmerli, W. D. (1989). Symptoms and treatment responses of generalized anxiety disorder patients with high versus low levels of cardiovascular complaints. *American Journal of Psychiatry, 146,* 854–859.

Hollander, E. (1993). Introduction. In E. Hollander (Ed.), *Obsessive–compulsive related disorders.* Washington, DC: American Psychiatric Press.

Hollander, E., DeCaria, C., Gully, R., Nitescu, A., Suckow, R. F., Gorman, J. M., Klein, D. F., & Liebowitz, M. R. (1991). Effects of chronic fluoxetine treatment on behavioral and neuroendocrine responses to meta-chlorophenylpiperazine in obsessive–compulsive disorder. *Psychiatry Research, 36,* 1–17.

Hollister, L. E. (1992). Panic disorder: Old wine in new bottles? *Integrative Psychiatry, 8,* 75–83.

Holt, C. S., Heimberg, R. G., Hope, D. A., & Liebowitz, M. R. (1992). Situational domains of social phobia. *Journal of Anxiety Disorders, 6,* 63–77.

Hope, D. A., & Heimberg, R. G. (1993). Social phobia and social anxiety. In D. H. Barlow (Ed.), *Clinical handbook of psychological disorders: A step-by-step treatment manual* (2nd ed., pp. 13–37). New York: Guilford Press.

Hornsveld, R.H.J., Kraaimaat, F. W., & van Dam-Baggen, R.M.J. (1979). Anxiety/discomfort and handwashing in obsessive–compulsive and psychiatric control patients. *Behaviour Research and Therapy, 17,* 223–228.

Horwath, E., Johnson, J., & Hornig, C. D. (1993). Epidemiology of panic disorder in African Americans. *American Journal of Psychiatry, 150,* 465–469.

Horwath, E., Wolk, S. I., Goldstein, R. B., Wickramaratne, P., Sobin, C., Adams, P., Lish, J. D., & Weissman, M. M. (1995). Is the comorbidity between social phobia and panic disorder due to familial cotransmission or other factors? *Archives of General Psychiatry, 52,* 574–582.

Hubbard, J., Realmuto, G. M., Northwood, A. K., & Masten, A. S. (1995). Comorbidity of psychiatric diagnoses with posttraumatic stress disorder in survivors of childhood trauma. *Journal of the American Academy of Child and Adolescent Psychiatry, 34,* 1167–1173.

Hudson, J. I., Pope, H. G., Yurgelun-Todd, D., Jonas, J. M., & Frankenburg, F. R. (1987). A controlled study of anorexia nervosa and obsessive nervosa. *British Journal of Psychiatry, 27,* 57–60.

Hwu, H., Yeh, E. K., & Chang, L. Y. (1989). Prevalence of psychiatric disorders in Taiwan defined by the Chinese Diagnostic Interview Schedule. *Acta Psychiatrica Scandinavica, 79,* 136–147.

Insel, T. R. (1992). Toward a neuroanatomy of obsessive–compulsive disorder. *Archives of General Psychiatry, 49,* 739–744.

Insel, T. R., & Akiskal, H. S. (1986). Obsessive–compulsive disorder with psychotic features: A phenomenologic analysis. *American Journal of Psychiatry, 143,* 1527–1533.

Insel, T. R., & Winslow, J. T. (1990). Neurobiology of obsessive–compulsive disorder. In M. A. Jenike, L. Baer, & W. E. Miniciello (Eds.), *Obsessive-compulsive disorders: Theory and management* (pp. 118–131). Chicago: Year Book Medical.

Janet, P. (1903). *Les obsessions et la psychasthenie [Obsessions and neurasthenia]* (Vol. 1). Paris: Alcan.

Johnson, J., Weissman, M. M., & Klerman, G. L. (1990). Panic disorder, comorbidity, and suicide attempts. *Archives of General Psychiatry, 47,* 805–808.

Kagan, J., Reznick, J. S., Snidman, N., Gibbons, J., & Johnson, M. O. (1988). Childhood derivatives of inhibition and lack of inhibition to the unfamiliar. *Child Development, 59,* 1580–1589.

Kagan, J., Snidman, N., & Arcus, D. M. (1992). Initial reactions to unfamiliarity. *Current Directions in Psychological Science, 1,* 171–174.

Karno, M., & Golding, J. (1991). Obsessive–compulsive disorder. In L. N. Robins & D. A. Regier (Eds.), *Psychiatric disorders in America: The Epidemiologic Catchment Area study* (pp. 204–219). London: Free Press.

Karno, M., Golding, J. M., Sorenson, S. B., & Burnam, M. A. (1988). The epidemiology of obsessive–compulsive disorder in five US communities. *Archives of General Psychiatry, 45,* 1094–1099.

Katon, W. (1994). Primary care–psychiatry panic disorder management module. In B. E. Wolfe & J. D. Maser (Eds.), *Treatment of panic disorder* (pp. 41–56). Washington, DC: American Psychiatric Press.

Keller, M. B., Yonkers, K. A., Warshae, M. G., Pratt, L. A., Gollan, J. K., Massion, A. O., White, K., Swartz, A. R., Reich, J., & Lavori, P. W. (1994). Remission and relapse in subjects with panic disorder and panic with agoraphobia: A prospective short-interval naturalistic follow-up. *Journal of Nervous and Mental Disease, 182,* 290–296.

Kendler, K. S., MacLean, C., Neale, M., & Kessler, K. C. (1991). The genetic epidemiology of bulimia nervosa. *American Journal of Psychiatry, 148,* 1627–1637.

Kendler, K. S., Neale, M. C., Kessler, R. C., Heath, A. C., & Eaves, L. J. (1992). The genetic epidemiology of phobias in women: The interrelations of agoraphobia, social phobia, situational phobia, and simple phobia. *Archives of General Psychiatry, 49,* 273–281.

Kessler, R. C., McDonagle, K., Zhao, S., Nelson, C., Hughes, M., Eshleman, S., Wittchen, H-U., & Kendler, K. S. (1994). Lifetime and 12-month prevalence of DSM-III psychiatric disorders in the United States: Results from the National Comorbidity Survey. *Archives of General Psychiatry, 51,* 8–19.

Khanna, S., & Channabasavanna, S. (1987). Towards a classification of compulsions in obsessive–compulsive neurosis. *Psychopathology, 20,* 23–28.

Klass, E. T., Di Nardo, P. A., & Barlow, D. H. (1989). DSM-III-R personality diagnoses in anxiety disorder patients. *Comprehensive Psychiatry, 30,* 251–258.

Klein, D. F. (1993). False suffocation alarms, spontaneous panics, and related conditions: An integrative hypothesis. *Archives of General Psychiatry, 50,* 306–317.

Klein, D. F., & Gorman, J. M. (1987). A model of panic and agoraphobic development. *Acta Psychiatrica Scandinavica, 76,* 87–95.

Klerman, G. L. (1992). Treatments for panic disorder. *Journal of Clinical Psychiatry, 53* (Suppl.), 14–19.

Kozak, M. J., & Foa, E. B. (1994). Obsessions, overvalued ideas, and delusions in obsessive–compulsive disorder. *Behaviour Research and Therapy, 32,* 343–353.

Kushner, M. G., Sher, K. J., & Beitman, B. D. (1990). The relation between alcohol problems and the anxiety disorders. *American Journal of Psychiatry, 147,* 685–695.

Kushner, M. G., Thomas, A. M., Bartels, K. M., & Beitman, B. D. (1992). Panic disorder history in the families of patients with angiographically normal coronary arteries. *American Journal of Psychiatry, 149,* 1563–1567.

Ladouceur, R., Rheaume, J., Freeston, M. H., Aublet, F., Jean, K., Lachance, S., Langlois, F., & de Pokomandy-Morin, K. (1995). Experimental manipulations of responsibility: An analogue test for models of obsessive–compulsive disorder. *Behaviour Research and Therapy, 33*, 937–946.

Lee, C. K., Kwak, Y. S., Yamamoto, J., Rhee, H., Kim, Y. S., Han, J. H., Choi, J. O., & Lee, Y. H. (1990). Psychiatric epidemiology in Korea: I. Gender and age differences in Seoul. *Journal of Nervous and Mental Disease, 178*, 242–246.

Levin, A. P., Schneier, F. R., & Liebowitz, M. R. (1989). Social phobia: Biology and pharmacology. *Clinical Psychology Review, 9*, 129–140.

Ley, R. (1985). Blood, breath, and fears: A hyperventilation theory of panic attacks and agoraphobia. *Clinical Psychology Review, 5*, 271–285.

Liebowitz, M. R. (1987). Social phobia. *Modern Problems of Pharmacopsychiatry, 22*, 141–173.

Liebowitz, M. R., Campeas, R., & Hollander, E. (1987). MAOIs: Impact on social behavior [Letter to the Editor]. *Psychiatry Research, 22*, 89–90.

Liebowitz, M. R., & Fyer, A. J. (1994). Diagnosis and clinical course of panic disorder with and without agoraphobia. In B. E. Wolfe & J. D. Maser (Eds.), *Treatment of panic disorder* (pp. 19–30). Washington, DC: American Psychiatric Press.

Liebowitz, M. R., Salmán, B. S., Jusino, C. M., Garfinkel, R., Street, L., Cárdenas, D. L., Silvestre, J., Fyer, A. J., Carrasco, J. L., Davies, S., Guarnaccia, P., & Klein, D. F. (1994). *Ataque de nervios* and panic disorder. *American Journal of Psychiatry, 151*, 871–875.

Livingston-Van Noppen, B., Rasmussen, S., Eisen, J., & McCartney, L. (1990). Family function and treatment in obsessive–compulsive disorder. In M. Jenike, L. Baer, & W. Minichiello (Eds.), *Obsessive–compulsive disorders: Theory and management* (pp. 325–340). Chicago: Year Book Medical.

Lo, W. H. (1967). A follow-up study of obsessional neurotics in Hong Kong Chinese. *British Journal of Psychiatry, 113*, 823–832.

Lovibond, P. F., & Rapee, R. M. (1993). The representation of feared outcomes. *Behaviour Research and Therapy, 31*, 595–608.

Ludwig, R. P., & Lazarus, P. J. (1983). Relationship between shyness in children and constricted cognitive control as measured by the Stroop Color–Word Test. *Journal of Consulting and Clinical Psychology, 51*, 386–389.

Lyonfields, J. D., Borkovec, T. D., & Thayer, J. F. (1995). Vagal tone in generalized anxiety disorder and the effects of aversive imagery and worrisome thinking. *Behavior Therapy, 26*, 457–466.

Mancuso, D. M., Townsend, M. H., & Mercante, D. E. (1993). Long-term follow-up of generalized anxiety disorder. *Comprehensive Psychiatry, 34*, 441–446.

Mannuzza, S., Fyer, A. J., Liebowitz, M. R., & Klein, D. F. (1990). Delineating the boundaries of social phobia: Its relationship to panic disorder and agoraphobia. *Journal of Anxiety Disorders, 4*, 41–59.

Margraf, J. (1993). Hyperventilation and panic disorder: A psychophysiological connection. *Advances in Behaviour Research and Therapy, 15*, 49–74.

Margraf, J., Ehlers, A., & Roth, W. T. (1988). Mitral valve prolapse and panic disorder: A review of their relationship. *Psychosomatic Medicine, 50*, 93–113.

Markowitz, J. S., Weissman, M. M., Ouellette, R., Lishe, J. D., & Klerman, G. L. (1989). Quality of life in panic disorder. *Archives of General Psychiatry, 46*, 984–992.

Marks, I. M. (1969). *Fears and phobias.* New York: Academic Press.

Marten, P. A., & Brown, T. A. (1993). Evaluation of the ratings comprising the associated symptom criterion of DSM-III-R generalized anxiety disorder. *Journal of Nervous and Mental Disease, 181*, 646–682.

Massion, A. O., Warshaw, M. G., & Keller, M. B. (1993). Quality of life and psychiatric morbidity in panic disorder and generalized anxiety disorder. *American Journal of Psychiatry, 150,* 600–607.

Mavissakalian, M. R., & Hamann, M. S. (1987). DSM-III personality disorders in agoraphobia: II. Changes with treatment. *Comprehensive Psychiatry, 28,* 356–361.

Mavissakalian, M. R., Hamann, M. S., Haidar, S. A., & de Groot, C. M. (1995). Correlates of DSM-III personality disorder in generalized anxiety disorder. *Journal of Anxiety Disorders, 9,* 103–115.

Mavissakalian, M. R., Hamann, M. S., & Jones, B. (1990). A comparison of DSM-III personality disorders in panic/agoraphobia and obsessive–compulsive disorder. *Comprehensive Psychiatry, 31,* 238–244.

McFall, M. E., & Wollersheim, J. P. (1979). Obsessive–compulsive neurosis: A cognitive behavioral formulation and approach to treatment. *Cognitive Therapy and Research, 3,* 333–348.

McNally, R. J. (1994). *Panic disorder: A critical analysis.* New York: Guilford Press.

Mellman, T. A., & Uhde, T. W. (1987). Obsessive–compulsive symptoms in panic disorder. *American Journal of Psychiatry, 12,* 1573–1576.

Mendlewicz, J., Papdimitriou, G., & Wilmotte, J. (1993). Family study of panic disorder: Comparison with generalized anxiety disorder, major depression and normal subjects. *Psychiatric Genetics, 3,* 73–78.

Mineka, S., & Zinbarg, R. (1995). Conditioning and ethological models of social phobia. In R. Heimberg, M. Liebowitz, D. Hope, & F. Schneier (Eds.), *Social phobia: Diagnosis, assessment and treatment* (pp. 134–162). New York: Guilford Press.

Myers, J. K., Weissman, M. M., Tischler, G. L., Holzer, C. E., III, Leaf, P. J., Orvachel, H., Anthony, J. D., Boyd, J. H., Burke, J. D., Jr., Kramer, M., & Stolzman, R. (1984). Six-month prevalence of psychiatric disorders in three communities: 1980–1982. *Archives of General Psychiatry, 41,* 959–967.

Neal, A., & Turner, S. (1991). Anxiety disorders research with African Americans. *Psychological Bulletin, 109,* 400–410.

Neligh, G., Baron, A. E., Braun, P., & Czarnecki, M. (1990). Panic disorder among American Indians: A descriptive study. *American Indian and Alaska Native Mental Health Research, 4,* 43–53.

Nickell, P. V., & Uhde, T. W. (1995). Neurobiology of social phobia. In R. Heimberg, M. Liebowitz, D. Hope, & F. Scheiner (Eds.), *Social phobia: Diagnosis, assessment and treatment* (pp. 113–133). New York: Guilford Press.

Noyes, R., Jr., Garvey, M. J., Cook, B. L., & Samuelson, L. (1989). Follow-up study of patients with panic disorder and agoraphobia with panic attacks treated with tricyclic antidepressants. *Journal of Affective Disorders, 16,* 249–257.

Noyes, R., Woodman, C., Garvey, M. J., & Cook, B. L. (1992). Generalized anxiety disorder vs. panic disorder: Distingishing characteristics and patterns of comorbidity. *Journal of Nervous and Mental Disease, 180,* 369–379.

Oberlander, E. L., Schneier, F. R., & Liebowitz, M. R. (1994). Physical disability and social phobia. *Journal of Clinical Psychopharmacology, 14,* 136–143.

Ohman, A. (1986). Face the beast and fear the face: Animal and social fears as prototypes for evolutionary analyses of emotion. *Psychophysiology, 23,* 123–145.

Ohman, A., Dimberg, U., & Ost, L. G. (1985). Animal and social phobias: Biological constraints on the learned fear response. In S. Reiss & R. Bootzin (Eds.), *Theoretical issues in behavior therapy* (pp. 123–175). New York: Academic Press.

Papp, L. A., Martinez, J. M., Klein, D. F., Coplan, J. D., & Gorman, J. M. (1995). Rebreathing tests in panic disorder. *Biological Psychiatry, 30,* 240–245.

Pauls, D. L., Alsobrook S. P., Goodman, W. K., Rasmussen, S. A., & Leckman, J. L. (1995). A family study of obsessive–compulsive disorder. *American Journal of Psychiatry, 152,* 76–84.

Pauls, D. L., Towbin, K. E., Leckman, J. G., Zahner, G.E.P., & Cohen, D. J. (1986). Gilles de la Tourette syndrome and obsessive–compulsive disorder: Evidence supporting an etiological relationship. *Archives of General Psychiatry, 43,* 1180–1182.

Pitman, R. K. (1987). A cybernetic model of obsessive–compulsive psychopathology. *Comprehensive Psychiatry, 28,* 334–343.

Pollard, C. A., & Henderson, J. G. (1988). Four types of social phobia in a community sample. *Journal of Nervous and Mental Disease, 176,* 440–445.

Potts, N.L.S., & Davidson, J.T.R. (1995). Pharmacological treatments: Literature review. In R. Heimberg, M. Liebowitz, D. Hope, & F. Scheiner (Eds.), *Social phobia: Diagnosis, assessment and treatment* (pp. 334–365). New York: Guilford Press.

Power, K. G., Simpson, R. J., Swanson, V., & Wallace, L. A. (1990). A controlled comparison of cognitive–behavior therapy, diazepam, and placebo, alone and in combination, for the treatment of generalized anxiety disorder. *Journal of Anxiety Disorders, 4,* 267–292.

Rachman, S. (1976). Obsessional–compulsive checking. *Behaviour Research and Therapy, 14,* 437–443.

Rachman, S. J. (1977). The conditioning theory of fear aquisition: A critical examination. *Behaviour Research and Therapy, 15,* 375–387.

Rachman, S., & de Silva, P. (1978). Abnormal and normal obsessions. *Behaviour Research and Therapy, 16,* 233–248.

Rachman, S., & Wilson, G. T. (1980). *The effects of psychological therapy.* Oxford, England: Pergamon Press.

Raj, B. A., Corvea, M. H., & Dagon, E. M. (1993). The clinical characteristics of panic disorder in the elderly: A retrospective study. *Journal of Clinical Psychiatry, 54,* 150–155.

Rapoport, J. L. (1986). Childhood obsessive–compulsive disorder. *Journal of Child Psychology and Psychiatry, 19,* 134–144.

Raskin, M., Peeke, H.V.S., Dickman, W., & Pinsker, H. (1982). Panic and generalized anxiety disorders. *Archives of General Psychiatry, 39,* 687–689.

Rasmussen, S., & Eisen, J. (1990). Epidemiology and clinical features of obsessive–compulsive disorder. In M. A. Jenike, L. Baer, & W. G. Minichiello (Eds.), *Obsessive–compulsive disorders: Theory and management* (pp. 10–27). Chicago: Year Book Medical.

Rasmussen, S., & Eisen, J. (1991). Phenomenology of obsessive–compulsive disorder. In J. Insel & S. Rasmussen (Eds.), *Psychobiology of obsessive–compulsive disorder* (pp. 743–758). New York: Springer-Verlag.

Rasmussen, S., & Tsuang, M. (1986). DSM-III obsessive–compulsive disorder: Clinical characteristics and family history. *American Journal of Psychiatry, 143,* 317–322.

Reed, G. F. (1985). *Obsessional experience and compulsive behavior.* Orlando, FL: Academic Press.

Reich, J., Noyes, R., & Troughton, E. (1987). Dependent personality disorder associated with phobic avoidance in patients with panic disorder. *American Journal of Psychiatry, 144,* 323–326.

Reich, J., Warshaw, M., Peterson, L. G., White, K., Keller, M., Lavori, P., & Yonkers, K. A. (1993). Comorbidity of panic and major depressive disorder. *Journal of Psychiatric Research, 27*(Suppl. 1), 23–33.

Reich, J., & Yates, W. (1988). Family history of psychiatric disorders in social phobia. *Comprehensive Psychiatry, 29,* 72–75.

Reimann, B. C., McNally, R. J., & Cox, W. M. (1992). The comorbidity of obsessive–compulsive disorder and alcoholism. *Journal of Anxiety Disorders, 6,* 105–110.

Riddle, M. A., Scahill, L., King, R., Hardin, M. T., Towbin, K. E., Ort, S. I., Leckman, J. F., & Cohen, D. J. (1990). Obsessive–compulsive disorder in children and adolescents: Phenomenology and family history. *Journal of the American Academy of Child and Adolescent Psychiatry, 29,* 776–772.

Riggs, D. S., Hiss, H., & Foa, E. B. (1992). Marital distress and the treatment of obsessive–compulsive disorder. *Behavior Therapy, 23,* 585–597.

Robertson, M. M., Trimble, M. R., & Lees, A. J. (1988). The psychopathology of the Gilles de la Tourette syndrome: A phenomenological analysis. *British Journal of Psychiatry, 152,* 383–390.

Rosenbaum, J. F., Pollock, R. A., Otto, M. W., & Pollack, M. H. (1995). Integrated treatment of panic disorder. *Bulletin of the Menninger Clinic, 59*(Suppl. A), A4–A26.

Roy-Byrne, P., Wingerson, D., Cowley, D., & Dager, S. (1993). Psychopharmacologic treatment of panic, generalized anxiety disorder, and social phobia. *Psychiatric Clinics of North America, 16,* 719–735.

Salkovskis, P. M. (1989). Cognitive–behavioural factors and the persistence of intrusive thoughts in obsessional problems. *Behaviour Research and Therapy, 27,* 677–682.

Sanderson, W. C., Di Nardo, P. A., Rapee, R. M., & Barlow, D. H. (1990). Syndrome comorbidity in patients diagnosed with a DSM-III-Revised anxiety disorder. *Journal of Abnormal Psychology, 99,* 308–312.

Schneier, F. R., Johnson, J., Hornig, C. D., Liebowitz, M. R., & Weissman, M. M. (1992). Social phobia: Comorbidity and morbidity in an epidemiological sample. *Archives of General Psychiatry, 49,* 282–288.

Schneier, F. R., Liebowitz, M. R., Beidel, D., Fyer, A. J., George, M. S., Heimberg, R. G., Holt, C. S., Klein, A. P., Levin, A. P., Lydiard, R. B., Mannuzza, S., Martin, L. Y., Nardi, A. E., Terrill, D. R., Spitzer, R. L., Turner, S. M., Uhde, T. W., Figueira, I. V., & Versiani, M. (1994). Social phobia. In T. A. Widiger, A. J. Frances, H. A. Pincus, R. Ross, M. B. First, & W. Davis (Eds.), *DSM-IV sourcebook* (Vol. 2, pp. 507–548). Washington, DC: American Psychiatric Press.

Shadick, R. N., & Borkovec, T. D. (1991, November). *Generalized anxiety disorder and comorbid personality disorders: Prevalence and treatment.* Paper presented at the annual meeting of the Association for the Advancement of Behavior Therapy, New York.

Shafran, R., Ralph, J., & Tallis, F. (1995). Obsessive–compulsive symptoms and the family. *Bulletin of the Menninger Clinic, 59,* 472–479.

Shear, M. K., Leon, A., & Spielman, S. (1994). Panic disorder: Directions for future research. In B. E. Wolfe & J. D. Maser (Eds.), *Treatment of panic disorder* (pp. 227–236). Washington, DC: American Psychiatric Press.

Shekim, W. O., Asarnow, R. F., Hess, E., & Zaucha, K. (1990). A clinical and demographic profile of a sample of adults with attention deficit hyperactivity disorder, residual state. *Comprehensive Psychiatry, 31,* 416–425.

Shioiri, T., Murashita, J., Kato, T., Fujii, K., & Takahashi, S. (1996). Characteristic clinical features and clinical course in 270 Japanese outpatients with panic disorder. *Journal of Anxiety Disorders, 10,* 163–172.

Simeon, D., Hollander, E., & Cohen, L. (1994). Obsessive–compulsive related disorders. In E. Hollander, J. Zohar, D. Marazziti, & B. Olivier (Eds.), *Current insights in obsessive–compulsive disorder* (pp. 53–63). New York: John Wiley & Sons.

Smail, P., Stockwell, T., Canter, S., & Hodgson, R. (1984). Alcohol dependence and phobic anxiety states. I. A prevalence study. *British Journal of Psychiatry, 144,* 53–57.

Solyom, L., Ledwidge, B., & Solyom, C. (1986). Delineating social phobia. *British Journal of Psychiatry, 149,* 464–470.

Starcevic, V., Uhlenhuth, E. H., Kellner, R., & Pathak, D. (1992). Patterns of comorbidity in panic disorder and agoraphobia. *Psychiatry Research, 42,* 171–183.

Stein, M. B., Heuser, I. J., Juncos, J. L., & Uhde, T. W. (1990). Anxiety disorders in patients with Parkinson's disease. *American Journal of Psychiatry, 147,* 217–220.

Steketee, G. (1990). Personality traits and disorders in obsessive compulsives. *Journal of Anxiety Disorders, 4,* 351–364.

Steketee, G. (1993). *Treatment of obsessive–compulsive disorder.* New York: Guilford Press.

Steketee, G. S., Quay, S., & White, K. (1991). Religion and guilt in OCD patients. *Journal of Anxiety Disorders, 5,* 359–367.

Stemberger, R. T., Turner, S. M., Beidel, D. C., & Calhoun, K. S. (1995). Social phobia: An analysis of possible developmental factors. *Journal of Abnormal Psychology, 104,* 526–531.

Strauss, C. C., & Last, C. G. (1993). Social and simple phobias in children. *Journal of Anxiety Disorders, 7,* 141–152.

Swedo, S., Rapoport, J., Leonard, H., Lenane, M. C., & Cheslow, D. L. (1989). Obsessive–compulsive disorder in children and adolescents. *Archives of General Psychiatry, 46,* 335–345.

Telch, M. J., Schmidt, N. B., Jaimez, T. L., Jacquin, K. M., & Harrington, P. J. (1995). Impact of cognitive–behavioral treatment on quality of life in panic disorder patients. *Journal of Consulting and Clinical Psychology, 63,* 823–830.

Thayer, J. F., Friedman, B. H., & Borkovec, T. D. (1996). Autonomic characteristics of generalized anxiety disorder and worry. *Biological Psychiatry, 39,* 255–266.

Townsley, R. (1992). *Social phobia: Identification of possible etiological factors.* Unpublished doctoral dissertation, University of Georgia, Athens.

Turner, S. M., Beidel, D. C., Borden, J. W., Stanley, M. A., & Jacob, R. G. (1991). Social phobia: Axis I and II correlates. *Journal of Abnormal Psychology, 100,* 102–106.

Turner, S. M., Beidel, D. C., Dancu, C. V., & Keys, D. J. (1986). Psychopathology of social phobia and comparison to avoidant personality disorder. *Journal of Abnormal Psychology, 95,* 389–394.

Turner, S. M., Beidel, D. C., & Nathan, R. S. (1985). Biological factors in obsessive–compulsive disorders. *Psychological Bulletin, 97,* 430–450.

Turner, S. M., Beidel, D. C., & Townsley, R. M. (1990). Social phobia: Relationship to shyness. *Behaviour Research and Therapy, 28,* 497–505.

Turner, S. M., Beidel, D. C., & Townsley, R. M. (1992). Social phobia: A comparison of specific and generalized subtypes and avoidant personality disorder. *Journal of Abnormal Psychology, 101,* 326–331.

Van Noppen, B., Steketee, G., McCorkle, B. H., & Pato, M. (1997). Group and multifamily behavioral treatment for obsessive–compulsive disorder: A pilot study. *Journal of Anxiety Disorders, 11,* 431–446.

Van Oppen, P., De Haan, E., Van Balkom, A.J.L.M., Spinhoven, P., Hoogduin, K., & Van Dyck, R. (1995). Cognitive therapy and exposure in vivo in the treatment of obsessive–compulsive disorder. *Behaviour Research and Therapy, 33,* 379–390.

Warren, R., & Zgourides, G. D. (1991). *Anxiety disorders: A rational–emotive perspective.* New York: Pergamon Press.

Warshaw, M. G., Massion, A. O., Peterson, L. G., Pratt, L. A., & Keller, M. B. (1995). Suicidal behavior in patients with panic disorder: Retrospective and prospective data. *Journal of Affective Disorders, 34,* 235–247.

Weiller, E., Boyer, P., Lepine, J. P., & Lecrubier, Y. (1994). Prevalence of recurrent brief depression in primary care. Special Issue: Recurrent brief depression. *European Archives of Psychiatry and Clinical Neuroscience, 244,* 174–181.

Weissman, M. (1990). The hidden patient: Unrecognized panic disorder. *Journal of Clinical Psychiatry, 51*(Suppl.), 5–8.

Weissman, M. (1994). Panic disorder: Epidemiology and genetics. In B. E. Wolfe & J. D. Maser (Eds.), *Treatment of panic disorder* (pp. 31–39). Washington, DC: American Psychiatric Press.

Weissman, M. M., Bland, R. C., Canino, G. J., Greenwald, S., Hwu, H-G., Lee, C. K., Newman, S. C., Oakley-Browne, M. A., Rubio-Stipec, M., Wickramaratne, P. J., Wittchen, H-U., & Yeh, E-K. (1994). The cross-national epidemiology of obsessive–compulsive disorder. *Journal of Clinical Psychiatry, 55,* 5–10.

Westling, D. E., & Ost, L. G. (1995). Cognitive bias in panic disorder patients and changes after cognitive behavioral treatments. *Behaviour Research and Therapy, 33,* 585–588.

Westphal, C. (1871). Die agoraphobie: Eine neuropathische erscheinung [Agoraphobia: A neuropathological manifestation]. *Archiv fur psychiatrie und Nervenkrankheiten, 3,* 138–171.

Widiger, T. A. (1992). Generalized social phobia versus avoidant personality disorder: A commentary on three studies. *Journal of Abnormal Psychology, 101,* 340–343.

Wittchen, H-U., & Essau, C. A. (1993). Epidemiology of panic disorder: Progress and unresolved issues. *Journal of Psychiatric Research, 27*(Suppl. 1), 47–68.

Wittchen, H-U., Zhao, S., Kessler, R. C., & Eaton, W. W. (1994). Generalized anxiety disorder in the National Comorbidity Survey. *Archives of General Psychiatry, 51,* 355–364.

Wolfe, B. E., & Maser, J. D. (Eds.). (1994). *Treatment of panic disorder: A consensus development conference.* Washington, DC: American Psychiatric Press.

Woodman, C. L. (1993). The genetics of panic disorder and generalized anxiety disorder. *Annals of Clinical Psychiatry, 5,* 231–239.

Woody, S., & Rachman, S. (1994). Generalized anxiety disorder (GAD) as an unsuccessful search for safety. *Clinical Psychology Review, 14,* 743–753.

Yonkers, K. A., Warshaw, M. G., Massion, A. C., & Keller, M. B. (1996). Phenomenology and course of generalized anxiety disorder. *British Journal of Psychiatry, 168,* 308–313.

Zohar, J., Insel, T. R., Berman, K. F., Foa, E. B., Hill, J. L., & Weinberger, D. R. (1989). Anxiety and cerebral blood flow during behavioral challenge: Dissociation of central from peripheral and subjective measures. *Archives of General Psychiatry, 46,* 505–510.

# Suggested Reading

Panic and Agoraphobic Disorders

Burrows, G. D., Roth, M., & Noyes, R. (Eds.). (1990). *Neurobiology of anxiety.* Amsterdam: Elsevier.

McNally, R. J. (1995). *Panic disorder: A critical analysis.* New York: Guilford Press.

Rachman, S., & Maser, J. D. (Eds.). (1988). *Panic: Psychological perspectives.* Hillsdale, NJ: Lawrence Erlbaum.

Walker, J. R., Norton, G. R., & Ross, C. A. (Eds.). (1991). *Panic disorder and agoraphobia: A comprehensive guide for the practitioner.* Pacific Grove, CA: Brooks/Cole.

## Social Phobia

Heimberg, R. G., Liebowitz, M. R., Hope, D. A., & Schneier, F. R. (Eds.). (1995). *Social phobia: Diagnosis, assessment and treatment.* New York: Guilford Press.

Turner, S. M., Beidel, D. C., & Townsley, R. M. (1992). Behavioral treatment of social phobia. In S. Turner, K. Calhoun, & H. Adams (Eds.), *Handbook of clinical behavior therapy* (2nd ed., pp. 13–37). New York: John Wiley & Sons.

## GAD

Barlow, D. H. (1988). *Anxiety and its disorders.* New York: Guilford Press.

Davey, G.C.L., & Tallis, F. (Eds.). (1994). *Worrying: Perspectives in theory, assessment, and treatment.* New York: John Wiley & Sons.

Markway, B. G., Carmin, C. N., Pollard, C. A., & Flynn, T. (1992). *Dying of embarrassment.* Oakland, CA: New Harbinger.

## OCD

Baer, L. (1991). *Getting control.* Boston: Little, Brown.

Foa, E., & Wilson, R. (1991). *Stop obsessing!* New York: Bantam Books.

Jenike, M., Baer, L., & Minichiello, W. (Eds.). (1990). *Obsessive–compulsive disorders: Theory and management* (2nd ed.). Chicago: Year Book Medical.

Pato, M. T., & Zohar, J. (Eds.). (1991). *Current treatments of obsessive–compulsive disorder.* Washington, DC: American Psychiatric Press.

Steketee, G., & White, K. (1990). *When once is not enough.* Oakland, CA: New Harbinger.

# Schizophrenia

John S. Brekke and Elizabeth S. Slade

I live in a closet. Unlike most closets, mine is invisible. No one else can see or touch it or even come inside to keep me company. Nevertheless, its imprisoning walls and terrifying darkness are very real.

The closet is schizophrenia, a major mental illness or, as some professionals now refer to it, a neurobiological disorder. I have suffered from schizophrenia for a good part of my adult life. It is treatable but it is as yet without a cure.

The first signs of schizophrenia may appear suddenly, but often, as in my case, the onset is insidious and gradual. Although I did not have schizophrenia as a child, I see now that certain aspects of my childhood experience might be seen in hindsight as prodromal to the illness itself. For example, a certain anguishing hypersensitivity revealed itself at an early age in kindergarten: My fear of touching the play money used to teach us about real money and my distaste for the texture and color of graham crackers and apple juice we ate at snack time were so intense that I hid in the coat closet to avoid them. A few years later, I remember walking the family dog each night and believing a fire hydrant was a miniature nun who spoke to me about St. Sebastian, suggesting to me that I, too, was to die a martyr. In high school, it became harder and harder to conceal my difficulties, and although I was a good student and earned my share of As and Bs, I became virtually mute during the school day. Because of this and my habit of staring straight ahead even when addressed directly, some of the other students took to calling me "the zombie" (Wagner, 1996).

* * *

I am a person with schizophrenia. I am also a college graduate with 27 hours toward a master's degree. I have published three articles in national journals and hold a full-time position as a technical editor for a major engineering–technical documentation corporation.

I have suffered from this serious mental illness for over 25 years. In fact, I can't think of a time when I wasn't plagued with hallucinations, delusions, and paranoia. At times, it feels like the operator in my brain just doesn't get the message to the right people. It can be very confusing to have to deal with different people in my head. When I become fragmented in my thinking, I start to have my worst problems. I have been hospitalized because of this illness many times, sometimes for as long as two to four months (Jordan, 1995).

Schizophrenia is one of the most perplexing and scientifically investigated mental disorders. The quotes that open this chapter provide a small glimpse into the world of schizophrenia. Although its causes are still unknown, those who struggle to cope with the disorder and those who provide support or treatment to people with schizophrenia are well aware of the suffering and challenges it presents. In this chapter, we will highlight some recent advances in the understanding of this disorder and discuss the clinical implications of this knowledge. First, we will define some critical concepts and provide background information about schizophrenia. We will then highlight findings in five areas and briefly discuss several areas where knowledge is rapidly emerging.

This chapter is based on several assumptions. First, the amount of published research on schizophrenia is enormous. Covering the years 1990–1996, the Medline database lists nearly 10,000 articles with schizophrenia as the main focus. Because of the sheer volume of publications, we have often relied on secondary sources, such as literature reviews and edited collections. Second, this chapter will take a selective look at this vast literature, focusing on those areas in which something like breakthrough knowledge has emerged that also has significant clinical implications. Third, given the structure of this book, the literature on the treatment of schizophrenia is covered in another chapter. Fourth, although there are still unresolved diagnostic dilemmas in identifying schizophrenia, there have been large leaps in establishing the reliability and validity of our diagnostic systems. Finally, the most viable models for understanding this disorder are multivariate and biopsychosocial in nature: They involve the interaction of diathesis and stress factors to explain the occurrence and course of the disorder (see Freeman, 1989; Nicholson & Neufeld, 1992; Yank, Bentley, & Hargrove, 1993, for useful reviews). Therefore, the knowledge that this chapter surveys ranges from genetics to cross-cultural factors.

## Background Concepts and Knowledge

Establishing a valid diagnostic category for a disorder requires scientific and clinical consensus in five areas: (1) phenomenology (signs, symptoms, and traits), (2) etiology, (3) course, (4) prognosis, and (5) treatment responsiveness (Millon, 1991). In each of these areas, schizophrenia, as it is currently understood, is marked by heterogeneity. In fact, the term "heterogeneity" is so often used to describe the character of this disorder that one might conclude that there are few nomothetic patterns to deal with. Therefore, before beginning to survey our breakthrough knowledge, we will present some definitions and background knowledge.

### CONCEPTUAL BACKGROUND

By diagnostic convention, schizophrenia is marked at some point by psychosis. *Psychosis* can be broadly defined as a dramatic disruption and impairment of reality testing. It typically involves one or more of the psychotic symptoms of hallucinations, delusions, thought disorder, or bizarre behavior.[1] A *hallucination* is defined as the sensory perception of something that is not actually there. Hallucinations can occur in all five sensory domains. Approximately 50 percent of those with schizophrenia have hallucinations, the vast majority of which are auditory (Cutting, 1990, 1995). *Delusions* are false beliefs that are entrenched and impervious to reality testing. They range from the bizarre ("my brain is in a jar on Mars") to the nonbizarre ("someone has tapped my phone"). According to Cutting, approximately 90 percent of people with schizophrenia have delusions at some point.

Formal thought disorder takes many forms in schizophrenia and manifests as disorganized speech. Commonly occurring thought disorders are loose associations, or *derailment*, where unrelated or weakly related topics are strung together in sentences or phases. *Tangentiality* is marked by an elaborated train of speech or thought that begins on one topic and ends on another one with no clear relationship between the two topics. *Illogicality* refers to presenting bizarre explanations for things or events that defy common logic or our understanding of the course of nature. *Incoherence* manifests as a breakdown in the grammatical structure of speech and can result in *word salad,* or words just being strung together without regard for their content. The poverty of content of speech refers to a considerable volume of speech that contains few ideas or little actual content. Some formal thought disorder has been found to occur in a majority of people with schizophrenia (Andreasen, 1979; Cutting, 1995).

Bizarre behavior in schizophrenia can manifest in a variety of ways such as very odd dressing, sexually inappropriate behavior, or unpredictable swearing or yelling. One type of bizarre behavior is called *catatonia* and is usually marked by its involuntariness and decreased reactivity to the environment. It ranges from the virtual absence of movement while maintaining consciousness (stupor), to repetitive movement of body parts (stereotypies), or the repetition of the movements of others (echopraxia). These catatonic symptoms occur in 5 percent to 10 percent of schizophrenic cases.

Hallucinations, delusions, thought disorder, and bizarre behavior are typically called the "positive symptoms." They represent an exaggeration or overpresence of normal functions. Schizophrenia also can be marked by certain negative symptoms, which have recently taken on diagnostic significance. These symptoms reflect the absence of certain functions that are normally present such as affect, speech, pleasure, feeling, or volition. Three negative symptoms are diagnostically inclusive for schizophrenia: alogia, flat affect, and avolition. More than 50 percent of people with schizophrenia will manifest one or more negative symptoms during some phase of the disorder (Cutting, 1995).

## EPIDEMIOLOGIC BACKGROUND

The epidemiologic identity of schizophrenia has been investigated with a variety of methods. Most notable among these are the Epidemiologic Catchment Area study (ECA) (Robins & Regier, 1991) and the National Comorbidity Survey (NCS) (Kessler et al., 1994), using population-based survey methods as well as birth

---

[1]It should be noted that in modern diagnostic terms, *reality* is defined in a sociocultural context in that certain experiences, such as hearing the voice of a dead relative, are not considered psychotic if they are culturally normative.

cohort studies (for example, Helgason & Magnusson, 1989). Birth cohort studies follow a randomly selected sample of people from birth into adulthood. These studies attempt to establish the frequency, distribution, and temporal variations of schizophrenia in a population and to establish its association with other conditions or risk factors. This knowledge contributes to understanding the etiology of schizophrenia and to developing strategies for preventing or controlling the disorder. Jablensky (1995) has provided a comprehensive review of the epidemiology of schizophrenia as it is currently understood (see Hafner & Heiden, 1997, for another review). We summarize below some of Jablensky's main conclusions, which are given as background facts about the disorder for this chapter.

The morbid risk for schizophrenia is about 1 percent. This means that approximately one out of every 100 people who survive through the entire risk period for schizophrenia (generally ages 18–55) will develop the disorder. The risk rate for men and women is about equal. Although some evidence suggests that there are nonrandom pockets of higher or lower incidence, no population has been found in which schizophrenia is rare or nonexistent. The mortality of people with schizophrenia is at least double the population average. This is due mostly to suicide.

Concerning the clinical phenomenology of schizophrenia, the age of onset before puberty is rare, although there is no upper age limit for onset. The average age of onset for men is about 23 years, with the peak onset occurring between ages 18 to 25. The average age of onset for women is about 27, with peaks occurring between ages 20 to 27 and after 35. The onset of the disorder is usually preceded by a premorbid handicap in cognition, language, and social competence that might appear early in life. The mode of onset can vary between acute and insidious, with acute onset being predictive of better outcome. The long-term course of the disorder is highly variable, with about one-third of cases falling into each of the following categories: recovered, cycle of relapses and remissions, and chronic deterioration. The course and outcome of schizophrenia are significantly better in developing countries than in Western industrialized societies.

Turning to risk factors, there is strong evidence for the heritability of the disorder, and the risk of schizophrenia increases with the number of genes shared with a person manifesting the disorder. Schizophrenia carries with it an excess of minor physical anomalies, and the incidence of schizophrenia fluctuates in association with exposure to influenza during months 3–6 of gestation.

Having established some foundation in terms of concepts relevant to schizophrenia as well as background epidemiologic knowledge, we turn to five areas in which there is significant new knowledge about schizophrenia, knowledge that also has important implications for social work practice. Some of these advances will elaborate on the background knowledge we have outlined above.

## Breakthrough Areas

### *COURSE AND OUTCOME OF SCHIZOPHRENIA*

Studies on the course and outcome of schizophrenia are integral to our understanding of the characteristics and uniqueness of the disorder as well as to establishing the effects of psychosocial factors and service interventions on the trajectory of the disorder. Although it is difficult to come to definitive conclusions from recent course studies because of some methodological considerations that will be addressed below, we include this section as a breakthrough for one important reason. Recent studies on the course of schizophrenia have challenged the once-common assumption that schizophrenia implies a chronic, deteriorating course encumbered with unremitting deficits in most psychosocial domains of functioning. These recent studies suggest much more variation in clinical and psychosocial outcome than was previously thought to exist (for reviews, see Angst, 1988; Harrow, Sands, Silverstein, & Goldberg, 1997; Johnstone, 1991; McGlashan, 1988; Möller & von Zerssen, 1995).

Before discussing the findings from these studies, several methodological issues need to be considered. First, the reliability and breadth of the diagnostic convention that is used in a study can have a significant influence on what the course of the disorder looks like. Unreliable diagnoses might include people who are false positive or exclude those who are false negative for schizophrenia from the sample. Similarly, a broader diagnostic convention might include people who have milder forms of the disorder or who would not be classified as having schizophrenia had narrower criteria been used. This could lead to a more benign course and outcome for the disorder in the aggregate. Most recent course studies have attempted to use clearly operationalized diagnostic criteria, but the breadth of the diagnostic convention can still be problematic for cross-study comparisons.

A second issue concerns how outcome is defined and measured. For example, categories such as "improved," "deteriorating," or "chronic" are descriptively attractive, but how the categories are constructed, which functional domains they reflect, and the conditions under which any person is placed in one of the categories can have a dramatic influence on what the course and outcome of any disorder looks like. Another concern is whether global or multidimensional measures are used. A global functional measure such as the Global Assessment Scale (Endicott, Spitzer, Fleiss, & Cohen, 1976) is attractive because of the ease of administration and analysis; however, there is evidence that it reflects more symptomatic than psychosocial outcome in schizophrenia (Brekke, 1992). Multidimensional measures such as the Level of Functioning Scale (Strauss & Carpenter, 1972) yield discrete scores in four functional domains (work, social, hospitalization, and symptoms). There is evidence that these outcome domains in schizophrenia are modestly related and have distinct trajectories over time (Carpenter & Strauss, 1991; Gaebel & Pietzcker, 1987; Strauss & Carpenter, 1972, 1977). Therefore, the outcome picture for schizophrenia is likely to vary on the basis of the outcome domain examined. Unfortunately, in this literature there is little established convention in any of these areas. Nonetheless, we would like to highlight certain findings.

Several retrospective studies have examined the psychosocial condition of people with schizophrenia 20 to 30 years after the onset of the disorder (Angst, 1988; Johnstone, 1991; McGlashan, 1988; Möller & von Zerssen, 1995). In general, these studies have found that up to one-third of people with schizophrenia are recovered; one-third are mildly or moderately impaired; and one-third have very poor outcomes. These findings suggest that up to 50 percent of people with the disorder have good to mild outcomes. It should be noted that across studies there can be wide variation in the percentage of people in each outcome category. So even though the outcome for schizophrenia is highly variable, ranging from good to poor, for most people schizophrenia is a lifetime disorder with some degree of impairment throughout life. Most of the functional impairment associated with the disorder occurs in the first five to 10 years of the disorder, with a leveling in the deterioration after that.

Typologies in the clinical course of the disorder also have been investigated (Harding, 1988; Marengo, 1994). There is considerable heterogeneity in course types including acute or insidious onset, static or undulating course (with linear and nonlinear trajectories), concluding with a range of functional outcomes. Several studies also have found that the outcome is worse for schizophrenia than for other major mental illnesses such as depression. Finally, it should be noted that this outcome picture needs to be balanced against a somewhat less favorable picture that comes from recent studies that have investigated a shorter follow-up period and that use more stringent outcome assessments (Möller & von Zerssen, 1995).

## POSITIVE AND NEGATIVE SYMPTOMS

Schizophrenia is a clinically heterogeneous disorder. It has been described in terms of subtypes based on age at onset, course, outcome, positive family history, and brain morphology (McGlashan & Fenton, 1992; Shore, 1987). Fluctuating subtype definitions make the concept of schizophrenia hard to understand, but they also reflect attempts to refine and improve our understanding of this multifaceted illness. The terms "positive" and "negative" were proposed by Crow (1980) to describe different clinical manifestations of schizophrenia, which he believed might represent different disease processes.

In Crow's (1980) model, the positive symptoms—delusions, hallucinations, and thought disorders—were posited to be the result of a biochemical imbalance, such as an excess of dopamine $D_2$ receptors, and would therefore be more likely to respond to antipsychotic medication. Conversely, the negative symptoms—affective flattening, alogia, and avolition—were thought to be associated with diffuse brain damage and would, therefore, respond poorly to somatic treatment.

The concept of a positive–negative dichotomy has had a profound effect on subsequent studies of schizophrenia (Andreasen, 1985; Andreasen, Flaum, Swayze, Tyrrell, & Arndt, 1990; Fenton & McGlashan, 1991; Kay, 1990; McGlashan & Fenton, 1992). Efforts to categorize the symptoms have led to the question of how and why a particular symptom manifestation should be classified as positive or negative. *Positive symptoms*, for example, have been described as "distortions or exaggerations of functions that are normally present but have been disinhibited" (Andreasen, Roy, & Flaum, 1995, p. 32). *Negative symptoms*, on the other hand, refer to aspects of functioning that normal people ordinarily have but are conspicuously absent in people with schizophrenia. Although people presenting with the illness have been categorized as having either predominantly positive or negative symptoms, the distinction also has been used dimensionally with no attempt to subtype people (Buchanan & Carpenter, 1994).

Cromwell (1993) described the trajectory of the positive and negative symptoms over the course of the disorder. What follows is an abridged version of that summary:

> During the premorbid period, negative symptoms may accrue. They are usually characterized as poor premorbid adjustment. These negative symptoms may persist into later phases when the condition becomes labeled a psychosis. During the acute phase, positive symptoms emerge. Both positive and negative symptoms become prominent and elevated. Although positive symptoms may be reduced after the acute period (or after any succeeding acute relapse episode), they tend not to disappear. Over 50 percent of patients with schizophrenia continue to have positive symptoms. Compared with negative symptoms, which tend to have an enduring course, positive symptoms are relatively unstable. Therefore, relapse episodes are characterized by the recurrence of positive symptoms. Among the positive symptoms,

hallucinations tend to be the most stable. Negative symptoms elevate as well during the acute period. They decrease at the end of the period but not completely. (p. 338)

More recent studies using factor analytic methods have produced results that suggest the division of positive and negative symptoms into two groups is an oversimplification (Andreasen et al., 1995). These studies have found that a three-factor model consisting of positive, disorganized, and negative symptoms might be more adequate (Brekke, DeBonis, & Graham, 1994; Buchanan & Carpenter, 1994; Peralta, deLeon, & Cuesta, 1992). In this model, the positive symptoms comprise delusions and hallucinations; the disorganized dimension comprises bizarre behavior, positive formal thought disorder, and inappropriate affect; and the negative symptoms consist of alogia, flat affect, and avolition. In terms of the association between the symptom factors and aspects of psychosocial functioning such as social and work performance, there is evidence to indicate that positive symptoms are weakly correlated with psychosocial performance, whereas negative and disorganized symptoms are significantly but modestly related to decrements in psychosocial functioning (Brekke et al., 1994; McGlashan & Fenton, 1992).

Current studies also are attempting to relate these symptom factors to neurobiological measures, including abnormal patterns in cerebral blood flow, and neurocognitive and psychophysiological measures (for example, Andreasen et al., 1990; Liddle, 1987; Liddle, Friston, Frith, & Frankowaik, 1992; Brekke, Raine, & Thomson, 1995). It is possible that this research will lead to the development of more specific interventions capable of targeting schizophrenia symptoms as they are uniquely expressed in a given person.

## GENETIC FACTORS

One of the most prominent trends in the genetic literature on schizophrenia has been the sophisticated reanalyses of family, twin, and adoption studies that emerged in the 1960s and 1970s (Shore, 1987). Many of the reanalyses have been motivated by challenges to the ways in which schizophrenia has been operationally defined. Recognizing this motivation, various investigators have sought to discover whether schizophrenia is really a familial condition once it has been defined using modern diagnostic conventions (McGuffin & O'Donovan, 1993).

Family studies are based on a simple idea: If the incidence of a disorder among the relatives of people with the same disorder is greater than that in the general population, the disorder is assumed to be genetic in origin (Rosenthal, 1971). Moreover, family studies attempt to demonstrate that the closer one is genetically to the affected person, or *proband,* the greater is the morbid risk of schizophrenia. It is generally accepted, for example, that the likelihood that a member of the general population will get the disease is 1 percent. This can be compared with figures compiled by Gottesman, McGuffin, and Farmer, (1987) and Kendler and Diehl (1993) in reviews of Western European genetic epidemiologic studies. Using standardized methods of assessment and explicitly operationalized diagnostic criteria, the authors looked at the occurrence of schizophrenia in the relatives of those already affected. The percentage ranged from 3.5 percent in nieces and nephews to 14.0 percent in dizygotic twins to 46.0 percent in monozygotic twins. Clearly, the risk of schizophrenia increases with the number of genes shared with a person manifesting the disorder.

Twin studies compare the concordance rate for schizophrenia in pairs of monozygotic twins with the rate in dizygotic twins (Pardes, Kaufmann, Pincus, & West, 1989). The underlying assumptions of these studies are that monozygotic twins share all the same genes, whereas dizygotic twins have only half their genes in common, and both types of twins share their prenatal and postnatal environments approximately to the same extent. As in early family studies, the early twin studies were not based on modern operationalized criteria. However, one of the larger series from the preoperational era (Gottesman & Shields, 1972) was sufficiently robust to lend itself to a reanalysis with modern diagnostic criteria. Farmer, McGuffin, and Gottesman (1987) studied 21 probands who had schizophrenia according to the criteria of the *Diagnostic and Statistical Manual of Mental Disorders* (3rd ed.) (DSM-III) (American Psychiatric Association [APA], 1980). They found that 48 percent of their monozygotic twins shared the disorder. There were 21 dizygotic probands, who had a concordance rate of only 10 percent. A later study (Onstad, Skre, Torgersen, & Kringlen, 1991) using DSM-III-R (APA, 1987) criteria, which looked at 31 monozygotic twins affected with the disorder, also revealed a concordance rate of 48 percent. The 21 dizygotic twins had a concordance rate of only 4 percent.

Torrey (1992) reviewed several twin studies conducted from 1953 to 1991. He included in the analysis only those in which zygosity could be determined with reasonable accuracy and looked at pairwise (as opposed to proband) concordance rates. Using the pairwise method, each twin pair is treated as a separate unit, and concordance is calculated as the percentage of pairs in which both pairs have the illness. His study revealed a concordance rate of 28 percent for monozygotic twins and 6 percent for dizygotic twins. Although his figures suggest that we may be overestimating the genetic contribution to schizophrenia, genetics remains the single most clearly defined etiologic factor in schizophrenia.

Adoption studies attempt to separate the contribution of nature and nurture by studying children raised away from their biological parents (Pardes et al., 1989). They offer compelling evidence for a genetic transmission of schizophrenia. A landmark study of people with schizophrenia who had been adopted early in life was conducted by Kety, Rosenthal, Wender, Schulsinger, and Jacobsen (1976). They compared the rate of schizophrenia among the biological and adoptive parents and found that 20.3 percent of 118 biological parents of adopted-away people with schizophrenia had schizophrenia spectrum disorder, compared with only 5.8 percent of 224 adoptive parents. Kendler and Gruenberg (1984) re-examined these results using stricter and more explicit criteria. Comparing diagnoses based on DSM-III in adoptees and relatives, schizophrenia and related disorders were significantly more common in the biological relatives (13.3 percent) of people with schizophrenia than in controls (1.3 percent).

A study underway by Wahlberg and associates (1997) is the first adoption study to use operational criteria in its original design. The nationwide Finnish study blindly compared matched-control adoptees with a sample of the adopted-away offspring of those with schizophrenia. One of the major goals of the study has been to examine the rearing environment of the adoptive family and assess its members' emotional health. Based on several assessment techniques, including semistructured interviews and the Family Rorschach, the families were assigned to five groups: healthy, mildly disturbed, neurotic, rigid–syntonic, and severely disturbed. Among the 155 index offspring, the percentage of both psychoses and other severe diagnoses was significantly higher than in the 186 matched control adoptees. This finding supports the genetic transmission hypothesis. Notable, however, is the finding that no seriously disturbed offspring were found in a healthy or mildly disturbed adoptive family regardless of genetic risk. This result suggests that genetic risk may be a necessary but not sufficient condition for developing schizophrenia. It might best be seen as a disorder that develops contingent on some environmental factor (a *stressor*) that must interact with a genetic predisposition (a *diathesis*).

Based on a variety of genetic transmission studies, Gottesman and colleagues (1987) and Kendler and Diehl (1993) concluded that approximately 70 percent to 75 percent of the variance in the liability to develop schizophrenia is under genetic control, but the remaining 25 percent to 30 percent is not.

Now we summarize several notions of the mode of transmission of schizophrenia. Because the pattern of genetic transmission of schizophrenia is currently unknown, several possible models have been considered. The simplest model proposes that a single defective gene predisposes a person to schizophrenia (Asherton, Mant, & McGuffin, 1995). This gene may have a highly variable expression, depending on the compounding effects of environmental factors, ranging from a severe form of the disorder to minor psychological abnormalities among relatives. This has been called a "Mendelian pattern" because the defective gene is either a dominant, recessive, or sex-linked gene. Under the polygenic model, genetic factors are assumed to be a result of the additive effects of several genes. It generates the hypothesis that schizophrenia is caused by a combination of a number of specific genes that interact with environmental factors, both biological and psychosocial (Gottesman et al., 1987). The mixed model suggests that the expression of a single major gene is altered by the interaction, or coaction with a number of other genes, each having a small effect on its own (Asherton et al., 1995).

Because most current models that attempt to explain the transmission and occurrence of schizophrenia combine a diathesis (a constitutional vulnerability) and a stressor (Kendler & Diehl, 1993), we now turn to an examination of the factors that might result from or interact with a genetically based diathesis to produce schizophrenia.

## NEURODEVELOPMENTAL FACTORS

The models for understanding how schizophrenia occurs have shifted dramatically in the past several years. The shift has been from viewing the disorder as arising from adult-onset cerebral pathology that would become more severe as the disorder progressed to viewing it as resulting from pathological neurodevelopment that occurs long before the illness manifests. Therefore, the neurodevelopmental model directs attention to the prenatal and perinatal stages of development (McGrath & Murray, 1995). The failure to find adult-onset cerebral changes concomitant with the occurrence of schizophrenia, combined with replicable findings of neurodevelopmental abnormalities, have fueled this change in perspective (Weinberger, 1995).

Several lines of evidence suggest that schizophrenia might best be described as a neurodevelopmental disorder. First, it has been suggested that disruptive intrauterine events could manifest in other realms of physical development. Therefore, the presence of minor physical anomalies (MPAs) among people with schizophrenia could be evidence of neurodevelopmental problems. There is some evidence that schizophrenia is marked by abnormalities such as limb length, fingerprint patterns, or head circumference (Green, Satz, & Christenson, 1994; Green, Satz, Gaier, Ganzell, & Kharabi, 1989). Although there are many methodological issues that need to be resolved in this area, various MPAs are also seen in other neurodevelopmental disorders.

Second, there is evidence that neurologic abnormalities are present in people before the onset of schizophrenia. These deficits occur in the areas of motor functioning, autonomic responsivity, and attention (Weinberger, 1995). These findings are suggestive of premorbid developmental problems in the brain. Third, a growing (if not always consistent) body of literature points to cerebral morphological deficits in schizophrenia, such as ventricular enlargement, reduced cerebral volume, and incomplete lateralization of the brain (Buchanan, Stevens, & Carpenter, 1997; Chua & McKenna, 1995). More important to the neurodevelopmental hypothesis is the growing evidence that these morphological problems predate the onset of the illness. Fourth, emerging evidence points to cerebral abnormalities in schizophrenia that are associated with the development and organization of cellular structures in the brain (*cytoarchitecture*) that are fixed during the second trimester of pregnancy. This final line of research is the most compelling with regard to the neurodevelopmental hypothesis of schizophrenia (Davis & Bracha, 1996; Weinberger, 1995).

If schizophrenia is associated with neurodevelopmental abnormalities, what might be the cause of the developmental insult? One body of literature finds an association between greater pregnancy and birth complications (PBCs) and an increased incidence of schizophrenia (Hultman, Ohman, Cnattingius, Wieselgren, & Lindstrom, 1997; McGrath & Murray, 1995). An association has been found between schizophrenia and PBCs such as low birthweight, prematurity, preeclampsia, prolonged labor, hypoxia, and fetal distress. However, the hypothesis that PBCs are linked to schizophrenia in adult life have not been unequivocally supported (Buka, Tsuang, & Lipsitt, 1993). It also is important to consider that the direction of the causal relationship is unclear. For example, it is possible that PBCs are more likely in fetuses that are neurodevelopmentally compromised in utero.

PBCs have been more consistently associated with schizophrenia in populations that are already genetically vulnerable to developing schizophrenia. These high-risk people, according to Olin and Mednick (1996), are identified as such if their parent, usually the mother, has the illness. In the Copenhagen High Risk Project, Mednick, Parnas, and Schulsinger (1987) followed 207 high-risk and 104 control children prospectively for 25 years. Those subjects who later developed schizophrenia experienced significantly more, and more severe, perinatal complications than those who did not develop the disorder. Consonant with that study's findings, Cannon, Mednick, and Parnas (1989), using a subsample of the Copenhagen subjects, found that delivery complications associated with periventricular damage increased the risk for genetically vulnerable people. These findings indicate that whatever the nature of the genetic predisposition, it was already expressed at the time of birth so that it could interact with the delivery complications (Olin & Mednick, 1996).

A second body of literature finds that exposure to influenza during the second trimester of pregnancy is possibly related to increases in the incidence of schizophrenia (Kunugi et al., 1995; McGrath, Pemberton, Welham, & Murray, 1994; Mednick, Machon, Huttunen, & Bonnet, 1988). It must be noted, however, that the cross-study replicability of these findings has been inconsistent (McGrath & Murray, 1995). Overall, these findings raise the specter of multiple environmental events that could interact with a genetic predisposition to schizophrenia to give rise to the disorder. The factors that have an effect between conception and birth may not be causes of schizophrenia but rather key events in a complex network of risk factors (McGrath & Murray, 1995).

A final issue concerning neurodevelopment involves the mechanisms of the delayed onset of the disorder. In other words, if the cerebral defect occurs during uterine or perinatal periods, then why does the disorder commonly manifest two decades later? Two possibilities are currently proposed (Weinberger, 1995). First, it is possible that there is a second pathological process that occurs around the time of the onset of the illness. Second, there might be an interaction between the neurodevelopmental defect and the normal developmental events that occur in early adulthood. A third possibility is suggested by recent studies on schizophrenia in childhood and adolescence (Rapoport et al., 1997; Zahn, Jacobsen, & Gordon, 1997). These studies suggest that there could be a progressive deterioration in brain functioning over time from childhood through adolescence that eventually results in the expression of schizophrenia.

## PSYCHOSOCIAL FACTORS

It has long been speculated that environmental factors may serve to potentiate or depotentiate genetic vulnerabilities in people at risk for or diagnosed with schizophrenia. These psychosocial factors can be related to the onset of the disorder or to the severity of its course and outcome over time. We will consider three factors: family interactions, life events, and culture.

### Family Interactions

Research over the past 25 years has revealed three types of intrafamilial dysfunction that are consistently associated with the onset and course of schizophrenia: communication deviance (CD), affective style (AS), and expressed emotion (EE) (Miklowitz, 1994; Miklowitz & Goldstein, 1993).

*Communication deviance* refers to unclear, unintelligible parent–child communication that interferes with the child's ability to develop logical thought and to perceive and process information accurately (Miklowitz & Goldstein, 1993). It is measured from the Thematic Apperception Test (TAT) and has been defined "as the degree to which the parent unconsciously acts in terms of his or her own needs without regard to the potentially conflicting needs of the child" (Karon & Widener, 1994, p. 48). It is speculated that in adulthood, this becomes manifest as the core symptoms of schizophrenia: disorders of thought and perception. *Affective style* refers to a relative's interactional behavior during problem-solving discussions, and negative AS refers to guilt-inducing, critical, or intrusive statements (Miklowitz, 1994).

Are high levels of CD and AS related to the onset of schizophrenia? This question was addressed by Goldstein (1987) in a 15-year study that looked at 64 disturbed but nonpsychotic adolescents who presented for treatment at a UCLA clinic in the mid- to late 1960s. Goldstein hypothesized that schizophrenia would be the likely outcome when certain patterns of adolescent disturbances and negative communication were present. Parents were administered a series of psychological assessments at baseline, including the TAT and an evaluation of their affective styles based on a direct interaction task. After 15 years, 28 percent of the adolescents in the study had developed schizophrenia or schizophrenia spectrum disorders that encompassed schizotypal and paranoid personality disorders. Children of parents who both scored high on CD and were identified as having a negative affective style were far more likely to have developed schizophrenia and related disorders at 15 years than those children of low-CD parents. Interestingly, the form of the adolescent problem had limited predictive value.

The conceptual framework of expressed emotion was developed in the late 1950s (Brown, 1959) following the observation that an emotionally charged family atmosphere was linked to rapid relapses among patients with schizophrenia. After a decade of development, the measure has led to extensive research, particularly in the past 10 to 15 years.

EE is rated from audiotaped interviews of involved family members who are asked open-ended questions covering a one-month period (Bebbington, Bowen, Hirsch, & Kuipers, 1995). They are asked to discuss the onset of problems, symptoms, coping responses, and other aspects of their relationship with affected people. The audiotapes are then rated not only for content but also for the emotional aspects of the communication, including pitch and emphasis. Frequency ratings are then made that cover five areas: the number of critical comments and positive remarks, global ratings of hostility, warmth, and emotional overinvolvement. There are now at least 26 prospective studies of the role of EE as a risk factor for relapse in schizophrenia. Bebbington and Kuipers (1994) analyzed aggregate data from 25 worldwide studies yielding a total of 1,346 cases. Regardless of gender or geographical location, EE was significantly related to relapse rates. The overall relapse rate for high-EE subjects was 50 percent; the relapse rate for low-EE cases was 21 percent.

It is important to remember three things when considering the findings on family risk factors. First, the causal relationships among these constructs has not been determined (Miklowitz, 1994). In other words, it is possible (even likely) that CD, AS, and EE in families is a product of stressful interactions between the ill child and the parents. For example, the stress of living with the ill child through the phases of the disorder could contribute to the difficult family environment as well as to the parents' behaviors. This observation suggests that an interactional model with bidirectional causality might be the most useful for understanding the mechanisms of family risk factors. Second, there is evidence that certain family environments can be protective and attenuate the risk for schizophrenia and that family involvement with the ill family member can facilitate improved patient functioning under certain conditions (Brekke & Mathiesen, 1995; Olin & Mednick, 1996). Third, aspects of family interaction such as CD, AS, and EE are amenable to therapeutic intervention and change (Miklowitz, 1994). Several studies suggest that actively engaging family members in treatment and rehabilitation can be important in relapse prevention (for reviews, see Dixon & Lehman, 1995; Penn & Mueser, 1996).

## Life Events

The effect of stressful life events and relapse also has been studied extensively in recent years, but the findings have been inconsistent (Bebbington et al., 1995). This inconsistency may be a result of the fact that life events are not equivalent and are therefore difficult to measure. Also, confounding any measurement is the person's previous experience and his or her unique susceptibility to a given event. Of interest, however, is a study conducted by Leff and Vaughn (1980), which looked at the combined effects of independent life events and the EE of key relatives. The patients were, for the most part, not taking medication. The authors found that the interaction of high-EE relatives and the experience of stressful life events was predictive of relapse. Conversely, those from low-EE households were more likely to withstand the impact of life events without relapse. In a later study, Leff, Kuipers, Berkowitz, Vaughn, and Sturgeon (1983) concluded that subjects on regular neuroleptic medication were protected from life event stress or high-EE stress but were likely to relapse if the two forms of stress occurred together. The tentative conclusion reached by Bebbington et al. (1995) is that life-event stress on its own is relatively unimportant in schizophrenia relapse. Perhaps the changes incurred through life events are not as important as the stress occasioned by living in a high-EE family.

## Culture

The international and cross-national studies on the course and outcome of schizophrenia find a significantly better outcome for the disorder in non-Western developing countries when compared with industrialized Western countries as well as a more benign symptom profile among immigrant ethnic groups from developing countries (Karno & Jenkins, 1993; Lefley, 1990; Lin & Kleinman, 1988). For example, Chandrasena (1987) found a lower prevalence of Schneiderian first-rank symptoms among psychotic inpatients who migrated to the West from developing countries compared with those native to the United Kingdom and Canada. Findings from multinational and longitudinal World Health Organization (WHO) studies have consistently demonstrated a better course and prognosis for patients in developing countries than in the industrialized countries (Craig, Siegel, Hopper, Lin, & Sartorius, 1997; Sartorius et al., 1986).

Despite methodological criticisms of the WHO studies (Cohen, 1992), Lin and Kleinman (1988) argued that the better prognosis in non-Western patients with schizophrenia constitutes the single most important finding in cross-cultural psychiatry. They hypothesized that the sociocentric nature of cultures in developing countries is the mediating mechanism related to better prognosis of the illness. In support of this hypothesis, there are two anecdotal studies that described highly sociocentric patterns in ethnic communities dealing with a mental illness (Perelberg, 1983; Swerdlow, 1992). A recent study in the United States, which compared cross-ethnic symptom differences among people with schizophrenia, found that higher levels of sociocentricity among ethnic groups mediated a more benign symptom profile for ethnic groups when compared with nonethnic groups (Brekke & Barrio, 1997). This provides evidence for a cultural mechanism that mollifies the severity of the clinical presentation of schizophrenia.

# Emerging Issues

Given the vast amount of research being conducted on schizophrenia, we would also like to highlight areas where findings and issues are emerging rapidly.

## COMORBIDITY WITH DRUG AND ALCOHOL ABUSE

The abuse of drugs and alcohol among people with schizophrenia (dual diagnosis) has emerged as a significant clinical issue for several reasons (Group for the Advancement of Psychiatry, 1992). First, the rates of substance use and the incidence of substance use disorders for people with schizophrenia is considerably higher than among their age-matched peers in the general population. Second, the use of alcohol and other drugs has been associated with poorer adjustment and treatment outcomes. It has been linked with wide array of psychosocial problems ranging from symptomatic exacerbation to homelessness and increased medical problems. Given the negative impact on the overall course and outcome of the disorder, as well as the alarming incidence of the problem, the development of effective treatment programs for patients with dual diagnoses has become a major priority (Bartels et al., 1993; Drake, Bartels, Teague, Noordsy, & Clark, 1993; Drake, McHugo, & Noordsy, 1993; Kosten & Ziedonis, 1997).

## SCHIZOAFFECTIVE DISORDER

Schizoaffective disorder combines a full presentation of both affective and schizophrenic features in a defined period of illness. Therefore, it does not meet criteria for either schizophrenia or a mood disorder. The estimates on the occurrence of the disorder suggest that its incidence is about one-half that of schizophrenia, which suggests that it is a significantly occurring disorder. Currently there is considerable controversy over whether it is a distinct disorder apart from either schizophrenia or mood disorders, whether it is a mixture of the two disorders, or whether it represents an artificial diagnostic distinction that lies on a continuum from schizophrenia to mood disorders (Tsuang, Levitt, & Simpson, 1995). The outcome of the disorder is generally better than for schizophrenia but worse than for the mood disorders.

## SCHIZOPHRENIA SPECTRUM PERSONALITY DISORDERS

The schizophrenia spectrum personality disorders are the schizotypal, schizoid, and paranoid personality disorders. In terms of symptomatology, these disorders can appear to be an attenuated version of schizophrenia but are distinct in that they do not incur any psychotic decompensation. An increasing body of evidence also suggests that these disorders are similar to schizophrenia in symptom structure, genetics, and pathophysiology (Raine, Lencz, & Mednick, 1995). As such, they are being studied to determine the factors that result in such a dramatic qualitative distinction between them and schizophrenia and what this may mean in terms of prevention or early intervention.

## NEUROCOGNITIVE DEFICITS

A growing body of literature suggests that people with schizophrenia have cognitive deficits in the areas of attention, memory, and the executive functions that require the organization and use of information to solve problems (Gold & Harvey, 1993; Goldberg & Gold, 1995; Levin, Yurgelun-Todd, & Craft, 1989). Although isolating these deficits can be helpful in determining the brain areas most affected by the disorder, there has been increasing interest in how these neurocognitive deficits are associated with psychosocial functioning in schizophrenia (Green, 1996) and how they might delimit responsiveness to psychosocial rehabilitation (Brekke, Raine, Ansel, Lencz, & Bird, 1997). Finally, the existence of these deficits has led to emerging interest in cognitive rehabilitation as a way to correct or attenuate the cognitive dysfunction and to provide an adjunct to traditional psychosocial interventions (Green, 1993, 1996).

## NEUROCHEMISTRY

The dopamine theory is the pre-eminent theory of schizophrenia and has generated enormous research (Carlsson, 1995; Owen & Simpson, 1995). In essence, the theory states that schizophrenia is associated with excessive dopaminergic activity in the central nervous system. Dopamine is a neurotransmitter that acts in a system of the brain important for cognition and emotion. Research suggests that the primary therapeutic activity of antipsychotic medications is their blockage of dopamine activity in the brain. After two decades of research, however, no unequivocal empirical evidence supports the dopamine hypothesis, yet its heuristic value remains enormous. A great amount of research continues on the neurochemical basis of schizophrenia. Recent research concerns a variety of dopamine receptors and the interaction of dopamine with other chemical systems in the brain, such as serotonin and amino acid neurotransmitters. It also is clear that neurochemical research in schizophrenia will benefit from attention to symptomatic subtypes and other aspects of heterogeneity in the disorder that might involve distinct neurochemical systems.

## NEUROPATHOLOGY AND BRAIN IMAGING

Studies on the neuropathology of schizophrenia attempt to find anatomical substrates of the disorder (Buchanan et al., 1997; Falki & Bogerts, 1995). Modern studies on schizophrenia focus on determinations of volume, cell counts, laterality measures, and investigations of glial cells, which are the cementing and supportive structures for the neurons. Studies over the past 15 years have revealed a multitude of morphological abnormalities in various brain structures of people with schizophrenia, yet none has been found that is characteristic, or pathognomonic, of schizophrenia. It should be noted that most of the anatomical changes associated with schizophrenia are subtle and (compared with other brain disorders) nondegenerative, suggesting a neurodevelopmental origin.

In the past two decades, great technological advances have been made in our ability to image the brain (Liddle, 1995). The macroscopic structures of the brain can be studied with X ray computed tomography (CT) or magnetic resonance imaging (MRI) techniques. Functional activity in the brain, such as blood flow, metabolism, and electrical activity, can be studied using photon emission tomography (PET), single photon emission computed tomography (SPECT), or brain electrical activity mapping (BEAM). These imaging techniques have contributed to the discovery of structural and functional deficits associated with schizophrenia. This research holds great promise for unlocking the nature of the brain abnormalities constitutive of schizophrenia.

## NEURODYNAMICS

Hoffman and McGlashan (1993) organized a body of articles around the theme of neurodynamics in schizophrenia. *Neurodynamics* "refers to interactions of large numbers of neurons that, in the short run, transform input information derived from their environments into meaningful output, and, in the long run, use this information to alter their own architectures" (p. 15). Neurodynamics involves the study of information processing, neural learning, neurodevelopment, and plasticity in neural structure and function. It has relevance to understanding the dynamic changes in cognition and brain structure that are associated with the vulnerability to the disorder, the emergence of psychosis, the organismic response to the disorder, and how the illness interacts with normal psychobiological processes. Waddington (1993) offered a synthesis of findings on the structural and functional deficits in schizophrenia from a neurodynamic perspective.

## Interactive Multifactorial Models

This chapter is based on the assumption that interactive biopsychosocial models are the most viable for understanding the occurrence, course, and outcomes of schizophrenia. Clearly, the revolution that has occurred in our understanding of the biological bases for mental disorders is extraordinary (for example, Andreasen, 1984). It is critical, however, to reiterate that the discovery of a singular or multifaceted biological basis for a disorder does not imply a unifactorial model for understanding the etiology, course, and outcome of that disorder. For example, as discussed above, there are genetic models that presuppose environmental stressors, which can be seen as nonbiologically based events that shape the genetic expression of a disorder. Therefore, the continued use and development of multifactorial models, such as the vulnerability–stress–protective factors model of schizophrenia (Goldstein, 1987; Nuechterlein et al., 1992), should be a central focus of schizophrenia research.

In this effort, social work is well situated to make contributions to the specification and testing of these models because of its history of using a biopsychosocial and ecological model, which is based on interactive and reciprocal causal mechanisms to explain social and psychological phenomena.

## Clinical Implications

Significant clinical implications emerge from this discussion of schizophrenia. We will outline the implications of each breakthrough area discussed above.

### COURSE AND OUTCOME

These findings have a number of implications for treatment providers' expectations of people with schizophrenia and for educating clients and family members. First, the prognosis for schizophrenia is better than has previously been thought. It is a disservice to clients and family members to state that the outcome will be unremittingly poor, because up to one-third of clients will experience a good to mildly dysfunctional long-term outcome. On the other hand, it also is likely that most people with schizophrenia will show some form of debilitation throughout their lives, and up to one-third will have poor outcomes. Differential outcome based on the functional domain examined also is likely, so poor outcomes in one functional domain, such as work, are not necessarily associated with poor outcomes in other functional domains. Therefore, clinicians should be encouraged to build on strengths or functional capacities that clients show in some psychosocial areas, even if they are incapacitated in others. Providers and clients should not predict long-term outcome from short-term outcomes. We also can expect that the majority of the debilitation will likely occur in the first five years of the disorder. Therefore, early intervention in both medication and psychosocial rehabilitation should be advocated. The course of the disorder also will show considerable heterogeneity across people, so an individualized approach based on a longitudinal perspective is crucial.

## SYMPTOMATIC PRESENTATION

Studies on symptomatic subtypes in schizophrenia suggest that there will be notable differences in clinical presentation among people. Some will show predominantly positive, negative, or disorganized symptoms, or combinations of all three. It also is likely that any person will experience different symptoms during various states and phases of the disorder over time. This suggests that clinicians must carefully attend to the symptom profile of each client across time.

The individualization of symptom expression has implications for treatment. There are growing efforts to target new medications to distinct symptom groups, although current medications are most effective with positive symptoms. The symptomatic profile of the client also has been discussed in terms of psychosocial interventions. People with negative symptoms often have more trouble getting started in social situations. They appear slow and are often poor communicators. Wing (1989) suggested that these patients should be offered a structured, emotionally neutral environment that makes only demands that can be understood and managed. Demands should be sufficient enough, however, to challenge patients to make the best of their assets. Clinicians involved in the counseling or psychosocial rehabilitation of these clients need to be sensitive to the level of stimulation in group situations. Overstimulating environments can be overwhelming, causing the patient with negative symptoms to retreat. At the same time, understimulating environments add to the environmental poverty, amplifying communication impairment and withdrawal. Those with positive symptoms, however, are not limited by the same deficits. They can be encouraged to cope with their symptoms, even if they cannot be eliminated. For example, although they may hear voices, they can learn to see them as an aspect of their illness. This possibility of putting positive symptoms in some perspective might be why they are not as strongly associated with decrements in psychosocial functioning as negative symptoms.

## GENETICS

The search for the genetic contribution of schizophrenia in family, twin, and adoption studies has clearly demonstrated *significant* genetic effects but *not exclusive* genetic effects. As Reiss, Plomin, and Hetherington (1991) pointed out, "What is often forgotten is that although the evidence for a genetic contribution to the etiology of the disorder is beyond dispute, no studies indicate that genetic effects account for all the variation between ill and not ill individuals" (p. 284).

Counseling related to genetic knowledge can begin before conception, during pregnancy, before the risk period for the disorder, or after it occurs. Before conception, people who have a positive family history and who want to take genetic risk into consideration for family planning can be given accurate information about transmission and genetic risk. During pregnancy, the importance of prenatal care and maintaining the mother's health can be emphasized. Strategies for reducing the likelihood of perinatal difficulties, such as careful planning with a physician, can be advocated. After birth and before the risk period for the disorder, parents can be sensitized to early detection of premorbid deficits that might portend schizophrenia. It should be emphasized that a healthy rearing environment can serve as a protective factor against the onset of schizophrenia. As yet, there are no clearly developed early intervention models, but we can educate the family as to which familial and nonfamilial factors can exacerbate or ameliorate the onset and course of the disorder.

Once the disorder occurs, the client and his or her family can be educated so as to reduce blame and focus on coping and protective factors such as treatment and rehabilitation. Clearly, social workers will have the opportunity to participate in the identification of at-risk children and offer support to families through education and counseling. However, throughout the counseling process, social workers will need to be especially sensitive to the distress that genetic knowledge may cause families.

## NEURODEVELOPMENT

Knowledge about neurodevelopmental factors in schizophrenia suggests that prevention through good prenatal and perinatal health care is essential. Neurodevelopmental models also indicate that intervention to prevent or ameliorate environmental stressors is important. These stressors can result from birth complications or from normal developmental events, such as making school transitions, establishing peer and dating relationships, and receiving emancipation from the home. Although we do not advocate sheltering at-risk people from normal developmental challenges, it is possible that they will need careful attention during these periods. Neurodevelopmental factors also can be part of a comprehensive explanation of the disorder to clients and family members.

## PSYCHOSOCIAL FACTORS

Findings strongly suggest that the onset and course of schizophrenia are not driven solely by biological determinants. It appears that people with schizophrenia and their families can benefit from learning about the effects of emotional elements and behaviors in their relationships as well as stressors and protective factors in their environments. Through counseling, social workers can assist families with addressing issues of communication and alleviating deleterious interaction patterns. Education about the disorder and its management is crucial. Many of these strategies are dealt with in family psychoeducation and behavioral intervention models available in the literature. However, mental health professionals should be cautioned against placing families in dichotomous categories of healthy and unhealthy and affixing blame on them for their children's disorder. Families are complex, and although it seems apparent that education and treatment hold one key, ultimately they may prove ineffective if the family feels labeled rather than empathically understood.

In terms of psychosocial treatment, Levin and Brekke (1993) found that within a rehabilitation program, a staff-to-client interactive milieu that was based on clarity of expectations and reduced emotional intensity facilitated clients' integration into their peer milieu. This outcome is reflective of the CD and EE findings in families. It suggests that a variety of interactive milieus in which clients participate should be engineered to avoid negative dynamics such as CD or EE. In this regard, clients also can be taught the techniques of stress management and cognitive interventions to remove or alleviate stressors that might prove overloading to them. The findings on culture can be used to design interventions that build on existing cultural strengths, such as sociocentric involvement, and to place cultural sensitivity as preeminent in clinicians' assessments and interventions. Perhaps this approach also is a transferable cultural mechanism, such that it might be possible to help others build sociocentric social structures.

Finally, the impact of psychosocial factors such as family interaction and culture should encourage the search for other salient psychosocial influences. At the microlevel, issues such as identity, self-concept, and subjective experience have been related to functional outcomes (Brekke, Levin, Wolkon, Sobel, & Slade, 1993; Strauss & Estroff, 1989; Warner, Taylor, Powers, & Hyman, 1989). Macro issues such as neighborhood and community factors also deserve attention as psychosocial stressors or protectors for people with schizophrenia.

## Conclusion

Schizophrenia is one of the most costly and debilitating mental disorders. Social workers provide a majority of the professional mental health treatment to people with schizophrenia. An accurate understanding of the biological, psychological, and social forces that shape the onset and course of this disorder is an essential ingredient in the care and treatment of this vulnerable population.

We began this chapter with remarks from two people who struggle with schizophrenia. Social workers must educate themselves as to the causes, courses, and outcomes of this disorder to the extent that scientific methods can reveal them. It also is essential that social workers allow themselves to be educated by those who live with the illness and whose voices can reveal the personal narrative and subjective truth of schizophrenia.

## References

American Psychiatric Association. (1980). *Diagnostic and statistical manual of mental disorders* (3rd ed.). Washington, DC: Author.

American Psychiatric Association. (1987). *Diagnostic and statistical manual of mental disorders* (3rd ed., rev.). Washington, DC: Author.

Andreasen, N. C. (1979). Thought, language, and communication disorders I: Clinical assessment of terms and evaluation of their reliability. *Archives of General Psychiatry, 36,* 1315–1321.

Andreasen, N. C. (1984). *The broken brain: The biological revolution in psychiatry.* New York: Harper & Row.

Andreasen, N. C. (1985). Positive vs. negative schizophrenia: A critical evaluation. *Schizophrenia Bulletin, 11,* 380–389.

Andreasen, N. C., Flaum, M., Swayze, V. M., Tyrrell, G., & Arndt, S. (1990). Positive and negative symptoms in schizophrenia: A critical reappraisal. *Archives of General Psychiatry, 47,* 615–621.

Andreasen, N. C., Roy, M. A., & Flaum, M. (1995). Positive and negative symptoms. In S. R. Hirsch & D. R. Weinberger (Eds.), *Schizophrenia* (pp. 28–45). Oxford, England: Blackwell Science.

Angst, J. (1988). European long-term follow-up studies of schizophrenia. *Schizophrenia Bulletin 14,* 501–513.

Asherton, P., Mant, R., & McGuffin, P. (1995). Genetics and schizophrenia. In S. R. Hirsch & D. R. Weinberger (Eds.), *Schizophrenia* (pp. 253–274). Oxford, England: Blackwell Science.

Bartels, S. J., Teague, G. B., Drake, R. E., & Clark, R. E. (1993). Substance abuse in schizophrenia: Service utilization and costs. Presentation to the 144th Annual Meeting of the American Psychiatric Association, 1991, New Orleans. *Journal of Nervous and Mental Disease, 181,* 227–232.

Bebbington, P. E., Bowen, J., Hirsch, S. R., & Kuipers, E. A. (1995). Schizophrenia and psychosocial stresses. In S. R. Hirsch & D. R. Weinberger (Eds.), *Schizophrenia* (pp. 587–604). Oxford, England: Blackwell Science.

Bebbington, P. E., & Kuipers, L. (1994). The predictive utility of expressed emotion in schizophrenia. *Psychological Medicine, 24,* 707–718.

Brekke, J. (1992). An examination of the relationships among three outcome scales in schizophrenia. *Journal of Nervous and Mental Disease, 180,* 162–167.

Brekke, J. S., & Barrio, C. (1997). Cross-ethnic symptom differences in schizophrenia: The influence of culture and minority status. *Schizophrenia Bulletin, 23,* 305–316.

Brekke, J., DeBonis, J., & Graham, J. (1994). A latent structure analysis of positive and negative symptoms in schizophrenia. *Comprehensive Psychiatry, 35,* 252–259.

Brekke, J., Levin, S., Wolkon, G., Sobel, G., & Slade, B. (1993). Psychosocial functioning and subjective experience in schizophrenia. *Schizophrenia Bulletin, 19,* 599–608.

Brekke, J., Long, J., Nesbitt, N., & Sobel, E. (1997). The impact of service characteristics on functional outcomes from community support programs for persons with schizophrenia: A growth curve analysis. *Journal of Consulting and Clinical Psychology, 65,* 464–475.

Brekke, J., & Mathiesen, S. (1995). Effects of parental involvement on the functioning of noninstitutionalized adults with schizophrenia. *Psychiatric Services, 46,* 1149–1155.

Brekke, J., Raine, A., & Thomson, C. (1995). Cognitive and psychophysiological correlates of positive, negative and disorganized symptoms in schizophrenia spectrum disorders. *Psychiatry Research, 57,* 241–250.

Brekke, J., Raine, A., Ansel, M., Lencz, T., & Bird, L. (1997). Neuropsychological and psychophysiological correlates of psychosocial functioning in schizophrenia. *Schizophrenia Bulletin, 23,* 19–28.

Brown, G. W. (1959). Experiences of discharged chronic schizophrenic mental hospital patients in various types of living group. *Milbank Memorial Fund Quarterly, 37,* 105–131.

Buchanan, R. W., & Carpenter, W. T. (1994). Domains of psychopathology: An approach to the reduction of heterogeneity in schizophrenia. *Journal of Nervous and Mental Disease, 182,* 193–204.

Buchanan, R. W., Stevens, J. R., & Carpenter, W. T. (1997). The neuroanatomy of schizophrenia: Editor's introduction. *Schizophrenia Bulletin, 23,* 365–367.

Buka, S. L., Tsuang, M. T., & Lipsitt, L. P. (1993). Pregnancy/delivery complications and psychiatric diagnosis: A prospective study. *Archives of General Psychiatry, 50,* 151–156.

Cannon, T. D., Mednick, S. A., & Parnas, J. (1989). Genetic and perinatal determinants of structural brain deficits in schizophrenia. *Archives of General Psychiatry, 46,* 883–889.

Carlsson, A. (1995). The dopamine theory revisited. In S. R. Hirsch & D. R. Weinberger (Eds.), *Schizophrenia* (pp. 379–400). Oxford, England: Blackwell Science.

Carpenter, W. T., & Strauss, J. S. (1991). The prediction of outcome in schizophrenia IV: Eleven-year follow-up of the Washington IPSS Cohort. *Journal of Nervous and Mental Disease, 179,* 517–525.

Chandrasena, R. (1987). Schneider's first rank symptoms: An international and interethnic comparative study. *Acta Psychiatrica Scandinavica, 76,* 574–578.

Chua, S. E., & McKenna, J. P. (1995). Schizophrenia—A brain disease? A critical review of structural and functional cerebral abnormality in the disorder. *British Journal of Psychiatry, 166,* 563–582.

Cohen, A. (1992). Prognosis for schizophrenia in the Third World: A re-evaluation of cross-cultural research. *Culture, Medicine and Psychiatry, 16,* 53–75.

Craig, T. J., Siegel, C., Hopper, K., Lin, S., & Sartorius, N. (1997). Outcome in schizophrenia and related disorder compared between developing and developed countries. *British Journal of Psychiatry, 170,* 229–233.

Cromwell, R. L. (1993). A summary view of schizophrenia. In R. L. Cromwell & C. R. Snyder (Eds.), *Schizophrenia* (pp. 335–349). New York: Oxford University Press.

Crow, T. J. (1980). Molecular pathology of schizophrenia: More than one disease process? *British Medical Journal, 280,* 66–68.

Cutting, J. (1990). *The right cerebral hemisphere and psychiatric disorders.* New York: Oxford University Press.

Cutting, J. (1995). Descriptive psychopathology. In S. R. Hirsch & D. R. Weinberger (Eds.), *Schizophrenia* (pp. 15–27). Oxford, England: Blackwell Science.

Davis, J. O., & Bracha, H. S. (1996). Prenatal growth markers in schizophrenia: A monozygotic co-twin control study. *American Journal of Psychiatry, 153,* 1166–1172.

Dixon, L. B., & Lehman, A. F. (1995). Family interventions for schizophrenia. *Schizophrenia Bulletin, 21,* 631–643.

Drake, R. E., Bartels, S. J., Teague, G. B., Noordsy, D. L., & Clark, R. E. (1993). Treatments of substance abuse in severely mentally ill patients. *Journal of Nervous and Mental Disease, 181,* 606–611.

Drake, R. E., McHugo, G. J., & Noordsy, D. L. (1993). Treatment of alcoholism among schizophrenic outpatients: 4-year outcomes. *American Journal of Psychiatry, 150,* 328–329.

Endicott, J., Spitzer, R. L., Fleiss, J. L., & Cohen, J. (1976). The Global Assessment Scale: A procedure for measuring overall severity of psychiatric disturbance. *Archives of General Psychiatry, 33,* 766–771.

Falkai, P., & Bogerts, B. (1995). The neuropathology of schizophrenia. In S. R. Hirsch & D. R. Weinberger (Eds.), *Schizophrenia* (pp. 275–292). Oxford, England: Blackwell Science.

Farmer, A. E., McGuffin, P., & Gottesman, I. I. (1987). Twin concordance for DSM-III schizophrenia: Scrutinizing the validity of the definition. *Archives of General Psychiatry, 44,* 634–641.

Fenton, W. S., & McGlashan, T. H. (1991). Natural history of schizophrenia subtypes: Positive and negative symptoms and long-term course. *Archives of General Psychiatry, 48,* 978–986.

Freeman, H. (1989). Relationship of schizophrenia to the environment. *British Journal of Psychiatry, 155*(Suppl. 5), 90–99.

Gaebel, W., & Pietzcker, A. (1987). Prospective study of course of illness in schizophrenia: Part II. Prediction of outcome. *Schizophrenia Bulletin, 13,* 299–305.

Gold, J. M., & Harvey, P. D. (1993). Cognitive deficits in schizophrenia. *Psychiatric Clinics of North America, 16,* 295–312.

Goldberg, T. E., & Gold, J. M. (1995). Neurocognitive deficits in schizophrenia. In S. R. Hirsch & D. R. Weinberger (Eds.), *Schizophrenia* (pp. 146–162). Oxford, England: Blackwell Science.

Goldstein, M. J. (1987). The UCLA high-risk project. *Schizophrenia Bulletin, 13,* 505–514.

Gottesman, I. I., McGuffin, P., & Farmer, A. E. (1987). Clinical genetics as clues to the "real" genetics of schizophrenia. (A decade of modest gains while playing for time.) *Schizophrenia Bulletin, 13,* 23–48.

Gottesman, I. I., & Shields, J. (1972). *Schizophrenia and genetics: A twin study vantage point.* New York: Academic Press.

Green, M. F. (1993). Cognitive remediation in schizophrenia: Is it time yet? *American Journal of Psychiatry, 150,* 178–187.

Green, M. F. (1996). What are the functional consequences of neurocognitive deficits in schizophrenia? *American Journal of Psychiatry, 153,* 321–330.

Green, M. F., Satz, P., & Christenson, C. (1994). Minor physical anomalies in schizophrenic patients, bipolar patients and their siblings. *Schizophrenia Bulletin, 20,* 433–440.

Green, M. F., Satz, P., Gaier, D. J., Ganzell, S., & Kharabi, F. (1989). Minor physical anomalies in schizophrenia. *Schizophrenia Bulletin, 15,* 91–99.

Group for the Advancement of Psychiatry. (1992). *Beyond symptom suppression: Improving long-term outcomes of schizophrenia.* Washington, DC: American Psychiatric Press.

Hafner, H., & Heiden, W. (1997). Epidemiology of schizophrenia. *Canadian Journal of Psychiatry, 42,* 139–151.

Harding, C. M. (1988). Course types in schizophrenia: An analysis of European and American studies. *Schizophrenia Bulletin, 14,* 633–643.

Harrow, M., Sands, J. R., Silverstein, M. L., & Goldberg, J. F. (1997). Course and outcome for schizophrenia versus other psychotic patients: A longitudinal study. *Schizophrenia Bulletin, 23,* 287–303.

Helgason, T., & Magnusson, H. (1989). The first 80 years of life: A psychiatric epidemiological study. *Acta Psychiatrica Scandinavica, 79*(Suppl. 348), 85–94.

Hoffman, R. E., & McGlashan, T. H. (1993). Neurodynamics and schizophrenia research: Editor's introduction. *Schizophrenia Bulletin, 19,* 15–19.

Hultman, C. M., Ohman, A., Cnattingius, S., Wieselgren, I., & Lindstrom, L. H. (1997). Prenatal and neonatal risk factors for schizophrenia. *British Journal of Psychiatry, 170,* 128–133.

Jablensky, A. (1995). Schizophrenia: The epidemiological horizon. In S. R. Hirsch & D. R. Weinberger (Eds.), *Schizophrenia* (pp. 206–252). Oxford, England: Blackwell Science.

Johnstone, E. C. (1991). Disabilities and circumstances of schizophrenic patients: A follow-up study. *British Journal of Psychiatry, 159*(Suppl. 3), 46.

Jordan, J. C. (1995). Schizophrenia: Adrift in an anchorless reality. *Schizophrenia Bulletin, 21,* 501–503.

Karno, M., & Jenkins, J. H. (1993). Cross-cultural issues in the course and treatment of schizophrenia. *Psychiatric Clinics of North America, 16,* 339–350.

Karon, B. P., & Widener, A. J. (1994). Is there really a schizophrenogenic parent? *Psychoanalytic Psychology, 11,* 47–61.

Kay, S. (1990). Significance of the positive–negative distinction in schizophrenia. *Schizophrenia Bulletin, 16,* 635–652.

Kendler, K. S., & Diehl, S. R. (1993). The genetics of schizophrenia: A current genetic–epidemiologic perspective. *Schizophrenia Bulletin, 19,* 261–285.

Kendler, K. S., & Gruenberg, A. M. (1984). An independent antigen of the Danish adoption study of schizophrenia, VI. *Archives of General Psychiatry, 41,* 555–564.

Kessler, R. C., McGonagle, K. A., Zhao, S., Nelson, C. B., Hughes, M., Eshleman, S., Wittchen, H-U., & Kendler, K. S. (1994). Lifetime and 12-month prevalence of DSM-III-R psychiatric disorders in the United States: Results from the National Comorbidity Survey. *Archives of General Psychiatry, 51*(8), 8–19.

Kety, S. S., Rosenthal, D., Wender, P. H., Schulsinger, F., & Jacobsen, B. (1976). Mental illness in the biological and adoptive families of individuals who have become schizophrenic. *Behavioral Genetics, 6,* 219–225.

Kosten, T. R., & Ziedonis, D. M. (1997). Substance abuse and schizophrenia: Editor's introduction. *Schizophrenia Bulletin, 23,* 181–186.

Kunugi, H., Nanko, S., Takei, N., Saito, K., Hayashi, N., & Kazamatsuri, H. (1995). Schizophrenia following in utero exposure to the 1957 influenza epidemic in Japan. *American Journal of Psychiatry, 1152,* 450–452.

Leff, J. P., Kuipers, L., Berkowitz, R., Vaughn, C. E., & Sturgeon, D. (1983). Life events, relatives expressed emotion and maintenance neuroleptics in schizophrenia relapse. *Psychological Medicine, 13,* 799–806.

Leff, J. P., & Vaughn, C. E. (1980). The interaction of life events and relative's expressed emotion in schizophrenia and depressive neurosis. *British Journal of Psychiatry, 136,* 146–153.

Lefley, H. P. (1990). Culture and chronic mental illness. *Hospital and Community Psychiatry, 41,* 277–286.

Levin, S., & Brekke, J. (1993). Factors related to integrating persons with chronic mental illness into a social milieu. *Community Mental Health Journal, 29,* 25–34.

Levin, S., Yurgelun-Todd, D., & Craft, S. (1989). Contributions of clinical neuropsychology to the study of schizophrenia. *Journal of Abnormal Psychology, 98,* 341–356.

Liddle, P. F. (1987). Schizophrenic syndrome, cognitive performance and neurological dysfunction. *Psychological Medicine, 17,* 49–57.

Liddle, P. F. (1995). Brain imaging. In S. R. Hirsch & D. R. Weinberger (Eds.), *Schizophrenia* (pp. 425–440). Oxford, England: Blackwell Science.

Liddle, P. F., Friston, K. J., Frith, C. D., & Frankowaik, R.S.J. (1992). Cerebral blood flow and mental processes in schizophrenia. *Journal of the Royal Society of Medicine, 85,* 224–226.

Lin, K. M., & Kleinman, A. M. (1988). Psychopathology and clinical course of schizophrenia: A cross-cultural perspective. *Schizophrenia Bulletin, 14,* 555–567.

Marengo, J. (1994). Classifying the courses of schizophrenia. *Schizophrenia Bulletin, 20,* 519–536.

McGlashan, T. H. (1988). A selective review of recent North American long-term follow-up studies of schizophrenia. *Schizophrenia Bulletin, 14,* 569–574.

McGlashan, T. H., & Fenton, T. H. (1992). The positive-negative distinction in schizophrenia: Review of natural history validators. *Archives of General Psychiatry, 49,* 63–72.

McGrath, J., & Murray, R. (1995). Risk factors for schizophrenia: From conception to birth. In S. R. Hirsch & D. R. Weinberger (Eds.), *Schizophrenia* (pp. 187–205). Oxford, England: Blackwell Science.

McGrath, J., Pemberton, M. R., Welham, J. L., & Murray, R. M. (1994). Schizophrenia and the influenza epidemics of 1954, 1957, and 1959, a southern hemisphere study. *Schizophrenia Research, 14,* 1–8.

McGuffin, P., & O'Donovan, M. C. (1993). Modern diagnostic criteria and models of transmission of schizophrenia. In R. L. Cromwell & C. R. Snyder (Eds.), *Schizophrenia.* (pp. 62–75). New York: Oxford University Press.

Mednick, S. A., Machon, R. A., Huttunen, M. O., & Bonnet, D. (1988). Adult schizophrenia following prenatal exposure to an influenza epidemic. *Archives of General Psychiatry, 45,* 189–192.

Mednick, S. A., Parnas, J., & Schulsinger, F. (1987). The Copenhagen high-risk project, 1962–1986. *Schizophrenia Bulletin, 13,* 485–495.

Miklowitz, D. J. (1994). Family risk indicators in schizophrenia. *Schizophrenia Bulletin, 20,* 137–149.

Miklowitz, D. J., & Goldstein, M. J. (1993). Mapping the intrafamilial environment of the schizophrenic patient. In R. L. Cromwell & C. R. Snyder (Eds.), *Schizophrenia* (pp. 313–332). New York: Oxford University Press.

Millon, T. (1991). Classification is psychopathology: Rationale, alternatives, standards. *Journal of Abnormal Psychology, 100*, 245–261.

Möller, H. J., & von Zerssen, D. (1995). Course and outcome of schizophrenia. In S. R. Hirsch & D. R. Weinberger (Eds.), *Schizophrenia* (pp. 106–127) Oxford, England: Blackwell Science.

Nicholson, I. R., & Neufeld, R.W.J. (1992). A dynamic vulnerability perspective on stress and schizophrenia. *American Journal of Orthopsychiatry, 62*, 117–130.

Nuechterlein, K. H., Dawson, M. E., Gitlin, M., Ventura, J., Goldstein, M. J., Snyder, K. S., Yee, C. M., & Mintz, J. (1992). Developmental processes in schizophrenic disorders: Longitudinal studies of vulnerability and stress. *Schizophrenia Bulletin, 18*, 387–425.

Olin, S. S., & Mednick, S. A. (1996). Risk factors of psychosis: Identifying vulnerable populations' premorbidity. *Schizophrenia Bulletin, 22*, 223–240.

Onstad, S., Skre, I., Torgersen, S., & Kringlen, E. (1991). Twin concordance for DSM-III-R schizophrenia. *Acta Psychiatrica Scandinavica, 83*, 395–402.

Owen F., & Simpson, M.D.C. (1995). The neurochemistry of schizophrenia. In S. R. Hirsch & D. R. Weinberger (Eds.), *Schizophrenia* (pp. 358–378). Oxford, England: Blackwell Science.

Pardes, H., Kaufmann, C. A., Pincus, H. A., & West, A. (1989). Genetics and psychiatry: Past discoveries, current dilemmas, and future directions. *American Journal of Psychiatry, 146*, 435–443.

Penn, D. L., & Mueser, K. T. (1996). Research update on the psychosocial treatment of schizophrenia. *American Journal of Psychiatry, 153*, 607–617.

Peralta, V., deLeon, J., & Cuesta, M. J. (1992). Are there more than two syndromes in schizophrenia? A critique of the positive-negative dichotomy. *British Journal of Psychiatry, 161*, 335–343.

Perelberg, R. J. (1983). Mental illness, family and networks in a London borough: Two cases studied by an anthropologist. *Social Science and Medicine, 17*, 481–491.

Raine, A., Lencz, T., & Mednick, S. (Eds.). (1995). *Schizotypal personality.* Cambridge, England: Cambridge University Press.

Rapoport, J. L., Giedd, J., Kumra, S., Jacobsen, L., Smith, A., Lee, P., Nelson, J., & Hamburger, S. (1997). Childhood-onset schizophrenia: Progressive ventricular change during adolescence. *Archives of General Psychiatry, 54*, 897–903.

Reiss, D., Plomin, R., & Hetherington, E. M. (1991). Genetics and psychiatry: An unheralded window on the environment. *American Journal of Psychiatry, 148*, 283–291.

Robins, L. N., & Regier, D. A. (Eds.). (1991). *Psychiatric disorders of America: The epidemiological catchment area study.* New York: Free Press.

Rosenthal, D. (1971). *The genetics of psychopathology.* New York: McGraw-Hill.

Sartorius, N., Jablensky, A., Korten, A., Ernberg, G., Anker, M., Cooper, J. E., & Day, R. (1986). Early manifestations and first-contact incidence of schizophrenia in different cultures. *Psychological Medicine, 16*, 909–928.

Shore, D. (1987). Special report: Schizophrenia. *Schizophrenia Bulletin, 13*, 1–15.

Strauss, J. S., & Carpenter, W. T. (1972). The prediction of outcome in schizophrenia: I. Characteristics of outcome. *Archives of General Psychiatry, 27*, 739–746.

Strauss, J. S., & Carpenter, W. T. (1977). The prediction of outcome in schizophrenia III: Five-year outcome and its predictors. *Archives of General Psychiatry, 34,* 159–163.

Strauss, J. S., & Estroff, S. E. (Eds.). (1989). Subjective experiences of schizophrenia and related disorders: Implications for understanding and treatment. *Schizophrenia Bulletin, 15,* 177–178.

Swerdlow, M. (1992). "Chronicity," "Nervios," and community care: A case study of Puerto Rican psychiatric patients in New York City. *Culture, Medicine, and Psychiatry, 16,* 217–235.

Torrey, E. F. (1992). Are we overestimating the genetic contribution to schizophrenia? *Schizophrenia Bulletin, 18,* 159–170.

Tsuang, M. T., Levitt, J. J., & Simpson, J. C. (1995). Schizoaffective disorder. In S. R. Hirsch & D. R. Weinberger (Eds.), *Schizophrenia* (pp. 46–57). Oxford, England: Blackwell Science.

Waddington, J. L. (1993). Neurodynamics of abnormalities in cerebral metabolism and structure in schizophrenia. *Schizophrenia Bulletin, 19,* 55–69.

Wagner, P. S. (1996). A voice from another closet. *Schizophrenia Bulletin, 22,* 399–401.

Wahlberg, E. K., Wynne, L. C., Oja, H., Keskitalo, P., Pykalainen, L., Lahti, I., Moring, J., Naarala, M., SOrri, A., Seitamaa, M., Laksy, K., Kolassa, J., Teinari, P. (1997). Gene–environment interaction in vulnerability to schizophrenia: Findings from the Finnish adoptive family study of schizophrenia. *American Journal of Psychiatry, 154,* 355–362.

Warner, R., Taylor, D., Powers, M., Hyman, J. (1989). Acceptance of the mental illness label by psychotic patients: Effects on functioning. *American Journal of Orthopsychiatry, 59,* 398–409.

Weinberger, D. R. (1995). Schizophrenia as a neurodevelopment disorder. In S. R. Hirsch & D. R. Weinberger (Eds.), *Schizophrenia* (pp. 293–323). Oxford, England: Blackwell Science.

Wing, J. K. (1989). The concept of negative symptoms. *British Journal of Psychiatry, 155* (Suppl. 7), 10–14.

Yank, G. R., Bentley, K. J., & Hargrove, D. S. (1993). The vulnerability-stress model of schizophrenia: Advances in psychosocial treatment. *American Journal of Orthopsychiatry, 63,* 55–69.

Zahn, T. P., Jacobsen, L. K., & Gordon, C. T. (1997). Autonomic nervous indicators of psychopathology in childhood-onset schizophrenia. *Archives of General Psychiatry, 54,* 904–912.

# Substance Use Disorders

Carl G. Leukefeld and Robert Walker

Social workers and mental health professionals tend to shy away from alcohol and drug abuse issues. In part, this avoidance may be related to national policies that have blended treatment with social control, thus creating a value conflict or role confusion for many professionals. This conflict also is complicated by stereotypes of substance abusers. In addition, alcohol and drug policies in the United States have vacillated between supply reduction and demand reduction activities. On the one hand, alcohol is a legally regulated substance with a system, which includes the Federal Bureau of Alcohol, Tobacco, and Firearms (ATF), for monitoring and enforcing its production, distribution, and use. Demand reduction activities for both alcohol and drugs include treatment, prevention, education, and research for both alcohol and drugs, which are driven by the U.S. Department of Health and Human Services and the U.S. Department of Education. Drugs, on the other hand, are controlled and regulated by the U.S. Food and Drug Administration, which oversees the development of safe compounds, whereas the control or supply reduction of illegal drugs is the responsibility of the U.S. Drug Enforcement Administration (DEA) and the Bureau of Customs. The DEA drug classification schedules differentiate by how drugs are distributed; drug effects, medical uses, and potential for abuse; and penalties for drug possession and trafficking.

Policy shifts between supply reduction and demand reduction are largely related to political forces. Demand reduction is the principal focus of this chapter. A balanced supply-and-demand reduction approach is needed because of the number of illegal substance abusers. However, political decision makers are now shifting funds to prisons because Americans want immediate solutions to problems such as substance abuse. But drug and alcohol abuse are chronic and relapsing disorders (Leukefeld & Tims, 1990), and there are no instant cures or quick fixes. We are now moving into a period of managed care that is expected to produce unprecedented changes in the treatment delivery system. This trend might have unforeseen consequences for the entire concept of demand reduction.

Support for this chapter was provided by grant No. R0-1DA10101 and No. U0-1DA08154 from the National Institute on Drug Abuse.

# Epidemiology

Estimates of alcohol and drug use in the general population come primarily from household data through the National Household Survey, school data from the High School Senior Survey, community data from the Epidemiologic Catchment Area (ECA) Survey, jail data from the Drug Use Forecasting (DUF) System, prison data from the Bureau of Justice Statistics, and emergency room data from the Drug Abuse Warning Network (Leukefeld, 1996). It should be noted that there is a striking difference in the level of substance use in the United States when information collected in jails, lock-ups, and prisons is compared with data from households, schools, and the general population. People who are arrested are placed in jails and lock-ups, and many people "pass through" these institutions. Prisons, on the other hand, are institutions where people are confined for greater periods of time. Prisons, jails, and lock-ups have higher concentrations of people who abuse drugs because there is a relationship between drugs and crime.

Since 1975, trends from the National Household Survey and the High School Senior Survey indicate almost similar peaks and declines in marijuana, cocaine, cigarette, and alcohol use. However, although overall trends are downward for people who reside in households and for students who remain in school, other indicators report increases in illegal drug use. Data from people who come into contact with emergency rooms, jails, detention centers, and prisons show sustained high-use patterns (Leukefeld, 1996; Leukefeld, Miller, & Hays, 1996).

## HOUSEHOLDS

The National Household Survey provides a picture of alcohol and other drug use in the general population for those ages 12 and older, both in and out of school (Substance Abuse and Mental Health Services Administration [SAMHSA], 1994). The survey was conducted biannually from 1975 until 1979, when it became triennial. Now it is done annually. Data show lifetime, annual, and past-month use rates for age groups 12–17, 18–25, 26–34, and 35 and older. The consumption of alcohol for 12- to 17-year-olds rose from 54 percent in 1974 to a high of 70 percent in 1979 and decreased to 46 percent in 1991. Consumption of alcohol increased for the 18- to 25-year-old group from 82 percent in 1974 to 90 percent in 1991, with a high of 95 percent in 1979. Alcohol consumption for those ages 26 and older increased from 73 percent in 1974 to 89 percent in 1991. The majority of both male and female respondents ages 12–21 who drank alcohol in the previous month indicated that they were current smokers (73 percent for males and 75 percent for females). In U.S. households, more than one-third (37 percent) of people ages 12 and older (more than 77 million people) self-reported using an illicit drug during their lifetimes (SAMHSA, 1994). These included 70 million people who reported using marijuana, 23 million who had tried cocaine, 18 million who had used hallucinogens, 4 million who had tried crack cocaine, and more than 2 million who had tried heroin. Current use for any illicit drug was at 5.6 percent, with most reported drug use decreasing among households. An overall decrease in both casual and heavy heroin use, as well as in cocaine use, also was noted from 1988 to 1993, with the exception of an increase in heavy heroin use from 1992 to 1993.

## SCHOOLS

Since 1975, the High School Senior Survey has collected data from approximately 16,000 seniors in a sample of about 130 public and private high schools across the country (Gall & Lucas, 1996; National Institute on Drug Abuse, 1994). Data from the High School Senior Survey is available for lifetime drug use (any drug use), drug use in the 12-month period before the survey, and current drug use (use in the 30-day period before the survey). The survey includes those students who remained in school (did not drop out) before their senior year and those attending school on the day of the survey. The survey has been criticized for underestimating drug-using behaviors because estimates suggest that about one-third of 18-year-olds are absent on the day of the survey or drop out of high school and that drug use rates for those people are higher. The proportion of seniors who reported ever using alcohol decreased from the high of 93 percent in 1980 to 87 percent in 1993. Alcohol use in the previous 12 months peaked in 1979 at 88 percent and decreased to 76 percent in 1993. When high school data are examined from 1991 to 1993, drug use among seniors increased slightly overall for any illicit drug use, from 44.1 percent in 1991 to 45.6 percent in 1994, but has been decreasing from a high of 65.6 percent in 1979. Overall drug use among seniors has been steadily decreasing from a high of 54.0 percent in 1979 to a low of 40.0 percent in 1992.

## JAILS AND PRISONS

Jails and prisons contain large numbers of drug abusers who are mostly urban poor and from ethnic groups. Drug use is confirmed by urine tests for 11 drugs collected in 24 city jails and lock-ups by the DUF and indicates that drug use is at a high level for those who come into contact with U.S. jails and lock-ups. DUF data indicate that 40 percent to 60 percent of arrestees were using one or more drugs other than alcohol at the time of their arrests (National Institute of Justice, 1993). For example, in 1993, 36 percent to 75 percent of men tested positive for drugs, with an average of 63 percent using at least one drug. The percentage of women who tested positive for any drug ranged from 45.0 percent to 79.0 percent, with an average of 67.5 percent in these 24 U.S. cities. Thus, about eight of every 10 men who were booked and almost seven of every 10 women who were booked in 1993 tested positive for illegal drugs.

Whereas the number of state prisoners increased by almost three times from 1979 to 1992, the number of inmates incarcerated for drug offenses increased from about 6 percent in 1979 to about 22 percent in 1992, with sentencing for drug possession shorter than for trafficking. A nationally representative sample of U.S. prison inmates reported that about 50 percent used drugs in the month before incarceration and about 80 percent of inmates used illicit drugs at least once (Bureau of Justice Statistics, 1991).

## EMERGENCY ROOMS

Hospital emergency room drug episodes increased about 14 percent, from more than 403,000 in 1988 to 466,897 in 1993, according to data collected by the Drug Abuse Warning Network (National Drug Control Strategy, 1995). These emergency room contacts are defined as episodes representing a single occurrence in which the use of a drug was revealed or detected. In 1993, the reasons given for going to emergency rooms for a drug-related contact were overdose, at 53 percent; chronic effects, at 11 percent; unexpected reactions, at 12 percent; seeking detoxification, at 10 percent; withdrawal, at 2 percent; and other or unknown reasons, at 12 percent. Deaths by drug-induced causes increased from 1979 to 1992. For females, the increase was 12 percent (from 3,445 to 3,937); for males, the increase was 53 percent (from 3,656 to 7,766) (Rouse, 1995).

## GENERAL POPULATION

The National Comorbidity Survey (NCS) is a probability sample ($N = 8,098$ respondents) of the noninstitutionalized U.S. civilian population that was conducted from September 1990 to February 1992. DSM-III-R lifetime and 12-month prevalence data are reported. Psychiatric disorders included are affective, anxiety, drug or alcohol abuse/dependence, nonaffective psychosis, and antisocial personality. The NCS estimates that approximately 52 million Americans ages 15 to 54, or 29.5 percent of the U.S. population, had some type of alcohol, drug abuse, or mental health disorder (Kessler et al., 1994). An estimated 20 million Americans, or 11.3 percent of the U.S. population, are estimated to abuse alcohol or drugs, or be dependent on alcohol or drugs. An estimated 8 million, or 4.5 percent of the U.S. population of 15- to 54-year-olds, have had a substance-related disorder[1] and a mental disorder within the past year. The proportion of the U.S. population with a history of dependence for tobacco is 24.1 percent ± 1.0 SE; for alcohol, 14.1 percent ± 0.7 SE; and for other drugs, 7.5 percent SE ± 0.4 percent (Anthony, Arria, & Johnson, 1995).

The ECA study provides information on the prevalence of the abuse of alcohol, other drugs, and mental disorders in the United States (Regier, Farmer, et al., 1990). The ECA study, an earlier study than the NCS, reported lower general population prevalence estimated rates for dependence and abuse. The ECA estimated the U.S. population prevalence rate for alcohol dependence at 13.5 percent and for other drug dependence and abuse at 6.1 percent.

Alcohol is associated with a number of problems. Those problems include accidents and crashes related to driving. Of those who report that they drink, about 40 percent report problems associated with being drunk more than twice per month. These problems were associated with age groups, with those ages 18 to 25 generally reporting the highest percentage of problems (Leukefeld, 1996; Rouse, 1995). Alcohol- and drug-involved traffic accidents are the leading cause of death among people under 25 years of age. Each year drugs and alcohol account for about 17,500 deaths from vehicle crashes (Centers for Disease Control and Prevention [CDC], 1994). However, fatal traffic crashes involving alcohol decreased for all drivers from 1980 to 1993; during that time period, the largest decrease was for the 16- to 20-year-old group, which went from 53 percent in 1980 to 27 percent in 1993 (Insurance Institute for Highway Safety, 1994).

## HIV/AIDS

The transmission of HIV and AIDS, for about one-third of those who are diagnosed with AIDS, is related to drug injection (CDC, 1994). Studies (DesJarlais,

---

[1]Unless otherwise noted, and consistent with the 4th edition of the *Diagnostic and Statistical Manual of Mental Disorders* (DSM-IV) (American Psychiatric Association, 1994), the term "substance-related disorder" is used in this chapter to refer to drug and alcohol abuse and dependence.

Friedman, & Stoneburner, 1988; Lange et al., 1988) have shown that from 70 percent to nearly 100 percent of injecting drug users share injection equipment, and through this behavior they place themselves, their sex partners, and children at high risk for contracting and transmitting HIV/AIDS. About three-fourths of AIDS cases that are transmitted from mother to child during pregnancy or childbirth (perinatal transmission) occur among children born to women who are abusing IV drugs or who are current or former sex partners of IV drug abusers (Chamberland, White, Lifson, & Sonders, 1987). Studies have examined the use of community outreach workers to distribute bleach for needle cleaning to control the spread of HIV and to educate drug abusers about HIV prevention. The educational approach has been tried in larger cities; however, this approach is incompatible with the "no-drug-use goals" of both drug treatment agencies and the justice system. The opposing goals of the two approaches has spawned considerable media attention.

## Biopsychosocial Approach

A biopsychosocial orientation integrates the essential dimensions of substance-related disorders into a conceptual model that can provide a framework for diagnosis, treatment, and prevention. The model has become the dominant paradigm for understanding addiction and the various methods of treatment because it encompasses essential aspects without necessary cause–effect assumptions (Donovan, 1986; 1988). The dual diagnosis movement also has heightened awareness of a biopsychosocial orientation, which integrates traditional disease-model thinking with other psychiatric and social models (Wallace, 1986). The American Psychiatric Association (APA, 1995) incorporated biopsychosocial dimensions for assessment and treatment of substance use disorders but, curiously, avoided the use of the term.

### BIOLOGICAL FACTORS

The biology of psychoactive substances is complex and varies from substance to substance. Our knowledge about the physiological effects of alcohol is extensive, whereas knowledge about short-term effects from other substances is less definitive. Alcohol use is associated with changes in hormonal secretion; damage to the liver; increased rates of cardiovascular disease; increased rates of gastrointestinal disease (including cancers); pancreatic disease; and damage to the kidney, lung, bone, skin, and other systems (Littrell, 1991). Cocaine is associated primarily with acute physiological phenomena, including respiratory distress and cardiovascular complications (Gold, 1992). The following discussion of biological factors will focus mostly on neurochemical dimensions because they are more closely associated with the addictive process and other psychiatric disorders.

The biological dimensions of substance-related disorders incorporate genetic factors and neurochemical mechanisms that can either explain or illustrate the mental and emotional functioning of people with substance-related disorders. The evidence of a genetic component to alcoholism has been formulated from twin and adoption studies designed to explore environmental and genetic determinants of alcoholism. These studies examine outcomes for identical and fraternal twins who were placed in separate homes as well as the different effects of alcoholic environments on adopted children with various levels of genetic inheritance. Although these studies are not definitive, there is strong evidence for a genetic predisposition toward alcoholism (Kendler, Neale, Heath, Kessler, & Evans, 1994; Littrell, 1991).

Heritability of dependence (not abuse) is most likely where the parental alcoholism and related symptoms are severe (Pickens et al., 1991). Whether the same statements can be made for other substances is less clear, but recent investigations seem to point toward some common heritable mechanisms for many disorders that co-occur with substance use. It is possible that addictive disorders, attention deficit disorder, food bingeing, marked traits of compulsivity, and impulsivity share a common genetically influenced chemical imbalance in the brain's reward mechanism processes (Blum, Cull, Braverman, & Comings, 1996). This research sets the stage for understanding comorbidity and co-occurrence of other disorders of mood, affect, and personality along with substance-related disorders. The neurochemical irregularities that seem to promote or contribute to addiction susceptibility also are implicated in some personality disorders, mood disorders, anxiety, and the impulse and compulsivity problems mentioned above.

Alcohol and other psychoactive drugs affect and are affected by different neurotransmitters, including dopamine, norepinephrine, and serotonin. The genetic coding for receptor cells for dopamine has been linked with alcoholism (Blum et al., 1990; Parsian et al., 1991), although there is continuing diversity of opinion about the causative relationships between genetic findings and alcohol. Dopamine is involved in the processes and content of thought as well as in activating the pleasure or reward centers of the brain. These limbic activations are perceived as pleasurable sensations or as desirable mental states. Alcohol, cocaine, and certain hallucinogens affect the receptivity or availability of dopamine in the brain and thus play a key role in brain reward mechanisms.

Norepinephrine is an excitatory neurotransmitter that is involved in the panic response. When norepinephrine is depleted or sensitivity to it has become diminished, depression may result. People with depression have high rates of anxiety and panic (Akiskal, 1990; Regier, Burke, & Burke, 1990). Fear causes the release of large amounts of norepinephrine with resultant psychological alertness and psychomotor activity including increased heart rate, accelerated respiration, and sweating. Cocaine and amphetamine produce these effects as well through their norepinephrine-like activity. The aftereffects of prolonged fearfulness can result in the exhaustion of norepinephrine, which can contribute to depressed mood. The aftereffects of withdrawal from cocaine and amphetamine can include features similar to depression. As with alcoholism, there tends to be a familial pattern with panic and other anxiety disorders (Merikangas, 1990). In addition, antisocial people with alcoholism have lower levels of norepinephrine in cerebral spinal fluid (CSF) and urinary norepinephrine output (Raine, 1993). Thus, genetic influences may be important in explaining these patterns.

Serotonin is a neurotransmitter that has been associated with feelings of satisfaction, contentment, and well-being. Reduced brain levels of serotonin are associated with depression, suicidality, and increased lethality of both suicidal and homicidal tendencies. People with diminished serotonin levels are often irritable and more violent than those with more normative levels (Goodwin & Jamison, 1990; Volavka, 1995). People with early-onset alcoholism have low levels of serotonin metabolites in their CSF, suggesting a fundamental disorder of neurotransmitter availability (Fils-Aime et al., 1996).

The findings described above highlight the significance of comorbidity of substance-related disorders with other psychiatric problems—particularly those associated with disturbances of social behavior. Neurotransmitter system irregularities also could be associated with multiple pathways of expression in behaving, thinking, and feeling. Thus, it is possible that this common vulnerability accounts for the overlap of some disorders with substance-related disorders. This also could help explain the serial nature of disorders that some addicted people go through when they attain abstinence but then experience panic disorder, depression, or obsessive–compulsive disorder.

## PSYCHOLOGICAL FACTORS

Psychological factors associated with substance use disorders are as complex as the biological and genetic factors. In addition to personal development issues, there are two psychological factors that appear to be important in current discussions of substance-related disorders: (1) the role of stress in abuse and dependence and (2) the cognitive structures of addicted or abusing people.

Does stress cause alcoholism? Common sense would say "yes," but Littrell's (1991) review of the literature in this area illustrates the complexity of the matter. Recent specific stressors appear to be related to increased alcohol consumption, but it also is clear that there are major differences between men and women with stressors and alcohol use (Littrell, 1991). Although relapse appears to be associated with stressful precipitants, stress reduction methods do not appear to prevent relapse (Shiffman, 1988). However, when a person with substance abuse or dependence believes that stress is related to alcohol or other drug use or experiences a perceived need for use, the relationship between stress and the substance takes on a new complexity. Consequently, stress plays into the person's expectations and can become an important variable in drug-taking behavior (Annis & Davis, 1988). The self-medication hypothesis of addiction suggests that the person uses substances selectively to reduce undesirable mental states and to relieve either acute or chronic emotional suffering (Brehm & Khantzian, 1992). Stress also emerges as a factor in comorbidity with various stress-related disorders, such as posttraumatic stress disorder (PTSD) and sexual abuse survival, and substance use disorders.

The cognitive processes associated with substance use disorders should be a major component of assessment and treatment. Cognitive functioning in the person with substance-related disorder can vary from normal—that is, indistinguishable from that of non-substance users—to profoundly impaired. The typical pattern includes a set of distortions that are seen as wrapped around the drug-taking experience. These beliefs stimulate drug-taking behavior and are used to rationalize the consequences for the person. There are any number of irrational and dysfunctional beliefs centered on drug taking and drinking. In fact, it has been suggested that this constellation of beliefs and automatic thoughts can be one of the most powerful sustainers of the addictive or abusive behavior (Beck, Wright, Newman, & Liese, 1993). Beck and associates pointed to the importance of focusing therapy on these beliefs as a way to change feelings and moods of a person with substance abuse. The thoughts elicit emotions that someone with substance abuse believes demand alteration through the only familiar and proven means known to the person—chemicals. The mood seems unendurable, so the person engineers an alteration toward a better mental state with drugs or alcohol.

## SOCIAL FACTORS

There is no question that social and cultural factors contribute substantially to drug-taking and alcohol-drinking behavior. Although it is difficult to measure the effects of large-scale economic events on substance-related disorders, evidence of a synergistic contribution exists. Economic losses can contribute to drug-taking behavior, and substance abuse can have far-reaching effects on the economy, including the cost of lost productivity and the considerable costs associated with crime and law enforcement and criminal justice.

When using the biopsychosocial model of substance use disorders, an appreciation of the relationship between culture and behavior is needed. The economic deprivation of the inner-city environment is clearly associated with the hidden economy of crack cocaine trafficking. The economic trends of the 1980s and 1990s have pointed toward increasing the wealth of those who are wealthy and increasing poverty for those who are less well off. This disfranchisement of the poor population leads to hopelessness and helplessness—emotions that fuel the potent, if transient, feelings of power that can initially be obtained with drug use. The loss of housing supports for poor people, less health care, loss of employment opportunities, and poor educational attainment for those who reside in the inner cities provides fuel for hopelessness (Johnson & Muffler, 1992). In research examining the stages of development into full-fledged crack cocaine use, young people provide constant evidence of their sociocultural poverty through diminished academic attainment, detachment from families, and engagement with drug-using peer groups (Kandel & Davies, 1996). This last feature—the close involvement with drug-using peers—can be a significant factor in developing drug prevention or treatment strategies because the peer group has such an intense influence on a person's behavior. The subculture and peer environment also can shape the choice of drugs or routes of administration (Johnson & Muffler, 1992). Without a change in peer socialization, recovery is usually a "long shot."

## A BIOPSYCHOSOCIAL APPROACH

At the most fundamental level, the biopsychosocial approach suggests that a substance-related disorder is supported by physiological and genetic components; distorted beliefs and ideas; and an environment that with the other two components stimulates and sustains dependence or abuse. When providing treatment, these three dimensions can guide the continuing focus of care; otherwise, recovery can be jeopardized. The three dimensions are interactive and interdependent. A substance-using person's thinking error can contribute to mishandling a social interaction that subsequently leads to a failure at work or in a relationship. The person's biogenetic vulnerabilities poorly prepare him or her for managing the powerful negative feelings this failure can elicit. It is this complex interplay of physiology, self, and the social world that makes substance use disorders difficult to treat or prevent with simplistic "one-size-fits-all" approaches.

## TREATMENT AND OTHER INTERVENTIONS

The biopsychosocial orientation helps provide a framework to guide treatment. Several modalities are commonly used in treating substance-related disorders. Treatment often begins with a concern expressed by the family, an employer, or a court. The actions taken by any of these concerned parties can result in the person being screened by a substance abuse professional to determine whether he or she has a disorder that might require treatment or other services. Following a screening, it is likely that the next step will be an intervention, in which the person is presented with his or her behaviors or is motivated as a part of pretreatment and then is offered treatment. Treatment might begin with detoxification, using the medical or social model, when a person cannot safely detoxify in a home setting. Following detoxification, the person is assessed again for continuing treatment needs. These might include residential or inpatient care, which is rare in the 1990s; intensive outpatient care; or traditional outpatient care. Throughout treatment, the client is referred to self-help programs to augment other treatment strategies. Upon discharge from residential care or as part of intensive outpatient care, self-help programs, such as Alcoholics Anonymous (AA) and Narcotics Anonymous become vital components of the person's recovery.

## Prevalence and Outcome Measures

Several sets of measures have been consistently used in the alcohol and other drug abuse areas in addition to outcome measures. Three measures have been incorporated in the literature, as noted above, to examine drug and alcohol use, abuse, and dependence. These measures are used by epidemiologists to report population and subpopulation prevalence and trends for use and abuse. (See the National Household Survey and High School Senior Survey findings presented above.) The three measures used in epidemiologic studies are (1) *current use,* defined as use in the past 30 days; (2) *past-year use,* or use in the previous 12 months; and (3) *lifetime use,* defined as use taking place at any point in the person's life. There also is a need to present community-level data for DSM-IV levels of abuse and dependence for alcohol and other drugs (APA, 1994). For example, these abuse and dependence diagnostic classifications are the kinds of data that can be used to examine treatment needs and to plan interventions that meet treatment deficits for alcohol and other drug abusers and dependency.

According to DSM-IV, the criteria for substance abuse and dependence include a maladaptive pattern of substance abuse leading to clinically significant impairment or distress, as manifested by three or more of seven criteria at any time in the same three months. The seven criteria in DSM-IV can be paraphrased as (1) tolerance, either a need for markedly increased amounts of the substance to achieve intoxication or markedly diminished effect with continued use of the same amount of the substance; (2) withdrawal, manifested as either characteristic withdrawal or the same or a closely related substance taken to relieve or avoid withdrawal symptoms; (3) taking the substance in larger amounts or for longer than intended; (4) persistent desire or unsuccessful efforts to cut down or control use; (5) spending a great deal of time in activities necessary to obtain the substance, use the substance, or recover from its effects; (6) giving up or reducing important social, occupational, or recreational activities because of substance use; and (7) using the substance despite knowledge that a persistent or recurring physical or psychological problem is likely to be caused or exacerbated by the substance.

The Addiction Severity Index (ASI) has been widely used by alcohol and drug practitioners and researchers to measure treatment outcome (McLellan, Luborsky, Woody, & O'Brien, 1980). The ASI is a structured 40-minute interview designed to assess severity in seven areas, including alcohol and drug use (both injection and noninjection), employment, criminal behavior, legal status, psychological status, physical health, and demographics. ASI ratings have been shown to provide reliable and valid measures of problem severity for both drug and alcohol users and sensitive measures for treatment change (Kosten, Rounsaville, & Kleber, 1987; McLellan et al., 1992). Similar outcome measures have been used in outcome studies, but they do not have the clinical utility of severity ratings that the ASI can provide. These studies include the Treatment Outcome Prospective Study and the Drug Abuse Reporting Program. Although the outcome measures are scaled similarly, the same scaling can differ.

Self-report data have been and are used in outcome and epidemiologic studies. This practice is not without discussion concerning the validity of self-report (see Amsel, Mandell, Mathias, Mason, & Lockerman, 1976; Feucht, Stephens, & Walker, 1994; Mieczkowski, Barzeley, Gropper, & Wish, 1991). Self-reported information related to alcohol and other drug use is collected confidentially, so individual names are not used. Much of the information also is collected anonymously; therefore, names are never asked. With confidentiality assurance, respondents generally will talk about their use of substances. However, it could be argued that the current rates of self-reported alcohol and other drug use are underreported because a certain percentage of respondents do not reveal their alcohol or illegal substance use.

To monitor current alcohol and other drug use, treatment programs, the criminal justice system, and other settings, including employee assistance programs, collect body fluids of possible substance users. Breath is used to test for the presence of alcohol, which also is found in blood. Urine is collected and analyzed using gas chromatography in a laboratory. Onsite testing kits for urine also are available and provide immediate information about the person's use of drugs. Hair can be collected and analyzed to determine the presence of a drug and when the drug was used (Baumgartner, Hill, & Bland, 1989).

## Family Issues

Family issues related to alcohol and drug dependence and use should incorporate concerns about the effects of drugs on the development of the fetus. The evidence suggests that the specific effects of intrauterine exposure to cocaine are difficult to delineate, but the risk of harm is sufficient to cause alarm (Volpe, 1992). Federal funding initiatives through the Center for Substance Abuse Prevention are focused on decreasing these effects through the use of demonstration models aimed at pregnant women who are at risk for substance use. The outcome of these programs is being assessed.

Clinical experience indicates that the entire family becomes involved when one member has a substance use disorder. The role of the family as a motivator and sustainer during recovery is considered to be important (Stanton & Heath, 1995). The family frequently must be assisted with promoting the successful participation of the dependent member in treatment. Some research suggests that family therapy is a most promising form of treatment (Kaufman, 1992), although there is considerable debate on the effectiveness of family therapy with substance use disorders (Edwards & Steinglass, 1995). The Edwards and Steinglass meta-analysis of 21 studies suggested that families are important motivators for the initiation of treatment but that family therapy is only marginally more effective than other modalities after the initial phase.

Minuchin's (1975) concepts of enmeshment and disengagement—concepts from the early period of family therapy development—are still widely accepted. In fact, clinical experience suggests that the typical substance abuser's family exhibits disorder in the system of relating among all members; hence the importance of engaging all members in treatment. Some practitioners favor using the concept of an "addictive family" to capture the complex interactions that arise with a substance-abusing member (Williams, 1996). Unfortunately, many of the treasured family concepts in the substance abuse field not only lack empirical evidence but also have been shown to be fraught with value judgments that can be problematic. The concept of codependency is an example. No empirical evidence supports the concept of codependency, and no attention is given to the gender biasing that is implied in its use (Anderson, 1994). The concept also ignores the power differential between men and women, and it incorporates the notion of blaming the victim (Anderson, 1994).

Teaching parenting skills and more effective ways of dealing with unconstructive behavior has been found to be helpful with adolescent substance abusers (Bailey, 1991). Little research, however, supports the effectiveness of family therapy for youths who abuse substances. Complications also are associated with the nosology of substance use disorders in adolescence. That is, adult nosological concepts often misrepresent and mislabel the phenomenon (Bukstein & Kaminer, 1994). Although the DSM-IV has attempted to capture selected familial disorder traits, there still is no generally accepted nosology of family disorders, and research is hampered by this lack of objective criteria.

## Comorbidity

Comorbidity of other mental and emotional disorders with substance use disorders has been addressed in a variety of ways. The emergence of addictionology initially discouraged comorbidity discussions because the concept seemed to promote interpretations of drug use and alcoholism as sequelae of other primary psychological factors. Addictionologists have expended considerable effort in the past decades to establish the primacy of substance use disorders. Discussions of comorbidity might seem to threaten those gains. Subsequently, the idea that purely psychological problems were the propelling force behind addiction has not been validated by research (Miller & Gold, 1991). The discussion has now taken on far greater complexity because of awareness of dual diagnosis conditions. The term "dual diagnosis" is used to capture the distinct nature of disorders and the independence of two or more simultaneously existing conditions (Miller, 1994).

One of the persistent problems inherent in causative explanations for dual diagnosis conditions was that whatever disorder was seen as primary became the focus of treatment, whereas the other or secondary disorder generally received scant attention. The failures of this simplistic model become apparent when substance use disorders are ignored in mental health clinics and when mental health problems are ignored in alcohol and other drug recovery centers.

Comorbidity models or dual diagnosis models have added considerable complexity to the understanding of the substance user. There are several terms used to capture the concept of dual diagnosis, including "co-occurrence," "comorbidity," and "coexistence," each of which has slightly different nuances. The possible interactions or features of comorbidity might be characterized with Widiger's (1989) conceptualization of comorbidity of personality and mood disorders. These conditions might be characterized by any of the following:

- They are distinct and separate conditions that simply occur simultaneously without interdependence.

- Mood disorders contribute to a need for self-medication and resulting abuse or dependence (Khantzian, 1985).
- Substance-related disorders might create circumstances that lead to mood disorders.
- There might be synergistic, mutually potentiating relationships between mental or emotional disorders and substance use disorders.
- Substance-related and other disorders might arise from common biological vulnerabilities that can be expressed in multiple pathways.
- Other psychiatric disorders might be accentuated and aggravated by substance use.

Several mental and emotional disorders are associated with substance-related disorders, including mood disorders, anxiety disorders, personality disorders, attention deficit or hyperactivity, schizophrenia, traumatic stress disorders, sexual abuse survivorship, eating disorders, closed-head injury, and other neurocognitive impairments. Although homelessness is not a diagnosis, it is a social condition that clearly creates additional vulnerability for alcohol and drug use and could be considered in our discussion of comorbidities.

Substance-related disorder comorbidity is more common and complex than many practitioners expect. Among people with an extensive history of alcohol disorder, there is a lifetime prevalence of 70 percent for at least one other mental or emotional disorder (Regier, Farmer, et al., 1990). Regier, Farmer, and colleagues reported the overall prevalence rates for any alcohol or drug use disorder or mental disorder to be 15.7 percent within a one-month span, 19.5 percent within six months, and 32.7 percent for a lifetime. The lifetime prevalence for any mental disorder, excluding alcohol or drug abuse, is estimated to be 22.5 percent.

## MOOD AND ANXIETY DISORDERS

A substantial literature exists on the comorbidity of substance-related disorders and mood disorders. Early studies have reported that 28 percent to 59 percent of people with alcoholism experience depression (Weissman et al., 1977). Recent research continues to show this relationship. The bifurcation of the alcohol-abusing population into two distinct groups largely consistent with Cloninger's (1987) Type I and Type II classification for males with alcoholism suggests a split on the depression variable. In other words, people with Type I demonstrate depressive symptom sets, and those with Type II exhibit antisocial behaviors (Epstein, Ginsburg, Hesselbrock, & Schwarz, 1994; Irwin, Schuckit, & Smith, 1990; Windle, 1994; Zucker, Ellis, & Fitzgerald, 1994). The co-occurrence of depression with alcoholism may be important for determining treatment pathways. In addition, the presence of mood disorder might be a distinguishing feature from the more resistive antisocial variant of male substance abuse and dependence. Women and girls with this antisocial variant, on the other hand, have high rates of depression and can represent yet a different treatment challenge (Mulder, Wells, Joyce, & Bushnell, 1994). The co-occurrence of depression and alcoholism signals the importance of thoroughly exploring the synergistic effects of one disorder with the other. For example, a person might attempt to relieve depression by drinking, but alcohol can contribute pharmacologically to depression. Clearly, the presence of another disorder complicates the treatment situation, but comorbidity does not necessarily affect relapse rates or recovery rates from mood disorder in spite of some evidence to the contrary (Hirshfield, Hasin, Keller, Endicott, & Wunder, 1994).

Mood disorders show a complex comorbidity with anxiety disorders (Maser & Cloninger, 1990). In addition, people with anxiety disorders, including the whole gamut of phobias, have increased vulnerability toward alcohol abuse or dependence (Kushner, Sher, & Beitman, 1990; Schuckit & Hesselbrock, 1994). The synergy of disorder maps multiple vulnerabilities: The anxious person is more likely to use alcohol, and the alcohol user is more likely to be anxious either because of predisposing factors or pharmacology alone. However, complexities increase when other comorbidities are added. Thus, the synergy of certain personality disorders (particularly B clusters) with both mood disorder and substance-related disorder is potent and of great concern in planning treatment (Walker, 1992).

## PERSONALITY DISORDERS

Substance-related disorders are often comorbid with personality disorders in treatment populations, with rates that range from 14 percent to 55 percent (Blume, 1989). Conversely, people with personality disorders are at high risk for substance-related disorder (Nagel, 1989; Vaillant, 1983). The association of antisocial personality disorder with alcoholism was discussed above and has been reiterated in a large-scale study of substance abusers in treatment (Flynn, Craddock, Luckey, Hubbard, & Dunteman, 1996). Other personality disorders are more evident in clinical samples of substance abusers and dependent groups, including borderline, narcissistic, avoidant, dependent, and schizotypal. However, no single personality type is associated with substance-related disorders (Allen & Frances, 1986).

Comorbidity of personality disorders with substance-related disorders has significant implications for treatment, and interventions likely will need to be dually focused throughout the length of treatment. There is a growing literature that identifies models for the simultaneous care of both disorders (Cohen & Levy, 1992; Evans & Sullivan, 1990). The development of cognitive approaches to both sets of disorders also provides the opportunity to meet both aspects of a person's treatment needs (Beck et al., 1990; Beck et al., 1993).

## ATTENTION DEFICIT DISORDERS

Attention deficit hyperactivity disorder (ADHD) in children has been associated with a variety of other disorders, including personality disorder, depression, and substance-related disorders (Biederman et al., 1996). The long-term outcome for ADHD children as adults is predicted by some of Biederman and associates' prospective (1996) and retrospective studies (Biederman, Newcorn, & Sprich, 1991). The person with ADHD has a vulnerability for mood disorders and personality disorders that provides another vulnerability for substance-related disorders as discussed above. Apart from studies of people with pre-existing ADHD who might progress to substance-related disorders, there is additional concern about drug use and its effects on concentration and attentive functioning. For example, heavy marijuana use is associated with residual neuropsychological effects even after abstinence, but it is unclear whether the attention problems are a result of drug residue in the brain or neurotoxic effects of the drug (Pope & Yurgelin-Todd, 1996). There are possible synergistic effects when people with ADHD use substances and experience increasing problems with attention focusing, concentration, and memory capacities.

### TRAUMA-RELATED DISORDERS

Trauma-related disorders (acute stress disorder and PTSD) are being identified as more common comorbidities with substance-related disorders. The two most visible expressions of PTSD in substance abuse treatment populations are Vietnam veterans and adult survivors of childhood sexual abuse or of rape at any age. Meichenbaum (1994) cited Green's report that 75 percent of Vietnam veterans with PTSD also have at least one other diagnosis, the most common being depression and substance abuse. Among veterans in substance abuse treatment who were assessed for dissociative symptoms, which are associated with traumatic events, 41 percent had elevated scores, suggesting the need for further evaluation (Dunn, Paolo, & Fleet, 1993). Another study found that 48 percent of women in eight substance abuse treatment facilities had histories of incest (Janiskowski & Glover, 1994). The cause-and-effect relationship between sexual abuse and substance-related disorders is still unknown. However, there is evidence that the presence of sexual trauma and PTSD in substance abusers complicates their recovery (Chiavaroi, 1992; Kolodner & Frances, 1993; Teets, 1995). These trauma-related disorders add complexity to the diagnosis and treatment of people with substance-related disorders, and they suggest a need for cross-training treatment providers in both areas (Zweben, Clark, & Smith, 1994). Attention should be paid to other domestic violence themes for people with substance abuse, because drugs and alcohol are often implicated with these problems.

### CLOSED-HEAD INJURY AND OTHER NEUROCOGNITIVE IMPAIRMENTS

Neurocognitive dysfunction and neuropsychological dysfunction have numerous causes, including genetic factors as well as traumatic injury and chemical toxicity. These disorders can occur in people with other comorbidities, making detection more difficult (Oepen et al., 1993). Antisocial behavior is associated with a higher comorbidity of closed-head injury and other neuropsychological deficits, primarily frontal lobe damage that results in diminished inhibition of impulses and aggression (Bowman, 1997; Raine, 1993; Volavka, 1995). Diminished abstracting ability and impaired emotional regulation are among the other features of neurocognitive damage found in people with substance abuse (Miller, 1990).

### HOMELESSNESS

Homelessness is not a comorbidity but is a social condition that brings with it a set of additional clinical complexities. More than 50 years ago, Straus (1946) began describing the comorbid features of homelessness and alcoholism. The characteristics of dependency on institutions, coupled with the poor self-regulating skills described in his profile, are valid today (Straus, 1974). Homeless men and women represent another variation in the population of alcohol- and drug-dependent people—not the paradigm of the disorder as is sometimes represented in the media.

# Future Priorities

The epidemiologic data presented at the beginning of this chapter describe the high level of alcohol and other drug use in the United States. Although this use is not the highest recorded level of drug use in this country, the use is at generally unacceptable levels. It also seems clear to many observers that drug use is a drain on our resources and is a factor in the expanding criminal justice system, particularly prisons (Leukefeld, 1996). More people are currently being arrested for drug violations and related crimes, particularly in large cities and urban areas. Many of the arestees are from communities of color and are male, especially African American males. We know little about this phenomenon. Some of these arrestees are criminals who happen to use drugs and others are drug users who commit crimes to obtain drugs for their own use.

Numerous challenges face the substance abuse field in the coming decade. What is the future of funded treatment and other interventions for substance-related disorders? The expansion of private inpatient services in the 1980s appears to have contracted with the advent of managed care and the increasing demands for evidence of positive treatment outcomes. With public-sector funding following the private sector into a managed care format, the future of funding for substance abuse treatment is questionable.

Public attitudes about substance abuse and dependence seem to be drifting toward a neomoralistic perspective in place of a sympathetic disease model. Public policy increasingly focuses on the link between crime and drug abuse. This perspective not only promotes the positive use of treatment for convicted offenders, but it also appears to convey an unintended overidentification of substance-related disorders with criminality. Also, there is question as to whether the traditional treatment approaches have value in compulsory contexts. AA attendance, for example, does not appear to have any effect on abstinence or reduction in substance use when it is compulsory (Montgomery, Miller, & Tonigan, 1995). Social work and related disciplines involved in substance abuse intervention need to remind the public and policymakers that criminal drug abusers are but one subpopulation and do not constitute the majority of substance-dependent people.

Research should continue to explore outcomes from different treatment approaches and, to the degree possible, control for variables outside treatment, such as natural maturational processes. This line of research is needed because many professionals share doubt about the effectiveness of treatment. Science, not anecdotally based beliefs, should be used to answer the question of what treatments work best.

Tobacco must receive greater emphasis in both prevention and treatment of substance-related disorders. Recent research suggests that mortality is more attributable to tobacco than to alcohol or other drugs (Hurt et al., 1996). Therefore, it seems logical that substance abuse treatment professionals become sensitized to the importance of treating nicotine addiction in concert with traditional drug addiction. Although research suggests that nicotine abstinence does not threaten other recovery gains (Hurt et al., 1994; Joseph, Nichol, & Anderson, 1993), many clinicians fear that attaining abstinence from alcohol is fragile enough without attempting simultaneous nicotine abstinence. However, nicotine might be the most potent of the gateway drugs that pave the way for addictive disease. Clearly, prevention efforts must be directed toward adolescents who seem particularly vulnerable to the appeal of tobacco use.

Finally, an unsettled clinical issue in the substance abuse field is the role of spiritual methods for recovery. Additional research should be focused on the use of meditation as a method of treating or preventing substance use disorders in people with high-risk factors for abuse or dependence. The spiritual elements of the African American community, both Christian and Muslim, may be effective in working with the African American drug abuser who is at high risk for violent death and incarceration. It may be time for the white-dominated professions to turn to the African American community and other communities not merely for assistance with outreach but also for guidance about recovery methods and related outcomes, because it is possible that current approaches are culturally inappropriate.

# References

Akiskal, H. S. (1990). Toward a clinical understanding of the relationship of anxiety and depressive disorders. In J. D. Maser & C. R. Cloninger (Eds.), *Comorbidity of mood and anxiety disorders* (pp. 597–610). Washington, DC: American Psychiatric Press.

Allen, M. H., & Frances, R. J. (1986). Varieties of psychopathology found in patients with addictive disorders: A review. In R. E. Meyer (Ed.), *Psychopathology and addictive disorders* (pp. 17–38). New York: Guilford Press.

American Psychiatric Association. (1994). *Diagnostic and statistical manual of mental disorders* (4th ed.). Washington, DC: Author.

American Psychiatric Association. (1995). *Practice guideline for treatment of patients with substance use disorders—Alcohol, cocaine, opioids.* Washington, DC: Author.

Amsel, Z., Mandell, W., Mathias, L., Mason, C., & Lockerman, I. (1976). Reliability and validity of self-reported illegal activities and drug use collection from narcotic addicts. *International Journal of the Addictions, 11,* 325–336.

Anderson, S. (1994). A critical analysis of the concept of codependency. *Social Work, 39,* 677–685.

Annis, H. M., & Davis, C. S. (1988). Assessment of expectancies. In D. M. Donovan & G. A. Marlatt (Eds.), *Assessment of addictive behaviors* (pp. 84–111). New York: Guilford Press.

Anthony, J. C., Arria, A. M., & Johnson, E. O. (1995). Epidemiology and public health issues for tobacco, alcohol and other drugs. In J. M. Oldham & M. B. Riba (Eds.), *Review of psychiatry* (Vol. 14, pp. 15–46). Washington, DC: American Psychiatric Press.

Bailey, G. W. (1991). Substance use and abuse. In J. M. Weiner (Ed.), *Textbook of child and adolescent psychiatry* (pp. 439–451). Washington, DC: American Psychiatric Press.

Baumgartner, W. A., Hill, V. A., & Bland, W. H. (1989). Hair analysis for drugs of abuse. *Journal of Forensic Science, 34,* 1433–1454.

Beck, A. T., Freeman, A., & Associates. (1990). *Cognitive therapy of personality disorders.* New York: Guilford Press.

Beck, A. T., Wright, F. D., Newman, C. F., & Liese, B. S. (1993). *Cognitive therapy of substance abuse.* New York: Guilford Press.

Biederman, J., Faraone, S., Milberger, S., Guite, J., Mick, E., Chen, L., Mennin, D., Marrs, A., Oulette, C., Moore, P., Spencer, T., Norman, D., Wilens, T., Kraus, I., & Perrin, J. (1996). A prospective 4-year follow-up study of attention-deficit hyperactivity and related disorders. *Archives of General Psychiatry, 53,* 437–446.

Biederman, J., Newcorn, J., & Sprich, S. (1991). Comorbidity of attention deficit hyperactivity disorder with conduct, depressive, anxiety and other disorders. *American Journal of Psychiatry, 148,* 564–577.

Blum, K., Cull, J. G., Braverman, E. R., & Comings, D. E. (1996). Reward deficiency syndrome. *American Scientist, 84,* 132–145.

Blum, K., Noble, E. P., Sheridan, P. J., Montgomery, A., Ritchie, T., Jagadeeswaran, P., Nogami, H., Briggs, A. H., & Cohn, J. B. (1990). Allelic association of human dopamine $D_2$ receptor gene in alcoholism. *JAMA, 263*, 2055–2060.

Blume, S. (1989). Dual diagnosis: Psychoactive substance abuse and the personality disorders. *Journal of Psychoactive Drugs, 21*, 139–144.

Bowman, M. L. (1997). Brain impairment in impulsive violence. In. C. D. Webster & M. A. Jackson (Eds.), *Impulsivity: Theory, assessment, and treatment* (pp. 116–141). New York: Guilford Press.

Brehm, N. M., & Khantzian, E. J. (1992). A psychodynamic perspective. In J. H. Lowinson, P. Ruiz, R. B. Millman, & J. G. Langrod (Eds.), *Substance abuse: A comprehensive textbook* (pp. 106–117). Baltimore: Williams & Wilkins.

Bukstein, O., & Kaminer, Y. (1994). The nosology of adolescent substance abuse. *American Journal on Addictions, 3*, 1–13.

Bureau of Justice Statistics. (1991). *Survey of state prison inmates* (Report No. NCJ-136949). Rockville, MD: Author.

Centers for Disease Control and Prevention. (1994). *Morbidity and Mortality Weekly Report, 43*, 861–865.

Chamberland, M., White, C., Lifson, A., & Sonders, T. J. (1987, June). *AIDS in heterosexual contacts: A small but interesting group of cases.* Presentation at the Third International Conference on AIDS, Washington, DC.

Chiavaroi, T. (1992). Rehabilitation from substance abuse in individuals with a history of sexual abuse. *Journal of Substance Abuse Treatment, 9*, 349–354.

Cloninger, C. R. (1987). Neurogenetic adaptive mechanisms in alcoholism. *Science, 236*, 410–416.

Cohen, J., & Levy, S. J. (1992). *The mentally ill chemical abuser: Whose client?* New York: Lexington Books.

DesJarlais, D. C., Friedman, S. R., & Stoneburner, R. L. (1988). HIV infections and intravenous drug use: Critical issues in transmission dynamics, infection outcomes and prevention. *Review of Infectious Diseases, 10*, 151–158.

Donovan, D. M. (1986). An etiologic model of alcoholism. *American Journal of Psychiatry, 143*, 1–11.

Donovan, D. M. (1988). Assessment of addictive behaviors: Implications of an emerging biopsychosocial model. In D. Donovan & G. Marlatt (Eds.), *Assessment of addictive behaviors* (pp. 3–50). New York: Guilford Press.

Dunn, G. E., Paolo, A. M., & Fleet, J. V. (1993). Dissociative symptoms in a substance abuse population. *American Journal of Psychiatry, 150*, 1043–1047.

Edwards, M. E., & Steinglass, P. (1995). Family therapy treatment outcomes for alcoholism. *Journal of Marital and Family Therapy, 21*, 475–509.

Epstein, E. E., Ginsburg, B. E., Hesselbrock, V. M., & Schwarz, J. C. (1994). Alcohol and drug abusers subtyped by antisocial personality and primary or secondary depressive disorder. In T. Babor, V. Hesselbrock, R. Meyer, & W. Shoemaker (Eds.), *Types of alcoholics: Evidence from clinical, experimental and genetic research* (pp. 41–56). New York: New York Academy of Sciences.

Evans, K., & Sullivan, J. M. (1990). *Dual diagnosis: Considering the mentally ill substance abuser.* New York: Guilford Press.

Feucht, T. E., Stephens, R. C., & Walker, M. (1994). Drug use among juvenile arrestees: A comparison of self-report, urinalysis and hair assay. *Journal of Drug Issues, 24*, 99–116.

Fils-Aime, M-L., Eckhardt, M. J., George, D. T., Brown, G. L., Mefford, I., & Linniola, M. (1996). Early-onset alcoholics have lower cerebrospinal fluid 5-hydroxyindole acetic acid levels than late-onset alcoholics. *Archives of General Psychiatry, 53,* 211–216.

Flynn, P. M., Craddock, S. G., Luckey, J. W., Hubbard, R. L., & Dunteman, G. H. (1996). Comorbidity of antisocial personality and mood disorders among psychoactive substance-dependent treatment clients. *Journal of Personality Disorders, 10,* 56–67.

Gall, T. L., & Lucas, D. M. (Eds.). (1996). *Statistics on alcohol, drug and tobacco use.* Detroit: Gale Research.

Gold, M. S. (1992). Cocaine (and crack): Clinical aspects. In J. H. Lowinson, P. Ruiz, R. B. Millman, & J. G. Langrod (Eds.), *Substance abuse: A comprehensive textbook* (2nd ed., pp. 205–221). Baltimore: Williams & Wilkins.

Goodwin, F. K., & Jamison, K. R. (1990). *Manic–depressive illness.* New York: Oxford University Press.

Hirshfield, R.M.A., Hasin, D., Keller, M. B., Endicott, J., & Wunder, J. (1994). Depression and alcoholism: Comorbidity in a longitudinal study. In J. D. Maser & R. C. Cloninger (Eds.), *Comorbidity of mood and anxiety disorders* (pp. 293–304). Washington, DC: American Psychiatric Press.

Hurt, R. D., Eberman, K. M., Croghan, I. T., Offord, K. P., Davis, L. J., Morse, R. M., Palmen, M. A., & Bruce, B. K. (1994). Nicotine-dependence treatment during inpatient treatment for other addictions: A prospective intervention trial. *Alcoholism: Clinical and Experimental Research, 18,* 867–872.

Hurt, R. D., Offord, K. P., Croghan, I. T., Gomez-Dahl, L., Kottke, T. E., Morse, R. M., & Melton, L. J. (1996). Mortality following inpatient addictions treatment. *JAMA, 275,* 1097–1103.

Insurance Institute for Highway Safety. (1994). *Alcohol fatality facts 1994.* Arlington, VA: Author.

Irwin, M., Schuckit, M., & Smith, T. L. (1990). Clinical importance of age at onset in Type 1 and Type 2 primary alcoholics. *Archives of General Psychiatry, 47,* 320–324.

Janiskowski, T. I., & Glover, N. M. (1994). Incest and substance abuse: Implications for treatment professionals. *Journal of Substance Abuse Treatment, 11,* 177–183.

Johnson, B. D., & Muffler, J. (1992). Sociocultural aspects of drug use and abuse in the 1990s. In J. H. Lowinson, P. Ruiz, R. B. Millman, & J. G. Langrod (Eds.), *Substance abuse: A comprehensive textbook* (2nd ed., pp. 118–137). Baltimore: Williams & Wilkins.

Joseph, A. M., Nichol, K. L., & Anderson, H. (1993). Effect of treatment for nicotine dependence on alcohol and drug treatment outcomes. *Addictive Behaviors, 18,* 635–644.

Kandel, D. B., & Davies, M. (1996). High school students who use crack and other drugs. *Archives of General Psychiatry, 53,* 71–80.

Kaufman, E. (1992). Family therapy: A treatment approach with substance abusers. In J. H. Lowinson, P. Ruiz, R. B. Millman, & J. G. Langrod (Eds.), *Substance abuse: A comprehensive textbook* (2nd ed., pp. 520–532). Baltimore: Williams & Wilkins.

Kendler, K. S., Neale, M. C., Heath, A. C., Kessler, R. C., & Evans, L. J. (1994). A twin study of alcoholism in women. *American Journal of Psychiatry, 151,* 707–715.

Kessler, R. C., McGonagle, K. A., Zhao, S., Nelson, C., Hughes, M., Eshleman, S., Wittchen H-U., & Kendler, K. S. (1994). Lifetime and 12-month prevalence of DSM-III-R psychiatric disorders in the United States: Results from the National Comorbidity Survey. *Archives of General Psychiatry, 51,* 8–19.

Khantzian, E. J. (1985). The self-medication hypothesis of addictive disorders: Focus on heroin and cocaine dependence. *American Journal of Psychiatry, 142,* 1259–1264.

Kolodner, G., & Frances, R. (1993). Recognizing dissociative disorders in patients with chemical dependency. *Hospital and Community Psychiatry, 44,* 1041–1043.

Kosten, T., Rounsaville, B., & Kleber, H. (1987). A 2.5-year follow-up of cocaine abuse among opioid addicts: Have our treatments helped? *Archives of General Psychiatry, 44,* 281–285.

Kushner, M. G., Sher, K. J., & Beitman, B. D. (1990). The relation between alcohol problems and the anxiety disorders. *American Journal of Psychiatry, 147,* 685–695.

Lange, W. R., Snyder, F. R., Lozovsky, D., Kaistha, V., Kaczanter, M. A., & Jaffee, J. M. (1988). Geographic distribution of human immunodeficiency virus markers in parenteral drug abusers. *American Journal of Public Health, 78,* 443–446.

Leukefeld, C. G. (1996). Introduction. In T. L. Gall & D. M. Lucas (Eds.), *Statistics on alcohol, drug and tobacco use* (pp. ix–xv). Detroit: Gale Research.

Leukefeld, C. G., Miller, T. W., & Hays, L. (1996). Drug use. In M. Mattaini & B. Thayer (Eds.), *Finding solutions to social problems: Behavioral analysis for social change* (pp. 373–396). Washington, DC: American Psychological Association.

Leukefeld, C. G., & Tims, F. M. (1990). Compulsory treatment for drug abuse. *International Journal of the Addictions, 26,* 621–640.

Littrell, J. (1991). *Understanding and treating alcoholism: An empirically based clinician's handbook for treatment of alcoholism.* Hillsdale, NJ: Lawrence Erlbaum.

Maser, J. D., & Cloninger, C. R. (1990). Comorbidity of anxiety and mood disorders: Introduction and overview. In J. D. Maser & C. R. Cloninger (Eds.), *Comorbidity of mood and anxiety disorders* (pp. 3–12). Washington, DC: American Psychiatric Press.

McLellan, T., Kushner, H., Metzger, D., Peters, R., Smith, I., Grissom, G., Pettinati, M., & Argerian, M. (1992). The fifth edition of the Addiction Severity Index. *Journal of Substance Abuse Treatment, 9,* 199–213.

McLellan, T., Luborsky, L., Woody, G., & O'Brien, C. (1980). An improved diagnostic instrument for substance abuse patients: The Addiction Severity Index. *Journal of Nervous and Mental Disease, 168,* 26–33.

Meichenbaum, D. (1994). *A clinical handbook/practical therapist manual for assessing and treating adults with post-traumatic stress disorder (PTSD).* Waterloo, Ontario: Institute Press.

Merikangas, K. R. (1990). Comorbidity for anxiety and depression: Review of family and genetic studies. In J. D. Maser & C. R. Cloninger (Eds.), *Comorbidity of mood and anxiety disorders* (pp. 331–348). Washington, DC: American Psychiatric Press.

Mieczkowski, T., Barzeley, D., Gropper, B., & Wish, E. (1991). Concordance of three measures of cocaine use in an arrestee population: Hair, urine, and self-report. *Journal of Psychoactive Drugs, 23,* 241–249.

Miller, L. (1990). Neuropsychodynamics of alcoholism and addiction: Personality, psychopathology, and cognitive style. *Journal of Substance Abuse Treatment, 7,* 31–49.

Miller, N. S. (1994). The interactions between coexisting disorders. In N. S. Miller (Ed.), *Treating coexisting psychiatric and addictive disorders: A practical guide.* Center City, MN: Hazelden.

Miller, N. S., & Gold, M. S. (1991). *Drugs of abuse: A comprehensive series for clinicians* (Vol. 2: Alcohol). New York: Plenum Medical Books.

Minuchin, S. (1975). *Families and family therapy.* Cambridge, MA: Harvard University Press.

Montgomery, H. A., Miller, W. R., & Tonigan, J. S. (1995). Does Alcoholics Anonymous involvement predict treatment outcome? *Journal of Substance Abuse Treatment, 12,* 241–252.

Mulder, R. T., Wells, J. E., Joyce, P. R., & Bushnell, J. A. (1994). Antisocial women. *Journal of Personality Disorders, 8,* 279–287.

Nagel, S. B. (1989). Addictive behaviors: Problems in treatment with borderline patients. In J. F. Masterson & R. Klein (Eds.), *Psychotherapy of the disorders of the self* (pp. 395–410). New York: Brunner/Mazel.

National Drug Control Strategy. (1995). *Strengthening communities' response to drugs and crime.* Washington, DC: U.S. Government Printing Office.

National Institute of Justice. (1993). *Drug use forecasting: 1993 annual report on adult arrestees: Drugs and crime in America's cities* (Report No. NCJ-147411). Rockville, MD: Author.

National Institute on Drug Abuse. (1994). *Monitoring the future study, 1975–1994: National high school senior drug abuse survey.* Rockville, MD: Author.

Oepen, G., Levy, M., Saemann, R., Harrington, A., Handren, M., Pinnone, L., Pollen, L., Ellison, J., & Boshes, R. (1993). A neuropsychological perspective on dual diagnosis. *Journal of Psychoactive Drugs, 25,* 129–133.

Parsian, A., Todd, R. D., Devor, E. J., O'Malley, K. L., Suarez, B. K., Reich, T., & Cloninger, C. R. (1991). Alcoholism and alleles of the human $D_2$ dopamine receptor locus. *Archives of General Psychiatry, 48,* 655–663.

Pickens, R. W., Svikis, D. S., McGue, M., Lykken, D. T., Heston, L. L., & Clayton, P. J. (1991). Heterogeneity in the inheritance of alcoholism. *Archives of General Psychiatry, 48,* 19–28.

Pope, H. G., & Yurgelin-Todd, D. (1996). The residual cognitive effects of heavy marijuana use in college students. *JAMA, 275,* 521–527.

Raine, A. (1993). *The psychopathology of crime: Criminal behavior as a clinical disorder.* San Diego: Academic Press.

Regier, D. A., Burke, J. D., & Burke, K. C. (1990). Comorbidity of affective and anxiety disorders in the NIMH Epidemiologic Catchment Area program. In J. D. Maser & C. R. Cloninger (Eds.), *Comorbidity of mood and anxiety disorders* (pp. 113–122). Washington, DC: American Psychiatric Press.

Regier, D. A., Farmer, M. E., Rae, D. S., Locke, B. Z., Keith, S. J., Judd, L. L., & Goodwin, F. K. (1990). Comorbidity of mental disorders with alcohol and other drug abuse: Results from the Epidemiologic Catchment Area (ECA) study. *JAMA, 264,* 2511–2518.

Rouse, B. A. (Ed.). (1995). *Substance abuse and mental health statistics sourcebook.* Washington, DC: U.S. Government Printing Office.

Schuckit, M. A., & Hesselbrock, V. (1994). Alcohol dependence and anxiety disorders: What is the relationship? *American Journal of Psychiatry, 151,* 1723–1734.

Shiffman, S. (1988). Behavioral assessment. In D. M. Donovan & G. A. Marlatt (Eds.), *Assessment of addictive behaviors* (pp. 139–188). New York: Guilford Press.

Stanton, M. D., & Heath, A. W. (1995). Family treatment of alcohol and drug abuse. In R. H. Mikesell, D-D. Lusterman, & S. H. McDaniel (Eds.), *Integrating family therapy: Handbook of family psychology and systems theory* (pp. 529–544). Washington, DC: American Psychological Association.

Straus, R. (1946). Alcohol and the homeless man. *Quarterly Journal of Studies on Alcohol, 7,* 360–404.

Straus, R. (1974). *Escape from custody: A study of alcoholism and institutional dependency as reflected in the life of a homeless man.* New York: Harper & Row.

Substance Abuse and Mental Health Services Administration, Office of Applied Studies. (1994). *National household survey on drug abuse population estimates 1993* (DHHS Pub. No. 94-3017). Washington, DC: Author.

Teets, J. M. (1995). Childhood sexual trauma of chemically dependent women. *Journal of Psychoactive Drugs, 27,* 231–238.

Vaillant, G. (1983). *The natural history of alcoholism.* Cambridge, MA: Harvard University Press.

Volavka, J. (1995). *Neurobiology of violence.* Washington, DC: American Psychiatric Press.

Volpe, J. J. (1992). Effect of cocaine upon the fetus. *New England Journal of Medicine, 327,* 399–407.

Walker, R. (1992). Substance abuse and B-cluster disorders I: Understanding the dual-diagnosis patient. *Journal of Psychoactive Drugs, 24,* 223–232.

Wallace, J. (1986). The other problems of alcoholics. *Journal of Substance Abuse Treatment, 3,* 163–171.

Weissman, M. M., Pottenger, M., Kleber, H., Ruben, H. L., Williams, D., & Thompson, W. D. (1977). Symptom patterns in primary and secondary depression: A comparison of primary depressives with depressed opiate addicts, alcoholics and schizophrenics. *Archives of General Psychiatry, 34,* 854–862.

Widiger, T. A. (1989). The categorical distinction between personality and affective disorders. *Journal of Personality Disorders, 3,* 77–91.

Williams, T. G. (1996). Substance abuse and addictive personality disorders. In F. W. Kaslow (Ed.), *Handbook of relational diagnosis and dysfunctional family patterns* (pp. 448–462). New York: John Wiley & Sons.

Windle, M. (1994). Coexisting problems and alcoholic risk among adolescents. In T. Babor, V. Hesselbrock, R. Meyer, & W. Shoemaker (Eds.), *Types of alcoholics: Evidence from clinical, experimental and genetic research* (pp. 157–164). New York: New York Academy of Sciences.

Zucker, R. A., Ellis, D. A., & Fitzgerald, H. E. (1994). Developmental evidence for at least two alcoholisms: I. Biopsychosocial variation among pathways into symptomatic difficulty. In T. Babor, V. Hesselbrock, R. Meyer, & W. Shoemaker (Eds.), *Types of alcoholics: Evidence from clinical, experimental and genetic research* (pp. 134–146). New York: New York Academy of Sciences.

Zweben, J. E., Clark, H. W., & Smith, D. E. (1994). Traumatic experiences and substance abuse: Mapping the territory. *Journal of Psychoactive Drugs, 26,* 327–344.

## Suggested Reading

Galanter, M., & Kleber, H. D. (Eds.). (1994). *Textbook of substance abuse treatment.* Washington, DC: American Psychiatric Press.

Lowinson, J. M., Ruiz, P., Millman, R. B., & Langrod, J. G. (Eds). (1992). *Substance abuse: A comprehensive textbook* (2nd ed.). Baltimore: Williams & Wilkins.

Oldham, J. M., & Riba, M. B. (Eds.). (1995). *Review of psychiatry* (Vol. 14, Section I, Substance Abuse). Washington, DC: American Psychiatric Press.

# Personality Disorders

Nancee Blum and Bruce Pfohl

Mental health professionals soon learn that there are more differences than similarities between people who share the same Axis I diagnosis. One person with a diagnosis of major depression may be extremely dependent and inhibited, whereas another may be very impulsive and irritable. One person with obsessive–compulsive disorder may maintain almost no friendships, whereas another is gregarious. Such differences are often referred to as "personality." The *Diagnostic and Statistical Manual of Mental Disorders* (4th ed.) (DSM-IV) (American Psychiatric Association [APA], 1994) defines *personality* as "enduring patterns of perceiving, relating to, and thinking about the environment and oneself that are exhibited in a wide range of social and personal contexts" (p. 630). When the personality traits constitute a rigid pattern of behavior leading to distress and impairment, a personality disorder may be present.

DSM-IV places personality diagnoses on a separate axis—Axis II—to emphasize the fact that personality may introduce additional liabilities and assets that are independent of the Axis I diagnosis. Data supporting the validity of some of the personality diagnoses in DSM-IV are limited. Even so, the personality diagnoses provide a useful lexicon for describing personality differences. For therapists, the individual criteria for a personality disorder can be used to identify long-term problems in interpersonal functioning that may need to be addressed in therapy. Although the personality diagnoses are presented as categorical diagnoses that are either present or absent, it is often useful to note personality traits on Axis II that may influence therapy even when full criteria for a disorder are not met.

DSM-IV divides the personality disorders into three clusters on the basis of descriptive similarities. People with cluster A characteristics (paranoid, schizoid, and schizotypal) often appear odd and eccentric; those with cluster B characteristics (histrionic, narcissistic, borderline, and antisocial) are described as dramatic, emotional, or erratic; and people with disorders in cluster C (avoidant, dependent, and obsessive–compulsive) often appear anxious or fearful. Although the clusters may be a useful tool for thinking about and remembering the personality disorders, empirical studies find that the actual distribution of diagnoses provides only weak support for the clusters (Fabrega, Ulrich, Pilkonis, & Mezzich, 1991). It is not hard to find people who simultaneously have two or more personality diagnoses from different clusters. In clinical practice, the clusters are often used as a diagnostic shorthand.

For example, patients who allow others to make most of their decisions, who are highly anxious in social situations, and who are overly sensitive to criticism may be described as having cluster C features.

# Categorical DSM-IV Personality Disorders

## PARANOID PERSONALITY DISORDER

Paranoid personality disorder is characterized by suspiciousness and a pervasive and unwarranted distrust of others such that their motives are interpreted as malevolent. People with this disorder assume that others will exploit, harm, or deceive them. They are likely to come into the medical care system not because they recognize their problems but rather because of litigation issues, such as a disability or malpractice claim.

These patients are often considered difficult to work with in psychotherapy because of their distrust of the therapist's motives, denial of difficulties, and reluctance to disclose personal information. There have been case reports on the successful treatment of paranoid personality disorder with cognitive therapy (Turkat, 1985; Turkat & Maisto, 1985; Williams, 1988), but there are no controlled studies of response to either psychotherapy or pharmacotherapy. The prevalence of paranoid personality disorder is reported to be 0.5 percent to 2.5 percent in the general population, 10 percent to 30 percent among those in inpatient psychiatric settings, and 2 percent to 10 percent in outpatient mental health clinics. In clinical samples, the disorder is diagnosed more frequently in males than females (APA, 1994).

## SCHIZOID PERSONALITY DISORDER

Schizoid personality disorder is characterized by detachment from social relationships and a restricted range of emotional expressiveness in interpersonal settings. People who have this disorder are apparently uncommon in clinical settings, and empirical data are limited (APA, 1994). Because people with this disorder are not distressed by the lack of social relationships, they will be likely to come to clinical attention for other reasons, such as an acute stressor or change in life circumstances. There are few data regarding either psychotherapy or pharmacotherapy in the treatment of schizoid personality disorder. Cognitive interventions, social skills training, and group therapy may be of some benefit (Kalus, Bernstein, & Siever, 1995). Schizoid personality disorder is diagnosed slightly more often in males than females.

## SCHIZOTYPAL PERSONALITY DISORDER

Schizotypal personality disorder is the third disorder in the so-called "odd cluster" of the DSM personality disorders and is distinguished from paranoid personality disorder and schizoid personality disorder by eccentricity and cognitive–perceptual distortions. The disorder shares the traits of suspiciousness with paranoid personality disorder as well as the social isolation of schizoid personality disorder. People with this disorder have social and interpersonal deficits marked by acute discomfort with and reduced capacity for close relationships, although they may be sufficiently motivated to interact with others so as to be widely known as eccentric. These people often come to the mental health setting because of problems in occupational and social functioning or referral by concerned members of the community. Schizo-typal personality disorder has been reported to occur in approximately 3 percent of the general population and may be slightly more common in males (APA, 1994).

## ANTISOCIAL PERSONALITY DISORDER

Antisocial personality disorder is characterized by a pervasive pattern of disregard for and violation of the rights of others that begins in childhood or early adolescence and continues into adulthood. Childhood conduct disorder behaviors involve a persistent pattern in which the basic rights of others or major age-appropriate societal rules are violated (for example, aggression to people and animals, destruction of property, and lying). People with antisocial personality disorder may come to the attention of clinicians because of depressed mood or substance abuse problems.

This diagnosis has been criticized for its emphasis on overt criminal acts rather than more general personality traits of psychopathy, contributing to an overdiagnosing of the disorder in prison and forensic institutions (Widiger & Corbitt, 1995). The overall prevalence of antisocial personality disorder in community samples is about 3 percent in males and 1 percent in females. Prevalence estimates in clinical settings vary from 3 percent to 30 percent, depending on the predominant characteristics of the populations being sampled. Even higher prevalence rates are associated with substance abuse treatment and prison settings (APA, 1994). The disorder is diagnosed much more frequently in males than in females, which partly may result from criteria that emphasize antisocial behaviors seen most often in males. Most research studies have been confined to male subjects (Widiger et al., 1996).

## BORDERLINE PERSONALITY DISORDER

Borderline personality disorder is characterized by instability in interpersonal relationships, self-image, affects, and control of impulsivity. People with borderline personality disorder account for a high proportion of hospital emergency room visits and inpatient hospitalizations because of suicidal threats, actions, or self-mutilating behaviors. Angry outbursts and suicidal behaviors often occur in response to seemingly minor stressors, such as a therapist announcing that he or she will be on vacation for a few days. An inexperienced clinician may experience extreme frustration when a patient rapidly changes from overdependence to angry rejection. Understanding the diagnosis as a disorder of emotion regulation has led to the development of more effective cognitive–behavioral therapies to teach emotion regulation and interpersonal skills. An important outcome has been the demonstration of a decrease in suicidal behaviors and in the use of high-intensity services such as emergency rooms and inpatient hospitalizations (Kehrer & Linehan, 1996; Linehan, Armstrong, Suarez, Allmon, & Heard, 1991; Linehan, Heard, & Armstrong, 1993).

Borderline personality disorder overlaps extensively with Axis I disorders, particularly mood disorders (Gunderson & Phillips, 1991), posttraumatic stress disorder (Gunderson & Sabo, 1993), and other personality disorders (Pfohl, Coryell, Zimmerman, & Stangl, 1986). The prevalence of borderline personality disorder is estimated at 2 percent of the general population, 10 percent in outpatient mental health clinics, and 20 percent among psychiatric inpatients. Among clinical populations with personality disorders, prevalence is estimated to be 30 percent to 60 percent. Borderline personality disorder is diagnosed predominantly (about 75 percent) in females (APA, 1994).

## HISTRIONIC PERSONALITY DISORDER

Histrionic personality disorder is characterized by excessive emotionality, a provocative interpersonal style, and attention-seeking behavior. In the clinical setting, the dramatic presentation may appear out of proportion to the actual seriousness of the medical or emotional problem. Attempts to control and obtain attention from others often take the form of exaggerated compliments, gifts, flirtatiousness, or requests for special treatment (for example, extra time during appointments). Patients with histrionic personality disorder may have numerous somatic complaints. Prevalence of histrionic personality disorder is estimated at 2 percent to 3 percent in general population studies and 10 percent to 15 percent in inpatient and outpatient mental health settings when assessed with a structured interview (APA, 1994).

## NARCISSISTIC PERSONALITY DISORDER

Narcissistic personality disorder is characterized by grandiosity, need for admiration, and lack of empathy. People with this disorder may become frustrated and angry when they do not get the recognition or special treatment they believe they deserve and may react with rage or counterattack. Such people are not likely to seek psychiatric help unless they have received a severe challenge to their sense of superiority. In the clinical setting, these patients often describe the many important people they know and imply that the clinician is not prestigious enough to treat them. Estimates of prevalence of narcissistic personality disorder range from 2 percent to 16 percent in clinical populations and less than 1 percent in the general population. Narcissistic personality disorder is diagnosed most often in males (50 percent to 75 percent) (APA, 1994).

The inclusion of narcissistic personality disorder in the DSM has been somewhat controversial because of its high comorbidity with other personality disorders (Livesley & Schroeder, 1991) and the lack of validation of the disorder through such external criteria as a specific etiological pathway, a specific course, or a specific treatment outcome (Gunderson, Ronningstam, & Smith, 1995).

## AVOIDANT PERSONALITY DISORDER

Avoidant personality disorder is characterized by social inhibition, feelings of inadequacy, and hypersensitivity to negative evaluation. People with this disorder are likely to avoid social or occupational situations that require interpersonal contact because of fear of criticism, disapproval, or rejection. In contrast to the criteria for many other personality disorders, people with avoidant personality disorder frequently have sufficient insight to provide the clinician with the symptoms necessary to make the diagnosis. The prevalence of avoidant personality disorder is between 0.5 percent to 1.0 percent in the general population and about 10.0 percent in outpatient mental health clinics (Widiger, 1991a). Avoidant personality disorder is diagnosed with equal frequency in males and females (APA, 1994).

The relationship between avoidant personality disorder and social phobia, generalized type on Axis I, is unclear, but there is some evidence that the two can be distinguished from one another. Millon and Martinez (1995) characterized avoidant personality disorder as a problem of relating to other people and social phobia as a problem of performing in social situations.

## DEPENDENT PERSONALITY DISORDER

Dependent personality disorder is characterized by an excessive need to be taken care of, which leads to submissive and clinging behavior and fears of separation. People with this disorder may come to the treatment setting following the loss of a relationship that previously supported them or when a relationship becomes increasingly emotionally or physically abusive. Suggestions that require more autonomous functioning may be rejected by patients because of their lack of confidence in their own ability. In some cases, these people may passively acquiesce to a plan to separate from an abusive partner, only to return to that person within a short time.

## OBSESSIVE–COMPULSIVE PERSONALITY DISORDER

Obsessive–compulsive personality disorder is characterized by preoccupation with perfectionism, mental and interpersonal control, and orderliness at the expense of flexibility, openness, and efficiency. There are data to suggest that this personality disorder is associated with less functional impairment than most of the other personality disorders (Nakao et al., 1992). To some extent, these traits may be adaptive in certain situations and occupations, and it is only when they reach the level of significant functional impairment with work and interpersonal relationships that they constitute a disorder. Prevalence estimates using systematic assessment, are 1 percent in community samples and 3 percent to 10 percent in people presenting to mental health clinics. The disorder is diagnosed about twice as often among males (APA, 1994).

Because of the similarity in names between obsessive–compulsive disorder (Axis I) and obsessive–compulsive personality disorder (Axis II), it is appropriate to comment on the possible overlap. The findings for studies using DSM-III and DSM-III-R criteria with clinical and structured interviews suggest that the majority of people with Axis I obsessive–compulsive disorder do not have Axis II obsessive–compulsive personality disorder (Baer et al., 1990). Most people with obsessive–compulsive personality disorder never develop obsessive–compulsive disorder (Pollak, 1987). Among patients with obsessive–compulsive disorder who have a personality disorder, several other personality disorders may be as common or more common than obsessive–compulsive personality disorder (Black, Noyes, Pfohl, Goldstein, & Blum, 1993).

# DSM-IV Appendix

In its appendix, the DSM-IV includes two additional criteria sets as disorders needing further study: depressive and passive–aggressive personality disorders.

## DEPRESSIVE PERSONALITY DISORDER

Depressive personality disorder is characterized by a pervasive pattern of depressive cognitions and behaviors. People with this disorder tend to brood and worry and may feel that they do not deserve enjoyment or pleasure. These people tend to judge others as harshly as they judge themselves. This pattern may occur with equal frequency in males and females (APA, 1994). Depressive personality disorder may be on a spectrum with the Axis I mood disorders (Akiskal, 1989), with family history, treatment response, and possibly etiology similar to the relationship between schizophrenia and schizotypal personality disorder. Clarification is needed on the relationship between depressive personality disorder and Axis I depressive disorders and Axis II personality disorders (Phillips, Gunderson, Hirschfeld, & Smith, 1990).

## PASSIVE–AGGRESSIVE PERSONALITY DISORDER

Passive–aggressive personality disorder (negativistic personality disorder) is characterized by a pervasive pattern of negativistic attitudes and passive resistance to demands for adequate performance in social and occupational situations. Resistance may take the form of procrastination, forgetfulness, stubbornness, and intentional inefficiency, particularly in response to tasks assigned by authority figures.

Passive–aggressive personality disorder was included in both DSM-III and DSM-III-R. The lack of data about the disorder led Blashfield, Sprock, and Fuller (1990) to suggest its deletion from Axis II. The criteria set in the appendix to DSM-IV is intended to represent a more broadly conceived negativistic personality disorder that has wider application than its World War II origins, when it was used to describe military personnel who expressed their opposition to authority figures indirectly through subversion rather than through more direct means (Millon & Radovanov, 1995).

## Alternative Conceptualizations of Personality

Controversy still exists about whether personality disorder is best conceptualized as a series of continuous dimensions or as the discrete categories used in the DSM (Widiger, 1991a). A major limitation of the categorical approach to personality disorder classification is its failure to reconcile with the extensive body of research that describes a number of reproducible personality traits that are distributed normally and independently in the general population (Digman, 1992). Most of the research is published in psychological rather than psychiatric journals, although psychiatrists are increasingly interested in determining whether a series of basic and independent personality trait dimensions can be detected in clinical populations (Cloninger, 1987; Heumann & Morey, 1990). The majority of these studies are based on data from self-rating questionnaires with a multiple-choice or true–false format.

Dimensional approaches to personality disorders have attempted to identify fundamental dimensions that underlie the entire range of normal and pathological personality functioning. The Eysenck (1970) Personality Inventory has been studied extensively in both normal and clinical populations. Three dimensions are identified: neuroticism, extroversion, and psychoticism. The NEO Personality Inventory (Costa & McCrae, 1990) assesses five major dimensions: neuroticism, extroversion, openness to experience, agreeableness, and constraint. The Temperament and Character Inventory (Cloninger, 1987) assesses four dimensions of temperament (novelty seeking, harm avoidance, reward dependence, and persistence) and three dimensions of character (self-directedness, cooperativeness, and self-transcendence).

There seems to be a developing consensus that these varied instruments represent slightly different approaches to measuring five or six basic personality dimensions (Digman, 1992; Widiger, 1991b). Although a dimensional approach may supplement or replace the categorical approach to making diagnoses on Axis II, several problems limit its immediate application. In many of the studies, most of the data have been collected on relatively normal populations rather than those seen in a psychiatric setting. Some of the instruments do not differentiate episodic Axis I–related state symptoms from more stable Axis II traits. Even those instruments that do focus on Axis II traits may be influenced by episodic fluctuations of Axis I disorders (Hirschfeld et al., 1983; Reich, Noyes, Coryell, & O'Gorman, 1986). In other cases, dimensional measures of personality have been shown to predict a less favorable outcome for an Axis I disorder, independent of the severity of the Axis I episode at the time of index evaluation (Kerr, Roth, Schapira, & Gurney, 1972; Noyes et al., 1990; Pfohl, Coryell, Zimmerman, & Stangl, 1987; Weissman, Prusoff, & Klerman, 1978).

# Etiology

## PSYCHOSOCIAL FACTORS

Some of the current personality disorder diagnoses are rooted in the psychoanalytic concepts of oral (dependent), anal (obsessive–compulsive), and phallic (histrionic) personality types. These anatomic references correspond to the psychosexual stage of development during which a "fixation" might develop, giving rise to the associated personality type (Auchincloss & Michels, 1983). Using factor analysis, several studies suggest that factors related to each personality type can be derived from clinical samples (Lazare, Klerman, & Armor, 1970; Torgersen, 1980). Verifying the fixation hypothesis has been less successful. In a review of more than a dozen studies that attempted to systematically assess anal character and childhood experience with toilet training, Pollak (1979) was unable to find any clear connection.

Analytic theories of the etiology of borderline personality run the gamut from overprotective mothering (Levy, 1943; Masterson, 1976) to maternal neglect (Gunderson & Englund, 1981; Guntrip, 1969). There is some empirical support for these explanations. Gunderson, Kerr, and Englund (1980) abstracted family interview information from patients diagnosed with borderline personality disorder and an equal number of "neurotics" and patients with paranoid schizophrenia. The diagnostic criteria were similar to those in DSM-III. Blind ratings of more than 72 family characteristics showed families of patients with borderline personality disorder to be distinguishable by "the rigid tightness of the marital bond to the exclusion of the attention, support, or protection of the children" (p. 27). The authors acknowledge methodological problems. However, similar results were obtained by Frank and Paris (1981). There has been some empirical support for the presence of overinvolved mothers and underinvolved fathers in borderline personality disorder (Soloff & Millward, 1983).

An association between borderline personality disorder and childhood sexual abuse has been stated repeatedly in the literature. This association has been supported more recently by systematic empirical studies that rely on patient self-report of emotional, physical, and sexual abuse in childhood (Herman, Perry, & van der Kolk, 1989; Ludolph et al., 1990; Zanarini, Gunderson, Marino, Schwartz, & Frankenburg, 1989).

Studies that investigate the relationship between parenting behavior and personality diagnoses are few and cannot be considered definitive. Future studies will need to consider a number of issues, including retrospective falsification of reported past behavior, the impact of the child's personality on parental behavior, and the possibility of genetic factors that might influence both parenting style and personality disorder in the offspring. Because the concordance rate for personality disorder among identical twins is not 100 percent, giving some attention to psychosocial factors makes sense. However, what those psychosocial factors might be or how much of the variance they might explain is unknown.

## FAMILIAL AND GENETIC RISK FACTORS

Available studies of familial and genetic associations in Axis II tend to be limited to a few specific personality disorders, namely, schizotypal, antisocial, and borderline personality disorders. The studies that do exist suggest that genetic factors are an important component of the risk for personality disorder just as they are for Axis I disorders. Some of the largest studies using twin methodology do not use categorical personality diagnoses but rather look at dimensional personality traits such as dependency, obsessiveness, hysteria, and neuroticism. These studies compare genetically identical (homozygous) twins with nonidentical (heterozygous) twins. For most personality traits, at least half the individual variation appears to be accounted for by genetic factors (Tellegen et al., 1988; Torgersen, 1980).

Schizotypal personality disorder has been shown to be genetically related to schizophrenia (Kendler, 1985; Siever, 1985). This conclusion is based on family studies showing that schizotypal personality disorder is more prevalent among first-degree relatives of people with schizophrenia than in the general population (Baron et al., 1985; Schulz et al., 1986; Soloff & Millward, 1983). No other personality disorder shows a similarly high rate of overlap with schizophrenia.

Adoption studies have demonstrated a higher risk for antisocial personality disorder in the offspring of men with antisocial behavior, even when the offspring are raised by adoptive parents without antisocial behavior (Cadoret, 1978; Cloninger, Sigvardsson, Bohman, & von Knorring, 1982). Some of these studies show that the adoptive environment also plays a role in the risk for antisocial personality disorder (Cadoret, Troughton, Bagford, & Woodworth, 1990).

Several studies have demonstrated that borderline personality disorder is more frequent among family members of people diagnosed with the disorder (Loranger, Oldham, & Tulis, 1982; Pope, Jonas, Hudson, Cohen, & Gunderson, 1983). The latter study also suggests some type of link between borderline personality disorder and major depression, although the reasons for this association are not clear. Additional studies using twin or adoption methodology are needed to help sort out the relevant environmental and genetic factors.

As with Axis I disorders, the goal is to eventually identify the specific genes that play a role in the etiology of personality disorders. Some researchers believe that genes controlling the activity of neurotransmitters are likely to account for personality differences (Cloninger, 1987; Siever & Davis, 1991). Finding such genes is not antithetical to the existence of environmental risk factors. In fact, the identification of specific genes should allow for greater statistical power in measuring the remaining portion of the variance that can be accounted for by environment.

## LONGITUDINAL COURSE AND OUTCOME

Over the past couple of decades, professionals and the general public have become more aware of the treatability of psychiatric disorders. We anticipate that people with diagnoses such as major depression, bipolar disorder, panic disorder, anorexia nervosa, and obsessive–compulsive disorder will improve with appropriate treatment and that in most cases they will live productive and satisfying lives. Professionals and the general public often do not hold the same optimism for people diagnosed as having antisocial, schizotypal, borderline, or dependent personality disorders. To some extent, this attitude is understandable. The DSM definition of personality disorder described above mentions longitudinal stability, but stability is relative, and increasing data support the idea that personality disorders, or at least problem behaviors associated with personality disorders, can improve with time and professional intervention.

Empirical studies of the longitudinal stability of personality over time generally fall into two categories: (1) studies of the general population using dimensional self-report measures of personality and (2) studies of clinical populations using categorical interview measures. McCrae and Costa (1990) published the results of a number of population-based personality assessments with test–retest intervals of up to 10 to 15 years. Test–retest correlations are generally greater than 0.70 for such dimensional measures as general activity, restraint, ascendance, sociability, emotional stability, friendliness, extroversion, openness, and conscientiousness. Group mean scores on these measures also show little change over an interval of 10 to 15 years.

In contrast, studies of clinical samples meeting criteria for specific personality disorders appear to show less stability over time. For example, when patients with borderline personality disorder are re-evaluated over 15 years, it appears that fewer than half still have this disorder (McGlashan, 1983). Follow-up studies of five years' duration or less yield only somewhat higher stabilities, in the 0.5 to 0.6 range (McDavid & Pilkonis, 1996). Follow-up studies also are available for antisocial personality disorder. One 16- to 45-year follow-up of people with antisocial personality disorder found that among those located for interview, fewer than half could still be identified as having the disorder (Black, Baumgard, & Bell, 1995). Similar results were reported in an older study of antisocial personality using a follow-up duration of nine years (Guze, 1976).

Overall, these results suggest sufficient stability in clinically significant personality traits to validate the DSM-IV concept of "enduring patterns of perceiving, relating to, and thinking about the environment and oneself," along with sufficient variability and attenuation in traits over time to support some degree of optimism about the potential for improvement. One explanation for improvement over time may be "regression to the mean." Because the clinical samples tend to start with people who are extremes on personality dimensions, there may be a tendency to shift toward normality over time. It also appears that specific interventions can accelerate the shift toward healthier personality functioning. Several controlled studies show that specific forms of psychotherapy can result in measurable improvements in less than a year (Linehan et al., 1993; Stevenson & Meares, 1992). Medications may also play a useful role in treating certain types of severe personality disorders even in the absence of Axis I disorders (Goldberg et al., 1986; Soloff, 1990; Soloff et al., 1993).

## Cultural Bias

More potential for cultural bias probably exists in the assessment of personality disorders than is the case for most of the Axis I disorders (Foulks, 1996). For example, letting parents decide who you should marry might be considered a sign of extreme dependency in many Western cultures, whereas this same behavior is the norm in some Eastern cultures. The tendency to be emotionally expressive is considered characteristic of some societies, whereas great emotional restraint is considered common in others. The potential for bias may be greatest when the mental health professional comes from a different culture from the person being assessed.

The DSM-IV describes two methods for reducing the effects of cultural bias. First, many of the criteria suggest rating people in the context of cultural background. For example, the criteria for schizotypal personality disorder mentions that beliefs are only considered "odd" if they are "inconsistent with cultural norms"

(APA, 1994, p. 645). A second safeguard is that the disorder "leads to clinically significant distress or impairment in social, occupational, or other important areas of functioning" (p. 630).

## Gender Bias

The DSM-III diagnostic criteria for histrionic (and dependent) personality disorder were criticized as stereotypical of feminine behavior the the extent that women are more likely to receive this diagnosis (Kaplan, 1983). When personality is assessed using structured interviews that require the interviewer to simply note the presence or absence of certain traits, it appears that the rate of diagnosis is not more frequent in women (Ford & Widiger, 1989; Reich, 1987; Zimmerman & Coryell, 1989). In contrast, when clinicians are asked to globally make a personality diagnosis, there does appear to be a bias. When Warner (1978) used identical clinical vignettes in which only the patient's stated gender varied, there was a significant tendency to diagnose histrionic personality disorder more often in women and antisocial personality disorder more often in men. This suggests that, although the criteria for histrionic personality disorder may not be gender biased, the application of the diagnosis may be.

Like histrionic personality disorder, the criteria for dependent personality disorder were criticized as biased toward diagnosing more women than men (Kaplan, 1983). The distribution of DSM-III personality disorders by gender was investigated by Kass, Spitzer, and Williams (1983) using clinicians' diagnoses without a standardized assessment procedure. Dependent personality disorder was diagnosed 2.5 to four times more often in women than in men. When standardized self-report and interview instruments were used, Reich (1987) found that the percentage of females diagnosed with the disorder reflected the percentage of females in the clinic. These findings suggest that clinician behavior rather than the diagnostic criteria may be more closely related to gender bias. Dependent personality disorder is among the most frequently reported personality disorders in mental health clinics (APA, 1994).

## What Remains to Be Done

In clinical samples, personality disorders often co-occur with Axis I disorders. More work is needed to examine the nature of this association. For example, do Axis II disorders predispose a person to an Axis I disorder or vice versa? Are there biological and psychosocial factors that may predispose to disorders on both axes? It also is important to learn more about how the presence of an Axis I disorder may bias or otherwise affect the diagnosis of a personality disorder. Some of these questions are best answered by longitudinal follow-up studies, using comprehensive structured interviews for Axis I and II to clarify the relationships between the two axes.

Comparisons of categorical versus dimensional approaches to assessing personality are needed to achieve a clearer understanding of how dimensional measures of personality disorders relate to the system of categorical personality disorder diagnoses and whether these two methods may be complementary. This understanding may move the field away from a view of these two methods as either–or.

Further studies of specific psychotherapeutic techniques for treating specific personality disorders are warranted, such as controlled studies of the use of structured, manual-based therapies (Bartels & Crotty, 1992; Linehan, 1993). Finally, more work needs to be done on the role of medications in treating some personality problems.

# References

Akiskal, H. S. (1989). Validating affective personality types. In L. Robins & J. Barrett (Eds.), *The validity of psychiatric diagnosis* (pp. 217–227). New York: Raven Press.

American Psychiatric Association. (1994). *Diagnostic and statistical manual of mental disorders* (4th ed.). Washington, DC: Author.

Auchincloss, E. L., & Michels, R. (1983). Psychoanalytic theory of character. In J. P. Frosch (Ed.), *Current perspectives on personality disorders* (pp. 1–17). Washington, DC: American Psychiatric Press.

Baer, L., Jenike, M. A., Ricciardi, J. N., II, Holland, A. D., Seymour, R. J., Minichiello, W. E., & Buttolph, M. L. (1990). Standardized assessment of personality disorders in obsessive–compulsive disorder. *Archives of General Psychiatry, 47,* 826–830.

Baron, M., Gruen, R., Rainer, J. D., Kane, J., Asnis, L., & Lord, S. (1985). A family study of schizophrenic and normal control probands: Implications for the spectrum concept of schizophrenia. *American Journal of Psychiatry, 142,* 447–454.

Bartels, N. E., & Crotty, T. D. (1992). *A systems approach to treatment: Borderline personality disorder skill training manual.* Wheaton, IL: E.I.D. Treatment Systems.

Black, D. W., Baumgard, C. H., & Bell, S. E. (1995). A 16- to 45-year follow-up of 71 men with antisocial personality disorder. *Comprehensive Psychiatry, 36,* 130–140.

Black, D., Noyes, R., Jr., Pfohl, B., Goldstein, R., & Blum, N. (1993). Personality disorder in obsessive–compulsive volunteers, psychiatrically normal controls, and their first-degree relatives. *American Journal of Psychiatry, 150,* 1226–1232.

Blashfield, R., Sprock, J., & Fuller, A. (1990). Suggested guidelines for including/excluding categories in the DSM-IV. *Comprehensive Psychiatry, 31,* 15–19.

Cadoret, R. J. (1978). Psychopathology in adopted-away offspring of biologic parents with antisocial behavior. *Archives of General Psychiatry, 35,* 176–184

Cadoret, R. J., Troughton, E., Bagford, J., & Woodworth, G. (1990). Genetic and environmental factors in adoptee antisocial personality. *European Archives of Psychiatric and Neurologic Sciences, 239,* 231–240.

Cloninger, C. R. (1987). A systematic method for clinical description and classification of personality variants. *Archives of General Psychiatry, 44,* 573–588.

Cloninger, C. R., Sigvardsson S., Bohman, M., & von Knorring, A. (1982). Predisposition to petty criminality in Swedish adoptees. *Archives of General Psychiatry, 39,* 1242–1247.

Costa, P. T., & McCrae, R. R. (1990). Personality disorders and the five-factor model of personality. *Journal of Personality Disorders, 4,* 362–371.

Digman, J. (1992). Personality structure: Emergence of the five-factor model. *Annual Review of Psychology, 41,* 417–440.

Eysenck, H. J. (1970). A dimensional system of psychodiagnosis. In S. R. Mahrer (Ed.), *New approaches to personality classification* (pp. 169–208). New York: Columbia University Press.

Fabrega H., Ulrich R., Pilkonis P., & Mezzich J. (1991). On the homogeneity of personality disorder clusters. *Comprehensive Psychiatry, 32,* 373–386.

Ford, M., & Widiger, T. (1989). Sex bias in the diagnosis of histrionic and antisocial personality disorders. *Journal of Consulting and Clinical Psychology, 67,* 301–305.

Foulks, E. F. (1996). Culture and personality disorders. In J. E. Mezzich, A. Kleinman, H. Fabrega, & D. L. Parron (Eds.), *Culture and psychiatric diagnoses: A DSM-IV perspective.* Washington, DC: American Psychiatric Press.

Frank, H., & Paris, J. (1981). Recollections of family experience in borderline patients. *Archives of General Psychiatry, 38,* 1031–1034.

Goldberg, S. C., Schulz, S. C., Schulz, P. M., Resnick, R. J., Hamer, R. M., & Friedel, R. O. (1986). Borderline and schizotypal personality disorders treated with low-dose thiothixene vs. placebo. *Archives of General Psychiatry, 43,* 680–686.

Gunderson, J. G., & Englund, D. W. (1981). Characterizing the families of borderlines: A review of the literature. *Psychiatric Clinics of North America, 4,* 159–168.

Gunderson, J. G., Kerr, J., & Englund, D. W. (1980). The families of borderlines: A comparative study. *Archives of General Psychiatry, 37,* 27–33.

Gunderson, J. G., & Phillips, K. A. (1991). Borderline personality disorder and depression: A current overview of the interface. *American Journal of Psychiatry, 148,* 967–975.

Gunderson, J. G., Ronningstam, E., & Smith, L. E. (1995). Narcissistic personality disorder. In W. J. Livesley (Ed.), *The DSM-IV personality disorders* (pp. 201–212). New York: Guilford Press.

Gunderson, J. G., & Sabo, A. (1993). Borderline personality disorder and PTSD: Conceptual, phenomenologic, and treatment distinctions. *American Journal of Psychiatry, 150,* 19–27.

Guntrip, H. (1969). *Schizoid phenomena, object relations, and the self.* New York: International Universities Press.

Guze, S. B. (1976). *Criminality and psychiatric disorder.* New York: Oxford University Press.

Herman, J. L., Perry, J. C., & van der Kolk, B. A. (1989). Childhood trauma in borderline personality disorder. *American Journal of Psychiatry, 146,* 490–495.

Heumann, K. A., & Morey, L. C. (1990). Reliability of categorical and dimensional judgments of personality disorder. *American Journal of Psychiatry, 147,* 498–500.

Hirschfeld, R.M.A., Klerman, G. L., Clayton, P. J., Keller, M. B., McDonald, S. P., & Larkin, B. H. (1983). Assessing personality: Effects of the depressive state on trait measurement. *American Journal of Psychiatry, 140,* 695–699.

Kalus, O., Bernstein, D. P., & Siever, L. J. (1995). Schizoid personality disorder. In W. J. Livesley (Ed.), *The DSM-IV personality disorders* (pp. 58–70). New York: Guilford Press.

Kaplan, M. (1983). A woman's view of DSM-III. *American Psychologist, 38,* 786–792.

Kass, F., Spitzer, R. L., & Williams, J.B.W. (1983). An empirical study of the issue of sex bias in the diagnostic criteria of DSM-III Axis II personality disorders. *American Psychologist, 38,* 799–801.

Kehrer, C. A., & Linehan, M. (1996). Interpersonal and emotional problem solving skills and parasuicide among women with borderline personality disorder. *Journal of Personality Disorders, 10,* 153–163.

Kendler, K. (1985). Diagnostic approaches to schizotypal personality disorder: A historical perspective. *Schizophrenia Bulletin, 11,* 538–553.

Kerr, T. A., Roth, M., Schapira, K., & Gurney, C. (1972). The assessment and prediction of outcome in affective disorders. *British Journal of Psychiatry, 121,* 167–174.

Lazare, A., Klerman, G., & Armor, D. J. (1970). Oral, obsessive and hysterical personality patterns: Replication of factor analysis in an independent sample. *Journal of Psychological Research, 7,* 275–279.

Levy, D. M. (1943). *Maternal overprotection.* New York: Columbia University Press.

Linehan, M. M. (1993). *Skills training manual for treating borderline personality disorder.* New York: Guilford Press.

Linehan, M. M., Armstrong, H. E., Suarez, A., Allmon, D., & Heard, H. L. (1991). Cognitive–behavioral treatment of chronically parasuicidal borderline patients. *Archives of General Psychiatry, 48,* 1060–1064.

Linehan, M. M., Heard, H. L., & Armstrong, H. E. (1993). Naturalistic follow-up of a behavioral treatment for chronically parasuicidal borderline patients. *Archives of General Psychiatry, 50,* 971–974.

Livesley, W. J., & Schroeder, M. L. (1991). Dimensions of personality disorder: The DSM-III-R cluster B diagnoses. *Journal of Nervous and Mental Disease, 179,* 320–328.

Loranger, A. W., Oldham, J. M., & Tulis E. H. (1982). Familial transmission of DSM-III borderline personality disorder. *Archives of General Psychiatry, 39,* 795–799.

Ludolph, P. S., Westen, D., Misle, B., Jackson, A., Wixom, J., & Wiss, C. (1990). The borderline diagnosis in adolescents: Symptoms and developmental history. *American Journal of Psychiatry, 147,* 470–476.

Masterson, J. (1976). *Psychotherapy of the borderline adult.* New York: Brunner/Mazel.

McCrae, R. R., & Costa, P. T., Jr. (1990). *Personality in adulthood.* New York: Guilford Press.

McDavid, J. D., & Pilkonis, P. A. (1996). The stability of personality disorder diagnoses. *Journal of Personality Disorders, 10,* 1–15.

McGlashan, T. (1983). The borderline syndrome. *Archives of General Psychiatry, 40,* 1311–1323.

Millon, T., & Martinez, A. (1995). Avoidant personality disorder. In W. J. Livesley (Ed.), *The DSM-IV personality disorders* (pp. 218–233). New York: Guilford Press.

Millon, T., & Radovanov, J. (1995). Passive–aggressive (negativistic) personality disorder. In W. J. Livesley (Ed.), *The DSM-IV personality disorders* (pp. 312–325). New York: Guilford Press.

Nakao, K., Gunderson, J. G., Phillips, K. A., Ranaka, N., Yorifugi, K., Takaishi, J., & Nishimura, T. (1992). Functional impairment in personality disorders. *Journal of Personality Disorders, 6,* 24–33.

Noyes, R., Reich, J., Christiansen, J., Suelzer, M., Pfohl, B., & Coryell, W. A. (1990). Outcome of panic disorder: Relationship to diagnostic subtypes and comorbidity. *Archives of General Psychiatry, 47,* 809–818.

Pfohl, B., Coryell, W., Zimmerman, M., & Stangl, D. (1986). DSM-III personality disorders: Diagnostic overlap and internal consistency of individual DSM-III criteria. *Comprehensive Psychiatry, 27,* 21–34.

Pfohl, B., Coryell, W., Zimmerman, M., & Stangl, D. (1987). Prognostic validity of self-report and interview measures of personality in depressed patients. *Journal of Clinical Psychiatry, 48,* 468–472.

Phillips, K. A., Gunderson, J. G., Hirschfeld, R.M.A., & Smith, L. E. (1990). A review of the depressive personality. *American Journal of Psychiatry, 147,* 830–837.

Pollak, J. M. (1979). Obsessive compulsive personality: A review. *Psychological Bulletin, 86,* 225–241.

Pollak, J. M. (1987). Relationship of obsessive–compulsive personality to obsessive–compulsive disorder: A review of the literature. *Journal of Psychology, 121,* 137–148.

Pope, H. G., Jonas, J., Hudson, J., Cohen, B. M., & Gunderson, J. G. (1983). The validity of DSM-III borderline personality disorder. *Archives of General Psychiatry, 40,* 23–30.

Reich, J. (1987). Sex distribution of DSM-III personality disorders in psychiatric outpatients. *American Journal of Psychiatry, 144,* 485–488.

Reich, J. H., Noyes, R., Coryell, W., & O'Gorman, T. (1986). The effect of state anxiety on personality measurement. *American Journal of Psychiatry, 143,* 760–763.

Schulz, P. M., Schulz, S. C., Goldberg, S. C., Ettigi, P., Resnick, R. J., & Friedel, R. O. (1986). Diagnoses of the relatives of schizotypal outpatients. *Journal of Nervous and Mental Disease, 174,* 457–463.

Siever, L. J. (1985). Biological markers in schizotypal personality disorder. *Schizophrenia Bulletin, 11,* 564–575.

Siever, L. J., & Davis, K. L. (1991). A psychobiological perspective on the personality disorders. *American Journal of Psychiatry, 148,* 1647–1648.

Soloff, P. H. (1990). What's new in personality disorders? An update on pharmacologic treatment. *Journal of Personality Disorders, 4,* 223–243.

Soloff, P. H., Cornelius J., Anselm, G., Nathan, S., Perel, J. M., & Ulrich, R. F. (1993). Efficacy of phenelzine and haloperidol in borderline personality disorder. *Archives of General Psychiatry, 50,* 377–386.

Soloff, P. H., & Millward, J. W. (1983). Psychiatric disorders in the families of borderline patients. *Archives of General Psychiatry, 40,* 37–44.

Stevenson, J., & Meares, R. (1992). An outcome study of psychotherapy for patients with borderline personality disorder. *American Journal of Psychiatry, 149,* 358–362.

Tellegen, A., Lykken, D. T., Bourchard, T. J., Jr., Wilcox, K. J., Segal, N. L., & Rich, S. (1988). Personality similarity in twins reared apart and together. *Journal of Personality and Social Psychology, 54,* 1031–1039.

Torgersen, S. (1980). The oral, obsessive and hysterical personality syndromes: A study of hereditary and environmental factors by means of the twin method. *Archives of General Psychiatry, 37,* 1272–1277.

Turkat, I. D. (1985). Paranoid personality disorder. In I. D. Turkat (Ed.), *Behavioral case formulation* (pp. 155–198). New York: Plenum Press.

Turkat, I. D., & Maisto, S. A. (1985). Application of the experimental method to the formulation and modification of the personality disorders. In D. H. Barlow (Ed.), *Clinical handbook of psychological disorders* (pp. 503–570). New York: Guilford Press.

Warner, R. (1978). The diagnosis of antisocial and hysterical personality disorders: An example of sex bias. *Journal of Nervous and Mental Disease, 166,* 839–845.

Weissman, M. M., Prusoff, B. A., & Klerman, G. L. (1978). Personality and the prediction of long-term outcome of depression. *American Journal of Psychiatry, 135,* 797–800.

Widiger, T. A. (1991a). DSM-IV reviews of the personality disorders: Introduction to special series, *Journal of Personality Disorders, 5,* 122–134.

Widiger, T. A. (1991b). Personality disorder dimensional models proposed for DSM-IV. *Journal of Personality Disorders, 5,* 386–398.

Widiger, T. A., Cadoret, R., Hare, R. D., Robins, L., Rutherford, M., Zanarini, M., Alterman, A., Apple, M., Corbitt, E. M., Forth, A., Hart, S. D., Kultermann, J., & Woody, G. (1996). DSM-IV antisocial personality disorder field trial. *Journal of Abnormal Psychology, 105,* 3–16.

Widiger, T. A., & Corbitt, E. M. (1995). Antisocial personality disorder. In W. J. Livesley (Ed.), *The DSM-IV personality disorders* (pp. 103–126). New York: Guilford Press.

Williams, J. (1988). Cognitive intervention for a paranoid personality disorder. *Psychotherapy, 25,* 570–575.

Zanarini, M. C., Gunderson, J. G., Marino, M. F., Schwartz, E. O., & Frankenburg, F. R. (1989). Childhood experiences of borderline patients. *Comprehensive Psychiatry, 30,* 18–25.

Zimmerman, M., & Coryell, W. (1989). DSM-III personality disorder diagnosis in a nonpatient sample. *Archives of General Psychiatry, 46,* 682–689.

# Stress-Related Disorders

Kathleen Ell and Eugene Aisenberg

Juan is a nine-year-old Hispanic child. Recently, his teacher noticed a downward shift in Juan's attention and school performance over a period of several weeks. Previously quite attentive to his schoolwork, Juan now failed to complete his homework, appeared to daydream during class, and demonstrated uncharacteristic aggressive behavior. The teacher brought this to the attention of Juan's mother. However, no reason for the shift in Juan's behavior was identified. Juan's behavior persisted, and he became increasingly aggressive. At a parent–teacher conference one month later, Juan's mother indicated that her son was acting with hostility toward his younger brother and sister. Almost in passing, she mentioned for the first time that three armed gunmen had robbed the family in their car two months earlier.

On learning of this robbery, the teacher encouraged the mother to seek counseling services for Juan, and the teacher provided a referral. During the intake, Juan revealed to the therapist that he had been present in the family car when his grandfather was pistol whipped and the family terrorized by three armed men while the car was stopped at a railroad crossing. His grandfather was hospitalized for a week due to the injuries he suffered. The robbery occurred three months before the initial intake. During the course of the assessment, Juan indicated that he was often afraid and jumped at strange noises. He revealed that presently he was experiencing difficulty sleeping and often awoke at night. His mother confirmed that she had to leave the light on all night and sit with her son for a half-hour before he could sleep.

During the course of play therapy, Juan began to reveal the contents of a recurring and frightful dream he has experienced since the traumatic incident. He also demonstrated aggressive behavior utilizing a police officer doll to shoot repeatedly at a thief in a market. Juan disclosed to the therapist that he had not spoken of his fear or anger to anyone since the robbery.

Stressful events are a normal part of human lives. Most people will encounter more than one serious psychosocial stressor in their lifetimes, but not all, or even most, will experience subsequent levels of distress or functional impairment that require professional intervention. For the majority of people, distress is temporary and responsive to individual coping strategies and the receipt of emotional and tangible supports from close network ties. Indeed, in different ways, many people will be strengthened as a result of coping with stressful experiences.

Given the universality of stressful events, when is stress-related response psychopathological? Under what conditions and in what ways does stress cause psychiatric disorder (Mazure, 1995)? Clinicians and researchers have long recognized that psychosocial stress can be a significant factor in psychopathology (Mazure & Druss, 1995). Stress-related pathology was described by Freud and has been represented in psychiatric nomenclature for most of this century (Wilson, 1995). Contemporary research has begun to address questions about the nature of the association between life stress and the biological processes involved in mental disorders (Breier, 1995; Dohrenwend, Shrout, Link, Skodol, & Stueve, 1995; Falsetti, Resnick, Dansky, Lydiard, & Kilpatrick, 1995; Hammen, 1995; Kim & Jacobs, 1995).

In fact, evidence that psychosocial stressors are implicated in many mental disorders, including depression, anxiety, personality, and substance abuse disorders, has led to calls for future research to assess the validity of excluding disorders that are recognizably precipitated by external stressors from their current classification status (for example, mood and anxiety disorders) within the *Diagnostic and Statistical Manual of Mental Disorders* (4th ed.) (DSM-IV) (American Psychiatric Association [APA], 1994) and establishing an independent classification system for all disorders precipitated by stressful events. To support these arguments, proponents point to the unique features and prevalence of stress-related depression found in studies of community populations, older people, adolescents (Brent et al., 1994; Karam, 1994; Monroe, Kupfer, & Frank, 1992), and those who are physically ill (Leigh, 1993; Snyder, Strain, & Wolf, 1990; von Ammon Cavanaugh, 1995); evidence that depression is common among people exposed to trauma (Davidson & Foa, 1991a; McFarlane & Yehuda, 1996); evidence that stressful events are implicated in triggering the onset of recurrent disorders (Kessler, in press); and evidence that chronic role-related stresses are a significant factor in the higher prevalence of depression among women (McGrath, Keita, Strickland, & Russo, 1990) and of psychiatric disorder among the socioeconomically disadvantaged (Dohrenwend et al., 1992).

The DSM has long included a category for disorders that arise in response to stress. Adjustment disorder was first specified in the DSM-III (APA, 1980), and etiologic and symptomatic criteria for posttraumatic stress disorder (PTSD) were first included there. To date, research on adjustment disorder has been scant; however, there has been a dramatic increase in research on extreme psychological trauma following exposure to traumatic events. It is now clear that a significant number of people suffer severe distress and functional impairment in the face of extraordinary or traumatic life events and that some people experience severe distress when coping with more common but highly stressful life events. In addition, more is known about the characteristics of their distress, including specific symptom patterns and frequent co-occurrence with other mental disorders.

Recent research on psychopathology following exposure to psychosocial stressors is clustered in five critical areas: (1) uncovering the prevalence and characteristics of traumatic psychosocial stressors that pose the greatest risk for acute and long-term distress and functional impairment; (2) identifying and classifying stress-related symptomatology and impairment criteria that characterize responses outside of normal stress response and that merit professional intervention; (3) identifying the unique characteristics of stress response and disorder among children and adolescents; (4) documenting the prevalence of stress-related disorders within the general population and among high-risk populations; and (5) identifying the duration, degree of impairment, and comorbidity of stress disorder.

Social workers inevitably encounter people experiencing life stress; therefore, the profession's interest in fostering and facilitating adaptive coping and in preventing, ameliorating, or treating the negative psychological and functional sequelae of stressful life experience is a central component of its mission (Ell, 1996). People coping with stress like, Juan in the case study, are well known to social work practitioners. Advances in research on stress-related mental disorder have been facilitated by collaborative discourse between researchers and clinicians working with people who are coping with a broad range of stressors, including domestic and community violence, human-made and natural disasters, life-threatening physical illness, severe grief reactions, and combat and war-related experience. This chapter reviews recent research on traumatic stress disorder and adjustment disorder following exposure to psychosocial stressors and calls attention to unique stress-related symptomatology reflected in pathological grief, disorders with postpartum onset, and brief psychotic disorder. Throughout the chapter, research on children and adolescents is highlighted. The chapter concludes with a discussion of the need for future research.

## Psychosocial Stressors: The Etiologic Factor

Human stress has been the subject of literary, philosophical, religious, and scientific discourse throughout human history. Particularly dramatic advances from the scientific examination of human stress have marked the latter half of this century. The universality of stressful human experience (Selye, 1976) has spurred significant lines of scientific inquiry on human stress response within the fields of biology (Weiner, 1994), psychology (Lazarus, 1966), sociology (Pearlin, 1989), epidemiology (Kessler, Sonnega, Bromet, Hughes, & Nelson, 1995), and social ecology (Aneshensel, 1992; Hobfoll, 1988; Mirowsky & Ross, 1989). Increasingly, medical and behavioral scientists also are examining interactional processes among biological, psychological, and social factors that characterize human stress experience (Mazure, 1995). Building on and contributing to knowledge developed from basic science, health and human services, researchers and practitioners are beginning to collaborate in research aimed at advancing knowledge about ways to prevent and treat the negative sequelae of exposure to life stressors (Freedy & Hobfoll, 1995; Snow & Kline, 1995).

Among the early forerunners of the current focus on traumatic stressors, Lindemann (1944) identified acute grief reactions following the Coconut Grove fire, and Tyhurst (1958) described reactions of previously healthy people to severe stress. Each advocated prompt intervention soon after the traumatic experience to effect a positive outcome. At the same time, other researchers and practitioners began to describe characteristics of human response to the extraordinary stressors associated with war-related experiences, such as being in combat, being a prisoner of war, or living in a concentration camp (Kinzie & Goetz, 1996; Wilson, Harel, & Kahana, 1988).

Paralleling the focus on traumatic life stress, Caplan (1964) drew attention to the emotional crises precipitated by universal life experience, including serious physical illness and developmental transitions such as birth, bereavement, divorce, and retirement. On the basis of studies of these normal human crises, Caplan defined a crisis as a temporary upset in the emotional homeostasis of the person, produced by hazardous events. He argued that human crises posed both developmental opportunities for people to expand coping repertoires and enhance personal mastery and control as well as risks of serious and long-term impaired psychological functioning. Caplan (1974) became a leading advocate for community-based preventive mental health services, an effort in which he was actively joined by social work researchers and practitioners (Ell, 1996; Parad, 1971; Parad & Parad, 1990).

## Children and Stress

Although children also encounter war, accidents, serious illness, and human-made and natural disasters, particularly disturbing is their exposure to parental abuse, domestic violence, family break-up, and community violence. Unfortunately, despite the obvious vulnerability of children, research on children affected by trauma is recent and relatively sparse (Tyano et al., 1996). Moreover, there is less consistency in the methods used in research examining etiologic factors in child PTSD development. This inconsistency is attributed to the lack of a trauma type to unify the study of PTSD in children as well as developmental factors. In contrast, early research on PTSD in adults developed around the study of reactions of men to combat and women to rape (Foy, Madvig, Pynoos, & Camilleri, 1996).

Research on children has frequently focused on single traumatic events: accidents (Stoddard, Norman, & Murphy, 1989), natural disasters (LaGreca, Silverman, Vernberg, & Prinstein, 1996; Lonigan, Shannon, Taylor, & Sallee, 1994; Newman, 1976; Shannon, Lonigan, Finch, & Taylor, 1994), school sniper attacks (Pynoos et al., 1987), or schoolbus kidnappings (Terr, 1981). Children living in war zones (Arroyo & Eth, 1985; Nader et al., 1993) or in urban communities likened to war zones (Garbarino, Kostelny, & Dubrow, 1991) also have been studied.

Despite the documented impact of domestic violence and sexual abuse on the psychological functioning of children, only recently has PTSD begun to be assessed in affected children as an important adverse outcome of both single-event and chronic trauma (Burton, Foy, Bwanausi, Johnson, & Moore, 1994; Famularo, Kinscherff, & Fenton, 1988; Goodwin, 1985; Green, 1985; Lyons, 1987; McLeer, Deblinger, Atkins, Foa, & Ralphe, 1988; Pynoos et al., 1987; Saigh, 1991; Silvern & Kaersvang, 1989). The nature of the traumatic event in instances of physical and sexual abuse of children is different from traditional types of trauma associated with childhood PTSD. First, parents are often the perpetrators of violence against the children in instances of abuse. Second, repeated exposure to the abuse over time is common (Green, 1993), increasing the likelihood of resulting psychopathology (McLeer, Callaghan, Henry, & Wallen, 1994).

## Posttraumatic Stress Disorder

Based on recent empirical research and clinical consensus (Davidson & Foa, 1991a), DSM-IV nomenclature identifies *acute stress disorder* (ASD) and PTSD as being precipitated by exposure to an

> extreme traumatic stressor involving direct personal experience of an event that involves actual or threatened death or serious injury, or other threat to one's physical integrity; or witnessing an event that involves death, injury, or a threat to the physical integrity of another person; or learning about unexpected or violent death, serious harm or threat of death or injury experienced by a family member or other close associate. (p. 424)

Traumatic events include being diagnosed with a life-threatening illness, severe transportation accidents, personal assault (sexual, physical attack, robbery, and mugging), being kidnapped, being taken hostage, being subjected to terrorism, torture, incarceration as a prisoner of war or in a concentration camp, natural or manmade disasters, and military combat. It is important to note that DSM-IV omits the DSM-III-R criterion that the stressor should lie outside usual human experience (Amaya-Jackson & March, 1995). The World Health Organization (WHO) (1993) defines the stressor criterion as a short- or long-lasting event that is of "an exceptionally threatening or catastrophic nature, which is likely to cause pervasive distress in almost anyone" (p. 147). Not surprisingly, characteristics of the stressors, including the degree of life threat posed by the event, its intensity, and its duration are factors in the occurrence of PTSD (Solomon et al., 1993; Ullman, 1995; Weisaeth, 1989). Although not currently included in DSM-IV criteria, PTSD symptoms have been observed in the absence of an identified single traumatic event but where a build-up of highly stressful events precedes symptom onset (Scott & Stradling, 1994). PTSD symptoms also are common among children abused over a long period of time.

Traumatic events can shatter basic assumptions and beliefs about personal vulnerability and about the basic social fabric of the world. Many, if not all, people experience a range of symptoms immediately following traumatic event exposure and should be considered to be at risk for experiencing a severe human crisis (Ullman, 1995). Some people suffer temporary functional impairment. Fortunately, most trauma survivors recover without long-standing impairment. In fact, the typical pattern following a traumatic experience is resolution of early symptoms without the development of severe and debilitating psychopathology (McFarlane & Yehuda, 1996; Newman, Kaloupek, & Keane, 1996).

Nonetheless, a significant minority of people exposed to traumatic or catastrophic events are at risk for prolonged levels of distress and impairment, signaling a need for preventive or treatment intervention. It is not uncommon for people to report a range of symptoms, such as re-experiencing, avoidance, and arousal (Ullman, 1995). Traumatic events frequently precipitate responses of intense fear, helplessness, or horror (APA, 1994). Children's responses to a traumatic event also may be expressed by disorganized or agitated behavior. Among children, the traumatic event may be persistently re-experienced by repetitive play in which themes or aspects of the trauma are expressed, by frightening dreams without recognizable content, and by trauma-specific re-enactment (APA, 1994). As previously noted, repeated exposure to traumatic stressors, as in child abuse or exposure to a series of highly stressful events over time, also increases the risk of resulting psychopathology (McLeer et al., 1994; Pelcovitz et al., 1994; Scott & Stradling, 1994). Although much has been learned about PTSD, many questions remain, making it highly likely that future research will refine current understanding (Tomb, 1994).

## *DIAGNOSTIC CRITERIA*

Although most people will experience symptoms following trauma exposure, specific symptom criteria that aid in assessing psychopathology are now included in the DSM-IV. Reactions following a traumatic event are categorized as a normal symptom course, ASD, or PTSD (Classen, Koopman, & Spiegel, 1993). A person is diagnosed as having ASD if he or she develops at least three of the characteristic anxiety, dissociative, and other symptoms within one month after exposure (symptoms include a subjective sense of numbing, detachment, or absence of emotional responsiveness; a reduction in awareness of surroundings; derealization; deperson-alization; dissociative amnesia; persistent re-experience of the event; marked avoid-ance of stimuli that arouse recollection; and marked anxiety and arousal). Symp-toms last at least two days but less than one month (APA, 1994; Koopman, Classen, Cardena, & Spiegel, 1995; Lundin, 1994). The ASD diagnosis is similar to the diag-nosis of acute stress reaction in the International Classification of Diseases (WHO, 1993).

PTSD features 17 symptoms in the DSM-IV, and these are divided into three clusters: (1) re-experiencing of the traumatic event (for example, nightmares or flashbacks), (2) avoidance and numbing (for example, avoiding trauma reminders or detachment from other people), and (3) increased arousal (for example, hypervigi-lance or irritability). People experiencing at least one re-experiencing symptom, three avoidance-numbing symptoms, and two arousal symptoms for at least one month are defined as meeting symptom criteria for PTSD. The disorder is labeled "acute" if symptoms persist for less than three months, "chronic" if they last three months or more, and "delayed" if symptoms first appear six months or more after the traumatic event.

A PTSD diagnosis for children was first specified in the DSM-III-R (APA, 1987). As a result, less is known about PTSD observed in children than in adults (Saigh, Green, & Korol, 1996). Although PTSD symptomatology in children resembles PTSD in adults, there are differences in their reactions to traumatic stress (Pynoos & Nader, 1993; Terr, 1981, 1983), and these vary with child and stressor-specific factors (Famularo, Kinscherff, & Fenton, 1990; Kendall-Tackett, Williams, & Finkel-hor, 1993; Nader, Stuber, & Pynoos, 1991).

PTSD is characterized in children by persistent re-experiencing of the trauma; recurring unpleasant or frightening nightmares; sudden feelings and actions associat-ed with a belief that the stressful event is still ongoing or occurring; intense psycho-logical stress when exposed to situations similar to those in which the trauma oc-curred; persistent symptoms of increased psychological arousal, including difficulty falling asleep, nightmares, incontinence, poor concentration, irritability, exaggerated startled responses, and increased physiological reactivity when exposed to stimuli reminiscent of the traumatizing event; aggressive behavior problems; moodiness; feelings of guilt; avoidance; psychological numbing of responsiveness; and increased or decreased arousal (Parker & Randall, 1996; Pynoos & Nader, 1993). Regression in developmental achievements also is common, including regression to thumb sucking or enuresis (Drell, Siegel, & Gaensbauer, 1993). Terr (1991) proposed that childhood PTSD may take two forms, revealing different symptomatology in chil-dren. Type I results from a single traumatic event and is characterized by classic re-experiencing phenomena. Type II results from either a series of traumatic events or from exposure to a prolonged stressor. It is characterized by dissociation, denial, and numbing.

Particularly noteworthy, recent findings refute the notion that toddlers and in-fants cannot be affected by trauma because of their limited perceptual or cognitive capacities or because they are too young to know or remember what has happened. In fact, traumatized toddlers and infants experience similar symptoms, including re-experiencing the traumatic events in various ways, such as repetitive play; numbing of responsiveness, avoidance of reminders of the traumatic occurrence, various manifestations of hyperarousal, hypervigilance, exaggerated startle responses, night-mares, developmental regressions, clinging behavior, the development of new fears that were absent before the stressor, and the development of aggressive behaviors that were not present before the trauma (Drell et al., 1993; Scheeringa, Zeanah, Drell, & Larrieu, 1995; Zeanah & Scheeringa, 1996).

## *EPIDEMIOLOGY*

### Traumatic Events

No absolute rates are available, but exposure to traumatic events in the lifetime of people in the United States is high (with wide-ranging estimates of as high as 93 percent of the population having been exposed at some time in their lives), depending on the nature of events included in prevalence studies (Breslau, Davis, Andreski, & Peterson, 1991; Green, 1994; Kilpatrick et al., 1996; Vrana & Lauterbach, 1994). Numerous community and national studies have focused on the experience of crime victimization and sexual assault, reporting rates of victimization to be higher among women and to approach 75 percent (Kilpatrick & Resnick, 1993; North, Smith, & Spitznagel, 1994a, 1994b). Reported child abuse rates from national samples revealed prevalences of up to 27 percent of women and 16 percent of men (Finkelhor, Hotaling, Lewis, & Smith, 1990).

In 1990, it was estimated that each year at least 3.3 million children witness physical and verbal abuse among adults in their homes (Jaffe, Wolfe, & Wilson, 1990). Researchers in Los Angeles estimated that children witness approximately 20 percent of the homicides committed in that city (Groves, Zuckerman, Marans, & Cohen, 1993). In 1991 at Boston City Hospital, one of every 10 children attending the pediatric primary care clinic witnessed a shooting or stabbing before the age of six. The average age of the children was 2.7 years (Groves et al., 1993). In their sample of 1,000 African American elementary and high school students, Shakoor and Chalmers (1991) found that nearly three in four reported witnessing at least one instance of someone being robbed, stabbed, shot, or killed. Nearly half of the students claimed to have directly experienced such violent events.

### Prevalence among Adults

It is premature to draw firm conclusions from existing epidemiologic data on PTSD (de Girolamo & McFarlane, 1996). Given the relative recency of the inclusion of PTSD in diagnostic nomenclature, it is likely that PTSD is underreported, underdiagnosed, and underestimated in the general population (Everly, 1995). Particularly disturbing is the lack of epidemiologic studies on the prevalence of PTSD in children and adolescents (Amaya-Jackson & March, 1995; McNally, 1996). Further confounding the ability to be conclusive about the prevalence of PTSD are problems associated with the timing and method of assessment (de Girolamo & McFarlane, 1996). Additional epidemiologic research is needed to more completely understand the prevalence and incidence of this human problem. Despite the lack of precise population estimates, there is sufficient evidence to alert practitioners that a significant number of people suffer serious symptomatology following traumatic exposure.

Estimates of the prevalence of PTSD vary depending on the measures used to detect the disorder. For example, Epidemiologic Catchment Area (ECA) studies using the Diagnostic Interview Schedule (DIS) found that only about 1 percent of the general adult population suffers from this disorder (Davidson & Fairbank, 1993; Davidson, Hughes, Blazer, & George, 1991; Helzer, Robins, & McEvoy, 1987).

However, subsequent data indicate higher general population prevalence, raising questions about the sensitivity of the DIS in measuring PTSD (Green, 1994). For example, Breslau and colleagues (1991) estimated the lifetime rate of PTSD in the general population to be 9 percent. Administering modified versions of the DSM-III-R PTSD module from the DIS and of the Composite International Diagnostic Interview (CIDI) to a representative national sample of 5,877 people ages 15 to 54, the National Comorbidity Study estimated lifetime prevalence of PTSD to be 7.8 percent (Kessler et al., 1995). Prevalence was higher among women and those previously married.

Studies of at-risk populations, that is, people who have been exposed to a specific traumatic event, indicate that from one-third to one-half of adults will suffer serious psychological impairment (de Girolamo & McFarlane, 1996; Green, 1994; Green & Lindy, 1994; Madakasira & O'Brien, 1987). For example, Breslau and colleagues (1991) found that life threat or witnessing the injury or death of another, as well as undergoing physical assault, produced lifetime PTSD rates of approximately 25 percent in young adults living in the Detroit area. Kilpatrick and Resnick (1993) reported that among women who had experienced aggravated assault or rape, 39 percent and 35 percent, respectively, developed PTSD.

Combat and war-related exposure account for a significant number of victims of PTSD (de Girolamo & McFarlane, 1996; Kessler et al., 1995; Kramer, Lindy, Green, Grace, & Leonard, 1994; Sutker, Uddo, Brailey, Allain, & Errera, 1994) as do crime victimization and domestic violence (Foa & Riggs, 1995; Kessler et al., 1995; Kim-Goh, Suh, Blake, & Hiley, 1995; McLeer et al., 1994; North, Smith, & Spitznagel, 1994a; Pelcovitz et al., 1994; Trappler & Friedman, 1996). Recent studies have shown PTSD prevalence rates among victims of a natural disaster ranging up to 59 percent (Green & Lindy, 1994; Madakasira & O'Brien, 1987; McFarlane, 1992; Steinglass & Gerrity, 1990) and rates among victims of a technological disaster (for example, nuclear power plant breakdown or plane crash) ranging from 5 percent to 80 percent (de Girolamo & McFarlane, 1996).

Variable PTSD rates of up to 50 percent are found among patients suffering a life-threatening physical illness and physical trauma (Blanchard et al., 1995; Bryant, 1996; Green, 1994; Kelly et al., 1995; Kutz, Shabtai, Solomon, Neumann, & David, 1994; Lloyd, 1993; Patterson, Carrigan, Questad, & Robinson, 1990; Vrana & Lauterbach, 1994) and among psychiatric patients with other baseline diagnoses (de Girolamo & McFarlane, 1996). Finally, PTSD symptoms are frequently observed among emergency service providers, including trauma counselors and observers of traumatic events (Brom & Kleber, 1989; Bryant & Harvey, 1996; Figley, 1995; Lesaca, 1996; Marmar, Weiss, Metzler, Ronfeldt, & Foreman, 1996; Smith & deChesney, 1994; Ursano, Fullerton, Kao, & Bhartiya, 1995).

### Prevalence among Children

Summarizing a range of studies, which used different instruments and sampled children of various ages, Saigh et al. (1996) reported that the prevalence of PTSD following the occurrence of sexual abuse is fairly constant among children in treatment settings, with approximate rates of one-third to one-half manifesting PTSD symptomatology. McLeer et al. (1994) reported that 42.3 percent of clinically referred children who had been sexually abused met the criteria threshold for a DSM-III-R PTSD diagnosis. Kiser, Heston, Millsap, and Pruitt (1991) reported that 55 percent of their sample of 163 abused children had PTSD. Forty-nine children of this sample had been sexually abused. Rates for physical abuse were much lower than for sexual abuse, up to 20 percent when the victimized children were examined independently (Saigh et al., 1996). Deblinger, McLeer, Atkins, Ralphe, and Foa (1989) reported rates of PTSD at 20 percent in psychiatric inpatient children who had been sexually abused, 7 percent for those who suffered physical abuse, and 10 percent in nonabused children.

Researchers have found that rates of PTSD are high in youths exposed to life-threatening events (Amaya-Jackson & March, 1995; Fairbank, Schlenger, Saigh, & Davidson, 1995; McNally, 1996). For example, Davidson and Smith (1990) reported that children under age 11 who experience a life-threatening event are three times more likely to develop PTSD. Burton and colleagues (1994) examined the relationship between traumatic exposure, family dysfunction, and posttraumatic stress symptoms in male juvenile offenders. They found that 24 percent of the subjects had full DSM-III-R PTSD. Hubbard, Realmuto, Northwood, and Masten (1995) examined PTSD symptoms in a sample of 59 Cambodian young adults who survived massive trauma as children in their homeland, including starvation, separation from parents, and death of parents. They reported that 24 percent of the sample met the DSM-III-R diagnostic criteria for PTSD at the time of their interview and that 59 percent met the criteria for lifetime diagnosis for PTSD. Following the Buffalo Creek natural disaster, the PTSD prevalence rate among children ages two to 15 was 37 percent (Green, Lindy, Grace, & Leonard, 1992).

## COURSE AND FUNCTIONAL IMPAIRMENT

Examination of PTSD course and functional impairment yields both good and bad news. As previously suggested, the majority of people never develop full-blown PTSD, and among those who do exhibit symptoms at the outset, symptoms are relatively short lived (Dahl, 1989; McFarlane & Yehuda, 1996). For example, there is evidence that over time, children recover from traumatic exposure (Green et al., 1994) and that PTSD generally resolves without specific intervention among patients with burns (Patterson et al., 1990). However, little is yet known about the course and degree of morbidity among the majority of people exposed to traumatic events who neither seek nor receive professional help. Therefore, many questions remain about the natural course of stress reaction in the absence of specific intervention.

PTSD course and accompanying functional impairment are increasingly the subject of research. Three characteristics of PTSD identified in the research to date are particularly important to health and human service providers: the high degree of comorbidity associated with PTSD symptomatology; its highly variable course and progression among different people and following different traumatic events, including unrecognized victims of trauma; and unique features of PTSD among children. Least understood is the pathogenesis of PTSD.

## COMORBIDITY

PTSD is commonly found to co-occur with other disorders and negative outcomes, including depression, suicide, substance abuse, antisocial personality disorder, sexual dysfunction, phobias, obsessive–compulsive disorder, physical illness, somatization, higher health service utilization, homelessness, and criminal behavior (Bullman &

Kang, 1996; Burton et al., 1994; Dansky et al., 1996; Davis & Breslau, 1994; Friedman, Schnurr, & McDonagh, 1994; Green, 1994; Gunderson & Sabo, 1993; Hubbard et al., 1995; Kramer et al., 1994; North et al., 1994b; Walker, Gelfand, Gelfand, Koss, & Katon, 1995). PTSD symptoms among women with breast cancer have been found to negatively affect quality of life (Cordova et al., 1995).

Depression and anxiety with PTSD are common among both adults and children (Yule & Udwin, 1991). Depressive-spectrum symptomatology ranging from simple demoralization to major depression is the most common secondary comorbidity with PTSD (Amaya-Jackson & March, 1995). Research also indicates an interactive relationship among PTSD symptoms, depressive symptoms, and separation anxiety disorder (Goenjian et al., 1995). Traumatized children frequently exhibit symptoms of disorders in addition to PTSD, and children with other disorders often have PTSD as an intercurrent diagnosis (Famularo, Kinscherff, & Fenton, 1992; Herzog, Keller, Sacks, Yeh, & Lavor, 1992; Pynoos & Nader, 1993). Among a sample of sexually abused children, the co-occurrence of PTSD with attention-deficit/hyperactivity disorder (ADHD) was found to be 23.1 percent; 15.4 percent of the sample had both PTSD and conduct disorder (CD); and 11.5 percent had PTSD, ADHD, and CD (McLeer et al., 1994). Not surprisingly, Bird, Gould, and Staghezza (1993) reported a strong positive correlation between impairment and comorbidity and found that children with significant comorbidity used mental health services more heavily than children with only one diagnosis.

Comorbidity complicates assessment and diagnosis and presumably accounts for undetected trauma exposure and related symptoms. For example, a significant problem has been the failure to properly differentiate between posttraumatic stress symptoms and grief reactions and to consider their interaction (Pynoos, 1992). Pynoos observed how PTSD complicates the grieving process by repeatedly directing attention to the traumatic circumstances of the death and the surrounding issues. Besides true comorbidity, PTSD symptoms are often confounded by spurious comorbidity resulting from overlap among symptom criteria.

## VARIABLE COURSE

PTSD is characterized by varying illness trajectories over time (Blank, 1994). Wide variability in PTSD course and outcomes is not surprising given that PTSD occurs following exposure to different types of trauma (McFarlane & Yehuda, 1996) and that the contexts of event exposure vary (Blank, 1994). The high degree of comorbidity also influences illness course (Bremner, Southwick, Darnell, & Charney, 1996). Thus, it also is not surprising that PTSD is found among a broad range of children and adults receiving aid from a range of clinical and human services systems. A significant number of patients with PTSD experience prolonged distress and dysfunction (Herman, 1992; McFarlane, 1992). Data from the National Comorbidity Survey show that more than one-third of people with an index episode of PTSD fail to recover even after many years (Kessler et al., 1995). In some cases, PTSD symptoms wax and wane over months and even years, presumably contributing to lack of detection. In other cases, acute symptoms recur if the person is subjected to retraumatization (Tomb, 1994). Recovery rates are better during the first year following exposure; however, people continue to have a 50 percent chance of recovery even after two years (Kessler et al., 1995).

People experiencing acute stress disorder do not necessarily progress to PTSD (Dahl, 1989). However, the presence of severe acute dissociative symptoms, represented by detachment from others and the physical environment, alterations in perceptions, and impairment in memory (Cardena & Spiegel, 1993), are high-risk indicators for developing PTSD (Bremner & Brett, 1997; Dancu, Riggs, Hearst-Ikeda, Shoyer, & Foa, 1996; Foa & Riggs, 1995; Shalev, Peri, Canetti, & Schreiber, 1996; Spiegel, Koopman, & Classen, 1994). Dissociation is believed to impede emotional processing of the trauma (Foa & Riggs, 1995), and clinicians should consider appropriate intervention.

## OUTCOMES AMONG CHILDREN

The experience of a traumatic event can be overwhelming, wounding a child's psyche and spirit with serious debilitating consequences. Although neglected in the early stress literature, the effects of traumatic events on children's lives have been receiving major attention in recent years (Fink, Bernstein, Handelsman, Foote, & Lovejoy, 1995; Giaconia et al., 1994; Shannon et al., 1994).

Among children and adolescents, severe life stressors, such as divorce, severe physical illness, sexual abuse, and death of a significant other have been related to behavioral problems and psychiatric disorder (Fink et al., 1995; Giaconia et al., 1994; Kovacs, Ho, & Pollock, 1995; Merry & Andrews, 1994; Shannon et al., 1994). This finding is not surprising, given that a child is less able to process the trauma and has less defined and less developed resources and adaptive coping mechanisms to assist in the regaining of equilibrium and well-being (Caplan, 1964). In addition, children bear the burden of being least able to voice their feelings and fears. As a result, a child exposed to trauma may be particularly vulnerable to emotional and developmental problems (Gaensbauer, 1996). PTSD also may impair the academic performance of children. In DSM-IV, functional impairment (for example, academic problems) is recognized as a diagnostic indicator of the disorder (Saigh et al., 1996).

Children with PTSD often demonstrate markedly diminished interest in previously enjoyed activities and sometimes lose previously acquired skills. They also may show evidence of restricted affect, which can accompany feelings of detachment or estrangement from others (Amaya-Jackson & March, 1995). Child victims of trauma may develop a shortened sense of the future and experience difficulty seeing themselves in meaningful future adult roles (Wallach, 1993). Trauma related to child abuse can significantly disrupt the development of children's affect regulation, self-system, peer relationships, and school adaptation (Cicchetti & Toth, 1995).

Both school-age children and preschoolers who are exposed to violence are less likely to explore their physical environment and play freely. They may show less motivation to master their environment. In addition, they may withdraw and appear depressed or become aggressive (Keane, 1996). Exposure to trauma interferes with a child's normal development of trust and with the later emergence of autonomy through exploration (Osofsky & Fenichel, 1994). Traumatic experiences can affect children's expectations about the world, their sense of safety and security, as well as their sense of personal integrity (Pynoos, Steinberg, & Goenjian, 1996).

The issue of undetected trauma exposure and its accompanying distress is particularly relevant to children. Children who perform poorly in school may be suffering from intrusive thoughts and concentration impairment that accompany PTSD. Failure to recognize the impact of PTSD on school performance can result in mistaken evaluation of the child and a failure to properly educate the child (McNally, 1996). Indeed, because PTSD can mimic a disruptive behavior disorder, it is crucial to rule out PTSD as a cause of deteriorating school performance, poor concentration, irritability, or aggression before making any other diagnosis of a child, especially one who has experienced or witnessed violence or a life-threatening event (Osofsky, 1995).

## PATHOGENESIS, RISK, AND PROTECTIVE FACTORS

### Adult Risk

Unfortunately, research on risk and protective factors that may explain the progression from normal stress-related symptoms to PTSD and the poorer outcomes among people has been sparse (McFarlane & Yehuda, 1996; Shalev et al., 1996). To date, factors that have been correlated with the onset and course of PTSD include characteristics of the stressor (Ullman, 1995); level and type of exposure, such as life threat and physical pain (March, 1993; McNally, 1993; Schreiber & Galai, 1993; Solomon et al., 1993; Weisaeth, 1989); previous history of trauma, such as sexual trauma (Kramer & Green, 1991; Resnick, Yehuda, Pitman, & Foy, 1995); use of, lack of access to, or rapid loss of social support (Hobfoll, 1991; Irwin, 1996; Kaniasty & Norris, 1993; Kramer & Green, 1991; North, Smith, McCool, & Lightcap, 1989); and a history of psychiatric disorder (Smith, North, McCool, & Shea, 1990). For example, women with a history of precombat sexual trauma reported greater PTSD symptomatology following combat exposure than women denying precombat abuse (Engel et al., 1993). Less is known about gender, age, racial–ethnic, and socioeconomic status influences on PTSD.

Although external psychosocial stressors are the primary precipitating factor in PTSD, there is compelling evidence of a biological basis (Pitman, 1993; Tomb, 1994). For example, researchers have identified the neurobiological response to the stressor that contributes to prolonged symptoms reported by patients with PTSD (Southwick, Bremner, Krystal, & Charney, 1994; Southwick, Krystal, Johnson, & Charney, 1995). Delayed onset of PTSD symptoms is frequently observed (Bland, O'Leary, Farinaro, Jossa, & Trevisan, 1996; Bremner et al., 1996; McFarlane, 1988; Rahe, 1988). However, more research is needed to confirm early findings regarding the pathogenesis of PTSD and risk and protective factors (Green, 1994; Ullman, 1995).

### Childhood Risk

Least studied is the role of risk and protective factors, associated mediating and moderating variables, and their interactions in the development of posttraumatic stress symptoms in youngsters (Green et al., 1991). Unique to childhood PTSD etiology is the positive correlation between children's symptoms and trauma-related symptoms in their parents. Trauma exposure severity and parental trauma-related distress have been found to be positively correlated with risk for childhood PTSD (Foy et al., 1996). Thus, when members of the same family are exposed to trauma or a traumatic event, it appears that the parents' PTSD symptomatology may serve as a powerful mediating factor in the development of children's symptoms. Therefore, it is crucial to evaluate the parents' reactions to the shared trauma in determining any increased risk for children (Foy et al., 1996). According to studies of the mother–child relationship during war, "the level of emotional upset displayed by the child's parents, not the war situation itself, was the most important factor in predicting the child's response to the war" (Garbarino, Dubrow, Kostelny, & Pardo, 1992, p. 54).

Parental factors and child symptomatology also are correlated. Parental factors that seem most closely related to symptomatology in children include mothers' and fathers' own PTSD symptoms, levels of general parental psychopathology, the presence or extent of denial concerning the child's symptomatology, and changes in family functioning that may exert a powerful indirect effect on the child's functioning and development (Famularo, Fenton, Kinscherff, Ayoub, & Barnum, 1994). For some parents and caregivers, the stress associated with violence exposure and coping with this stressor affect their ability to parent their child as well as the child's capacity to form positive attachment relationships (Osofsky & Fenichel, 1994). Many parents or caregivers find it difficult to provide their children with support, love, and affection in a consistent manner when they live in a state of apprehension or anxiety generated by chronic domestic or community violence (Wallach, 1993). In research conducted with children up to age three who have been exposed to trauma and diagnosed with symptoms of PTSD, two types of distorted parent–child relationships have been identified: (1) role reversal—the child becomes the comforter or caretaker of the parent—and (2) the parental child—the child is given or assumes duties and responsibilities beyond his or her capacity (Scheeringa et al., 1995).

In evaluating and treating children exposed to trauma, it is important to understand certain factors that may contribute to the severity of response to the traumatic event: intensity, proximity, familiarity, and developmental status of the child (Zeanah & Scheeringa, 1996). Witnessing a shooting is a much more intense experience than seeing someone get pushed in the schoolyard. Proximity to the traumatic incident strongly increases the intensity of a child's response to the traumatic event, as does familiarity with the victim or perpetrator. Also, the developmental status of children will affect their responses and ability to cope (Zeanah & Scheeringa, 1996).

Findings with respect to gender differences in PTSD severity are inconclusive. In studies reporting significant differences, however, females reported higher distress scores and appeared to be more vulnerable than males (Foy et al., 1996; Yule & Canterbury, 1994). Vernberg, LaGreca, Silverman, and Prinstein (1996) found that girls report more distress following natural disasters than do boys. In their study, Curle and Williams (1996) substantiated that girls reported higher levels of anxiety and depression and higher scores on the intrusion scale of the Impact of Events Scale (IES) following a nonfatal bus accident. Such findings should be interpreted with caution because possible differences in lifetime trauma exposure between boys and girls were not controlled in these studies (Foy et al., 1996).

Other factors, such as personal characteristics and the duration of the traumatic event, also play a significant role in the level of stress experienced by the child exposed to trauma (Rosenthal & Levy-Shiff, 1993). Also, the degree of exposure is strongly correlated with risk for PTSD in children (Amaya-Jackson & March, 1995). Ethnicity and intelligence have been examined in a few studies of childhood PTSD (Burton et al., 1994; Nader, Pynoos, Fairbanks, & Frederick, 1990). The findings are consistent in revealing nonsignificance for these variables however, further research is needed to determine whether low intelligence may constitute a risk factor for chronic PTSD in children (McNally & Shin, 1995). Lower socioeconomic status and the presence of parental emotional problems are associated with an increased risk for PTSD in children who were burn victims (Stoddard et al., 1989).

Protective factors include positive interactions, attachment, relationships with parents or caregivers, and access to positive role models. Effective coping patterns, caring educational and community programs, and availability of social support also serve to buffer and protect a child in the face of traumatic stressors (Werner, 1995).

Research highlights the importance for children to establish and enjoy a close bond with at least one competent and emotionally stable person who is attuned to their needs (Werner, 1995). A principal determinant of the resiliency of a child is associated with the child's ability to make relationships and to make use of caring people in the environment (Wallach, 1993).

## DIAGNOSTIC AND SCREENING TOOLS

### Assessing Adults

The significant prevalence of trauma in the general and clinical population, the wide range of stressors known to precede PTSD, the disorder's known effects on and interactions with impaired functioning and distress, the likelihood of delayed symptom onset and protracted symptom duration, and the potential that trauma is obscured by comorbid conditions converge to alert practitioners to routinely assess clinical populations for trauma history and symptomatology (Davis & Breslau, 1994; Eilenberg, Fullilove, Goldman, & Mellman, 1996; Walker, Torkelson, Katon, & Koss, 1993). For example, adults who have experienced child abuse may present with symptoms long after the initial experience, and retraumatization also can trigger acute symptoms.

Unfortunately, many issues remain speculative regarding the assessment and diagnosis of PTSD, setting an agenda for future study. Practitioners are particularly challenged when making a differential diagnosis. Nevertheless, several lines of research are beginning to provide useful practice guidelines (Blank, 1994). The development of diagnostic and screening tools has been especially useful to practitioners (for an extensive review, see Newman et al., 1996).

Clinically administered assessment tools have been developed to assist in detecting and diagnosing PTSD (Allen, 1994; Hendrix, Anelli, Gibbs, & Fournier, 1994; Marmar et al., 1996; Neal, Busuttil, Herapath, & Strike, 1994). The Impact of Events Scale (IES) (Horowitz, Wilner, & Alvarez, 1979) is a 15-item self-report questionnaire measuring two dimensions of PTSD—trauma-related intrusion and avoidance. The PTSD Symptom Scale–Interview Version (PSS) is a 17-item clinician-administered scale that has been validated with rape victims (Foa, Riggs, Dancu, & Rothbaum, 1993). The Mississippi Scale for Combat-Related Posttraumatic Stress Disorder measures self-reported symptoms of posttraumatic stress in veteran populations (Keane, Caddell, & Taylor, 1988). A civilian form of the Mississippi Scale was subsequently developed and found to have high internal consistency (Vreven, Gudanowski, King, & King, 1995) and the validity and reliability of a Spanish version have been established (Norris & Perilla, 1996).

The utility of existing symptom inventories and diagnostic instruments, such as the DIS and the Symptom Checklist-90-R, has been reported (Weathers et al., 1996). The Purdue Post-Traumatic Stress Scale (PTSS) is an easily administered, 15-item self-report instrument based on DSM-III diagnostic criteria (Hendrix et al., 1994). The Self-Rating Traumatic Stress Scale (SR-TSS) (Davidson, 1995) assesses the severity and frequency of 17 items corresponding to DSM-III-R symptoms of PTSD. Measuring a complex of symptoms associated with the long-term effects of sexual abuse, the Trauma Symptom Checklist-40 (TSC–40) yields six subscales: Dissociation, Anxiety, Depression, Sexual Abuse Trauma Index, Sexual Problems, and Sleep Disturbances (Elliot & Briere, 1992). The TSC–40 also has been validated among psychiatric inpatients (Zlotnick et al., 1996).

Several instruments have been used to assess dissociative symptoms. The Stanford Acute Stress Reaction Questionnaire (SASRQ) assesses dissociative reactions in five areas: psychic numbing, depersonalization, derealization, amnesia, and stupor (Koopman et al., 1995). The Dissociative Experiences Scale (DES) is a 28-item questionnaire to assess the frequency and intensity of a range of dissociative experiences (Bernstein & Putnam, 1986).

Computerized tools also are being developed (Franklin, Nowicki, Trapp, Schwab, & Petersen, 1993; Neal et al., 1994). Although no adequately validated assessment tool is currently available to assist practitioners in identifying ASD among trauma survivors (Koopman et al., 1995), preliminary research is underway to develop a measure (Cardena & Spiegel, 1993).

## Assessing Children

Because of their developmental capacity, young children and infants are not able to report many of the symptoms of PTSD (Bingham & Harmon, 1996). This highlights the fact that PTSD is not easily or commonly diagnosed in this age group if the strict DSM criteria are applied. In addition, the rapid and complex developmental changes experienced by the infant pose further diagnostic challenges (Scheeringa et al., 1995).

Given the wide range of verbal skills and varying ability in children of different ages to reveal and express their internal experiences, assessment tools are needed that will be both sensitive and specific to the diverse representations of traumatic responses in children (Keane, 1996). This is especially crucial with regard to physical and sexual abuse of children, in which problems related to discovery, disclosure, and validation complicate the study of abuse-related PTSD in children (Foy et al., 1996). Although children may remember the trauma, they frequently experience difficulty in discussing it and often refuse to acknowledge that which they have previously described (Parker & Randall, 1996).

Although parents generally are good evaluators of children's externalizing behaviors, they tend to be less adequate in assessing their child's internalizing symptoms (Costello & Angold, 1988). Also, mothers' judgments about their children's symptoms are highly related to their own level of distress and willingness to believe their children (Everson, Hunter, Runyon, Edelsohn, & Coulter, 1989; Newberger, Geremy, Waternaux, & Newberger, 1993). Thus, parents may downplay or deny the impact of traumatic life experiences on their children. As a result, there is often a weak association between parent and children's reports of symptoms and behaviors. Ideally, therefore, assessments should be obtained from multiple sources, including the children, their parents, and the children's teachers (Kendall-Tackett et al., 1993).

Efforts to more precisely delineate the specific objective features of traumatic experiences associated with more severe posttraumatic reactions in children have led to the following considerations when conducting an assessment: age and developmental level of the child; the child's pre-existing temperament and personality; exposure to direct life threat; injury to self, including the extent of physical pain; witnessing a mutilating injury or death, especially of a family member or friend; hearing unanswered screams for help and cries of distress; smelling noxious odors; being trapped or without assistance; proximity to violent threat; unexpectedness and duration of the experience; extent of violent force and the use of a weapon or injurious object; number and nature of threats during a violent episode; witnessing atrocities; the relationship of the assailant or perpetrator to the victims; use of physical coercion; violation of the physical integrity of the child; degree of brutality and malevolence; family home environment; family's response to trauma; and available support systems. These factors are strongly associated with the onset, severity, and persistence of PTSD in children and, therefore, should be assessed when evaluating children (Green, 1993; Pynoos et al., 1996).

The diagnostic instruments used to determine childhood PTSD status and severity are not uniform and vary widely in quality. Saigh (1989) developed the Children's Posttraumatic Stress Disorder Inventory (CPTSDI). It is a structured interview for diagnosing DSM-III-R PTSD. The Revised Children's Manifest Anxiety Scale (RCMAS) (Reynolds & Richmond, 1978) also has been used to measure PTSD in children. A widely used instrument for diagnosing childhood PTSD is the Post-Traumatic Stress Disorder Reaction Index (PTSD–RI) (Frederick, 1985, 1986; Pynoos et al., 1987), a 20-item instrument that adults can complete as a self-report measure and which can be administered to children as a structured interview. Schwarzwald, Weisenberg, Waysman, Solomon, and Klingman (1993) updated the interview to ensure coverage of all DSM-III-R PTSD symptoms. Nader and Pynoos (1989) developed the Child Post-Traumatic Stress Disorder Inventory: Parent Inventory (CPTSD–I), a structured interview for questioning parents about symptoms exhibited by their traumatized children. It covers PTSD symptoms, associated features, personality traits, and history of traumatic events. The IES (Horowitz et al., 1979) also has been used as a measure of PTSD in children, although it is widely used as a measure of posttraumatic symptoms in adults. It includes subscales for intrusion and avoidance. However, the IES may fail to distinguish between PTSD and grief in children who have lost a friend or family member.

The Diagnostic Interview Schedule for Children, Version 4.0 (DISC–4.0) is a highly structured diagnostic interview instrument for use by trained lay interviewers to ascertain the most common diagnoses defined by the DSM-IV. The DISC–4.0 interview is based on earlier versions and is designed to be administered to children ages nine to 17 and their parents. It samples nonclinically referred children and adolescents and is designed for use in large-scale epidemiologic studies (Schaffer et al., 1996). It also contains subscales that measure childhood PTSD (Prudence Fisher, Executive Secretary, National Institute of Mental Health, DISC Editorial Board, personal communication, November 10, 1996). The Trauma Symptom Checklist for Children (TSCC) is a self-report measure of PTSD and related symptomology. It is intended for use in evaluating children who have experienced traumatic events such as witnessing violence, physical or sexual abuse, victimization by peers, and natural disasters (Briere, 1996). The Childhood Trauma Interview also is available to aid practitioners in identifying childhood trauma (Fink et al., 1995).

## Adjustment Disorder

*Adjustment disorder* is currently defined in the DSM-IV as being precipitated by "an identifiable psychosocial stressor or stressors" other than bereavement and including a single event, such as "termination of a romantic relationship" or multiple stressors, such as "marked business difficulties and marital problems." "Stressors may be recurrent . . . or continuous" (for example, living in a crime-ridden neighborhood), and "some stressors may accompany specific developmental events" (such as going to school, leaving the parental home, getting married, becoming a parent, failing to attain occupational goals, or retirement) (p. 623). It is important to note that these stressors are part of everyday life and interpersonal relationships (Al-Ansari & Matar, 1993).

Adjustment disorder includes heterogeneous symptoms and degrees of impairment and is used only when criteria for a more specific disorder are not met. To date, research on adult and childhood adjustment disorder is scant and focuses mostly on people with physical illness (Fabrega, Mezzich, & Mezzich, 1987). Consequently, far less is known about the epidemiology, course, or outcomes of adjustment disorder than about PTSD.

## DIAGNOSTIC CRITERIA

According to the DSM-IV,

> The essential feature of an adjustment disorder is the development of clinically significant emotional or behavioral symptoms . . . indicated either by marked distress that is in excess of what would be expected given the nature of the stressor, or by significant impairment in social or occupational [academic] functioning [within three months after the onset of the stressor]. AD [adjustment disorder] must resolve within six months of the termination of the stressor (or its consequences). However, the symptoms may persist for a prolonged period (i.e., longer than six months) if they occur in response to a chronic stressor (e.g., a chronic disabling general medical condition) or to a stressor that has enduring consequences (e.g., the financial and emotional difficulties resulting from a divorce). (p. 623)

Subtypes of adjustment disorder are classified according to predominant symptoms: with depressed mood, with anxiety, with mixed anxiety and depressed mood, with conduct disturbance, with mixed disturbance of emotions and conduct, and unspecified. Symptoms are no longer described as maladaptive but rather as clinically significant (Newcorn & Strain, 1995).

According to DSM-IV criteria, the dimensions on which PTSD and adjustment disorders differ are stressor and symptom variability. A child experiencing only limited difficulty in daily social or school functioning following an extreme stressor would receive a diagnosis of an adjustment disorder. A youngster exhibiting symptoms consistent with PTSD in response to a stressor that is not extreme also would receive a diagnosis of adjustment disorder (Lating, Zeichner, & Keane, 1995). Among adults and children and adolescents with adjustment disorder, the development of depressive symptoms alone is less characteristic. Recent studies found that among children and adolescents with adjustment disorder and among adults with physical illness, the majority presented with mixed emotional or mixed emotional and behavioral symptoms (Newcorn & Strain, 1995).

## EPIDEMIOLOGY

Given its defining features, it is not surprising that adjustment disorder is particularly prevalent, with estimates up to 50 percent, among people with physical illness (Alexander, Dinesh, & Vidyasagar, 1993; Carroll, Kathol, Noyes, Wald, & Clamon, 1993; Oxman, Barrett, Freeman, & Manheimer, 1994; Perez-Jimenez, Gomez-Bajo, Lopez-Castillo, Salvador, & Garcia, 1994; Pollock, 1992; Popkin, Callies, Colon, & Stiebel, 1990; Razavi & Stiefel, 1994; Shima, Kitagawa, Kitamura, Fujinawa, & Watanabe, 1994; Silverstone, 1996; Sullivan, Weinshenker, Mikail, & Bishop,

1995). Adjustment disorder also has been reported among refugees (Hinton et al., 1993).

Epidemiologic studies of adjustment disorder in children are rare. Within psychiatric clinic populations, Doan and Petti (1989) found a rate of 7 percent among child patients attending day units. Mezzich, Fabrega, Coffman, and Haley (1989) reported a rate of 16 percent among all youngsters under age 18 seen for evaluation at the Western Psychiatric Institute, with male and female patients being equally affected. A prevalence rate of 7.6 percent, determined by a cutoff score of 70 on the Children's Global Assessment Scale (CGAS), was found in a study of Puerto Rican children and adolescents (Bird et al., 1988). Among pediatric patients sampled from four different clinic sites, 25 percent to 65 percent of those who presented with psychiatric disturbance were diagnosed as having adjustment disorder (Newcorn & Strain, 1995).

## FUNCTIONAL IMPAIRMENT AND PROGNOSIS

Because research has been sparse, much remains to be clarified about the pathogenesis, progression, and time span between the onset of the stressor and the onset of a maladaptive reaction or its duration (Kovacs et al., 1995). The DSM-IV applies the diagnosis of adjustment disorder when the onset of symptoms presents within three months of the advent of the stressor and when symptoms do not persist longer than six months following the stressor (or its consequences). Adjustment disorder is regarded as acute if persisting less than six months and is considered chronic if enduring six months or longer (Newcorn & Strain, 1995).

Prognosis among people who are medically ill is good, with the majority of patients recovering without specific psychiatric intervention but benefiting from supportive intervention (Kathol & Wenzel, 1992). Group interventions reviewed in chapter 13 of this book are examples of effective supportive therapies. Ninety percent of the children who had adjustment disorder in a study examining the psychological adjustment of children after the acute onset of diabetes mellitus recovered after nine months (Newcorn & Strain, 1995). However, evidence suggests that the course of adjustment disorder extends beyond six months for a significant number of patients (Andreasen & Wasek, 1980; Cantwell & Baker, 1989; Despland, Monod, & Ferrero, 1995; Newcorn & Strain, 1995). Indeed, establishing appropriate temporal criteria in adjustment disorder has been a persistent problem (Newcorn & Strain, 1995).

High rates of self-harm have been found among people diagnosed with adjustment disorder (Vlachos, Bouras, Watson, & Rosen, 1994). In a five-year follow-up of 100 patients with adjustment disorder, 79 percent of adults were well at follow-up, whereas only 57 percent of adolescents were well and 13 percent of adolescents developed schizophrenia, schizoaffective disorder, major depression, bipolar disorder, antisocial personality, alcoholism, and substance abuse disorder (Andreasen & Hoenk, 1982). Adjustment disorder among children with end-stage renal disease has been related to poor relationships with peers at school (Fukunishi & Kudo, 1995) and to subsequent psychopathology among youths with new-onset diabetes (Kovacs et al., 1995). It is not clear, however, if poor outcomes observed among children and adolescents with adjustment disorder result from the disorder itself, the frequent existence of comorbidity, or problems in research design (Newcorn & Strain, 1995).

## COMORBIDITY

By definition, adjustment disorder is a residual diagnosis, so that it is only diagnosed when the disturbance does not meet criteria for another specific Axis I disorder and is not merely an exacerbation of a pre-existing Axis I or Axis II disorder. Among people who are physically ill, mixed-type adjustment disorder and major depression and anxiety are common. Comorbidity with some psychiatric disorders is high (for example, Mok & Watler, 1995). Adjustment disorder also is found to co-occur with substance abuse and suicidality (Greenberg, Rosenfeld, & Ortega, 1995). Children with adjustment disorder have been found to have a variety of comorbid disorders (Bukstein, Glancy, & Kaminer, 1992; Kovacs, Gatsonis, Pollock, & Parrone, 1994; Newcorn & Strain, 1995).

Studies of adjustment disorder using structured diagnostic instruments have reported a fairly high level of comorbidity (Kovacs et al., 1994). In a mixed group of children, adolescents, and adults, approximately 70 percent of the patients with adjustment disorder had at least one additional Axis I diagnosis (Newcorn & Strain, 1995). In a study of correlates of depressive disorders in children, 45 percent of those with adjustment disorder with depressed mood also had another disorder (Newcorn & Strain, 1995).

## DIAGNOSTIC AND ASSESSMENT ISSUES

Because adjustment disorder is commonly presented as a mixed type and with depression (Despland et al., 1995), differentiating adjustment disorder from major depression, anxiety, or personality disorders is difficult (Schatzberg, 1990). This is particularly true among people who are medically ill (Kathol & Wenzel, 1992; Snyder et al., 1990; von Ammon Cavanaugh, 1995). Adjustment disorder may present with subthreshold pathology in one or several symptom domains, further complicating diagnosis. Given the heterogeneity of this disorder, no single treatment intervention is appropriate for the disorder. Treatment strategies that may be considered include a range of psychodynamic, behavioral, pharmacological, and supportive psychological interventions (Biederman, 1990; Newcorn & Strain, 1995).

# Additional Stress-Related Symptomatology

## PATHOLOGICAL BEREAVEMENT

Bereavement is a part of normal human experience. Nonetheless, some people suffer extraordinary stress following a loss event (Horowitz, Bonanno, & Holen, 1993). The nature, duration, and severity of symptoms distinguish pathologic grief from normal grief (Kim & Jacobs, 1995). Although not classifying pathological bereavement as a specific disorder, DSM-IV calls attention to the presence of symptoms that are uncharacteristic of a normal grief reaction, including

> 1) guilt about things other than actions taken or not taken by the survivor at the time of the death; 2) thoughts of death other than the survivor feeling that he or she would be better off dead or should have died with the deceased person; 3) morbid preoccupation with worthlessness; 4) marked psychomotor retardation; 5) prolonged and marked functional impairment; and

> 6) hallucinatory experiences other than thinking that he or she hears the
> voice of, or transiently sees the image of, the deceased person. (pp. 684–685)

When observing these reactions, the practitioner is alerted to consider specific interventions, including the use of medication.

The stress associated with bereavement has long been a subject of research (Kim & Jacobs, 1995; Lindemann, 1944). Among questions to be addressed in further research are whether symptoms of pathologic grief are different from depressive or anxiety disorders and thus should be specified as a distinct disorder (Karam, 1994; Kim & Jacobs, 1995) and whether specific interventions are most effective for different types of grief reactions.

## POSTPARTUM ONSET

The DSM-IV identifies a new specifier for mood disorder, namely with postpartum onset (APA, 1994). This specifier is to be applied when the full criteria are met for a mood disorder episode, including major depression; manic or mixed episode in major depressive disorder; bipolar I disorder, or bipolar II disorder; or brief psychotic disorder. The onset of disorder should occur within four weeks postpartum. This diagnosis should alert practitioners to the possibility that occasionally a mother will experience a severe stress reaction that requires professional intervention both for herself and to reduce any risk to the well-being of the baby. In some cases, postpartum onset is accompanied by psychotic symptomatology, in which case the diagnosis is brief psychotic disorder.

The body of relevant research in this area is relatively small (Bell, Land, Milnes, & Hassanyeh, 1994). A recent analysis of existing research raised questions about whether postpartum depression might more appropriately be classified as an adjustment disorder (Whiffen, 1991). There also is evidence that depressive symptoms are common among African American pregnant teenagers and postpartum adolescents (Barnet, Joffe, Duggan, Wilson, & Repke, 1996) but may indicate dysphoria rather than a disorder (Affonso et al., 1992). A community study of 1,559 childbearing women screened six weeks postpartum using the Edinburgh Postnatal Depression Scale (Boyce, Stubbs, & Todd, 1993) estimated postpartum depression to be approximately 6 percent (Zelkowitz & Milet, 1995). Another study reported variable prevalence between 7 percent and 14 percent, depending on the time of assessment (Pop, Essed, deGeus, vanSon, & Komproe, 1993). Past psychiatric history has been shown to be an important prognostic indicator of long-term outcome, as are previous stressful life events (Kumar et al., 1993). Data also suggest that maternal depression is a risk factor for child abuse (Scott, 1992).

## BRIEF PSYCHOTIC DISORDER WITH MARKED STRESSORS

Brief psychotic disorder is a relatively rare diagnosis and has not been the subject of research. As defined in DSM-IV, it applies in the presence of one or more of the following symptoms: delusions, hallucinations, disorganized speech, or grossly disorganized or catatonic behavior. Symptoms must last one day to 30 days, with eventual return to premorbid level of functioning, and the episode is not better diagnosed as a mood disorder with psychotic features, schizoaffective disorder, or schizophrenia, nor is it the result of the direct physiological effects of a substance. Brief psychotic disorder with marked stressors applies when the episode follows an event that would be markedly stressful to almost anyone in similar circumstances in the person's culture.

## Future Research Priorities

In contrast to the research reviewed, far less research has been conducted on and thus less is known about individual differences in vulnerability to stress and stress modifiers, the nature of progression from normal stress response to disorder and the course of stress disorders over time, overlapping and differential stress-related symptom presentation as in substance abuse or mood disorder and the interface between PTSD and other mental disorders (Davidson & Foa, 1991b; Gunderson & Sabo, 1993; Schottenfeld & Cullen, 1985), and preventing and treating stress-related disorders (Ramsay, 1990). It is hoped that growing awareness of the scope of the problem and its potential toll on human lives will spur a significant increase in basic research and intervention and treatment studies to address these knowledge gaps.

To date, few studies have systematically evaluated the effectiveness of interventions for people with PTSD (Gerrity & Solomon, 1996; Johnson et al., 1996; Richards, Lovell, & Marks, 1994). People seeking treatment for PTSD symptoms also frequently present with other distress, such as depression, dysfunctional coping, problems in interpersonal relationships, and other life problems. Thus, practitioners are challenged to use combined treatments and interventions, including pharmacotherapy, that are targeted to multiple problems as well as specific symptoms. Future research is needed to confirm the effectiveness of approaches currently widely used by practitioners (Lundin, 1994; McFarlane, 1994; Meichenbaum, 1994; Sutherland & Davidson, 1994). For example, there is evidence that many patients remain symptomatic but that exposure techniques and cognitive reworking of PTSD memories are critical elements in effective treatment (McFarlane, 1994) and that people with acute stress disorder require supportive and behavioral treatments to reduce symptoms. In the case of PTSD, the use of cognitive treatments, at times in combination with medication for associated depression and anxiety, are recommended. For example, cognitive–behavioral treatments, including those that use live and imaginal exposure techniques, are increasingly used to treat PTSD (Mancoske, Standifer, & Cauley, 1994; Richards et al., 1994). Few studies have examined interventions for family members (Allen & Bloom, 1994; Nelson & Wright, 1996).

Population-based preventive interventions target at-risk people, assuming that although not everyone needs treatment, most would benefit from immediate information and support (Brom & Kleber, 1989). Critical-incident debriefing, open-ended support groups, stress inoculation, and psychoeducational and coping-skills training interventions are examples of strategies used by social workers and other mental health practitioners to enhance people's ability to respond to stressful life events and reduce the likelihood of their experiencing an overwhelming crisis or PTSD. These interventions generally include outreach to targeted populations in schools, workplaces, hospitals, and community disaster sites.

Forms of critical–incident debriefing have been developed for use with primary and secondary victims (Armstrong, Lund, McWright, & Tichenor, 1995; Bell, 1995). The latter include people who have observed the trauma, such as family members, fellow employees or students, military personnel (Armfield, 1994), and emergency workers, including mental health personnel. In critical–incident stress debriefing, crisis intervention groups are the method of choice (Wollman, 1993). Interventions are frequently provided by social workers in teams. Communitywide intervention programs are used in the face of natural disasters (Kaniasty & Norris, 1993; Wright, Ursano, Bartone, & Ingraham, 1990). Debriefing interventions are provided for victims and for observers, such as members of a military unit who have witnessed the death or severe injury of a colleague, and rescuers such as firefighters, police, and other emergency personnel (Bell, 1995; Brom & Kleber, 1989; Smith & deChesney, 1994). Notwithstanding their wide application by social workers and other mental health professionals, few of these interventions have been rigorously evaluated.

Well-controlled treatment outcome data also are lacking for childhood PTSD (Finkelhor & Berliner, 1996). As in the case of PTSD in adults, few studies have evaluated the effectiveness of interventions for children suffering from PTSD, and little is known about gender and cultural influences on the assessment of PTSD (Allen, 1994). The literature reflects numerous unsubstantiated case reports and theories of treatment based wholly on clinical experience. However, there is a general consensus that a cornerstone of treatment of children presenting with PTSD symptoms involves helping the child re-experience the trauma and its meaning in the context of a safe and supportive environment (Pynoos, 1990). Saigh (1992) reported the efficacy of cognitive behavioral psychotherapy intervention in treating children exposed to single-incident trauma. Also, Deblinger and colleagues (1989) have shown that this intervention benefits children with PTSD resulting from the trauma of sexual abuse. Family and group therapy interventions as well as play therapy also are deemed appropriate (Donnelly, Maletic, & March, 1996). It is likely that because posttraumatic responses tend to be multifaceted, the treatment goals should address multiple facets of the disorder, including behavioral, affective, and cognitive aspects (Ribbe, Lipovsky, & Freedy, 1995).

When establishing treatment goals for a traumatized child, it is crucial to take into account the chronicity of the trauma, the level of the child's exposure, and the personal characteristics of the child, including his or her developmental level, gender, and social support systems (Ribbe et al., 1995). In addition, treatment of childhood PTSD should include an educational component. Providing information regarding PTSD helps children understand its symptoms as well as natural responses to trauma. This process reduces children's fears, helps normalize the therapy, and assures children that their symptoms are understandable to the therapist and others. Also, educational efforts should be directed to the parents or caregivers to assist them in understanding the nature of the child's experience, his or her symptoms and feelings, as well as their own feelings.

Efficacy and effectiveness studies of intervention for adjustment disorder also are sparse. However, supportive interventions, such as those used in groups of patients with cancer (see chapter 13), have been found to be effective in reducing symptoms and enhancing quality of life.

Research on stress-related disorders among different cultural groups has been rare (Abueg & Chun, 1996; Al-Ansari & Matar, 1993; Collins, Dimsdale, & Wilkins, 1992; Hinton et al., 1993; Hough, Canino, Abueg, & Gusman, 1996; Marsella, Friedman, & Spain, 1996; Norris, 1992; Penk & Allen, 1991). As a result, little is known about racial and ethnic influences on the assessment or treatment of PTSD (Allen, 1994). For example, it is not known whether symptoms present differently among different racial and ethnic groups, or has health care–seeking behaviors, health beliefs, and clinical decision making vary among diverse cultural groups (Ell & Castenada, in press; Frueh, Smith, & Libet, 1996; Keane, Kaloupek, & Weathers, 1996; Kirmayer, 1996; Manson et al., 1996). Other relevant questions include determining the ways in which perceptions of traumatic events and psychosocial stressors vary among different cultural groups (Green, 1996). Culturally influenced preferences for treatment also merit study (DiNicola, 1996; Rosenheck & Fontana, 1996), as do sociopolitical influences on trauma exposure (Allen, 1996; Gusman et al., 1996; Howard, 1996; Robin, Chester, & Goldman, 1996; Root, 1996).

As previously noted, future studies are needed on the relationship between enduring PTSD symptoms and other types of disorders, such as personality disorder (Gunderson & Sabo, 1993). The long-term effects of childhood trauma on personality development and psychological functioning are not yet clearly understood.

Particularly important to social work practitioners is the need for practice-based studies of implementing screening for stress-related disorders among populations served by social workers, development and evaluation of practice guidelines for intervention with people identified to be at high risk or already symptomatic, and evaluation of interventions within different services systems.

## Conclusion

The rapidly growing body of mental health research on human response to stress provides social workers with critical knowledge on which to base their clinical decision making and intervention strategies as they aim to prevent or reduce suffering following exposure to traumatic and universal stressors. The research reviewed in this chapter has significantly advanced understanding of the serious psychological and functional consequences of stress exposure for many people, many of whom are likely to be served by social workers across a wide range of human services systems. The prevalence and characteristics of traumatic psychosocial stressors that pose the greatest risk for distress and functional impairment are now better understood. Symptom and impairment criteria for professional intervention have been clarified, and the unique characteristics of stress response and disorder among children and adolescents have been highlighted. The problem of lack of detection or hidden trauma has been uncovered, and significant progress is being made in developing screening and diagnostic tools to assist practitioners. The opportunity for social workers to make significant contributions to future research on intervention stands as a major challenge to practitioners and researchers.

## References

Abueg, F. R., & Chun, K. M. (1996). Traumatization stress among Asians and Asian Americans. In A. J. Marsella, M. J. Friedman, E. T. Gerrity, & R. M. Scurfield (Eds.), *Ethnocultural aspects of posttraumatic stress disorder: Issues, research, and clinical applications* (pp. 285–300). Washington, DC: American Psychological Association.

Affonso, D. D., Lovett, S., Paul, S., Sheptak, S., Nussbaum, R., Newman, L., & Johnson, B. (1992). Dysphoric distress in childbearing women. *Journal of Perinatology, 12,* 325–332.

Al-Ansari, A., & Matar, A. M. (1993). Recent stressful life events among Bahraini adolescents with adjustment disorder. *Adolescence, 28,* 339–346.

Alexander, P. J., Dinesh N., & Vidyasagar, M. S. (1993). Psychiatric morbidity among cancer patients and its relationship with awareness of illness and expectations about treatment outcome. *Acta Oncologica, 32,* 623–626.

Allen, I. M. (1996). PTSD among African Americans. In A. J. Marsella, M. J. Friedman, E. T. Gerrity, & R. M. Scurfield (Eds.), *Ethnocultural aspects of posttraumatic stress disorder: Issues, research, and clinical applications* (pp. 209–238). Washington, DC: American Psychological Association.

Allen, S. N. (1994). Psychological assessment of post-traumatic stress disorder. Psychometrics, current trends, and future directions. *Psychiatric Clinics of North America, 17,* 327–349.

Allen, S. N., & Bloom, S. L. (1994). Group and family treatment of post-traumatic stress disorder. *Psychiatric Clinics of North America, 17,* 425–427.

Amaya-Jackson, L., & March, J. S. (1995). Posttraumatic stress disorder. In J. S. March (Ed.), *Anxiety disorders in children* (pp. 276–300). New York: Guilford Press.

American Psychiatric Association. (1980). *Diagnostic and statistical manual of mental disorders* (3rd ed.). Washington, DC: Author.

American Psychiatric Association. (1987). *Diagnostic and statistical manual of mental disorders* (3rd ed., rev.). Washington, DC: Author.

American Psychiatric Association. (1994). *Diagnostic and statistical manual of mental disorders* (4th ed.). Washington, DC: Author.

Andreasen, N. C., & Hoenk, P. R. (1982). The predictive value of adjustment disorders: A follow-up study. *American Journal of Psychiatry, 139,* 584–590.

Andreasen, N. C., & Wasek, P. (1980). Adjustment disorder in adolescents and adults. *Archives of General Psychiatry, 37,* 1166–1170.

Aneshensel, C. S. (1992). Social stress: Theory and research. *Annual Review Sociology, 18,* 15–38.

Armfield, F. (1994). Preventing post-traumatic stress disorder resulting from military operations. *Military Medicine, 159,* 739–746.

Armstrong, K. R., Lund, P. E., McWright, L. T., & Tichenor, V. (1995). Multiple stressor debriefing and the American Red Cross: The East Bay Hills fire experience. *Social Work, 40,* 83–90.

Arroyo, W., & Eth, S. (1985). Children traumatized by Central American warfare. In S. Eth & R. Pynoos (Eds.), *Post-traumatic stress disorder in children* (pp. 103–120). Washington, DC: American Psychiatric Press.

Barnet, B., Joffe, A., Duggan, A. K., Wilson, M. D., & Repke, J. T. (1996). Depressive symptoms, stress and social support in pregnant and postpartum adolescents. *Archives of Pediatric and Adolescent Medicine, 148,* 64–69.

Bell, A. J., Land, N. M., Milnes, S., & Hassanyeh, F. (1994). Long-term outcome of postpartum psychiatric illness requiring admission. *Journal of Affective Disorders, 31,* 67–70.

Bell, J. L. (1995). Traumatic event debriefing: service delivery designs and the role of social work. *Social Work, 40,* 36–43.

Bernstein, E. M., & Putnam, F. W. (1986). Development, reliability, validity of a dissociation scale. *Journal of Nervous and Mental Disease, 174,* 727–737.

Biederman, J. (1990). The diagnosis and treatment of adolescent anxiety disorders. *Journal of Clinical Psychiatry, 51,* 20–26.

Bingham, R. D., & Harmon, R. J. (1996). Traumatic stress in infancy and early childhood: Expression of distress and developmental issues. In C. R. Pfeffer (Ed.), *Severe stress and mental disturbance in children* (pp. 499–532). Washington, DC: American Psychiatric Press.

Bird, H. R., Canino, G., Rubio-Stipec, M., Gould, M. S., Ribera, J., Sesman, M., Woodbry, M., Huestas-Godman, S., Pagan, A., Sanchez-Lacay, A., & Moscoso, M.

(1988). Estimates of the prevalence of childhood maladjustment in a community survey in Puerto Rico. *Archives of General Psychiatry, 45,* 1120–1126.

Bird, H. R., Gould, M. S., & Staghezza, B. M. (1993). Patterns of diagnostic comorbidity in a community sample of children aged 9 through 16 years. *Journal of the American Academy of Child and Adolescent Psychiatry, 32,* 361–368.

Blanchard, E. B., Hickling, E. J., Vollmer, A. J., Loos, W. R., Buckley, T. C., & Jaccard, J. (1995). Short-term follow-up of post-traumatic stress symptoms in motor vehicle accident victims. *Behavior Research and Therapy, 33,* 369–377.

Bland, S. H., O'Leary, E. S., Farinaro, E., Jossa, F., & Trevisan, M. (1996). Long-term psychological effects of natural disasters. *Psychosomatic Medicine, 58,* 18–24.

Blank, A. S. (1994). Clinical detection, diagnosis, and differential diagnosis of post-traumatic stress disorder. *Psychiatric Clinics of North America, 17,* 351–383.

Boyce, P., Stubbs, J., & Todd, A. (1993). The Edinburgh postnatal depression scale: Validation for an Australian sample. *Australian and New Zealand Journal of Psychiatry, 27,* 472–476.

Breier, A. (1995). Stress, dopamine, and schizophrenia: Evidence for a stress-diathesis model. In C. M. Mazure (Ed.), *Does stress cause psychiatric illness?* (pp. 67–86). Washington, DC: American Psychiatric Press.

Briere, J. (1996). *Trauma symptom checklist for children (TSCC).* Odessa, FL: Psychological Assessment Resources.

Bremner, J. D., & Brett, E. (1997). Trauma-related dissociative states and long-term psychopathology in posttraumatic stress disorder. *Journal of Traumatic Stress, 10,* 37–49.

Bremner, J. D., Southwick, S. M., Darnell, A., & Charney, D. S. (1996). Chronic PTSD in Vietnam combat veterans: Course of illness and substance abuse. *American Journal of Psychiatry, 155,* 369–375.

Brent D. A., Perper, J. A., Moritz, G., Liotus, L., Schweers, J., & Canobbio, R. (1994). Major depression or uncomplicated bereavement? A follow-up of youth exposed to suicide. *Journal of the American Academy of Child and Adolescent Psychiatry, 33,* 231–239.

Breslau, N., Davis, G. C., Andreski, P., & Peterson, E. (1991). Traumatic events and posttraumatic stress disorders in an urban population of young adults. *Archives of General Psychiatry, 48,* 216–222.

Brom, D., & Kleber, R. J. (1989). Prevention of post-traumatic stress disorders. *Journal of Traumatic Stress, 2,* 335–351.

Bryant, R. A. (1996). Predictors of post-traumatic stress disorder following burn injury. *Burn, 22,* 89–92.

Bryant, R. A., & Harvey, A. G. (1996). Posttraumatic stress reactions in volunteer firefighters. *Journal of Traumatic Stress, 9,* 51–61.

Bukstein, O. G., Glancy, L. J., & Kaminer, Y. (1992). Patterns of affective comorbidity in a clinical population. *Journal of the American Academy of Child and Adolescent Psychiatry, 31,* 1041–1045.

Bullman, T. A., & Kang, H. N. (1996). The risk of suicide among wounded Vietnam veterans. *American Journal of Public Health, 86,* 662–667.

Burton, D., Foy, D., Bwanausi, C., Johnson, J., & Moore L. (1994). The relationship between traumatic exposure, family dysfunction, and post-traumatic stress symptoms in male juvenile offenders. *Journal of Traumatic Stress, 7,* 83–93.

Cantwell, D. P., & Baker, L. (1989). Stability and natural history of DSM-III childhood diagnoses. *Journal of the American Academy of Child and Adolescent Psychiatry, 28,* 691–700.

Caplan, G. (1964). *Principles of preventive psychiatry.* New York: Basic Books.

Caplan, G. (1974). *Support systems and community mental health*. New York: Basic Books.

Cardena, E., & Spiegel, D. (1993). Dissociative reactions to the Bay Area earthquakes. *American Journal of Psychiatry, 150,* 474–478.

Carroll, B. T., Kathol, R. G., Noyes, R., Wald, T. G., & Clamon, G. H. (1993). Screening for depression and anxiety in cancer patients using the hospital anxiety and depression scale. *General Hospital Psychiatry, 15,* 69–74.

Cicchetti, D., & Toth, S. L. (1995). A developmental psychopathology perspective on child abuse and neglect. *Journal of the American Academy of Child and Adolescent Psychiatry, 34,* 541–565.

Classen, C., Koopman, C., & Spiegel, D. (1993). Trauma and dissociation. *Bulletin of the Menninger Clinic, 57,* 178–194.

Collins, D., Dimsdale, J. E., & Wilkins, D. (1992). Consultation/liaison psychiatry utilization patterns in different cultural groups. *Psychosomatic Medicine, 54,* 240–245.

Cordova, M. J., Andrykowski, M. A., Kenady, D. E., McGrath, P. C., Sloan, D. A., & Redd, W. H. (1995). Frequency and correlates of posttraumatic-stress-disorder-like symptoms after treatment for breast cancer. *Journal of Consulting and Clinical Psychology, 63,* 981–986.

Costello, E., & Angold, A. (1988). Scales to assess child and adolescent depression: Checklists, screens, and nets. *Journal of the American Academy of Child and Adolescent Psychiatry, 27,* 357–363.

Curle, C. E., & Williams, C. (1996). Posttraumatic stress reactions in children—Gender differences in the incidence of trauma reactions at 2 years and examination of factors influencing adjustment. *British Journal of Clinical Psychology, 35,* 297–309.

Dahl, S. (1989). Acute response to rape: A PTSD variant. *Acta Psychiatrica Scandinavica, 80,* 355–362.

Dancu, C. V., Riggs, D. S., Hearst-Ikeda, D., Shoyer, B. G., & Foa, E. B. (1996). Dissociative experiences and posttraumatic stress disorder among female victims of criminal assault and rape. *Journal of Traumatic Stress, 9,* 253–267.

Dansky, B. S., Brady, K. T., Saladin, M. E., Killeen, T., Becker, S., & Roitzsch, J. (1996). Victimization and PTSD in individuals with substance use disorders: Gender and racial differences. *American Journal of Drug and Alcohol Abuse, 22,* 75–93.

Davidson, J. (1995). *Self-Rating Traumatic Stress Scale*. Durham, NC: Duke University Medical Center.

Davidson, J.R.T., & Fairbank, J. A. (1993). The epidemiology of posttraumatic stress disorder. In J.R.T. Davidson & E. B. Foa (Eds.), *Posttraumatic stress disorder: DSM-IV and beyond* (pp. 147–169). Washington, DC: American Psychiatric Press.

Davidson, J.R.T., & Foa, E. B. (1991a). Diagnostic issues in posttraumatic stress disorder: Considerations for the DSM-IV. *Journal of Abnormal Psychology, 100,* 346–355.

Davidson, J.R.T., & Foa, E. B. (1991b). Refining criteria for posttraumatic stress disorder. *Hospital and Community Psychiatry, 42,* 259–261.

Davidson, J.R.T., Hughes, D., Blazer, D. G., & George, L. (1991). Post-traumatic stress disorder in the community: An epidemiological study. *Psychological Medicine, 21,* 713–721.

Davidson, J.R.T., & Smith, R. (1990). Traumatic experiences in psychiatric outpatients. *Journal of Traumatic Stress, 3,* 459–475.

Davis, G. C., & Breslau, N. (1994). Post-traumatic stress disorder in victims of civilian trauma and criminal violence. *Psychiatric Clinics of North America, 17,* 289–299.

Deblinger, E., McLeer, S. V., Atkins, M. S., Ralphe, D., & Foa, E. (1989). Post-traumatic stress in sexually abused, physically abused, and nonabused children. *Child Abuse and Neglect, 13,* 403–408.

de Girolamo, G., & McFarlane, A. C. (1996). The epidemiology of PTSD: A comprehensive review of the international literature. In A. J. Marsella, M. J. Friedman, E. T. Gerrity, & R. M. Scurfield (Eds.), *Ethnocultural aspects of posttraumatic stress disorder: Issues, research, and clinical applications* (pp. 33–85). Washington, DC: American Psychological Association.

Despland, J. N., Monod, L., & Ferrero, F. (1995). Clinical relevance of adjustment disorder in DSM-III-R and DSM-IV. *Comprehensive Psychiatry, 36,* 454–460.

DiNicola, V. F. (1996). Ethnocultural aspects of PTSD and related disorders among children and adolescents. In A. J. Marsella, M. J. Friedman, E. T. Gerrity, & R. M. Scurfield (Eds.), *Ethnocultural aspects of posttraumatic stress disorder: Issues, research, and clinical applications* (pp. 389–414). Washington, DC: American Psychological Association.

Doan, R. J., & Petti, T. A. (1989). Clinical and demographic characteristics of child and adolescent partial hospital patients. *Journal of American Academy of Child and Adolescent Psychiatry, 28,* 66–69.

Dohrenwend, B. P., Levav, I., Shrout, P. E., Schwartz, S., Nevah, G., Link, B. G., Skodol, A. E., & Stueve, A. (1992). Socioeconomic status and psychiatric disorders: The causation-selection issue. *Science, 255,* 946–952.

Dohrenwend, B. P., Shrout, P. E., Link, B. G., Skodol, A. E., & Stueve, A. (1995). Life events and other possible psychosocial risk factors for episodes of schizophrenia and major depression: A case-control study. In C. M. Mazure (Ed.), *Does stress cause psychiatric illness?* (pp. 43–66). Washington, DC: American Psychiatric Press.

Donnelly, C. L., Maletic, V., & March, J. S. (1996). Anxiety disorders in children and adolescents. In D. Parmellee (Ed.), *Child and adolescent psychiatry* (pp. 97–119). St. Louis: C. V. Mosby.

Drell, M. J., Siegel, C. H., & Gaensbauer, T. J. (1993). Post-traumatic stress disorder. In C. H. Zeanah (Ed.), *Handbook of infant mental health* (pp. 291–304). New York: Guilford Press.

Eilenberg, J., Fullilove, M. T., Goldman, R. G., & Mellman, L. (1996). Quality and use of trauma histories obtained from psychiatric outpatients through mandated inquiry. *Psychiatric Services, 47,* 165–169.

Ell, K. (1996). Crisis theory. In F. J. Turner (Ed.), *Social work treatment: Interlocking theoretical approaches* (4th ed., pp. 168–190). New York: Free Press.

Ell, K., & Castenada, I. (in press). Health care seeking behavior. In S. Loue (Ed.), *Handbook of immigrant health.* New York: Plenum Press.

Elliot, D., & Briere, J. (1992). Sexual abuse trauma among professional women: Validating the Trauma Symptom Checklist–40 (TSC–40). *Child Abuse and Neglect, 16,* 391–398.

Engel, C. C., Engel, A. L., Campbell, S. J., McFall, M. E., Russo, J., & Katon, W. (1993). Posttraumatic stress disorder symptoms and precombat sexual and physical abuse in Desert Storm veterans. *Journal of Nervous and Mental Disease, 181,* 683–688.

Everly, G. S. (1995). An integrative two-factor model of post-traumatic stress. In G. S. Everly & J. M. Lating (Eds.), *Psychotraumatology* (pp. 27–48). New York: Plenum Press.

Everson, M. D., Hunter, W. M., Runyon, D. K., Edelsohn, G. A., & Coulter, M. L. (1989). Maternal support following disclosure of incest. *American Journal of Orthopsychiatry, 59,* 197–207.

Fabrega, H., Mezzich, J. E., & Mezzich, A. C. (1987). Adjustment disorder as a marginal or transitional illness category in DSM-III. *Archives of General Psychiatry, 44,* 567–572.

Fairbank, J. A., Schlenger, W. E., Saigh, P. A., & Davidson, J. R. (1995). An epidemiologic profile of post-traumatic stress disorder: Prevalence, comorbidity, and risk factors.

In M. J. Friedman, D. S. Charney, & A. Y. Deutch (Eds.), *Neurobiological and clinical consequences of stress* (pp. 415–427). Philadelphia: Lippincott-Raven.

Falsetti, S. A., Resnick, H. S., Dansky, B. S., Lydiard, B., & Kilpatrick, D. G. (1995). The relationship of stress to panic disorder: Cause or effect? In C. M. Mazure (Ed.), *Does stress cause psychiatric illness?* (pp. 111–148). Washington, DC: American Psychiatric Press.

Famularo, R., Kinscherff, R., & Fenton, T. (1988). Propranolol treatment for children with acute posttraumatic stress disorder. *American Journal of Diseases of Children, 142*, 1244–1247.

Famularo, R., Kinscherff, R., & Fenton, T. (1990). Symptom differences in acute and chronic presentation of childhood post-traumatic stress disorder. *Child Abuse and Neglect, 14*, 439–444.

Famularo, R., Kinscherff, R., & Fenton, T. (1992). Psychiatric diagnoses of maltreated children: Preliminary findings. *Journal of the American Academy of Child and Adolescent Psychiatry, 31*, 863–867.

Famularo, R., Fenton, T., Kinscherff, R., Ayoub, C., & Barnum, R. (1994). Maternal and child posttraumatic stress disorder in cases of child maltreatment. *Child Abuse and Neglect, 18*, 27–36.

Figley, C. R. (1995). *Compassion fatigue: Coping with secondary traumatic stress disorder in those who treat the traumatized.* New York: Brunner/Mazel.

Fink, L. A., Bernstein, D., Handelsman, L., Foote, J., & Lovejoy, M. (1995). Initial reliability and validity of the childhood trauma interview: A new multidimensional measure of childhood interpersonal trauma. *American Journal of Psychiatry, 152*, 1329–1335.

Finkelhor, D., & Berliner, L. (1996). Research on the treatment of sexually abused children: A review and recommendations. *Journal of the American Academy of Child and Adolescent Psychiatry, 34*, 1408–1423.

Finkelhor, D., Hotaling, G., Lewis, I. A., & Smith, C. (1990). Sexual abuse in a national survey of adult men and women: Prevalence, characteristics, and risk factors. *Child Abuse and Neglect, 14*, 19–28.

Foa, E. B., & Riggs, D. S. (1995). Posttraumatic stress disorder following assault: Theoretical considerations and empirical findings. *Current Directions in Psychological Science, 4*, 61–65.

Foa, E. B., Riggs, D. S., Dancu, C. V., & Rothbaum, B. O. (1993). Reliability and validity of a brief instrument for assessing post-traumatic stress disorder. *Journal of Traumatic Stress, 6*, 459–474.

Foy, D., Madvig, B. T., Pynoos, R. S., & Camilleri, A. J. (1996). Etiologic factors in the development of posttraumatic stress disorder in children and adolescents. *Journal of School Psychology, 34*, 133–145.

Franklin, C., Nowicki, J., Trapp, J., Schwab, A. J., & Petersen, J. (1993). A computerized assessment system for brief, crisis-oriented youth services. *Families in Society, 74*, 602–616.

Frederick, C. J. (1985). Children traumatized by catastrophic situations. In S. Eth & R. S. Pynoos (Eds.), *Post-traumatic stress disorder in children* (pp. 73–99). Washington, DC: American Psychiatric Press.

Frederick, C. J. (1986). Post-traumatic stress disorder and child molestation. In A. W. Burgess & C. R. Hartman (Eds.), *Sexual exploitation of patients by health professionals* (pp. 133–142). New York: Praeger

Freedy, J. R., & Hobfoll, S. E. (Eds.). (1995). *Traumatic stress from theory to practice*. New York: Plenum Press.

Friedman, M. J., Schnurr, P. P., & McDonagh, C. A. (1994). Post-traumatic stress disorder in the military veteran. *Psychiatric Clinics of North America, 17,* 265–277.

Frueh, B. C., Smith, D. W., & Libet, J. M. (1996). Racial differences on psychological measures in combat veterans seeking treatment for PTSD. *Journal of Personality Assessment, 66,* 41–53.

Fukunishi, I., & Kudo, H. (1995). Psychiatric problems of pediatric end-stage renal failure. *General Hospital Psychiatry, 17,* 32–36.

Gaensbauer, T. (1996). Developmental and therapeutic aspects of treating infants and toddlers who have witnessed violence. In J. D. Osofsky & E. Fenichel (Eds.), *Islands of safety: Assessing and Treating Young Victims of Violence* (pp. 15–20). Washington, DC: Zero to Three/National Center for Clinical Infant Programs.

Garbarino, J., Dubrow, N., Kostelny, K., & Pardo, C. (1992). *Children in danger*. San Francisco: Jossey-Bass.

Garbarino, J., Kostelny, K., & Dubrow, N. (1991). *No place to be a child: Growing up in a war zone*. Lexington, MA: Lexington Books.

Gerrity, E. T., & Solomon, S. D. (1996). The treatment of PTSD and related stress disorders: Current research and clinical knowledge. In A. J. Marsella, M. J. Friedman, E. T. Gerrity, & R. M. Scurfield (Eds.), *Ethnocultural aspects of posttraumatic stress disorder: Issues, research, and clinical applications* (pp. 87–104). Washington, DC: American Psychological Association.

Giaconia, R. M., Reinherz, H. Z., Silverman, A. B., Pakiz, B., Frost, A. K., & Cohen, E. (1994). Ages of onset of psychiatric disorders in a community population of older adolescents. *Journal of the American Academy of Child and Adolescent Psychiatry, 33,* 706–717.

Goenjian, A. K., Pynoos, R. S., Steinberg, A. M., Najarian, L. M., Asarnow, I., Ghurabi, M., & Fairbanks, L. A. (1995). Psychiatric comorbidity in children after the 1988 earthquake in Armenia. *Journal of the American Academy of Child and Adolescent Psychiatry, 34,* 1174–1184.

Goodwin, J. (1985). Post-traumatic symptoms in incest victims. In S. Eth & R. S. Pynoos (Eds.), *Post-traumatic stress disorder in children* (pp. 157–168). Washington, DC: American Psychiatric Press.

Green, A. H. (1985). Children traumatized by physical abuse. In S. Eth & R. S. Pynoos (Eds.), *Post-traumatic stress disorder in children* (pp. 135–154). Washington, DC: American Psychiatric Press.

Green, B. L. (1993). Disasters and posttraumatic stress disorder. In J.R.T. Davidson & E. B. Foa (Eds.), *Posttraumatic stress disorder: DSM-IV and beyond* (pp. 75–97). Washington, DC: American Psychiatric Association.

Green, B. L. (1994). Psychosocial research in traumatic stress: An update. *Journal of Traumatic Stress, 7,* 341–362.

Green, B. L. (1996). Cross-national and ethnocultural issues in disaster research. In A. J. Marsella, M. J. Friedman, E. T. Gerrity, & R. M. Scurfield (Eds.), *Ethnocultural aspects of posttraumatic stress disorder: Issues, research, and clinical applications* (pp. 341–362). Washington, DC: American Psychological Association.

Green, B. L., Grace, M. C., Vary, M. G., Kramer, T. L., Gleser, G. C., & Leonard, A. C. (1994). Children of disaster in the second decade. *Journal of the American Academy of Child and Adolescent Psychiatry, 33,* 71–79.

Green, B. L., Korol, M., Grace, M. C., Vary, M. G., Leonard, A. C., Gleser, G. C., & Smitson-Cohen, S. (1991). Children and disaster: Age, gender, and parental effects on PTSD symptoms. *Journal of the American Academy of Child and Adolescent Psychiatry, 30,* 945–951.

Green, B. L., & Lindy, J. D. (1994). Post-traumatic stress disorder in victims of disasters. *Psychiatric Clinics of North America, 17,* 301–309.

Green, B. L., Lindy, J. D., Grace, M. C., & Leonard, A. C. (1992). Chronic posttraumatic stress disorder and diagnostic comorbidity in a disaster sample. *Journal of Nervous and Mental Disease, 180,* 760–766.

Greenberg, W. M., Rosenfeld, D. N., & Ortega, E. A. (1995). Adjustment disorder as an admission diagnosis. *American Journal of Psychiatry, 152,* 459–461.

Groves, B. M., Zuckerman, B., Marans, S., & Cohen, D. J. (1993). Silent victims: Children who witness violence. *JAMA, 269,* 262–264.

Gunderson, J. G., & Sabo, A. N. (1993). The phenomenological and conceptual interface between borderline personality disorder and PTSD. *American Journal of Psychiatry, 150,* 19–27.

Gusman, F. D., Stewart, J., Young, B. H., Riney, S. J., Abueg, F. R., & Blake, D. D. (1996). A multicultural developmental approach for treating trauma. In A. J. Marsella, M. J. Friedman, E. T. Gerrity, & R. M. Scurfield (Eds.), *Ethnocultural aspects of posttraumatic stress disorder: Issues, research, and clinical applications* (pp. 439–458). Washington, DC: American Psychological Association.

Hammen, S. L. (1995). Stress and the course of unipolar and bipolar disorders. In C. M. Mazure (Ed.), *Does stress cause psychiatric illness?* (pp. 87–110). Washington, DC: American Psychiatric Press.

Helzer, J., Robins, L., & McEvoy, L. (1987). Post-traumatic stress disorder in the general population: Findings of the Epidemiologic Catchment Area Survey. *New England Journal of Medicine, 31,* 1630–1634.

Hendrix, C. C., Anelli, L. M., Gibbs, J. P., & Fournier, D. G. (1994). Validation of the Purdue Post-Traumatic Stress Scale on a sample of Vietnam veterans. *Journal of Traumatic Stress, 7,* 311–318.

Herman, J. L. (1992). Complex PTSD: A syndrome in survivors of prolonged and repeated trauma. *Journal of Traumatic Stress, 5,* 377–391.

Herzog, D. B., Keller, M. B., Sacks, N. R., Yeh, C. J., & Lavor, P. W. (1992). Psychiatric comorbidity in treatment-seeking anorexics and bulimics. *Journal of the American Academy of Child and Adolescent Psychiatry, 31,* 810–818.

Hinton, W. L., Chen, Y. C., Du, N., Tran, C. G., Lu, F. G., & Miranda, J. (1993). DSM-III-R disorders in Vietnamese refugees: Prevalence and correlates. *Journal of Nervous and Mental Disease, 181,* 113–122.

Hobfoll, S. (1988). *The ecology of stress.* New York: Hemisphere.

Hobfoll, S. E. (1991). Traumatic stress: A theory based on rapid loss of resources. *Anxiety Research, 4,* 187–197.

Horowitz, M. J., Bonanno, G. A., & Holen, A. (1993). Pathological grief. *Psychosomatic Medicine, 55,* 260–273.

Horowitz, M. J., Wilner, N., & Alvarez, W. (1979). Impact of Events Scale: A measure of subjective stress. *Psychosomatic Medicine, 41,* 209–218.

Hough, R. L., Canino, G. J., Abueg, F. R., & Gusman, F. D. (1996). PTSD and related stress disorders among Hispanics. In A. J. Marsella, M. J. Friedman, E. T. Gerrity, & R. M. Scurfield (Eds.), *Ethnocultural aspects of posttraumatic stress disorder: Issues, research, and clinical applications* (pp. 301–328). Washington, DC: American Psychological Association.

Howard, D. E. (1996). Searching for resilience among African-American youth exposed to community violence: Theoretical issues. *Journal of Adolescent Health, 18,* 254–262.

Hubbard, J., Realmuto, G. M., Northwood, A. K., & Masten, A. S. (1995). Comorbidity of psychiatric diagnoses with posttraumatic stress disorder in survivors of childhood trauma. *Journal of the American Academy of Child and Adolescent Psychiatry, 34,* 1167–1173.

Irwin, H. J. (1996). Traumatic childhood events, perceived availability of emotional support, and the development of dissociative tendencies. *Child Abuse and Neglect, 20,* 701–707.

Jaffe, P., Wolfe, D., & Wilson, S. (1990). *Children of battered women: Issues in child development and intervention planning.* Newbury Park, CA: Sage Publications.

Johnson, D. R., Rosenheck, R., Fontana, A., Lubin, H., Charney, D., & Southwick, S. (1996). Outcome of intensive inpatient treatment for combat-related posttraumatic stress disorder. *American Journal of Psychiatry, 153,* 771–777.

Kaniasty, K., & Norris, F. H. (1993). A test of the social support deterioration model in the context of natural disaster. *Journal of Personality and Social Psychology, 64,* 395–408.

Karam, E. G. (1994). The nosological status of bereavement-related depressions. *British Journal of Psychiatry, 165,* 48–52.

Kathol, R. G., & Wenzel, R. P. (1992). Natural history of symptoms of depression and anxiety during inpatient treatment on general medicine wards. *Journal of General Internal Medicine, 7,* 287–293.

Keane, T. M. (1996). Clinical perspectives on stress, traumatic stress, and PTSD in children and adolescents. *Journal of School Psychology, 34,* 193–197.

Keane, T. M., Caddell, J. M., & Taylor, K. L. (1988). Mississippi Scale for Combat-Related Posttraumatic Stress Disorder: Three studies in reliability and validity. *Journal of Consulting and Clinical Psychology, 56,* 85–90.

Keane, T. M., Kaloupek, D. G., & Weathers, F. W. (1996). Ethnocultural considerations in the assessment of PTSD. In A. J. Marsella, M. J. Friedman, E. T. Gerrity, & R. M. Scurfield (Eds.), *Ethnocultural aspects of posttraumatic stress disorder: Issues, research, and clinical applications* (pp. 183–208). Washington, DC: American Psychological Association.

Kelly, B., Raphael, B., Smithers, M., Swanson, C., Reid, C., McLeod, R., Thomson, D., & Walpole, E. (1995). Psychological responses to malignant melanoma: An investigation of traumatic stress reactions to life-threatening illness. *General Hospital Psychiatry, 17,* 126–134.

Kendall-Tackett, K. A., Williams, L. M., & Finkelhor, D. (1993). Impact of sexual abuse on children: A review and synthesis of recent empirical studies. *Psychological Bulletin, 113,* 164–180.

Kessler, R. C. (in press). The effects of stressful life events on depression. *Annual Review of Psychology.*

Kessler, R. C., Sonnega, A., Bromet, E., Hughes, M., & Nelson, C. B. (1995). Posttraumatic stress disorder in the National Comorbidity Survey. *Archives of General Psychiatry, 52,* 1048–1060.

Kilpatrick, D., & Resnick, H. (1993). PTSD associated with exposure to criminal victimization in clinical and community populations. In J.R.T. Davidson & E. B. Foa (Eds.), *Post-traumatic stress disorder: DSM-IV and beyond* (pp. 113–143). Washington, DC: American Psychiatric Press.

Kilpatrick, D. G., Resnick, H. S., Freedy, J. R., Pelcovitz, D., Resnick, P., Roth, S., & van der Kolk, B. (1996). The posttraumatic stress disorder field trial: Evaluation of the

PTSD construct: Criteria A through E. In T. A Widiger, A. J. Frances, H. A. Pincus, M. B. First, R. Ross, & W. Davis (Eds.), *DSM-IV sourcebook* (Vol. II). Washington, DC: American Psychiatric Association.

Kim, K., & Jacobs, S. (1995). Stress of bereavement and consequent psychiatric illness. In C. M. Mazure (Ed.), *Does stress cause psychiatric illness?* (pp. 187–220). Washington, DC: American Psychiatric Press.

Kim-Goh, M., Suh, C., Blake, D. D., & Hiley, Y. B. (1995). Psychological impact of the Los Angeles riots on Korean-American victims: Implications for treatment. *American Journal of Orthopsychiatry, 65,* 138–146.

Kinzie, J. D., & Goetz, R. R. (1996). A century of controversy surrounding posttraumatic stress syndromes: The impact on DSM-III and DSM-IV. *Journal of Traumatic Stress, 9,* 159–179.

Kirmayer, L. J. (1996). Confusion of the senses: Implications of ethnocultural variations in somatoform and dissociative disorders for PTSD. In A. J. Marsella, M. J. Friedman, E. T. Gerrity, & R. M. Scurfield (Eds.), *Ethnocultural aspects of posttraumatic stress disorder: Issues, research, and clinical applications* (pp. 131–164). Washington, DC: American Psychological Association.

Kiser, L. J., Heston, J., Millsap, P. A., & Pruitt, D. B. (1991). Physical and sexual abuse in childhood: Relationships with post-traumatic stress disorder. *Journal of the American Academy of Child and Adolescent Psychiatry, 30,* 776–783.

Koopman, C., Classen, C., Cardena, E., & Spiegel, D. (1995). When disaster strikes, acute stress disorder may follow. *Journal of Traumatic Stress, 8,* 29–46.

Kovacs, M., Gatsonis, C., Pollock, M., & Parrone, P. L. (1994). A controlled prospective study of DSM-III adjustment disorder in childhood: Short-term prognosis and long-term predictive validity. *Archives of General Psychiatry, 51,* 535–541.

Kovacs, M., Ho, V., & Pollock, M. H. (1995). Criterion and predictive validity of the diagnosis of adjustment disorder: A prospective study of youths with new-onset insulin-dependent diabetes mellitus. *American Journal of Psychiatry, 152,* 523–528.

Kramer, T. L., & Green, B. L. (1991). Posttraumatic stress disorder as an early response to sexual assault. *Journal of Interpersonal Violence, 6,* 160–173.

Kramer, T., Lindy, J. D., Green, B. L., Grace, M. C., & Leonard, A. C. (1994). The comorbidity of post-traumatic stress disorder and suicidality in Vietnam veterans. *Suicide and Life-Threatening Behavior, 24,* 58–67.

Kumar, R., Marks, M., Wieck, A., Hirst, D., Campbell, I., & Checkley, S. (1993). Neuroendocrine and psychosocial mechanisms in post-partum psychosis. *Progress in Neuro-Psychopharmacology and Biological Psychiatry, 17,* 571–579.

Kutz, I., Shabtai, H., Solomon, Z., Neumann, M., & David, D. (1994). Post-traumatic stress disorder in myocardial infarction. *Israel Journal of Psychiatry and Related Sciences, 31,* 48–56.

LaGreca, A. M., Silverman, W. K., Vernberg, E. M., & Prinstein, M. J. (1996). Symptoms of posttraumatic stress in children after Hurricane Andrew: A prospective study. *Journal of Consulting and Clinical Psychology, 64,* 712–723.

Lating, J. M., Zeichner, A., & Keane, T. M. (1995). Psychological assessment of PTSD. In G. S. Everly & J. M. Lating (Eds.), *Psychotraumatology: Key papers and core concepts in the post-traumatic stress* (pp. 103–127). New York: Plenum Press.

Lazarus, R. S. (1966). *Psychological stress and the coping process.* New York: McGraw-Hill.

Leigh, H. (1993). Physical factors affecting psychiatric conditions. *General Hospital Psychiatry, 15,* 155–159.

Lesaca, T. (1996). Symptoms of stress disorder and depression among trauma counselors after an airline disaster. *Psychiatric Services, 47,* 424–426.

Lindemann, E. (1944). Symptomatology and management of acute grief. *American Journal of Psychiatry, 101,* 141–148.

Lloyd, G. G. (1993). Psychological problems and the intensive care unit: Need for greater awareness during and after admission. *British Medical Journal, 307,* 458–459.

Lonigan, C. J., Shannon, M. P., Taylor, A. J., & Sallee, F. R. (1994). Children exposed to disaster: II. Risk factors for the development of post-traumatic symptomatology. *Journal of the American Academy of Child and Adolescent Psychiatry, 33,* 94–105.

Lundin, T. (1994). The treatment of acute trauma: Post-traumatic stress disorder prevention. *Psychiatric Clinics of North America, 17,* 385–391.

Lyons, J. A. (1987). Posttraumatic stress disorder in children and adolescents: A review of the literature. *Journal of Developmental and Behavioral Pediatrics, 8,* 349–356.

Madakasira, S., & O'Brien, K. F. (1987). Acute posttraumatic stress in victims of a natural disaster. *Journal of Nervous and Mental Disease, 175,* 286–290.

Mancoske, R. J., Standifer, D., & Cauley, C. (1994). The effectiveness of brief counseling services for battered women. *Research on Social Work Practice, 4,* 53–63.

Manson, S., Beals, J., O'Nell, T., Piasecki, J., Bechtold, D., Keane, E., & Jones, M. (1996). Wounded spirits, ailing hearts: PTSD and related disorders among American Indians. In A. J. Marsella, M. J. Friedman, E. T. Gerrity, & R. M. Scurfield (Eds.), *Ethnocultural aspects of posttraumatic stress disorder: Issues, research, and clinical applications* (pp. 255–284). Washington, DC: American Psychological Association.

March, J. S. (1993). What constitutes a stressor? The criterion A issue. In J.R.T. Davidson & E. B. Foa (Eds.), *Posttraumatic stress disorder: DSM-IV and beyond* (pp. 37–54). Washington, DC: American Psychiatric Press.

Marmar, C. R., Weiss, D. S., Metzler, T. J., Ronfeldt, H. M., & Foreman, C. (1996). Stress responses of emergency services personnel to the Loma Prieta earthquake Interstate 880 freeway collapse and control traumatic incidents. *Journal of Traumatic Stress, 9,* 63–85.

Marsella, A. J., Friedman, M. J., & Spain, E. H. (1996). Ethnocultural aspects of PTSD: An overview of issues and research directions. In A. J. Marsella, M. J. Friedman, E. T. Gerrity, & R. M. Scurfield (Eds.), *Ethnocultural aspects of posttraumatic stress disorder: Issues, research, and clinical applications* (pp. 105–130). Washington, DC: American Psychological Association.

Mazure, C. M. (Ed.). (1995). *Does stress cause psychiatric illness?* Washington, DC: American Psychiatric Press.

Mazure, C. M., & Druss, B. G. (1995). A historical perspective on stress and psychiatric illness. In C. M. Mazure (Ed.), *Does stress cause psychiatric illness?* (pp. 1–42). Washington, DC: American Psychiatric Press.

McFarlane, A. C. (1988). The longitudinal course of posttraumatic morbidity: The range of outcomes and their predictors. *Journal of Nervous and Mental Disease, 176,* 30–39.

McFarlane, A. C. (1992). Avoidance and intrusion in posttraumatic stress disorder in the victims of a natural disaster. *Journal of Nervous and Mental Disease, 180,* 439–445.

McFarlane, A. C. (1994). Individual psychotherapy for post-traumatic stress disorder. *Psychiatric Clinics of North America, 17,* 393–408.

McFarlane, A. C., & Yehuda, R. (1996). Resilience, vulnerability, and the course of post-traumatic reactions. In B. A. van der Kolk, A. C. McFarlane, & L. Weisaeth (Eds.), *Traumatic stress: The effects of overwhelming experience on mind, body, and society* (pp. 155–179). New York: Guilford Press.

McGrath, E., Keita, G. P., Strickland, B. R., & Russo, N. F. (1990). *Women and depression: Risk factors and treatment issues.* Washington, DC: American Psychological Association.

McLeer, S. L., Callaghan, M., Henry, D., & Wallen, J. (1994). Psychiatric disorders in sexually-abused children. *Journal of the American Academy of Child and Adolescent Psychiatry, 33,* 313–319.

McLeer, S. V., Deblinger, E., Atkins, M. S., Foa, E. B., & Ralphe, D. (1988). Post-traumatic stress disorder in sexually abused children. *Journal of the American Academy of Child and Adolescent Psychiatry, 27,* 650–654.

McNally, R. J. (1993). Stressors that produce posttraumatic stress disorder in children. In J.R.T. Davidson & E. B. Foa (Eds.), *Posttraumatic stress disorder: DSM-IV and beyond* (pp. 57–74). Washington, DC: American Psychiatric Press.

McNally, R. J. (1996). Assessment of posttraumatic stress disorder in children and adolescents. *Journal of School Psychology, 34,* 147–161.

McNally, R. J., & Shin, L. M. (1995). Association of intelligence with severity of posttraumatic stress disorder symptoms in Vietnam combat veterans. *American Journal of Psychiatry, 152,* 936–938.

Meichenbaum, D. (1994). *A clinical handbook/practical therapist manual for assessing and treating adults with post-traumatic stress disorder (PTSD).* Waterloo, Ontario: Institute Press.

Merry, S. N., & Andrews, L. K. (1994). Psychiatric status of sexually abused children 12 months after disclosure of abuse. *Journal of the American Academy of Child and Adolescent Psychiatry, 33,* 939–944.

Mezzich, J. E., Fabrega, H., Jr., Coffman, G. A., & Haley, R. (1989). DSM-III disorders in a large sample of psychiatric patients: Frequency and specificity of diagnoses. *American Journal of Psychiatry, 146,* 212–219.

Mirowsky, J., & Ross, C. E. (1989). *Social causes of psychological distress.* New York: Aldine de Gruyter.

Mok, H., & Watler, C. (1995). Brief psychiatric hospitalization: Preliminary experience with an urban short-stay unit. *Canadian Journal of Psychiatry, 40,* 415–417.

Monroe, S. M., Kupfer, D. J., & Frank, E. (1992). Life stress and treatment course of recurrent depression: Response during index episode. *Journal of Consulting and Clinical Psychology, 60,* 718–724.

Nader, K., & Pynoos, R. S. (1989). *Child Post-Traumatic Stress Disorder Inventory: Parent Inventory.* Unpublished manuscript.

Nader, K., Pynoos, R., Fairbanks, L., & Frederick, C. (1990). Children's PTSD reactions one year after a sniper attack at their school. *American Journal of Psychiatry, 147,* 1526–1530.

Nader, K., Pynoos, R. S., Fairbanks, L., Frederick, C., Al-Ajeel, M., & Al-Asfour, A. (1993). A preliminary study of PTSD and grief among the children of Kuwait following the Gulf Crisis. *British Journal of Clinical Psychology, 32,* 407–416.

Nader, K., Stuber, M., & Pynoos, R. (1991). Posttraumatic stress reactions in preschool children with catastrophic illness: Assessment needs. *Comprehensive Mental Health Care, 1,* 223–239.

Neal, L. A., Busuttil, W., Herapath, R., & Strike, P. W. (1994). Development and validation of the Computerized Clinician Administered Post-Traumatic Stress Disorder Scale-1-Revised. *Psychological Medicine, 24,* 701–706.

Nelson, B. S., & Wright, D. W. (1996). Understanding and treating post-traumatic stress disorder symptoms in female partners of veterans with PTSD. *Journal of Marital and Family Therapy, 4,* 455–467.

Newberger, C. M., Geremy, I. M., Waternaux, C. M., & Newberger, E. H. (1993). Mothers of sexually abused children: Trauma and repair in longitudinal perspective. *American Journal of Orthopsychiatry, 63,* 92–102.

Newcorn, J. H., & Strain, J. (1995). Adjustment disorder in children and adolescents. *Journal of the American Academy of Child and Adolescent Psychiatry, 31,* 318–326.

Newman, C. J. (1976). Children of disaster: Clinical observations at Buffalo Creek. *American Journal of Psychiatry, 133,* 306–312.

Newman, E., Kaloupek, D. G., & Keane, T. M. (1996). Assessment of posttraumatic stress disorder in clinical and research settings. In B. A. van der Kolk, A. C. McFarlane, & L. Weisaeth (Eds.), *Traumatic stress: The effects of overwhelming experience on mind, body, and society* (pp. 242–278). New York: Guilford Press.

Norris, F. H. (1992). Epidemiology of trauma: Frequency and impact of different potentially traumatic events on different demographic groups. *Journal of Consulting and Clinical Psychology, 2,* 409–418.

Norris, F. H., & Perilla, J. L. (1996). The Revised Civilian Mississippi Scale for PTSD: Reliability, validity, and cross-language stability. *Journal of Traumatic Stress, 9,* 285–298.

North, C. S., Smith, E. M., McCool, R. E., & Lightcap, P. E. (1989). Acute postdisaster coping and adjustment. *Journal of Traumatic Stress, 2,* 353–360.

North, C. S., Smith, E. M., & Spitznagel, E. L. (1994a). Posttraumatic stress disorder in survivors of a mass shooting. *American Journal of Psychiatry, 151,* 82–88.

North, C. S., Smith, E. M., & Spitznagel, E. L. (1994b). Violence and the homeless: An epidemiologic study of victimization and aggression. *Journal of Traumatic Stress, 7,* 95–110.

Osofsky, J. D. (1995). The effects of exposure to violence on young children. *American Psychologist, 50,* 782–785.

Osofsky, J. D., & Fenichel, E. (Eds.). (1994). *Hurt, healing, and hope: Caring for infants and toddlers in violent environments.* Arlington, VA: Zero to Three/National Center for Clinical Infant Programs.

Oxman, T. E., Barrett, J. E., Freeman, D. H., & Manheimer, E. (1994). Frequency and correlates of adjustment disorder related to cardiac surgery in older patients. *Psychosomatics, 35,* 557–568.

Parad, H. J. (1971). Crisis intervention. In R. Morris (Ed.-in-Chief), *Encyclopedia of social work* (16th ed., Vol. 1, pp. 196–202). Washington, DC: National Association of Social Workers.

Parad, H. J., & Parad, L. G. (1990). *Crisis intervention.* Milwaukee: Families International.

Parker, J., & Randall, P. (1996). Post-traumatic stress disorder in children: The social work challenge. *Journal of Social Work Practice, 10,* 71–81.

Patterson, D. R., Carrigan, L., Questad, K. A., & Robinson, R. (1990). Post-traumatic stress disorder in hospitalized patients with burn injuries. *Journal of Burn Care and Rehabilitation, 11,* 181–184.

Pearlin, L. I. (1989). The sociological study of stress. *Journal of Health and Social Behavior, 30,* 241–256.

Pelcovitz, D., Kaplan, S., Goldenberg, B., Mandel, F., Lehane, J., & Guarrera, J. (1994). Post-traumatic stress disorder in physically abused adolescents. *Journal of the American Academy of Child and Adolescent Psychiatry, 33,* 305–312.

Penk, W., & Allen, I. (1991). Clinical assessment of post-traumatic stress disorders (PTSD) among American minorities who served in Vietnam. *Journal of Traumatic Stress, 4,* 41–67.

Perez-Jimenez, J. P., Gomez-Bajo, G. J., Lopez-Castillo, J. J., Salvador, R. M., & Garcia, T. V. (1994). Psychiatric consultation and post-traumatic stress disorder in burn patients. *Burns, 20,* 532–536.

Pitman, R. K. (1993). Biological findings in posttraumatic stress disorder: Implications for DSM-IV classification. In J.R.T. Davidson & E. B. Foa (Eds.), *Posttraumatic stress disorder: DSM-IV and beyond* (pp. 173–189). Washington, DC: American Psychiatric Press.

Pollock, D. (1992). Structured ambiguity and the definition of psychiatric illness: Adjustment disorder among medical inpatients. *Social Science and Medicine, 35,* 25–35.

Pop, V. J., Essed, G. G., deGeus, C. A., vanSon, M. M., & Komproe, I. H. (1993). Prevalence of post partum depression—Or is it post-puerperium depression? *Acta Obstetricia et Gynecologica Scandinavica, 72,* 354–358.

Popkin, M. K., Callies, A. L., Colon, E. A., & Stiebel, V. (1990). Adjustment disorders in medically ill inpatients referred for consultation in a university hospital. *Psychosomatics, 31,* 410–414.

Pynoos, R. S. (1990). Posttraumatic stress disorder in children and adolescents. In B. D. Garfinkel, G. A. Carlson, & E. B. Weller (Eds.), *Psychiatric disorders in children and adolescents* (pp. 48–63). Philadelphia: W. B. Saunders.

Pynoos, R. S. (1992). Grief and trauma in children and adolescents. *Bereavement Care, 11,* 2–10.

Pynoos, R. S., Frederick, C., Nader, K., Arroyo, W., Steinberg, A., Eth, S., Nunez, F., & Fairbanks, L. (1987). Life threat and posttraumatic stress in school-age children. *Archives of General Psychiatry, 44,* 1057–1063.

Pynoos, R. S., & Nader, K. (1993). Issues in the treatment of post-traumatic stress in children and adolescents. In J. Wilson & B. Raphael (Eds.), *The international handbook of traumatic stress syndromes* (pp. 535–549). New York: Plenum Press.

Pynoos, R. S., Steinberg, A. M., & Goenjian, A. (1996). Traumatic stress in childhood and adolescence: Recent developments and current controversies. In B. A. van der Kolk, A. C. McFarlane, & L. Weisaeth (Eds.), *Traumatic stress: The effects of overwhelming experience on mind, body, and society* (pp. 331–368). New York: Guilford Press.

Rahe, R. H. (1988). Acute versus chronic psychological reactions to combat. *Military Medicine, 153,* 365–372.

Ramsay, R. (1990). Invited review: Post-traumatic stress disorder: A new clinical entity? *Journal of Psychosomatic Research, 34,* 355–365.

Razavi, D., & Stiefel, F. (1994). Common psychiatric disorders in cancer patients: Adjustment disorders and depression disorders. *Supportive Care in Cancer, 2,* 223–232.

Resnick, H. S., Yehuda, R., Pitman R. K., & Foy, D. W. (1995). Effects of previous trauma on acute plasma cortisol level following rape. *American Journal of Psychiatry, 152,* 1675–1677.

Reynolds, C. R., & Richmond, B. O. (1978). What I think and feel: A revised measure of children's manifest anxiety. *Journal of Abnormal Child Psychology, 6,* 271–280.

Ribbe, D. P., Lipovsky, J. A., & Freedy, J. R. (1995). Posttraumatic stress. In A. R. Eisen, C. A. Kearney, & C. E. Schaefer (Eds.), *Clinical handbook of disorders in children and adolescents* (pp. 317–356). Northvale, NJ: Jason Aronson.

Richards, D. A., Lovell, K., & Marks, I. M. (1994). Post-traumatic stress disorder: Evaluation of a behavioral treatment program. *Journal of Traumatic Stress, 7,* 669–680.

Robin, R. W., Chester, B., & Goldman, D. (1996). Cumulative trauma and PTSD in American Indian communities. In A. J. Marsella, M. J. Friedman, E. T. Gerrity, & R. M. Scurfield (Eds.), *Ethnocultural aspects of posttraumatic stress disorder: Issues, research, and clinical applications* (pp. 239–254). Washington, DC: American Psychological Association.

Root, M. P. (1996). Women of color and traumatic stress in "domestic captivity": Gender and race as disempowering statuses. In A. J. Marsella, M. J. Friedman, E. T. Gerrity, & R. M. Scurfield (Eds.), *Ethnocultural aspects of posttraumatic stress disorder: Issues, research, and clinical applications* (pp. 363–387). Washington, DC: American Psychological Association.

Rosenheck, R., & Fontana, A. (1996). Ethnocultural variations in service use among veterans suffering from PTSD. In A. J. Marsella, M. J. Friedman, E. T. Gerrity, & R. M. Scurfield (Eds.), *Ethnocultural aspects of posttraumatic stress disorder: Issues, research, and clinical applications* (pp. 483–504). Washington, DC: American Psychological Association.

Rosenthal, M., & Levy-Shiff, R. (1993). Threat of missile attacks in the Gulf War: Mothers' perceptions of young children's reactions. *American Journal of Orthopsychiatry, 63*, 241–254.

Saigh, P. A. (1989). The validity of DSM-III posttraumatic stress disorder classification as applied to children. *Journal of Abnormal Psychology, 98*, 89–192.

Saigh, P. A. (1991). The development of posttraumatic stress disorder following four different types of traumatization. *Behavior Research and Therapy, 14*, 247–275.

Saigh, P. A. (1992). History, current nosology, and epidemiology. In P. A. Saigh (Ed.), *Posttraumatic stress disorder: A behavioral approach to assessment* (pp. 1–27). Boston: Allyn & Bacon.

Saigh, P. A., Green, B. L., & Korol, M. (1996). The history and prevalence of posttraumatic stress disorder with special reference to children and adolescents. *Journal of School Psychology, 34*, 107–131.

Schaffer, D., Fisher, P., Dulcan, M. K., Davies, M., Piacentini, J., Schwab-Stone, M. E., Lahey, B. B., Bourdon, K., Jensen, P. S., Bird, H. R., Canino, G., & Reiger, D. A. (1996). The NIMH Diagnostic Interview Schedule for Children Version 2.3: Description, acceptability, prevalence rates, and performance in the MECA Study. *Journal of the American Academy of Child and Adolescent Psychiatry, 35*, 865–877.

Schatzberg, A. F. (1990). Anxiety and adjustment disorder: A treatment approach. *Journal of Clinical Psychiatry, 51*, 20–24.

Scheeringa, M. S., Zeanah, C. H., Drell, M. J., & Larrieu, J. A. (1995). Two approaches to the diagnosis of posttraumatic stress disorder in infancy and early childhood. *Journal of the American Academy of Child and Adolescent Psychiatry, 34*, 191–200.

Schottenfeld, R. S., & Cullen, M. R. (1985). Occupation-induced posttraumatic stress disorders. *American Journal of Psychiatry, 142*, 198–202.

Schreiber, S., & Galai, G. T. (1993). Uncontrolled pain following physical injury as the core-trauma in the post-traumatic stress disorder. *Pain, 54*, 107–110.

Schwarzwald, J., Weisenberg, M., Waysman, M., Solomon, Z., & Klingman, A. (1993). Stress reaction of school-age children to the bombardment by SCUD missiles. *Journal of Abnormal Psychology, 102*, 404–410.

Scott, D. (1992). Early identification of maternal depression as a strategy in the prevention of child abuse. *Child Abuse and Neglect, 16*, 345–358.

Scott, M. J., & Stradling, S. G. (1994). Post-traumatic stress disorder without the trauma. *British Journal of Clinical Psychology, 33*, 71–74.

Selye, H. (1976). *The stress of life.* New York: McGraw-Hill.

Shakoor, B. H., & Chalmers, C. (1991). Co-victimization of African-American children who witness violence: Effects on cognitive, emotional and behavioral development. *Journal of the National Medical Association, 83*, 233–238.

Shalev, A. Y., Peri, T., Canetti, M. A., & Schreiber, S. (1996). Predictors of PTSD in injured trauma survivors: A prospective study. *American Journal of Psychiatry, 153,* 219–225.

Shannon, M. P., Lonigan, C. J., Finch, A. J., & Taylor, C. M. (1994). Children exposed to disaster. *Journal of the American Academy of Child and Adolescent Psychiatry, 33,* 80–93.

Shima, S., Kitagawa, Y., Kitamura, T., Fujinawa, A., & Watanabe, Y. (1994). Poststroke depression. *General Hospital Psychiatry, 16,* 286–289.

Silvern, L., & Kaersvang, L. (1989). The traumatized children of violent marriages. *Child Welfare, 68,* 421–436.

Silverstone, P. H. (1996). Prevalence of psychiatric disorders in medical inpatients. *Journal of Nervous and Mental Disease, 184,* 43–51.

Smith, C. L., & deChesney, M. (1994). Critical incident stress debriefings for crisis management in post-traumatic stress disorders. *Medicine & Law, 13,* 185–191.

Smith, E. M., North, C. S., McCool, R. E., & Shea, J. M. (1990). Acute post-disaster psychiatric disorders: Identification of persons at risk. *American Journal of Psychiatry, 147,* 202–206.

Snow, D. L., & Kline, M. L. (1995). Preventive interventions in the workplace to reduce negative psychiatric consequences of work and family stress. In C. M. Mazure (Ed.), *Does stress cause psychiatric illness?* (pp. 221–270). Washington, DC: American Psychiatric Press.

Snyder, S., Strain, J. J., & Wolf, D. (1990). Differentiating major depression from adjustment disorder with depressed mood in the medical setting. *General Hospital Psychiatry, 12,* 159–165.

Solomon, Z., Laor, N., Weiler, D., Muller, U. F., Hadar, O., Waysman, M., Koslowsky, M., Ben Yakar, M., & Bleich, A. (1993). The psychological impact of the Gulf War: A study of acute stress in Israeli evacuees. *Archives of General Psychiatry, 50,* 320–321.

Southwick, S. M., Bremner, J. D., Krystal, J. H., & Charney, D. S. (1994). Psychobiologic research in post-traumatic stress disorder. *Psychiatric Clinics of North America, 17,* 251–264.

Southwick, S. M., Krystal, J. H., Johnson, D. R., & Charney, D. S. (1995). Neurobiology of post-traumatic stress disorder. In G. S. Everly & J. M. Lating (Eds.), *Psychotraumatology: Key papers and core concepts in the post-traumatic stress* (pp. 49–72). New York: Plenum Press.

Spiegel, D., Koopman, C., & Classen, C. (1994). Acute stress disorder and dissociation. *Australian Journal of Clinical and Experimental Hypnosis, 22,* 11–23.

Steinglass, P., & Gerrity, E. (1990). Natural disasters and post-traumatic stress disorder: Short-term versus long-term recovery rates in two affected communities. *Journal of Applied and Social Psychiatry, 20,* 1746–765.

Stoddard, F. J., Norman, D. K., & Murphy, J. M. (1989). A diagnostic outcome study of children and adolescents with severe burns. *Journal of Trauma, 29,* 471–477.

Sullivan, M. J., Weinshenker, B., Mikail, S., & Bishop, S. R. (1995). Screening for major depression in the early stages of multiple sclerosis. *Canadian Journal of Neurological Sciences, 22,* 228–231.

Sutherland, S. M., & Davidson, J. R. (1994). Pharmacotherapy for post-traumatic stress disorder. *Psychiatric Clinics of North America, 17,* 409–423.

Sutker, P. B., Uddo, M., Brailey, K., Allain, A. N., & Errera, A. (1994). Psychological symptoms and psychiatric diagnoses in Operation Desert Storm troops serving graves registration duty. *Journal of Traumatic Stress, 7,* 159–171.

Terr, L. C. (1981). Psychic trauma in children: Observations following the Chowchilla school bus kidnapping. *American Journal of Psychiatry, 138,* 14–19.

Terr, L. C. (1983). Chowchilla revisited: The effects of psychic trauma four years after a school bus kidnapping. *American Journal of Psychiatry, 140,* 1543–1550.

Terr, L. C. (1991). Childhood traumas: An outline and overview. *American Journal of Psychiatry, 148,* 10–20.

Tomb, D. A. (1994). The phenomenology of post-traumatic stress disorder. *Psychiatric Clinics of North America, 17,* 237–250.

Trappler, B., & Friedman, S. (1996). Posttraumatic stress disorder in survivors of the Brooklyn bridge shooting. *American Journal of Psychiatry, 153,* 705–707.

Tyano, S., Iancu, J., Solomon, Z., Sever, J., Goldstein, I., Touviana, Y., & Bleich, A. (1996). Seven-year follow-up of child survivors of a bus-train collision. *Journal of the American Academy of Child and Adolescent Psychiatry, 35,* 365–373.

Tyhurst, J. S. (1958). The role of transitional states—including disaster—in mental illness. In Walter Reed Army Institute of Research (Ed.), *Symposium on preventive and social psychiatry* (pp. 58–81). Washington, DC: U.S. Government Printing Office.

Ullman, S. E. (1995). Adult trauma survivors and post-traumatic stress sequelae: An analysis of reexperiencing, avoidance and arousal criteria. *Journal of Traumatic Stress, 8,* 151–159.

Ursano, R. J., Fullerton, C. S., Kao, T. C., & Bhartiya, V. R. (1995). Longitudinal assessment of posttraumatic stress disorder and depression after exposure to traumatic death. *Journal of Nervous and Mental Disease, 183,* 36–42.

Vernberg, E. M., LaGreca, A. M., Silverman, W. K., & Prinstein, M. J. (1996). Prediction of posttraumatic stress symptoms in children after Hurricane Andrew. *Journal of Abnormal Psychology, 105,* 237–248.

Vlachos, I. O., Bouras, N., Watson, J. P., & Rosen, B. K. (1994). Deliberate self-harm referrals. *European Journal of Psychiatry, 8,* 25–28.

von Ammon Cavanaugh, S. (1995). Depression in the medically ill. Critical issues in diagnostic assessment. *Psychosomatics, 36,* 48–59.

Vrana, S., & Lauterbach, D. (1994) Prevalence of traumatic events and post-traumatic psychological symptoms in a nonclinical sample of college students. *Journal of Traumatic Stress, 7,* 289–302.

Vreven, D., Gudanowski, D., King, L., & King, D. (1995). The civilian version of the Mississippi PTSD Scale: A psychometric evaluation. *Journal of Traumatic Stress, 8,* 91–110.

Walker, E. A., Gelfand, A. N., Gelfand, M. D., Koss, M. P., & Katon, W. J. (1995). Medical and psychiatric symptoms in female gastroenterology clinic patients with histories of sexual victimization. *General Hospital Psychiatry, 17,* 85–92.

Walker, E. A., Torkelson, N., Katon, W. J., & Koss, M. P. (1993). The prevalence of sexual trauma in a primary care clinic. *Journal of the American Board of Family Practice, 6,* 465–471.

Wallach, L. B. (1993). Helping children cope with violence. *Young Children, 48,* 4–11.

Weathers, F. W., Litz, B. T., Keane, T. M., Herman, D. S., Steinberg, H. R., Huska, J. A., & Kraemer, H. C. (1996). The utility of the SCL-90–R for the diagnosis of war-zone related posttraumatic stress disorder. *Journal of Traumatic Stress, 9,* 111–127.

Weiner, H. (1994). The revolution in stress theory and research. In R. P. Liberman & J. Yager (Eds.), *Stress in psychiatric disorders* (pp. 1–36). New York: Springer.

Weisaeth, L. (1989). The stressors and the post-traumatic stress syndrome after an industrial disaster. *Acta Psychiatrica Scandinavica, 80,* 25–37.

Werner, E. E. (1995). Resilience in development. *Current Directions in Psychological Science, 4,* 81–85.

Whiffen, V. E. (1991). The comparison of postpartum with non-postpartum depression: A rose by any other name. *Journal of Psychiatry and Neuroscience, 16,* 160–165.

Wilson, J. P. (1995). The historical evolution of PTSD diagnostic criteria: From Freud to DSM-IV. In G. S. Everly & J. M. Lating (Eds.), *Psychotraumatology: Key papers and core concepts in the post-traumatic stress* (pp. 9–26). New York: Plenum Press.

Wilson, J. P., Harel, Z., & Kahana, B. (Eds.). (1988). *Human adaptation to extreme stress: From the Holocaust to Vietnam.* Cleveland: Cleveland State University.

Wollman, D. (1993). Critical-incident stress debriefing and crisis groups: A review of the literature. *Groups, 17,* 70–83.

World Health Organization. (1993). *The ICD-10 classification of mental and behavior disorders: Diagnostic criteria for research.* Geneva: Author.

Wright, K. M., Ursano, R. J., Bartone, P. T., & Ingraham, L. H. (1990). The shared experience of catastrophe: An expanded classification of the disaster community. *American Journal of Orthopsychiatry, 60,* 35–42.

Yule, W., & Canterbury, R. (1994). The treatment of post traumatic stress disorder in children and adolescents. *International Review of Psychiatry, 6,* 141–151.

Yule, W., & Udwin, O. (1991). Screening child survivors for post-traumatic stress disorders: Experiences from the "Jupiter" sinking. *British Journal of Clinical Psychology, 30,* 131–138.

Zeanah, C. H., & Scheeringa, M. (1996). Evaluation of posttraumatic symptomatology. In J. D. Osofsky & E. Fenichel (Eds.), *Islands of safety: Assessing and treating young victims of violence* (pp. 9–14). Washington, DC: Zero to Three/National Center for Clinical Infant Programs.

Zelkowitz, P., & Milet, T. H. (1995). Screening for post-partum depression in a community sample. *Canadian Journal of Psychiatry, 40,* 80–86.

Zlotnick, C., Shea, M. T., Begin, A., Pearlstein, T., Simpson, E., & Costello, E. (1996). The validation of the Trauma Symptom Checklist–40 (TSC–40) in a sample of inpatients. *Child Abuse and Neglect, 20,* 503–510.

# Mental Health Treatment and Services Research

# Background of Services and Treatment Research

Enola K. Proctor and Arlene Rubin Stiffman

Twenty years ago, the President's Commission on Mental Health launched mental health services research by seeking to answer three questions: (1) how people with mental illness in the United States were being served, (2) the extent to which they were underserved, and (3) who was affected by underservice (White House, 1977). Accurate documentation of prevalence of mental disorders was the first step in understanding how well services are delivered to those in need (Regier, Goldberg, & Taube, 1978). Research based on the initial epidemiologic studies has now documented convincingly the widespread and often unmet need for mental health treatment (Cleary, 1990). Research also has revealed that the consequences of untreated mental disorders and ineffective treatment include long-lasting disability; loss of productivity for the individual, community, and economy; and distress to people in need and those with whom they live, work, or interact. Many questions remain, however, about how to provide the highest quality of care to people with mental disorders. As stated in the 1991 National Plan of Research to Improve Services by the National Institute of Mental Health (NIMH),

> With any illness, but especially with . . . disorders that endure and disable people, providing the right medication is essential, but not enough. A full range of services attending to rehabilitation, independent living, and enhanced quality of life is needed. Finding ways to improve the standard of care and ways to provide it through better organization and financing of services are compelling public health needs . . . the quality of life of people with severe mental disorders can be improved by making the delivery of services an object of rigorous scientific inquiry to determine what works, and by assuring that the results are applied to systems of care throughout the nation. (p. vii)

## Mental Health Services: Overview and Research Agenda

The complexity of mental health services research stems from several factors. First, people with mental disorders receive care from a number of disparate service providers, organizations, and sectors of care (Regier et al., 1978). Second, studies may focus on individual patient encounters, organizational change, state and federal funding, or longitudinal outcomes of mental health consumers. Finally, unlike many other fields, mental health services research involves the scientific focus of several disciplines, including psychiatry, psychology, health economics, epidemiology, sociology, political science (Hargreaves, Catalano, Hu, & Cuffel, 1994) and, increasingly, social work.

Studies of mental health differ widely in their aims and methodology. The three major types are (1) efficacy (experimental outcome) studies, (2) effectiveness (naturalistic outcome) studies, and (3) studies of organizational function and structure.

Efficacy studies examine the impact of well-defined treatments under tightly controlled conditions, such as the implementation of interventions by highly skilled clinicians or by use of comprehensive treatment protocols under the close supervision of experts. These studies typically focus on testing causal paths between the services and the ultimate outcome of interest (Hargreaves et al., 1994). Like the counterpart in medical or mental health treatment studies, the usual design is the randomized services trial. However, efficacy studies in mental health services typically examine complex packages of treatments.

In contrast, effectiveness studies evaluate mental health services interventions in the naturalistic circumstances of care. Burns (1994) noted that, "There is not a protected setting in which to test an intervention such as case management, which, by definition, calls for 'real world' coordination of services by multiple human service agencies" (p. 254). Effectiveness studies address issues of access, often examining the use or nonuse of mental health services as well as services in sectors of care other than specialty mental health. One of the major challenges for effectiveness studies is exploring the needs of specific populations, such as children and adolescents, elderly people, and members of ethnic groups. Other challenges include evaluating the quality of care and the extent to which peoples' needs for care are effectively met.

Methodologically, researchers conducting effectiveness studies struggle with the challenge of ensuring fidelity—that is, the accuracy with which the treatment program is implemented (Brekke, 1987; McGrew, Bond, Dietzen, & Salyers, 1994). This is particularly difficult when the interventive program comprises multiple components, as in the case of assertive community treatment (see chapter 15) and multisystemic therapy programs (see chapters 14 and 16). Effectiveness studies need to better address both short- and long-term outcomes and use meaningful outcome indicators, such as symptoms, functional status, and quality of life.

A third type of mental health services study addresses the organization and functioning of mental health services systems (for example, children's services studies discussed in chapter 14). Variations in the financing, organization, and administration of the system; its structure, capacity, and methods of delivery; and its response to innovation or change in policy or financing (for example, funding level, managed competition, or health care reform) are of particular interest. Organizational studies typically address the effect of such factors on the level of services use by community residents (Hargreaves et al., 1994). Studies by the Robert Wood Johnson Foundation (Goldman, Morrissey, & Ridgely, 1994) exemplify this type of research in their examination of changes in the financing and organization of several cities' mental health services delivery systems. Organizational studies also may address coordination of care, an issue of increasing importance to consumers of mental health services. Yet coordination of care remains a challenge to attain, given the episodic and short-term use of inpatient care and the delivery of mental health services in several "nonspecialty" sectors of care, such as general medicine, child welfare, paid social services, and education.

To ensure its relevance to policy and practice, mental health services research must address access to care, quality of services, effectiveness of services, and cost-effectiveness of services delivery systems. After a brief overview of the documented need for care, this chapter reviews what is known and what still needs to be known about each of these issues.

## Prevalence of Mental Disorders and the Need for Care

National epidemiologic studies have demonstrated a widespread need for mental health services. In the 1980s, the Epidemiologic Catchment Area (ECA) studies found that between one-fifth and one-quarter of adults met the criteria for at least one mental health disorder (Leaf & Bruce, 1989; Robins & Regier, 1991). In the 1990s, the congressionally mandated National Comorbidity Survey (NCS) found even higher rates, with nearly 50 percent of respondents reporting at least one lifetime disorder and almost 30 percent reporting at least one disorder in the past 12 months (Kessler et al., 1994). The most common disorders were major depression, alcohol dependence, and phobias. Need was further found to be highly concentrated in the one-sixth of the population (14 percent) who had a history of three or more comorbid disorders.

Widespread need also has been documented in specific subpopulations, such as children and adolescents or elderly people. For children and adolescents, the estimated rates of need vary widely, depending on the instrument, the reporter, and how need is defined. For example, need can be defined as clinically significant symptoms, as meeting the criteria of the *Diagnostic and Statistical Manual of Mental Disorders*, 4th ed. (DSM-IV) (Stiffman & Cunningham, 1990), as functional status, or as impairment (John, Offord, Boyle, & Racine, 1995). Nevertheless, most studies relying on diagnostic criteria have found that between 14 percent and 25 percent of U.S. youths have a mental health problem (Boyle & Offord, 1988; Costello, Costello, et al., 1988; Offord et al., 1987), with recent findings based on combined youth and parent reports as high as 50 percent (Schaffer et al., 1996).

Similarly, studies show that up to 15 percent of elderly people who live in the community have depressive symptoms (Blazer, Hughes, & George, 1987), with 1 percent meeting DSM criteria for major depression and 2 percent meeting criteria for dysthymia (Weissman, Leaf, Bruce, & Florio, 1988). The prevalence of major depression is much higher among elderly people in treatment settings: 11 percent for those in hospitals (Koenig, Meador, Cohen, & Blazer, 1988) and 12 percent for those in nursing homes (Parmelee, Katz, & Lawton, 1989).

Rates of need may vary by ethnicity, gender, or socioeconomic status. Evidence is mixed regarding rates of mental disorders among people of color and other members of ethnic groups in the United States, particularly African Americans. The ECA data showed only modest differences by race. When the ECA rates were corrected for age, gender, socioeconomic status, and marital status, black and white Americans did not differ in prevalence of schizophrenia, antisocial disorders, affective disorder, drug dependence, or panic disorder. However, alcoholism, phobic disorders, generalized anxiety disorder, and somatization disorder were more common among African American respondents (Adebimpe, 1994). In contrast, African Americans in the

NCS had statistically significantly lower prevalences of affective disorders, substance use disorders, and lifetime comorbidity than did the white subjects. The NCS found no disorder to be more prevalent among African Americans than white people (Blazer, Kessler, McGonagle, & Swartz, 1994; Kessler et al., 1994). However, the NCS found that Hispanic respondents had statistically significantly higher prevalences of affective disorders and comorbidity than did white respondents but that they did not differ from the white subjects in rates of anxiety and alcohol use disorders (Kessler et al., 1994).

Comparing men and women, both the ECA and NCS studies found that women had higher prevalence of affective disorders and anxiety disorders and that men had higher rates of substance abuse and antisocial personality disorders. Epidemiologic surveys also have been consistent in finding that mental disorders decline with increases in income and education (Kessler et al., 1994).

The prevalence studies discussed above defined need by using the most stringent standard—that of meeting diagnostic criteria for a specific mental disorder. Need for mental health services also can be defined by major disabling symptoms (Leaf & Bruce, 1989). Recent studies have addressed need when symptoms are below the threshold for diagnostic disorder. People who do not meet the criteria for a disorder may have more symptoms than those who do meet the criteria, and they may be more functionally disabled (Stiffman, Earls, & Chueh, 1992). The ECA study found need rates of 15 percent by use of DSM criteria and 16 percent by use of symptoms, but only 3 percent by use of self-appraisal of mental health or self-reported disability (Kessler et al., 1994; Leaf et al., 1988; Regier et al., 1993). If need for mental health services begins with functional impairment rather than with diagnosis or symptoms, then actual need for services might differ greatly from that indicated by level of symptoms or diagnostic category. For example, a youth whose conduct disrupts others in school is more likely to be labeled as needing mental health services than a youth whose quiet depression does not affect others. Teachers might rate the former most in need, but the latter might be more likely to self-report need (Cohen, Kasen, Brook, & Struening, 1991).

Need for mental health services also might be defined as being at risk for mental health problems. For example, people who live in a dysfunctional or violent environment are more prone to engage in violent behaviors, which most mental health professionals define as indicating a need for services. Also, need may be defined by legal or political criteria. Within school systems, need for mental health services is often defined by being labeled severely emotionally disordered (SED); in many school systems, need is presumed not to exist without that label (Knitzer, 1982).

## Access to Care and Patterns in Mental Health Services Delivery

### DEFINING AND MEASURING MENTAL HEALTH SERVICES

As noted before, to understand patterns and problems in the use of mental health services, researchers must grapple with the noted complexity of mental health services. The literature reflects tremendous diversity in defining mental health services. For example, mental health services can be defined by the type of provider, the type of service rendered (George, 1990), or by the person who receives such services. In defining mental health services by the provider, one confronts a problem: Mental health services are delivered by mental health professionals (psychiatrists, psychologists, social workers, and so forth), by non–mental health professionals (primary care physicians), and by nonprofessionals (peer or self-help groups). Furthermore, all of these providers may occasionally deliver services that are considered outside the scope of mental health services, such as social or supportive services. If the goal is to help a person function more effectively and those services accomplish this, then do the services become, by definition, mental health services? Should the prescribing of psychotropic medications, regardless of reason, be viewed as a mental health services provision (George, 1990)?

A similar problem occurs with the definition of mental health services by the person who receives the services. As noted above, it is not always clear who needs mental health services. Those who need them may not always be those who meet strict criteria for mental illness.

This chapter uses the broadest possible definition of mental health services. Consistent with current trends in mental health services research, mental health services are defined as "any and all services provided for the purpose of the identification, diagnosis, and treatment of mental health problems" (George, 1990, p. 306).

## WHO USES MENTAL HEALTH SERVICES, AND WHO ARE THE UNDERSERVED?

A number of theoretical models have guided studies concerned with use and underuse of mental health services. However, only a few of these models were developed for this purpose; most were developed to explain generic behaviors. Three theoretical models, derived primarily from the social psychological literature, have been widely discussed and used. One of the best known is the Theory of Reasoned Action (Fishbein & Azjen, 1975), which asserts that attitudes, values, and motivation predict behavior. Janz and Becker (1984) used some of the same elements in their Health Belief Model, which suggests that people engage in a cost–benefit analysis based on the perceived threat of illness and the belief that a particular behavior (such as seeking health services) will reduce or eliminate that threat. Although Janz and Becker contended that their theory is supported, other studies found only weak support for certain key variables. Questions have been raised concerning the role of perceived susceptibility (Zapka, McCusker, Stoddard, & Morrison, 1990) and the roles of perceived personal risk, knowledge about prevention, and faith in that knowledge (Stiffman, Dore, Cunningham, & Earls, 1995).

Recently, Bandura's (1986) social learning theory has been combined with the theories cited above to explain health-related behavior. Like Janz and Becker, Bandura suggested that the behaviors of people are influenced by rewards. Bandura added the concept that behaviors are learned by experience and the observation of modeling by others and further stated that efficacy in regard to health-related preventive behaviors is learned and that self-efficacy in obtaining health services is an important mediator of preventive knowledge.

Despite their potential usefulness in explaining health risk behaviors, these theories confront a number of problems when dealing with mental health behaviors, any of which may serve to negate their explanatory predictive power. The mental health problems that should lead people to seek mental health services may, in fact, impair judgment (Zapka et al., 1990); be paired with potent drives, such as abuse or dependence (Bandura, 1986); be accompanied by irrational beliefs or values; or be influenced by others' cultural beliefs (Leaf, Bruce, & Tischler, 1986). Janz and Becker (1984) stressed that their model (and by implication other related models) may be inapplicable to behaviors that have a habitual or physiological drive component, are inhibited by economic or environmental factors, or do not have prevalent cues to action.

In contrast to these psychological models, the Andersen (1995) model is a system model designed to explain health behavior. It accounts for both individual self-determination and for the system in which the person operates. According to this model, the use of health services depends on three concepts: need factors, predisposing factors, and enabling factors. Andersen posited that need is the most important determinant of use. Predisposing factors include sociodemographic variables, ethnicity, health beliefs, and values. In the first two concepts, the Andersen model includes the two primary variables used in the social psychological theories. The truly unique determinants of the Andersen model are enabling factors: accessibility, availability, affordability, and acceptability.

Accessibility of services is a large but potentially modifiable barrier to mental health services. Access may be a particular problem with mental health services because patients may lack transportation or may not be able to seek help without people in their social network knowing about their problems. Availability also is a major issue because services are often differentially available in rural compared with urban areas (Kelleher, Taylor, & Rickert, 1992), both for different types of mental problems and for different age groups. Mental health services are notoriously expensive and often not covered by insurance, which leads to issues of affordability (Frank & McGuire, 1986; Frank & Morlock, 1994; Padgett, Patrick, Burns, Schlesinger, & Cohen, 1993). Finally, acceptability of mental health services may vary according to age cohort, ethnicity, education, and cultural background (Gibbs, 1990; Sussman, Robins, & Earls, 1987).

The Andersen model was specifically developed to understand why people use health services, evaluate equitable access to health care, and develop policies to promote such access. In this respect it differs dramatically from the aforementioned psychological theories that were adapted to the use of health care. The original Andersen (1968) model has gone through considerable revision, with the latest (1995) model featuring the recursive nature of health services use, outcomes, and multiple influences on services use. It is, therefore, a model that is particularly appropriate for understanding mental health services use. Moreover, it is the model used most frequently in studies of services use.

Studies of services use consistently demonstrate a wide gap between the experience of mental health problems and the receipt of services. Both the ECA studies and the NCS found high levels of unmet need. Very few people who met criteria for a mental disorder had obtained professional help for the disorder (Kessler et al., 1994; Regier et al., 1993). According to Kessler and colleagues (1994), even among those experiencing multiple (three or more) disorders in the past year, only one-third received any treatment (p. 12).

Several subgroups of the population appear to have particularly high rates of unmet need. With respect to children and adolescents, the gap between need and demand for mental health services is considerable (Burns, 1991). In studies of adolescents using consolidated mental and physical health services, fewer than 24 percent of those who met at least one criterion a for disorder had brought their symptoms to the attention of the health professional (Earls, Robins, Stiffman, & Powell, 1989; Stiffman, Earls, Robins, & Jung, 1988) Similarly, in the recent Methods for

Epidemiology of Child and Adolescent Mental Disorders Study (MECA), only approximately one-third of the children and adolescents who met at least one criterion for diagnosis received services (Leaf et al., 1996). In a review of the literature, Tuma (1989) found that although 20 percent of young children needed mental health services, only 5 percent received them. Unfortunately, children with high rates of environmental risk factors are most likely to have mental health problems and least likely to request or demand services (Saxe, Cross, & Silverman, 1988).

Elderly adults are at particular risk for unmet need because they are less likely than younger adults to use mental health services (Leaf et al., 1988; Wells, Golding, Hough, Burnam, & Karno, 1988). Even among those who use services (that is, those who had at least one contact with a mental health professional), elderly adults use specialty mental health services at lower levels (Padgett, Patrick, Burns, & Schlesinger, 1994). Only about one-third of elderly people with psychiatric disorders receive care from mental health specialists (Burns & Taube, 1990).

Rates of unmet need also vary by urban or rural status. Even among those who need mental health services, people living in rural areas are least likely to use such services. Those living in large urban areas have a greater likelihood of using mental health services, and the level of use rises with increasing urbanization (Human & Wasem, 1991; Rost, Smith, & Taylor, 1993; Taube & Rupp, 1986). These urban–rural differences in rates of use are often echoed by ethnic or cultural differences (Gibbs, 1990; Hoberman, 1992; Office of Technology Assessment, 1991; Raniseski & Sigelman, 1992; Rogler & Cortes, 1993).

Underuse of mental health care has many negative consequences, including subsequent use of higher levels of mental health services (Burns & Taube, 1990) and medical services (Leaf, 1994). For example, elderly people with mental disorders use health services at higher levels (Torian, Davidson, Fulop, Sell, & Fillit, 1992) and are more likely to be hospitalized as a result of an emergency room visit (Thienhaus, Rowe, Woellert, & Hillard, 1988).

Services research based on the Andersen model helps explain rates of unmet need and underuse of mental health care. Although most research based on the Andersen model has been on physical health care rather than mental health care, the results have been remarkably consistent. Research not using the Andersen model, but relying on constructs also used in it, has yielded findings consistent with the direction of effects predicted from the Andersen model. Need has been the most powerful predictor of services use in all studies based on the Andersen model (Andersen, 1975; Hulka & Wheat, 1985; Wolinsky & Coe, 1984). Studies consistently show that the heaviest users of mental health services are those with the most severe disabilities (Bartsch, Shern, Coen, & Wilson, 1995; Hibbard & Pope, 1986; Leaf et al., 1988; Taube, Goldman, Burns, & Kessler, 1988).

Enabling and predisposing factors primarily have been found to influence use of discretionary services (that is, those that are optional or not required) after researchers controlled for need. However, the overall variance explained by these variables is typically very low (less than 5 percent) (Branch et al., 1981). For people of color and other members of minority groups, need remains the highest predictor of services use even for discretionary use of services (Padgett et al. 1993, 1994; Wolinsky et al., 1989; Wolinsky & Johnson, 1992). Predisposing factors related to greater use of services are high socioeconomic status for use of mental health specialists (Wells, Manning, Duan, Newhouse, & Ware, 1986) and female gender for services seeking but not service volume (Leaf et al., 1985; Leaf & Bruce, 1987). Among the enabling factors shown to be associated with use of mental health services are geographic location, particularly rural compared with urban (Sommers, 1989); perception of barriers to services (Leaf et al., 1985); and health insurance coverage (Crow, Smith, McNamee, & Piland, 1994; Padgett et al., 1993). The cost of services also is closely related to their use. For example, even small copayments result in use of fewer outpatient services (Frank & McGuire, 1986), and people in more generous insurance plans use more services (Wells, Keeler, & Manning, 1990). Thus, the research literature supports the Andersen model in that need, enabling, and predisposing factors all have some relation to services use.

## SECTORS OF CARE

The ECA studies, in addition to pioneering the extent of need, also provided the first systematic evidence about sources of care. These studies revealed that people who received care for mental disorders did so from a variety of professionals, in a variety of settings (or "sectors") of care. Few people were found to have received care from specialty mental health providers. ECA data showed that only about one-third of all visits for mental health reasons were actually to mental health specialists. Over the course of one year, only 21 percent of those with mental disorders were seen in the specialty mental health sector; 54 percent were seen exclusively in the general medical sector; 3 percent were seen in the general hospital inpatient sector; and 22 percent were seen in human services agencies (Regier et al., 1993). These findings led Regier and colleagues to characterize the U.S. mental health services system as a "largely unorganized," "de facto" system comprising four major sectors.

Although many, if not most, people receive care outside the specialty mental health sector, far more is known about care within the specialty sector. For example, a household survey of almost 18,000 people, the National Medical Care Utilization and Expenditure Survey (NMCUES), revealed that approximately two-thirds of all outpatient mental health visits (and two-thirds of the total expenditures) were to psychiatrists or psychologists in private practice. People with mental disorders were more likely to see psychiatrists, and psychiatrists' patients were more likely to be hospitalized (Taube, Burns, & Kessler, 1984). However, these results are based only on insurance claims data, so they reflect only purchased, reimbursable services rather than a full array of indirect and direct care.

Use of specialty mental health services varies with gender, race, and age. Women diagnosed with a mental disorder are more likely to see mental health professionals than are men. ECA data indicate that African Americans were more likely than white people to rely on friends and relatives for help with mental health problems (Sussman et al., 1987). Also, those African Americans diagnosed with mental disorders who seek professional help are more likely to turn to their clergy (44.0 percent) than to mental health professionals (11.1 percent) (Brown, Ahmed, Gary, & Milburn, 1995). Differences in sector use according to race are evident among men: white men are more likely to use specialty mental health services, but African American men are more likely to be incarcerated (Gibbs, 1990).

Elderly people underuse specialty mental health services, even after discharge to community care following hospitalization for a psychiatric disorder. For example, postdischarge services use by elderly clients is spread across mental health, general medical, and formal aging sectors of care. However, the bulk of care is provided by family and friends, with heavy reliance on providers in the medical sector (Proctor, Morrow-Howell, & Dore, 1996).

Children and adolescents in particular are likely to receive mental health services through the nonspecialty sectors because specialty mental health services and treatment designed for them are relatively rare. Youths with mental illness using specialty services are often served the context of adult mental health services. For example, in St. Louis there is no specific provider for adolescent drug abuse services and only a few providers in the entire state of Missouri. Existing mental health specialty services for children and youths range from crisis care in psychiatric hospital wards or intensive residential treatment to talks with a school counselor, teacher, or primary care physician. Some levels of specialty care appear plentiful, as indicated by the many empty beds in adolescent psychiatric wards, but other levels of care are overburdened. Providers report difficulty in finding residential care for teenagers and dealing with the large caseloads carried by school counselors and social workers. Of all adolescents receiving specialty mental health care, two-thirds receive outpatient care, approximately one-fourth receive inpatient care, 8 percent use a residential treatment center, and 3 percent receive partial hospitalization (Burns, Taube, & Taube, 1990).

Nonspecialty services play a key role in identifying people who need mental health services. Access to specialty mental health treatment is often dependent on contact with professionals in nonspecialty sectors of care. Other public sectors or providers, often social workers, are key to expediting the receipt of mental health services (LeCroy & Ashford, 1992). Mechanic, Angel, and Davies (1991) identified four public sectors equipped to function as gateways to mental health services. In addition to the health sector, these gateways include the drug and alcohol abuse, criminal justice, and educational sectors of care. These gateway sectors may provide services themselves or connect the person to services (Lourie & Katz-Leavy, 1991). Social services agencies or providers are often the first to have a person in need of mental health services. They must accurately identify the problem, provide the services they can, and then refer the person in need to other specialty mental health services (Feldman & Stiffman, 1984; LeCroy & Ashford, 1992).

Population-specific gateways include formal aging services for elderly clients and child welfare or educational services for children and adolescents. Adults are most likely to consult primary health care providers about mental health problems (Leaf et al., 1985; Morlock, 1990), yet primary care providers may be unable to either detect mental disorders in a patient or provide adequate services to those with such disorder (Leaf, 1994). This has led to efforts to develop screening and interview procedures to enable primary care physicians to better diagnose specific mental disorders. One example is the Primary Care Evaluation of Mental Disorders (PRIME-MD) (Spitzer et al., 1995).

Teachers are most likely to be consulted for children's emotional or behavioral problems (Chang, Warner, & Weissman, 1988; Costello, Burns, Costello, Dulcan, & Brent, 1988; Costello, Farmer, Angold, Burns, & Erkanli, 1997), with primary health care providers coming second (Cohen et al., 1991). Despite the acceptance of the role of primary care physicians as the gatekeepers to mental health services for children and adolescents, studies have shown that they often fail to identify youths' mental health needs. Fewer than 8 percent of youths with mental health problems receive services or referrals from their primary health care source (Earls et al., 1989; Stiffman et al., 1988). Other studies of pediatricians or primary health care providers also have found high rates of underidentification of need (Costello, Burns, et al., 1988; Costello et al., 1997). One study showed that 83 percent of children who met diagnostic criteria had not been identified by their pediatricians as having mental health problems (Dulcan et al., 1990). For children and adolescents, rates of services provision through the juvenile justice or child welfare systems appear to be even lower (less than 1 percent) than services through the educational or primary health care sectors (Costello et al., 1997). However, this differential use of services may vary depending on the structure of the services sector. For example, Stiffman and colleagues found that in St. Louis, where the juvenile justice system has its own diagnostic and treatment unit, the juvenile justice system provided the most services (Stiffman, Chen, Elze, Dore, & Cheng. 1997).

Important questions regarding sectors of care await further study. For specific populations, better descriptive information (what services are used and from which sectors?) and critical analysis (what factors are associated with use of one sector rather than another?) are needed. Some people appear to use only one sector—such as the general medical sector, the mental health specialty sector, or informal providers (Pescosolido, Wright, Alegria, & Vera, 1995). Others rely on a combination or sequence of providers (Proctor et al., 1996). Thus, important issues, albeit rarely addressed in services studies, are understanding configurations of care, patterns of care, or various combinations of services across multiple sectors (George, 1992), as well as exploring the relationship between those patterns of care and treatment outcomes.

## LEVELS AND EPISODES OF CARE

Mental health services are offered in different levels of care, as well as by different sectors of care. George (1990) identified five levels of clinical care, from most to least restrictive: inpatient, residential treatment, residential supportive, partial care, and outpatient services. Level of care in mental health services delivery has shifted markedly over the past three decades (Grob, 1987).

Several dramatic trends are apparent. First, with respect to hospital care, the type of treatment facilities providing mental health care has changed; patient populations in state and county mental hospitals have declined, and the numbers of patients in psychiatric units of general hospitals have grown. The number of psychiatric units in short-term general hospitals doubled between 1952 and 1962, and by 1977, inpatient episodes in general hospital psychiatric units exceeded those in state mental hospitals (Goldman & Skinner, 1990). A second and related change has been the rapid rise in the number of episodes of care. Episodes of care provided by mental health facilities grew from 1.7 million in 1955 to 8.6 million in 1990 (Redick, Witkin, Atay, & Manderscheid, 1991). Over the past 20 years, more mental health organizations have been established and are operating at higher staffing levels. Redick and colleagues found that private psychiatric hospitals and federally funded community mental health centers increased their number of full-time staff between 1978 and 1980, as did private psychiatric hospitals, residential treatment centers for emotionally disturbed children, and multiservice mental health organizations. Third, the locus of care has changed from inpatient- to outpatient-based treatment. Although the rate of inpatient episodes per 100,000 population increased by 5.9 percent between 1955 and 1977, the rate for outpatient episodes increased by 900 percent (Goldman, Adams, & Taube, 1983). The number of clients served in community mental health agencies grew by more than one-third between 1990 and 1993 ("Law Places 36 Month Limit," 1994). The trend toward community-based care also is evident for adolescents. A 1986 NIMH survey showed that of all adolescents receiving mental health services, more than two-thirds received outpatient care, fewer than one-fourth received inpatient care, 8 percent received care through a residential treatment center, and 3 percent received partial hospitalization (Burns et al., 1990). Elderly people, however, remain disproportionately likely to receive mental health care in institutional settings (Thienhaus et al., 1988).

These shifts were prompted by an unusual convergence of several factors. First, exposés of conditions within public mental hospitals (Dain, 1976; Freedman, 1967) and an alarming report on the situation for children in some public mental hospitals (Rivera, 1972) prompted wide public concern. A second important factor was the development of effective psychotropic medication. For the first time, the symptoms of those who were most severely ill were sufficiently controlled so that they could function on a day-to-day basis. A third factor was the filing of lawsuits claiming civil liberties on behalf of involuntarily hospitalized patients. Finally, the locus of services delivery was affected by regulatory and funding factors, particularly Medicare and Medicaid coverage of mental health services in nonpublic facilities.

These factors led to a nationwide movement toward deinstitutionalization and promotion of treatment in the least-restrictive setting (Mechanic, 1990). The new assumption was that all mental hospital care was, at best, nonproductive and, at worst, actually damaging (Mechanic, 1986). It was further assumed that residence within a community would promote people's mental health. These factors and attitudes led to the present situation in which psychiatric hospitals care for only patients with the most acute symptoms. Hospitalization is now reserved for those who might harm themselves or others or for those who require inpatient assessment or regulation of medications. Moreover, in accordance with the parallel trend in physical health services and, in part, as an effort to reduce cost of care, length of hospital stays has been shortened. Both discharge planning and actual discharge occur as soon as possible—typically, as soon as the patient begins to tolerate and benefit from medication. Patients are then left to complete stabilization and begin recovery in the community. These treatment trends, along with evidence that incomplete recovery increases the likelihood of relapse, underscore the importance of community-based care.

The move to community care and the least-restrictive setting has not been uniformly positive (Mechanic, 1986). Deinstitutionalization and living in the least-restrictive setting meant that many patients with chronic problems were moved into the community without the supportive care they needed. This problem helped draw attention to the evaluation of mental health services in terms of quality of care, outcome attainment, extent of unmet need, and coordination of services across levels and sectors of care.

# Ensuring Quality of Care

## DEFINING QUALITY OF MENTAL HEALTH SERVICES

Payers and regulators of health and mental health services are increasingly turning to services researchers for help in defining, assessing, and ensuring the quality of care (Berwick, 1989). Concerned by evidence of wide variability in provider practices, health care purchasers demanded that the health care industry develop and implement methods for quality assurance reviews. Similarly, purchasers of mental health services have asked for evidence that the services they pay for meet standards for quality. Quality is a concern of services providers and advocates for people with mental illness as well: Quality may be affected by recent moves to limit services use through managed care and by legally mandated practices to use the least-restrictive settings of care (Segal, Watson, & Akutsu, 1996).

*Quality* is defined as the extent to which care meets predefined standards of good or acceptable care. Defining and measuring the quality of care are referred to as "quality assessment," and efforts to evaluate, certify, or improve the quality of care are referred to as "quality assurance" (Wells & Brook, 1990). This definition of quality, of course, leads to the question of what constitutes good or acceptable care. Quality is best judged in terms of outcome attainment. However, Wells and Brook have noted that this approach to defining and judging quality is dependent on evidence linking specific processes or interventions to treatment outcomes, such as reduction in symptomatology, empirical quality of life, and increased satisfaction.

Relatively little is known about the quality of mental health services. Pending the accumulation of that knowledge, mental health services researchers have defined and measured quality in different ways. For several years and in response to the need for accreditation of hospitals and services agencies, good or acceptable care has been assessed only in terms of structural or use characteristics (Steinwachs, 1990). For example, time on a waiting list, percentage of clients provided with a thorough assessment, and number of telephone rings until a call is answered have served as indicators of quality for mental health organizations. Through their quality assurance reviews, agencies have evaluated whether the standards of care accepted and valued by a particular services site are, in fact, met for the clients they serve.

## TREATMENT GUIDELINES AND QUALITY OF CARE

Good or acceptable care also has been evaluated in terms of the actual treatments or interventions delivered. In the absence of outcome data indicating effective care (Ellwood, 1988), quality has been defined by professional consensus. For example, Norquist et al. (1995) addressed the quality of care for depressed elderly clients using traditional components of quality care, such as thoroughness of medical and psychiatric examination and the appropriateness of admission to acute care (that is, appropriateness of level of care for patient need). Concerns remain that quality varies for subgroups of patients, in particular for people of color and members of other ethnic groups. For example, Segal, Bola, and Watson (1996) found that African Americans seeking treatment in psychiatric emergency services received statistically significantly more psychiatric medications than other patients, although clinicians devoted significantly less time to evaluating African American patients.

Professional consensus also has been used to formulate protocols and treatment guidelines. For example, guidelines for the treatment of depression have been developed by the NIMH Consensus Conferences, the Agency for Health Care Policy and Research (AHCPR), and the APA. To date, these guidelines have been targeted only to primary care physicians and psychiatrists, not to other professional groups. However, as noted above, professional consensus without evidence of effectiveness is inadequate for describing quality of care. Too much mental health services research to date has focused on simply monitoring services delivery and receipt of care. Yet research on quality of care, including outcomes, will be increasingly important in mental health research—particularly in studies of managed care.

## EFFECTIVENESS OF CARE

Several factors have heightened concern over the effectiveness of mental health services in recent years. First, widespread concern over the rising costs of health care has led the purchasers of care (that is, insurers and managed care companies) to question the quality and effectiveness of services, including mental health services. Second, the increasing availability of alternative sites, sources, and types of care encourages providers, consumers, and purchasers to demand evidence of the effectiveness of treatment. Third, studies of health and mental health services show important variations in the way specific conditions are managed, which are due, in all likelihood, to the lack of knowledge concerning the most effective practice for specific disorders (Clinton, McCormick, & Besteman, 1994). When care for the same disorder varies widely as a function of the individual preferences of the practitioner or as a function of geographic region, those who provide, manage, and pay for services become increasingly eager for standards of care.

Within mental health services, the efficacy of pharmacologic treatment was one of the first targets of empirical study. (Chapter 11 in this book reviews recent developments in psychopharmacology and its effectiveness.) During the 1980s, psychosocial treatments also became the focus of effectiveness studies. The importance of psychosocial interventions for people with serious and persistent mental illness is supported by a growing body of empirical evidence. For example, when combined with medication, individual and family psychoeducation and social skills training contribute to tenure in the community and personal and social adjustments (Hogarty et al., 1991). Effectiveness studies also have indicated the importance of attending to clients' more broadly defined social concerns (Perreault, Rogers, Leichner, & Sabourin, 1996).

The growing emphasis on effectiveness research is evident among all mental health and associated disciplines, including social work. For example, a review (Glisson, 1995) of social work publications in mental health between 1977 and 1988 revealed a doubling in the proportion of articles assessing intervention effectiveness or outcome. As discussed in other chapters of this book, effectiveness research in mental health services addresses a continuum of types of care, from single treatments to entire systems of service, and there are pressing issues for research on the effectiveness of mental health treatment and services.

## ENSURING THAT NEEDS ARE MET

Virtually all people with mental disorders have needs for care, although the nature and number of needs varies considerably. Some needs derive from the psychiatric disorder itself. These include the need for counseling, socialization, medication and medication monitoring, and leisure activities (Solomon, Gordon, & Davis, 1984). Others derive from comorbid medical conditions and include needs for physician attention and ongoing treatment, especially medications. Finally, some people with psychiatric impairment—elderly and persistently mentally ill people, for example—require assistance with activities of daily living.

A pressing agenda for mental health services research is determining how well these needs are met. For people with serious and persistent mental disorders, the concern is focused on the coordination of care across episodes of acute, postacute, and outpatient care. Effective community care must provide a range of needed services, appropriate and responsive to client needs, directly through referral or indirectly through contracts or other linkage arrangements.

Although the focus of care has shifted to the community, almost 1.5 million adults are admitted to inpatient facilities for psychiatric treatment annually (Koslowe, Rosenstein, Milazzo-Sayre, & Manderscheid, 1991). There are many studies of the outcome of psychiatric hospitalization but no clear consensus on how to define improvement (Pfeiffer, O'Malley, & Shott, 1996).

Although only a few studies have addressed patients' postacute needs, their findings confirm the prevalence of need and raise concerns. In a study of aftercare for 138 admissions to a geriatric unit of a state psychiatric hospital, Clark and Travis (1994) found that 76.6 percent of patients had three or more services needs. Younger adults with mental disorders (Solomon & Davis, 1985) discharged from acute care to community care have considerable unmet needs. Many people are unable to maintain positive functioning outside acute care settings. For example, they often deteriorate when they fail to continue their medication regimen. Further study is needed on the extent to which community and institutional care meet peoples' needs. Findings of such studies can inform psychiatric discharge planning, planning for community care, and reimbursement policies for postacute care.

The needs of the families of those with mental disorders also should be addressed. Because of gaps in existing services, people with severe disorders must often depend on care provided by their family members. Family members have become the primary caregivers to two-thirds of people with long-term illness (Lefley, 1995; NIMH, 1991; Proctor et al., 1996). Studies must evaluate how well needs for care are met by family and friends, and at what cost to people and society; in addition they must evaluate such family outcomes as burden, relationship problems, knowledge of mental illness, and ability to deal with behavior disturbances (Tessler, 1995).

## EVALUATING OUTCOME ATTAINMENT

Studies have convincingly demonstrated the wide range of problems and disabilities experienced by people with mental disorders. Accordingly, mental health services researchers increasingly understand that the policy impact and effectiveness of services should be evaluated in terms of the attainment of different types or domains of outcomes (Spitzer et al., 1995; Wells et al., 1989). Outcome studies should include subjective well-being and functional status. Far beyond the core disabling affective and cognitive symptoms, mental illness often impairs a person's ability to carry out activities of daily living, form and sustain meaningful social relationships, fulfill family roles, enjoy recreation, and work productively.

Rosenblatt and Attkisson (1993) identified four outcome domains for assessing mental health services: (1) clinical status—indicators of psychopathology and symptomatology, including physical, emotional, cognitive, and behavioral indicators; (2) functional status—indicators of ability to fulfill social and role functions, interpersonal relationships, and employment; (3) life satisfaction and fulfillment—indicators of well-being, vitality, and personal fulfillment; and (4) welfare and safety—self-injurious behavior or abuse, neglect, or violence against the person with mental disorders. Studies are needed to determine the relationships between various outcome domains, such as quality of life, physical well-being, symptomatology, and role functioning (NIMH, 1991). In addition, the validity and sensitivity of existing measures, particularly with special populations such as children, families, members of ethnic groups, and homeless people, need to be further addressed.

Given the consensus that mental health services need to address multiple outcomes, it is not surprising that services are often provided through complex treatment "packages" (Rosen & Proctor, 1978) that comprise varied interventions. For example, it has been established that relapse is less frequent when schizophrenic patients receive combinations of family psychoeducation, social skills training, and psychotropic medications (Hogarty et al., 1986), and studies also have shown the value of family psychosocial skills training (Hogarty et al., 1991). Similarly, as discussed in chapter 15, the assertive community treatment program of continuous, comprehensive, and highly flexible community care includes a full range of medical, psychosocial, and rehabilitation services delivered by community-based teams, 24 hours per day, seven days per week (Marx, Test, & Stein, 1973).

Such treatment packages, which are more and more the approaches of choice in mental health services, require the services of a wide range of mental health professionals, paraprofessionals, and lay caregivers. Studies of providers showed that social workers are more likely than psychiatrists and psychologists to provide such treatments as case management, psychoeducation, home-based services, group and family therapy, and discharge planning (Haber & McCall, 1989; Mayer & Rubin, 1983). Other chapters in this book detail recent breakthroughs in the use and effectiveness of such multifaceted interventions as psychoeducation, group treatment, community-based treatment models, and case management.

## COORDINATION OF CARE ACROSS SERVICES AND SERVICE SECTORS

Researchers have contended that mental health delivery systems are not systems at all but are an uncoordinated set of programs within the community, with patients linked to inappropriate or ineffective services or to no services at all (Morrissey, Tausig, & Lindsey, 1985). The need for collaboration between providers of mental health services and providers of related social, health, and financial support services is a consistent theme in the literature (Friedman, 1989). More and more frequently, providers of mental health services have attempted to coordinate their system into a full-fledged network (Morrissey, Hall, & Lindsey, 1982). Despite those attempts, there are few connections from sector to sector. The flow of resources among the different sectors that serve populations with emotional disorders has never been centrally coordinated (NIMH, 1990). Rather, this flow has depended largely on voluntary understandings and agreements concerning financing and transfer of clients (Frank & Morlock, 1994). Coordination has been attenuated because of multiple sources of authority and funding, conflicting objectives, differences in staff orientations and ideologies, and the perceived cost of coordination efforts. Services delivery agencies are often reluctant to give up any of their power or autonomy to the coordinators.

Despite the call for coordination, there is no strong evidence that better coordination of services results in better outcomes (Goldman et al., 1994). There is evidence, however, that better coordination among treatment facilities influences the care provided. The lack of coordination and integration between services precludes continuity of care (Mechanic & Aiken, 1987). People who need mental health services often have multiple problems that can seldom be dealt with in only one services setting. Therefore, it is vitally important to coordinate and integrate services over time across multiple providers in multiple sectors and through multiple types of services. This move to services integration is now a central theme in a number of services research programs.

The Child and Adolescent Service System Program (CASSP) provided funds to states to help them coordinate all services for children and adolescents by enhancing communication between providers from different services sectors and agencies (Stroul, 1985; Stroul & Friedman, 1986). Although the effectiveness of such programs has not been evaluated, acceptance of the concept has continued to spread and has spun off many integrated services programs, such as family preservation services (Goldman, 1988).

Ventura County, California, integrated mental health services to track escalating mental health costs (Jordan & Hernandez, 1990; Rosenblatt & Attkisson, 1993). As a result, integration of organization and funding of services for children ensures that children in the juvenile justice or educational sectors are screened for mental health problems. Once again, however, this attempt at coordination has not been evaluated.

From 1986 to 1991 the Robert Wood Johnson Foundation funded a nine-city demonstration project to increase integration of services and continuity of care. Although the results of their evaluation indicated increased integration and continuity, there was no indication of improvement in quality of life for the adult patients who participated in the project (Goldman et al., 1994; Lehman, Postrado, Roth, McNary, & Goldman, 1994).

Finally, a project at Fort Bragg, North Carolina (jointly supported by NIMH and the U.S. Army), provided a full continuum of coordinated specialty mental health care for families. This care included transportation, wraparound services, and comprehensive intake assessments. Like the Robert Wood Johnson study, increased coordination and integration was demonstrated, but better client outcomes were not. However, the Fort Bragg study did demonstrate that with better organization, the cost of services for achieving similar outcomes could be vastly reduced (Bickman, Bryant, & Summerfelt, 1993; Bickman et al., 1995).

These services integration programs and similar ones demonstrate that the mental health services community recognizes the wide range of social, welfare, and rehabilitative services required in mental health services. The move toward integrated community care is particularly important for social workers, who have always understood the necessity of providing those in need with a supportive environment to enhance their functioning.

## *COST AND COST-EFFECTIVENESS OF MENTAL HEALTH SERVICES*

Cost and financing for mental health services are major issues for future planning and policy development. This is particularly true because, as discussed above, escalating costs have triggered a move toward monitoring those costs and providing the least-expensive alternative services. Costs of and payments for mental health services have already undergone dramatic changes (Bickman & Dokecki, 1989). For example, in the 1950s, only about 50 percent of private insurance plans covered short-term inpatient mental health care, and only 38 percent covered any outpatient care. By the 1980s, 99 percent of health insurance plans covered hospitalization for mental health problems and 90 percent covered outpatient care (Tsai, Reedy, Bernacki, & Lee, 1988). With this growth in payer responsibility for covering mental health services came attempts to develop policies to regulate those costs. To understand such cost issues, it is necessary to understand how mental health services are financed. Figure 9-1 illustrates the transfer of goods and services (expanded from McGuire, 1990).

In the simplest possible arrangement, a client purchases goods delivered by a provider. However, most mental health services are funded through insurance. The smaller of the triangles in the figure shows the relationship between insurance payer, provider, and client. Clients (or their employers) pay an insurer a premium, then the health insurance pays for mental health services. When clients need services

FIGURE **9-1**

## Cost Issues for Mental Health Services

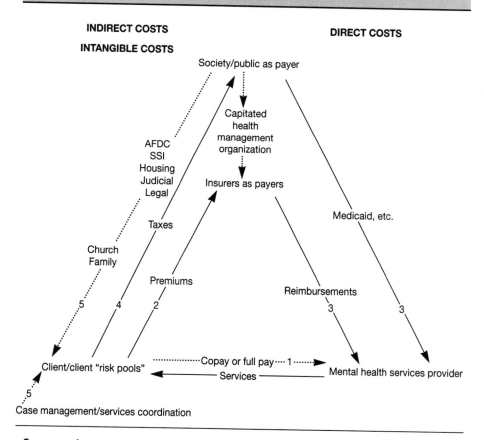

**Summary of cost containment procedures**

*Arrow 1*   Contain demand by requiring higher copayments or full out-of-pocket payments.

*Arrow 2*   Contain demand or use by raising insurance premiums or refusing to insure.

*Arrow 3*   Contain services costs by limiting reimbursement to particular kinds of services or for short duration of care.

*Arrow 4*   Contain need by manipulating risk pools so that the proportion of risky to nonrisky people is low.

*Arrow 5*   Contain need for more costly services by providing preventive, supportive, or low-cost services.

NOTES: AFDC = Aid to Families with Dependent Children; SSI = Supplemental Security Income.
SOURCE: Expanded from McGuire, T. G. (1990). Financing and reimbursement for mental health services. In C. A. Taube, D. M. Mechanic, & A. A. Hohmann (Eds.), *New directions for mental health services* (pp. 87–111). New York: Hemisphere.

from a provider, the provider delivers those services, and the insurer then reimburses the provider.

However, in our society, not all people or all services are covered by private insurance. The figure also has a larger triangle to include society or the public as a payer for services. In this case, services are reimbursed through Medicaid or other public funds to the provider. However, unlike the situation for private insurance, that same client may or may not have paid toward the public insurance—rather, a public pool of citizens has paid for it through taxes (McGuire, 1990).

As social workers are so well aware, clients with mental health needs also frequently require other services in addition to mental health services. Therefore, in the larger triangle, the figure shows indirect services provided by society to people with mental disorders. These may be legal or judicial services or public housing (Hu & Hausman, 1994). This arrow also represents costs to society of mental illness—for example, costs attributable to increased need for Aid to Families with Dependent Children (AFDC; now called Temporary Assistance for Needy Families [TANF]) or Supplemental Security Income (SSI) by people with mental illness. Some of these societal costs are borne also by nonprofit institutions, such as community centers or churches, and a large part are borne by the immediate or extended family of the client with mental health problems.

A major policy issue for mental health services concerns the need for cost containment, which is achieved by regulating the flow of direct and indirect services and costs along the two triangles shown in Figure 9-1. Basically, cost containment policy is directed at controlling both the demand for and the use of services.

Attempts to control demand and use through private insurance (the smaller triangle) is largely based on three factors (each shown on a different side of the triangle): (1) copayment or deductibles paid by the client (the copayments required for most mental health services are 50 percent, in contrast to 20 percent for physical health care; Tsai et al., 1988), (2) increases in individual premiums or denial of insurance by the insurer of the client, and (3) restricted or capped reimbursement levels or services from the insurer to the provider (Frank & McGuire, 1986).

Attempts to regulate demand and use in the public sector (the larger triangle) have focused largely on the development of health maintenance organizations (HMOs) that rely on capitated payment (Ellis & McGuire, 1988). That is, the HMO receives a specific amount for each client, whether or not that client needs or uses services. Consequently, the HMO benefits when fewer clients need, demand, or use services (Shortell, Gillies, & Devers, 1995). This group of clients is called their "risk pool." If the risk pool includes people who need, demand, and use many services, the HMO cannot survive financially. Therefore, the HMO responds by distributing the risk pool across a wide population of healthy people, reimbursing only for services known to be effective, emphasizing less costly early interventions, and providing cost-effective services.

The policy demands for cost containment necessitate new cost-effectiveness practices and research. It appears that the demands for cost containment might cause social workers to play an increasing role in mental health services (Berkman et al., 1990). If research demonstrates that particular types of services and treatments are as effective or more effective when provided by low-cost providers such as social workers, it would be in the payers' best interest to have those low-cost providers deliver the services. Most of the indirect services provided to clients with mental health problems (such as any welfare programs, legal and judicial services, and housing services) have always been an integral part of the mission of social work

(Warrick, Netting, Christianson, & Williams, 1992). Because such indirect services enable clients to live within a community and avoid use of the most expensive residential or hospital services, it benefits payers to see that these services are provided. There is some evidence that case management (or, more accurately, services coordination) lowers the total costs of services to people with mental illness (Hu & Jerrell, 1991; Jerrell & Hu, 1989) and reduces use of more expensive, medically oriented services (Berkman et al., 1990). Also, continuous, intensive case management has been shown to be effective in stabilizing patients in the community, although savings in hospital costs often are offset by increased costs of community care (Borland, McRae, & Lycan, 1989). The convergence of all of these issues augurs well for the future of social workers' roles in mental health services, and it challenges all providers to demonstrate the cost-effectiveness of their services.

## Directions and Trends

As this chapter has shown, the development of an adequate knowledge base to guide the delivery of mental health services is a formidable, pressing challenge. Mental health services research is an underdeveloped field (NIMH, 1991). Only a few investigators fully grasp the complex factors that affect the delivery of mental health services and have sufficient training to address such factors in their studies. According to NIMH (1991), "The development of the field requires a critical mass of researchers who can examine important issues and the creation of training environments that will attract talented investigators." (p. 58).

Social work was designated as one of the four core mental health professions in the federal legislation that established NIMH, and social workers are the largest professional group of mental health services providers (Redick et al., 1991). Yet social workers are insufficiently represented among mental health researchers. This underinvolvement is in part a result of the breadth of the profession's mission and its wide range of practice areas, which limits the number of social work researchers who focus their research on mental health (Task Force Report on Social Work Research, 1991). Further, training support for doctoral education in social work has been limited, and those few established social work researchers who do focus on mental health have worked in relatively insular environments. Social work researchers in mental health require stronger connections to other services researchers, to disciplines that inform and guide services research, and to sources of funding (Proctor, 1996).

Such problems are being mitigated by several recent developments. To date, funding from NIMH has established social work research development centers at seven universities. These centers enhance the support for mental health research in schools of social work and promote research on pressing mental health issues.

Given social work's historic leadership in providing services to people with mental disorders, the focus of these centers on service delivery issues is not surprising. Social work is uniquely familiar with clients, families, community dynamics, and the impact of organizational factors. This familiarity should ensure that studies conducted by social work researchers will address important questions and incorporate critical social and contextual factors in their conception, design, and implementation. The knowledge derived from these studies will likely produce clearer understanding of the services needs of vulnerable populations, including children, elderly and poor people, and people of color and members of ethnic groups. It also should produce a fuller picture of the roles of the various sectors in providing care and gateway providers in ensuring access to that care, the effect of differing services configurations on outcomes, and the impact on services of evolving cost containment policies.

# References

Adebimpe, V. R. (1994). Race, racism, and epidemiological surveys. *Hospital and Community Psychiatry, 45,* 27–31.

Andersen, R. (1968). *A behavioral model of families' use of health services.* Chicago: University of Chicago, Center for Health Administration Studies.

Andersen, R. (1975). Health service distribution and equity. In R. Andersen, J. Kravits, & O. W. Anderson (Eds.), *Equity in health services: Empirical analyses of public policy* (pp. 9–31). Cambridge, MA: Ballinger.

Andersen, R. M. (1995). Revisiting the behavioral model and access to medical care: Does it matter? *Journal of Health and Social Behavior, 36,* 1–10.

Bandura, A. (1986). *Social foundations of thought and action: A social cognitive theory.* Englewood Cliffs, NJ: Prentice Hall.

Bartsch, D. A., Shern, D. L., Coen, A. S., & Wilson, N. Z. (1995). Service needs, receipt, and outcomes for types of clients with serious and persistent mental illness. *Journal of Mental Health Administration, 22,* 388–402.

Berkman, B., Bonander, E., Rutchick, R., Silverman, P., Kemler, B., Marcus, L., & Isaacson-Rubinger, M. J. (1990). Social work in health care: Directions in practice. *Social Science and Medicine, 31,* 19–26.

Berwick, D. M. (1989). Health services research and quality of care: Assignments for the 1990s. *Medical Care, 27,* 763–771.

Bickman, L., Bryant, D., & Summerfelt, W. T. (1993). *Final report of the quality study of the Fort Bragg Evaluation Project.* Nashville, TN: Vanderbilt University, Center for Mental Health Policy.

Bickman, L., & Dokecki, P. R. (1989). Public and private responsibility for mental health services. *American Psychologist, 44,* 1133–1137.

Bickman, L., Guthrie, P. R., Foster, E. M., Lambert, E. W., Summerfelt, W. T., Breda, C. S., & Heflinger, C. A. (1995). *Evaluating managed mental services: The Fort Bragg experiment.* New York: Plenum Press.

Blazer, D. G., Hughes, D. C., & George, L. K. (1987). The epidemiology of depression in an elderly community population. *Gerontologist, 27,* 281–287.

Blazer, D. G., Kessler, R. C., McGonagle, K. A., & Swartz, M. S. (1994). The prevalence and distribution of major depression in a national comorbidity sample: The National Comorbidity Survey. *American Journal of Psychiatry, 151,* 979–986.

Borland, A., McRae, J., & Lycan, C. (1989). Outcomes of five years of continuous intensive case management. *Hospital and Community Psychiatry, 40,* 369–376.

Boyle, M. H., & Offord, D. R. (1988). Prevalence of childhood disorder, perceived need for help, family dysfunction and resource allocation for child welfare and children's mental health services in Ontario. *Canadian Journal of Behavioral Science, 20,* 374–388.

Branch, L., Jetter, A., Evashwick, C., Polansky, M., Rowe, G., & Diehr, P. (1981). Toward understanding elders' health service utilization. *Journal of Community Health, 7,* 80–92.

Brekke, J. S. (1987). The model-guided method for monitoring program implementation. *Evaluation Review, 11,* 281–299.

Brown, D. R., Ahmed, F., Gary, L. E., & Milburn, N. G. (1995). Major depression in a community sample of African Americans. *American Journal of Psychiatry, 152*, 373–378.

Burns, B. (1991). Mental health service use by adolescents in the 1970s and 1980s. *Journal of the American Academy of Child and Adolescent Psychiatry, 17*, 144–150.

Burns, B., & Taube, C. A. (1990). Mental health services in general medical care and nursing homes. In B. Fogel, A. Furino, & G. Gottlieb (Eds.), *Protecting minds at risk* (pp. 63–84). Washington DC: American Psychiatric Press.

Burns, B., Taube, C. A., & Taube, J. E. (1990). *Use of mental health sector services by adolescents: 1975, 1980, 1986* (NTIS No. PB 91–154 344/AS; Paper prepared under contract for the Carnegie Council on Adolescent Development and the Carnegie Corporation of New York, for the Office of Technology Assessment, U.S. Congress, Washington, DC). Springfield, VA: National Technical Information Service.

Burns, B. J. (1994). The challenges of child mental health services research. *Journal of Emotional and Behavioral Disorders, 2*, 254–259.

Chang, G., Warner, V., & Weissman, M. M. (1988). Physicians' recognition of psychiatric disorders in children and adolescents. *American Journal of Diseases of Children, 142*, 736–739.

Clark, W. G., & Travis, S. S. (1994). Elderly admissions to a state psychiatric hospital: Cohort characteristics, after-care needs, and discharge destinations. *Journal of Gerontological Social Work, 21*, 101–115.

Cleary, P. D. (1990). The need and demand for mental health services. In C. A. Taube, D. Mechanic, & A. A. Hohmann (Eds.), *New directions for mental health services* (pp. 161–184). New York: Hemisphere.

Clinton, J. J., McCormick, K., & Besteman, J. (1994). Enhancing clinical practice: The role of practice guidelines. *American Psychologist, 49*, 30–33.

Cohen, P., Kasen, S., Brook, J. S., & Struening, E. L. (1991). Diagnostic predictors of treatment patterns in a cohort of adolescents. *Journal of the American Academy of Child and Adolescent Psychiatry, 30*, 989–993.

Costello, E. J., Farmer, E.M.Z., Angold, A., Burns, B. J., & Erkanli, A. (1997). Psychiatric disorders among American Indian and white youth in Appalachia: The Great Smoky Mountains Study. *American Journal of Public Health, 87*, 827–832.

Costello, E. J., Burns, B. J., Costello, A. J., Dulcan, M., & Brent, D. (1988). Service utilization and psychiatric diagnosis in pediatric primary care: The role of the gatekeeper. *Pediatrics, 82*, 435–441.

Costello, E. J., Costello, A. J., Edelbrock, C., Burns, B. J., Dulcan, M. K., Brent, D., & Janiszewski, S. (1988). Psychiatric disorders in pediatric primary care: Prevalence and risk factors. *Archives of General Psychiatry, 45*, 1107–1116.

Crow, M. R., Smith, H. L., McNamee, A. H., & Piland, N. F. (1994). Considerations in predicting mental health care use: Implications for managed care plans. *Journal of Mental Health Administration, 21*, 5–23.

Dain, N. (1976). From colonial America to bicentennial America: Two centuries of vicissitudes in the institutional care of mental patients. *Bulletin of the New York Academy of Medicine, 52*, 1179–1196.

Dulcan, M. K., Costello, E. J., Costello, A. J., Edelbrock, C., Brent, D., & Janiszewski, S. (1990). The pediatrician as gatekeeper to mental health care for children: Do parents' concerns open the gate? *Journal of the American Academy of Child and Adolescent Psychiatry, 29*, 453–458.

Earls, F., Robins, L. N., Stiffman, A. R., & Powell, J. (1989). Comprehensive health care for high-risk adolescents: An evaluation study. *American Journal of Public Health, 79,* 999–1005.

Ellis, R. P., & McGuire, T. G. (1988). Insurance principles and design of prospective payment systems. *Journal of Health Economics, 7,* 215–237.

Ellwood, P. (1988). Outcomes management—A technology of patient experience. *JAMA, 318,* 1549–1556.

Feldman, R. A., & Stiffman, A. R. (1984). Traditional community agencies and the prevention of mental illness. *International Social Work,* 8–19.

Fishbein, M., & Azjen, I. (1975). *Belief, attitude, intention and behavior: An introduction to theory and research.* Reading, MA: Addison-Wesley.

Frank, R. G., & McGuire, T. G. (1986). A review of studies of the impact of insurance on the demand and utilization of specialty mental health services. *Health Services Research, 21,* 241–265.

Frank, R. G., & Morlock, L. L. (1994). *Coordination of mental health services: Organizational and financial considerations.* Report prepared for the Milbank Memorial Fund.

Freedman, A. M. (1967). Historical and political roots of the Community Mental Health Centers Act. *American Journal of Orthopsychiatry, 37,* 486–494.

Friedman, R. M. (1989). Service system research: Implications of a systems perspective. In P. E. Greenbaum, R. M. Friedman, A. Duchinowski, K. Kutash, & S. Silver (Eds.), *Conference proceedings: Children's mental health services and policy. Building a research base* (pp. 1–5). Tampa: Mental Health Institute.

George, L. K. (1990). Definition, classification, and measurement of mental health services. In C. A. Taube, D. Mechanic, & A. A. Hohmann (Eds.), *New directions for mental health services* (pp. 303–319). New York: Hemisphere.

George, L. K. (1992). Community and home care for mentally ill adults. In J. E. Birren, R. B. Sloane, G. D. Cohen, N. R. Hooyman, B. D. Lebowitz, M. H. Wykle, & D. E. Deutschman (Eds.), *Handbook of mental health and aging* (pp. 793–813). San Diego: Academic Press.

Gibbs, J. T. (1990). Mental health issues of African-American adolescents: Implications for policy and practice. In A. R. Stiffman & L. E. Davis (Eds.), *Ethnic issues and adolescent mental health* (pp. 21–52). Newbury Park, CA: Sage Publications.

Glisson, C. (1995). The state of the art of social work research: Implications for mental health. *Research on Social Work Practice, 5,* 205–222.

Goldman, H. H., Adams, N. H., & Taube, C. A. (1983). Deinstitutionalization: The data demythologized. *Hospital and Community Psychiatry, 34,* 129–134.

Goldman, H. H., Morrissey, J. P., & Ridgely, M. S. (1994). Evaluating the Robert Wood Johnson Foundation Program on Chronic Mental Illness. *Milbank Quarterly, 72,* 37–47.

Goldman, H. H., & Skinner, E. A. (1990). Specialty mental health services: Research on specialization and differentiation. In C. A. Taube, D. Mechanic, & A. A. Hohmann (Eds.), *New directions for mental health services* (pp. 23–38). New York: Hemisphere.

Goldman, S. K. (1988, October). *Series on community-based services for children and adolescents who are severely emotionally disturbed.* Washington, DC: CASSP Technical Assistance Center, Georgetown University Child Development Center.

Grob, G. (1987, April). *The politics of mental health policy in post-World War II America.* Paper presented at the meeting of the Organization of American Historians, Philadelphia.

Haber, S., & McCall, N. (1989). Use of nonphysician providers in the Medicare program: Assessment of the direct reimbursement of clinical social workers demonstration project. *Inquiry, 26,* 158–169.

Hargreaves, W., Catalano, R., Hu, T. W., & Cuffel, B. (1994). *A concept of mental health services research*. Unpublished manuscript, Institute for Mental Health Services Research, Berkeley.

Hibbard, J. H., & Pope, C. R. (1986). Age differences in the use of medical care in an HMO. *Medical Care, 24,* 52–66.

Hoberman, H. M. (1992). Ethnic minority status and adolescent mental health services utilization. *Journal of Mental Health Administration, 19,* 246–267.

Hogarty, G. E., Anderson, C. M., Reiss, D. J., Kornblith, S. J., Greenwald, D. P., Javna, C. P., & Madonia, M. J. (1986). Family psychoeducation, social skills training, and maintenance chemotherapy in the aftercare treatment of schizophrenia, I: One-year effects of a controlled study on relapse and expressed emotion. *Archives of General Psychiatry, 43,* 633–642.

Hogarty, G. E., Anderson, C. M., Reiss, D. J., Kornblith, S. J., Greenwald, D. P., Ulrigh, R. F., & Carner, M. (1991). Family psychoeducation, social skills training and maintenance chemotherapy in the aftercare treatment of schizophrenia. *Archives of General Psychiatry, 48,* 340–347.

Hu, T., & Hausman, J. W. (1994). *Cost effectiveness of community based care for individuals with mental health problems.* Unpublished manuscript.

Hu, T., & Jerrell, J. (1991). Cost effectiveness of alternative approaches in treating severely mentally ill in California. *Schizophrenia Bulletin, 17,* 461–468.

Hulka, B. S., & Wheat, J. R. (1985). Patterns of utilization: The patient perspective. *Medical Care, 23,* 438–460.

Human, J., & Wasem, C. (1991). Rural mental health in America. *American Psychologist, 46,* 232–239.

Janz, N. K., & Becker, M. H. (1984). The Health Belief Model: A decade later. *Health Education Quarterly, 11,* 1–47.

Jerrell, J. M., & Hu, T. W. (1989). Cost effectiveness of intensive clinical and case management compared with an existing system of care. *Inquiry, 26,* 224–234.

John, L. H., Offord, D. R., Boyle, M. H., & Racine, Y. A. (1995). Factors predicting use of mental health and social services by children 6–16 years old: Findings from the Ontario Child Health Study. *American Journal of Orthopsychiatry, 65,* 76–86.

Jordan, D. D., & Hernandez, M. (1990). The Ventura planning model: A proposal for mental health reform. *Journal of Mental Health Administration, 17,* 26–47.

Kelleher, K. J., Taylor, J. L., & Rickert, V. I. (1992). Mental health services for rural children and adolescents. *Clinical Psychology Review, 12,* 841–852.

Kessler, R. C., McGonagle, K. A., Zhao, S., Nelson, C. B., Hughes, M., Eshleman, S., Wittchen, H-U., & Kendler, K. S. (1994). Lifetime and 12-month prevalence of DSM-III-R psychiatric disorders in the United States: Results from the National Comorbidity Study. *Archives of General Psychiatry, 51,* 8–19.

Knitzer, J. (1982). *Unclaimed children.* Washington, DC: Children's Defense Fund.

Koenig, H. G., Meador, K. G., Cohen, H. J., & Blazer, D. G. (1988). Detection and treatment of major depression in older medically ill hospitalized patients. *International Journal of Psychiatry in Medicine, 18,* 17–31.

Koslowe, P. A., Rosenstein, M. J., Milazzo-Sayre, L. J., & Manderscheid, R. W. (1991). *Characteristics of persons serviced by private psychiatric hospitals. United States, 1986* (Mental Health Statistical Note 201). Rockville, MD: National Institute of Mental Health.

Law places 36-month limit on SSI, SSKI benefits to substance abusers, tightens SSDI requirements [News & Notes]. (1994). *Hospital and Community Psychiatry, 45,* 1051–1052.

Leaf, P. J. (1994). Psychiatric disorders and the use of health services. In J. Miranda, A. A. Hohmann, C. C. Attkisson, & D. B. Larson (Eds.), *Mental disorders in primary care* (pp. 377–401). San Francisco: Jossey-Bass.

Leaf, P. J., Alegria, M., Cohen, P., Goodman, S. H., Horwitz, S. M., Hoven, C. W., Narrow, W. E., Vaden-Kiernan, M., & Regier, D. A. (1996). Mental health service use in the community and schools: Results from the four-community MECA study. *Journal of the American Academy of Child and Adolescent Psychiatry, 35,* 889–897.

Leaf, P. J., & Bruce, M. L. (1987). Gender differences in the use of mental health related services: A re-examination. *Journal of Health and Social Behavior, 28,* 171–183.

Leaf, P. J., & Bruce, M. L. (1989, May–June). *The use of multiple indicators of need in predicting use of mental health services in the specialty and general medical sectors.* Paper presented at the World Psychiatric Association Section of Epidemiology and Community Psychiatry Symposium on Psychiatric Epidemiology and Primary Health Care, Toronto.

Leaf, P. J., Bruce, M. L., & Tischler, G. L. (1986). The differential effect of attitudes on the use of mental health services. *Social Psychiatry, 21,* 167–192.

Leaf, P. J., Bruce, M. L., Tischler, G. L., Freeman, D. H., Weissman, M. M., & Myers, J. K. (1988). Factors affecting the utilization of specialty and general medical mental health services. *Medical Care, 26,* 9–26.

Leaf, P. J., Livingston, M. M., Tischler, G. L., Weissman, M. M., Holzer, C. E., & Myers, J. I. (1985). Contact with health professionals for the treatment of psychiatric and emotional problems. *Medical Care, 23,* 1322–1337.

LeCroy, C. W., & Ashford, J. B. (1992). Children's mental health: Current findings and research directions. *Social Work, 28,* 13–20.

Lefley, H. P. (1995, September). *The family experience with mental illness: Applications in designing programs for families and consumers.* Keynote address, National Institute of Mental Health, Center for Mental Health Services Workshop, Designing Programs for Families and Consumers Based on Research on the Family Experience with Severe Mental Illness, Washington University, St. Louis.

Lehman, A. F., Postrado, L. T., Roth, D., McNary, S. W., & Goldman, H. H. (1994). Continuity of care and client outcomes in the Robert Wood Johnson Foundation Program on Chronic Mental Illness. *Milbank Quarterly, 72,* 105–122.

Lourie, I. S., & Katz-Leavy, J. (1991). New directions for mental health services for families and children. *Families in Society, 72,* 277–285.

Marx, A. J., Test, M. A., & Stein, L. J. (1973). Extrahospital management of severe mental illness. *Archives of General Psychiatry, 29,* 505–511.

Mayer, J. B., & Rubin, G. (1983). Is there a future for social work in HMOs? *Health & Social Work, 8,* 283–289.

McGrew, J. H., Bond, G. R., Dietzen, L., & Salyers, M. (1994). Measuring the fidelity of implementation of a mental health program model. *Journal of Consulting and Clinical Psychology, 62,* 670–678.

McGuire, T. G. (1990). Financing and reimbursement for mental health services. In C. A. Taube, D. Mechanic, & A. A. Hohmann (Eds.), *New directions for mental health services* (pp. 87–111). New York: Hemisphere.

Mechanic, D. (1986). The challenge of chronic mental illness: A retrospective and prospective view. *Hospital and Community Psychiatry, 37,* 891–896.

Mechanic, D. (1990). Introduction. The evolution of mental health services and mental health services research. In C. A. Taube, D. Mechanic, & A. A. Hohmann (Eds.), *New directions for mental health services* (pp. 1–7). New York: Hemisphere.

Mechanic, D., & Aiken, L. H. (1987). Improving the care of patients with chronic mental illness. *New England Journal of Medicine, 317,* 1634–1638.

Mechanic, D., Angel, R., & Davies, L. (1991). Risk and selection processes between the general and the specialty mental health sectors. *Journal of Health and Social Behavior, 32,* 49–64.

Morlock, L. (1990). Recognition and treatment of mental health problems in the general health care sector. In C. A. Taube, D. Mechanic, & A. A. Hohmann (Eds.), *New directions for mental health services* (pp. 39–61). New York: Hemisphere.

Morrissey, J. P., Hall, R. H., & Lindsey, M. (1982). *Interorganizational relations: A sourcebook of measures for mental health programs* (Series BN, No. 2). Washington, DC: U.S. Government Printing Office.

Morrissey, J. P., Tausig, M., & Lindsey, M. (1985). *Network analysis methods for mental health services system research: A comparison of two community support systems* (Series BN, No. 8). Washington, DC: U.S. Government Printing Office.

National Institute of Mental Health. (1991). *Caring for people with severe mental disorders: A national plan of research to improve services* (DHHS Publication No. ADM 91–1762). Washington, DC: U.S. Government Printing Office.

National Institute of Mental Health, National Advisory Mental Health Council. (1990). *National plan for research on child and adolescent mental disorders* (DHHS Publication No. ADM 90–1683). Rockville, MD: U.S. Government Printing Office.

Norquist, G., Wells, K. B., Rogers, W. H., Davis, L. M., Kahn, K., & Brook, R. (1995). Quality of care for depressed elderly patients hospitalized in the specialty psychiatric units or general medical wards. *Archives of General Psychiatry, 52,* 695–701.

Office of Technology Assessment. (1991). *Adolescent health* (Vol. II). Washington, DC: U.S. Government Printing Office.

Offord, D. R., Boyle, M. H., Szatmari, P., Rae-Grant, N. I., Links, P. S., Cadman, D. T., Byles, J. A., Crawford, J. W., Blum, H. M., Byrne, C., Thomas, H., & Woodward, C. A. (1987). Ontario Child Health Study: II. Six-month prevalence of disorder and rates of service utilization. *Archives of General Psychiatry, 44,* 832–836.

Padgett, D. K., Patrick, C., Burns, B. J., & Schlesinger, H. J. (1994). Women and outpatient mental health services: Use by black, Hispanic, and white women in a national insured population. *Journal of Mental Health Administration, 21,* 347–360.

Padgett, D. K., Patrick, C., Burns, B. J., Schlesinger, H. J., & Cohen, J. (1993). The effect of insurance benefit changes on use of child and adolescent outpatient mental health services. *Medical Care, 31,* 96–110.

Parmelee, P. A., Katz, I. R., & Lawton, M. P. (1989). Depression among institutionalized aged: Assessment and prevalence estimation. *Journal of Gerontology, 44,* M22–M29.

Perreault, M., Rogers, W. L., Leichner, P., & Sabourin, S. (1996). Patients' requests and satisfaction with services in an outpatient psychiatric setting. *Psychiatric Services, 47,* 287–292.

Pescosolido, B., Wright, E. R., Alegria, M., & Vera, M. (1995, February). *Formal and informal utilization patterns among the poor with mental health problems in Puerto Rico* (Indiana Consortium for Mental Health Services Research Paper Series, Paper No. 3). Bloomington: Indiana University Department of Sociology.

Pfeiffer, S., O'Malley, D. S., & Shott, S. (1996). Factors associated with the outcome of adults treated in psychiatric hospitals: A synthesis of findings. *Psychiatric Services, 47,* 263–269.

Proctor, E. K. (1996). Research and research training in social work: Climate, connections, and competencies. *Research on Social Work Practice, 6,* 366–378.

Proctor, E. K., Morrow-Howell, N., & Dore, P. (1996, July). *Functional dependency among elderly geropsychiatric patients discharged home after acute care.* Paper presented at the 10th NIMH International Conference on Mental Health Programs in the General Health Care Sector, Bethesda, MD.

Raniseski, J. M., & Sigelman, C. K. (1992). Conformity, peer pressure, and adolescent receptivity to treatment for substance abuse: A research note. *American Journal of Psychiatry, 150,* 185–194.

Redick, R. W., Witkin, M. J., Atay, J. E., & Manderscheid, R. W. (1991). *Outpatient care programs of mental health organizations, United States, 1988* (Mental Health Statistical Note). Washington, DC: U.S. Government Printing Office.

Regier, D. A., Goldberg, I. D., & Taube, C. A. (1978). The de facto U.S. mental health services system. *Archives of General Psychiatry, 35,* 685–693.

Regier, D. A., Narrow, W. E., Rae, D. S., Manderscheid, R. W., Locke, B. Z., & Goodwin, F. K. (1993). The de facto U.S. mental and addictive disorders service system: Epidemiologic Catchment Area prospective 1-year prevalence rates of disorders and services. *Archives of General Psychiatry, 50,* 85–94.

Rivera, G. (1972). *Willowbrook: A report on how it is and why it doesn't have to be that way.* New York: Random House.

Robins, L. N., & Regier, D. A. (Eds.). (1991). *Psychiatric disorders in America.* New York: Free Press.

Rogler, L. H., & Cortes, D. E. (1993). Help-seeking pathways: A unifying concept in mental health care. *American Journal of Psychiatry, 150,* 554–561.

Rosen, A., & Proctor, E. K. (1978) Specifying the treatment process: The basis of effectiveness research. *Journal of Social Service Research, 2,* 25–43.

Rosenblatt, A., & Attkisson, C. C. (1993). Integrating systems of care in California for youth with severe emotional disturbance: III. Answers that lead to questions about out-of-home placements and the AB377 Evaluation Project. *Journal of Child & Family Studies, 2,* 119–141.

Rost, K. M., Smith, G. R., & Taylor, J. L. (1993). Rural-urban differences in stigma and the use of care for depressive disorders. *Journal of Rural Health, 9,* 57–62.

Saxe, L., Cross, T., & Silverman, N. (1988). Children's mental health: The gap between what we know and what we do. *American Psychologist, 43,* 800–807.

Schaffer, D., Fisher, P., Dulcan, M. K., Davies, M., Piacentini, J., Schwab-Stone, M. E., Lahey, B. B., Bourdon, K., Jensen, P. S., Bird, H. R., Canino, G., & Regier, D. A. (1996). The NIMH Diagnostic Interview Schedule for Children Version 2.3: Description, acceptability, prevalence rates, and performance in the MECA study. *Journal of the American Academy of Child and Adolescent Psychiatry, 35,* 865–877.

Segal, S. P., Bola, J. R., & Watson, M. A. (1996). Race, quality of care, and antipsychotic prescribing practices in psychiatric emergency services. *Psychiatric Services, 47,* 282–286.

Segal, S. P., Watson, M. A., & Akutsu, P. D. (1996). Quality of care and use of less restrictive alternatives in the psychiatric emergency service. *Psychiatric Services, 47,* 623–627.

Shortell, S. M., Gillies, R. R., & Devers, K. J. (1995). Reinventing the American hospital. *Milbank Quarterly, 73,* 131–160.

Solomon, P. L., & Davis, J. M. (1985). Meeting community service needs of discharged psychiatric patients. *Psychiatric Quarterly, 57,* 11–17.

Solomon, P. L., Gordon, B. H., & Davis, J. M. (1984). Differentiating psychiatric readmissions from nonreadmissions. *American Journal of Orthopsychiatry, 54,* 426–435.

Sommers, I. (1989). Geographic location and mental health services utilization among the chronically mentally ill. *Community Mental Health Journal, 25,* 132–144.

Spitzer, R. L., Kroenke, K., Linzer, M., Hahn, S. R., Williams, J.B.W., deGruy, F. V., Brody, D., & Davies, M. (1995). Health related quality of life in primary care patients with mental disorders. Results from the PRIME-MD 1000 study. *JAMA, 274,* 1511–1517.

Steinwachs, D. M. (1990). Patterns of care methodologies: Utility for assessing costs and outcomes of mental health care. In C. A. Taube, D. Mechanic, & A. A. Hohmann (Eds.), *New directions for mental services* (pp. 185–197). New York: Hemisphere.

Stiffman, A. R., Chen, Y. W., Elze, D., Dore, P., & Cheng, L. C. (1997). Adolescents' and providers' perspectives on the need for and use of mental health services. *Journal of Adolescent Health, 21,* 335–342.

Stiffman, A. R., & Cunningham, R. (1990, October). *Epidemiology of child and adolescent mental illness.* Paper presented at the Conference on Child and Adolescent Mental Health, sponsored by the National Association of Deans and Directors of Schools of Social Work, Berkeley, CA.

Stiffman, A. R., Dore, P., Cunningham, R., & Earls, F. (1995). Person and environment in HIV risk behavior change between adolescence and young adulthood. *Health Education Quarterly, 22,* 233–248.

Stiffman, A. R., Earls, R., & Chueh, H. J. (1992). Predictive modeling of change in depressive disorder and counts of depressive symptoms in urban youths. *Journal of Research on Adolescence, 2,* 295–316.

Stiffman, A. R., Earls, F., Robins, L. N., & Jung, K. G. (1988). Problems and help-seeking in high-risk adolescent patients of health clinics. *Journal of Adolescent Health Care, 9,* 305–309.

Stroul, B. A. (1985). *Child and adolescent service system program state needs assessment materials.* Washington, DC: CASSP Technical Assistance Center, Georgetown University Child Development Center.

Stroul, B. A., & Friedman, R. M. (1986). *A system of care for children and youth with severe emotional disturbances* (rev. ed.). Washington, DC: CASSP Technical Assistance Center, Georgetown University Child Development Center.

Sussman, L. K., Robins, L. N., & Earls, F. (1987). Treatment-seeking for depression by African-American and white Americans. *Social Science Medicine, 24,* 187–196.

Task Force Report on Social Work Research. (1991). *Building social work knowledge for effective services and policies: A plan for research development.* Washington, DC: National Institute of Mental Health.

Taube, C. A., Burns, B. J., & Kessler, L. (1984). Patients of psychiatrists and psychologists in office-based practice: 1980. *American Psychologist, 39,* 1435–1447.

Taube, C. A., Goldman, H. H., Burns, B. J., & Kessler, L. G. (1988). High users of outpatient mental health services: I. Definition and characteristics. Center for Advanced Study in Behavioral Sciences Conference on Health Care Service Delivery (1984, Stanford, California). *American Journal of Psychiatry, 145,* 19–24.

Taube, C. A., & Rupp, A. (1986). The effect of Medicaid on access to ambulatory mental health care for the poor and near-poor under 65. *Medical Care, 24,* 677–686.

Tessler, R. C. (1995, September). *The family experience with mental illness: Implications for designing programs.* Paper presented at the National Institute of Mental Health, Center for Mental Health Services Workshop, Designing Programs for Families and Consumers Based on Research on the Family Experience with Severe Mental Illness, Washington University, St. Louis.

Thienhaus, O. J., Rowe, C., Woellert, P., & Hillard, J. R. (1988). Geropsychiatric emergency services: Utilization and outcome predictors. *Hospital and Community Psychiatry, 39,* 1301–1305.

Torian, L., Davidson, E., Fulop, G., Sell, L., & Fillit, H. (1992). The effect of dementia on acute care in a geriatric medical unit. *International Psychogeriatrics, 4,* 231–239.

Tsai, S. P., Reedy, S. M., Bernacki, E. J., & Lee, E. S. (1988). Effects of curtailed insurance benefits on use of mental health care. *Medical Care, 26,* 430–440.

Tuma, J. M. (1989). Mental health services for children: The state of the art. *American Psychologist, 44,* 188–189.

Warrick, L. H., Netting, F. E., Christianson, J. B., & Williams, F. G. (1992). Hospital-based case management: Results from a demonstration. *Gerontologist, 32,* 781–788.

Weissman, M. M., Leaf, P. J., Bruce, M. L., & Florio, L. (1988). The epidemiology of dysthymia in five communities: Rates, risks, comorbidity, and treatment. 140th Annual Meeting of the American Psychiatric Association (1987, Chicago, Illinois). *American Journal of Psychiatry, 145,* 815–819.

Wells, K. B., & Brook, R. H. (1990). The quality of mental health services: Past, present, and future. In C. A. Taube, D. Mechanic, & A. A. Hohmann (Eds.), *New directions for mental health services* (pp. 203–224). New York: Hemisphere.

Wells, K. B., Golding, J. M., Hough, R. L., Burnam, M. A., & Karno, M. (1988). Factors affecting the probability of use of general and medical health and social/community services for Mexican Americans and non-Hispanic whites. *Medical Care, 26,* 441–452.

Wells, K. B., Keeler, E., & Manning, W. G. (1990). Patterns of outpatient mental health care over time: Some implications for estimates of demand and for benefit design. *Health Services Research, 24,* 773–789.

Wells, K. B., Manning, W. G., Duan, N., Newhouse, J. P., & Ware, J. E. (1986). Sociodemographic factors and the use of outpatient mental health services. *Medical Care, 24,* 75–85.

Wells, K. B., Stewart, A., Hays, R. D., Burnam, M. A., Rogers, W., Daniels, M., Berry, S., Greenfield, S., & Ware, J. (1989). The functioning and well-being of depressed patients: Results from the Medical Outcomes Study. *JAMA, 262,* 914–919.

White House. (1977, February 17). *Executive Order No. 11973—President's Commission on Mental Health.* Washington, DC: Office of the White House Press Secretary.

Wolinsky, F. D., Aguirre, B. E., Fann, L. J., Keith, V. M., Arnold, C. L., Niederhauser, J. C., & Dietrich, K. (1989). Ethnic difference in the demand for physician and hospital utilization among older adults in major American cities: Conspicuous evidence of considerable inequalities. *Milbank Quarterly, 67,* 412–449.

Wolinsky, F. D., & Coe, R. M. (1984). Physician and hospital utilization among noninstitutionalized elderly adults: An analysis of the Health Interview Survey. *Journal of Gerontology, 39,* 334–341.

Wolinsky, F. D., & Johnson, R. J. (1992). Widowhood, health status, and the use of health services by older adults: A cross-sectional and prospective approach. *Journal of Gerontology, 47,* S8–S16.

Zapka, J. G., McCusker, J., Stoddard, A. M., & Morrison, C. (1990). Psychosocial factors and AIDS-related behavior of homosexual men: Measurement and associations. *Evaluation & the Health Professions, 13,* 283–297.

# Short-term Treatment:
## Models, Methods, and Research

Sophia F. Dziegielewski, John P. Shields, and Bruce A. Thyer

The efficacy and effectiveness of psychotherapy in general, and of social case-work in particular, have long been a subject of controversy and debate (Fischer, 1973, 1976; Segal, 1972). Although the number of methodologically credible outcome studies on social work practice in mental health was sparse a few decades ago, the number of such studies being published is growing at an exponential rate (Gorey, 1996; Gorey, Thyer, & Pawluck, in press), and the profession is now in a better position to determine the effectiveness of various models of intervention.

A considerable body of research conducted by social workers and others now exists on the effectiveness of planned short-term therapies (STTs). With the advent of managed care and practice guidelines, it seems clear that the provision of effective STTs is the wave of the future (Dziegielewski, 1996). Although "managed care" often means simply reducing the number of visits authorized for reimbursement for particular mental health or substance abuse problems, among progressive firms, managed care implies careful pretreatment assessments (including but not limited to the diagnosis of mental disorders), the use of structured inventories of patient functioning, the design and competent implementation of a treatment plan based on assessed risk or problem, and the monitoring of clinical outcomes using structured outcome measurement tools, including patient satisfaction. If credible data show clinically meaningful improvements, then authorization for additional therapy sessions is more likely than in cases lacking such data. To advance effective and high-quality treatment, professional organizations (for example, the American Psychiatric Association, the American Psychological Association, and NASW), the federal government, and managed care firms are developing clinical practice guidelines. Practice guidelines identify approved therapies for particular problems, treatment decision algorithms, and treatment protocols. To the extent that practice guidelines are firmly grounded in the empirical research literature and clinical consensus, they have the potential to significantly improve mental health services and patient outcomes. If, however, practice guidelines are primarily derived from fiscal or self-interested disciplinary considerations, they have great potential to reduce clinical effectiveness and even harm patients (Persons, Thase, & Crits-Christoph, 1996).

The issue of the efficacy of STTs is an old one for social workers. More than 65 years ago, noted social work educator and practitioner Jessie Taft (1933) wrote about the dynamics of time and time limits as important elements in social work practice with mental health clients. Wattie (1973) conducted a quasi-experimental comparison of short-term and long-term treatments provided to 140 families by social workers and found that STT yielded results equivalent to those produced by conventional therapy. The STT that was tested was one indigenous to social work, developed by Reid and Shyne (1969), and it later evolved into what is now known as "task-centered practice."

Apart from external contingencies imposed by managed care companies and practice guidelines, research funding has led the profession toward the adoption and practice of STTs. Studies of planned STTs have found them to be not only effective (Bloom, 1992a) but as effective as longer-term or conventional therapies (Koss & Shiang, 1994), whereas longer-term or conventional therapies are often not effective for the types of clients' problems seen by social workers (Fischer, 1976; Segal, 1972; Stuart, 1970). In addition, many clients specifically request STTs, and many social workers prefer to provide these intentionally planned therapies. Research also has shown that short-term psychotherapy may actually accelerate treatment efficacy as a function of the client and therapist agreeing on the length of treatment (Reynolds et al., 1996).

## What Is STT?

### *DEFINITION*

In common with other approaches, the objective of SSTs is to reduce negative symptoms and bring about positive changes in a client's behavior and life circumstances. In general, STT involves mutually agreed-on and specific personal and behavioral change goals and methods to achieve these aims over an explicitly defined period. To date, there are three general types of STT: traditional, intermittent, and a combination of both. All follow the same rules and procedures. However, in traditional STT, people practice in a closed therapeutic time frame (for example, two months). In intermittent therapy, sessions are spread out over time or occur only as needed. The combination of traditional STT and intermittent approaches is often used when continued follow-up is indicated.

Bloom (1992b) provided a good summary of the characteristics of planned SST:

> Short-term psychotherapy ranges in length from a minimum of one interview to a maximum of around 20 interviews, with an average duration of about six sessions. Few people talk about therapies longer than 20 interviews as short-term, although the upper limit is not fully agreed upon. Five fundamental components, other than actual duration, usually characterize planned short-term psychotherapy: (a) prompt intervention, (b) a relatively high level of therapist activity, (c) establishment of specific but limited goals, (d) the identification and maintenance of a clear focus, and (e) the setting of a time limit. (p. 157)

Although many approaches fall under the umbrella of STT, there can be subtle and not-so-subtle differences among them. For example, STT models can be somewhat different from traditional crisis intervention strategies. In crisis intervention the strategy is generally to help the person achieve a homeostatic balance or return to equilibrium (Roberts & Dziegielewski, 1995). In STT, the progress of the client can (and often does) go beyond resuming homeostasis to result in new and better coping styles and patterns of behavior. Therefore, although most crisis therapies are brief, brief treatments are not solely provided to clients in crisis. Many clients seek brief treatment for long-term problems, not just crisis situations.

## DIFFERENCES FROM LONG-TERM THERAPY

Some major differences exist between STT and long-term therapy. One difference primarily concerns the way in which the client is viewed. From a short-term perspective, the client is seen as a basically healthy person who is interested in increasing personal effectiveness and promoting positive interpersonal change (Budman & Gurman, 1988; Roberts & Dziegielewski, 1995). The goals of brief therapy are usually mutually defined by the client and the therapist (Wells, 1994). This approach is different from traditional psychotherapies, in which the goal (for example, insight) is often first defined and known (for example, insight) by the therapist and later shared with the client (Budman & Gurman, 1988). Goals in planned STT are concretely defined and many times address current problems in the client's day-to-day life circumstances (Epstein, 1995). This process differs from long-term therapy, in which reported memories of what happened long ago or recently are primarily worked through during the treatment sessions themselves (Budman & Gurman, 1988).

In brief treatment, the practitioner is seen as active and assumes a consultative role with the client. Client insight is not considered essential or necessary for treatment progress. Also, termination is discussed early in the therapeutic environment (Wells, 1994). Frequently, specific limits and a time for termination are agreed on during the first session. This approach contrasts with long-term therapies, in which termination is rarely discussed or determined in advance.

## ROLE OF THE SOCIAL WORKER

In STT the practitioner's role differs in several ways from the therapist's role in longer, more traditional approaches. First, the therapist is expected to be very active and directive; he or she must help the client at all times focus on the determined goals. The therapist also must encourage the client to go beyond the bounds of the therapy session and include real-life homework assignments and different forms of bibliotherapy (reading materials, see later in this chapter) to accompany the intervention. In addition, the therapist must convince the client not only that the client is competent and capable of change but also that the therapist is capable of helping him or her to achieve change.

The social worker must help the client establish specific but limited goals. The social work profession has long realized the importance of goal setting. With the advent of managed care, however, operationally and behaviorally defining goals is increasingly emphasized. Social workers must establish an atmosphere in which goals and the specific objectives for meeting them are viewed as realistic, obtainable, and measurable. In this environment a written or oral contract may be prepared to describe a mutual agreement to achieve specified objectives (Hepworth & Larsen, 1993). Finally, the social worker establishes time limits for the duration of treatment (usually agreed on in the first session) that are specifically identified and contracted. If an extension is needed, it is usually recontracted for only a specific purpose.

# Varieties of STT

The different STTs have developed from a variety of sources. Some were largely derived from particular theories of human behavior (for example, interpersonal psychotherapy, rational emotive behavior therapy); others evolved from empirical research findings that lacked an adequate theoretical formulation but yielded practice applications (such as exposure therapy for anxiety disorders). Additional sources have been practice wisdom and technical eclecticism (such as task-centered practice) and various philosophical perspectives (for example, constructivist therapy, solution-focused therapy). Regardless of their origin, SSTs are focused on producing meaningful changes in the objective and social realities of clients' lives and as such, are amenable to empirical research aimed at investigating the value of these approaches in treating mental disorder, reducing psychosocial problems, and improving client functioning and well-being.

To categorize SSTs is difficult because their assumptions and boundaries blur, sometimes differences are more apparent than real, and superficial similarities mask discordant views. Many treatments not expressly derived from brief therapy turn out to be effective as SSTs. Moreover, the literature on the subject is vast and growing, which makes reviewing the field a complicated task. However, in turning to the literature on brief therapies in mental health, a number of major approaches stand out. This chapter briefly describes those central themes in STTs.

## *INTERPERSONAL PSYCHOTHERAPY*

Interpersonal psychotherapy (IPT) is one of the better-researched forms of STT for mental disorders. A professional social worker, Myrna Weissman, MSW, PhD, was involved in its development (Klerman, Weissman, Rounsaville, & Chevron, 1984). Persons (1993) described the method:

> Interpersonal therapy, which draws upon the ideas of Adolph Meyer, John Bowlby, and Harry Stack Sullivan, emphasizes the importance of the depressed person's interpersonal environment. The goal of treatment is to alleviate symptoms by helping the patient become more effective in dealing with interpersonal losses and stresses. In contrast with more traditional psychodynamic therapies, it is time limited, deals with current—not past—relationships, and is concerned with interpersonal—not intrapsychic—phenomena. (pp. 305–306)

The approach has been used with individual clients, couples, and families. Therapy guidelines in the treatment manual (Klerman et al., 1984) reflect IPT's original formulation as a time-limited outpatient treatment for depressed clients. IPT has fees shown to be effective in controlled studies that have been reviewed and summarized elsewhere (Friedlander, 1993; Weissman, 1994). Clinical manuals have been developed to extend the approach beyond the treatment of depression (Crits-Cristoph & Barber, 1991; Levenson, 1995; Messer & Warren, 1995; Molnos, 1995).

IPT treatment generally addresses the present situation, and a focus on the "here and now" is usually assumed—that is, recent interpersonal events are emphasized, linking the stressful events to the client's current mood. Therapists are seen as active and supportive—a contributing factor to therapeutic gains (Rounsaville et al., 1987).

The IPT process is usually conceptualized as occurring in three phases. In the first phase (usually from one to three sessions), an assessment and intervention plan are devised. Assessment includes a diagnostic evaluation and psychiatric history. Particular attention is paid to changes in relationships proximal to the onset of symptoms. The client's interpersonal situation is highlighted, and focus is directed toward interpersonal problem areas such as grief, role disputes, role transitions, or deficits. Concentrating on one of these interpersonal areas helps the social worker identify problems in the interpersonal and social context that need to be addressed.

The middle phase of treatment is the goal-oriented phase, in which the actual treatment strategy is applied. Treatment is directly related to the identified interpersonal problem. For example, if it is a role dispute or conflict with a significant other, treatment would begin with clarifying the nature of the dispute. Options to resolve the dispute are considered. If resolution does not appear possible, strategies or alternatives to replace it are considered.

In the final phase of treatment, summarization and personal incorporation of therapeutic strategy are highlighted. This will help the client generalize treatment strategies learned in the clinical setting to situations or symptoms that may arise in the future. It is important to note that the therapist cannot expect to solve all the issues involved in an interpersonal conflict. Therefore, at times the elements of treatment are intended to get the client to acknowledge and actively seek changes, although these changes might not be complete by the end of the treatment sessions.

Landmark work on the effectiveness of IPT in the treatment of depression was conducted by the National Institute of Mental Health (NIMH) in the Treatment of Depression Collaborative Research Program (Elkin, 1994). This exhaustive study, the largest and most sophisticated ever undertaken in the evaluation of psychotherapy, examined the relative effectiveness of IPT, cognitive–behavioral treatment, antidepressant medication treatments and clinical management, and placebo medication and clinical management. The results are complex, leading to controversy and debate about their implications (Elkin, 1994; Persons, 1993). Neither form of psychotherapy was as effective as medication, but both STTs (which lasted 16 to 20 sessions) were superior to placebo. According to Persons (1993), "Results of this important study are discouraging for the psychotherapies. Perhaps the placebo condition was a powerful one. However, psychotherapists would like to think that their active treatments, based on specific mechanisms, are more effective than nonspecific placebos" (p. 309).

Apart from the NIMH collaborative project however, several studies have found that IPT is an effective treatment for depressed people (Weissman, 1984; Weissman & Akiskal, 1984; Weissman, Jarrett, & Rush, 1987; Weissman, Klerman, Prusoff, Sholomskas, & Padian, 1981). Weissman and Klerman (1989) have provided a summary of the technique and its supportive evidence, in which they noted, "In two clinical trials with ambulatory nonbipolar major depressives, we have demonstrated that for acute treatment, IPT as compared with nonscheduled treatment was more efficacious for symptom reduction and later for enhancing social functioning, and was about equal to tricyclics for symptom reduction" (p. 1872).

More recent reviews and clinical trials (Frank, 1991; Reynolds et al., 1997; Spinelli, 1997) support the efficacy of IPT as a treatment for some depressed people. Variants of IPT have been developed to treat depression in elderly patients (Miller et al., 1994; Sholomskas, Chevron, Prusoff, & Berry, 1983) and in HIV-positive patients. It also has been used to treat clients who abuse cocaine (Rounsaville, Gawin, & Kebler, 1985). A shorter-term version of IPT, interpersonal counseling (IPC), has been shown to be effective with minor depression (Klerman et al., 1987), with older adults (Mossey et al., 1996), and with cancer patients (Alter et al., 1996).

Training opportunities for acquiring skills in IPT are not yet widely available, which is perhaps the major drawback of this approach. To some extent, however, the available treatment manuals make up for this lack.

## COGNITIVE–BEHAVIORAL THERAPIES

Although it enjoys widespread currency, the term "cognitive–behavioral therapy" (CBT) is actually a misnomer because it is based on the misperception that behavior excludes the phenomenon of cognition. The reality is that for at least 50 years contemporary behaviorism has included cognitive (mental) events as part of its subject matter. For example, B. F. Skinner wrote extensively on such topics as thinking, self-control, self-talk, and emotions (Thyer, 1992). Early behavior therapies, such as systematic desensitization, were concerned with altering pathological affective reactions and the dysfunctional ways in which people talked to themselves. *The Social Work Dictionary* defined *behavior* as "any action or response by an individual, including observable activity, measurable physiological changes, cognitive images, fantasies, and emotions" (Barker, 1995, p. 33).

To contend that traditional mainstream behavior therapy ignored cognition or affect is simply wrong. Instead it attempts to explain or account for overt behavior, affect, and thoughts in terms of one's learning history. This is perhaps the most important theoretical distinction between behavior analysis and therapy and other psychotherapies, most of which rely on some variant of the hypothesis that behavior and affect are caused by what one thinks. The former is an environmental determinism, the latter a mental one (Thyer & Myers, 1997, 1998).

Clinicians and researchers operating from the position that how we think and what we say to ourselves is, to a large extent, a determinant of how we act and what we feel have developed STTs for a wide variety of disorders. Because these so-called cognitive approaches incorporate and extend, but do not repudiate, the learning theory foundations of behavior therapy, they have been collectively labeled as CBTs. Aaron Beck and Albert Ellis stand out as founders of a major school of CBT, as discussed below.

### Beck's Contributions to CBT

Aaron Beck was a psychodynamically trained psychiatrist who, in the 1960s, developed an etiologic theory of depression that led him to apply rather different approaches to its treatment. According to Beck, entering the social world presents events that create the basis for the development of early childhood experiences. These experiences are transformed into what a person believes to be true within certain limits or conditions. The schema that develops is the cognitive structure that organizes experience and behavior (Beck & Freeman, 1990). Schemas involve the ways in which people view certain aspects of their lives, including relationship aspects such as adequacy and the ability of others to love them. Once these schemas have been formulated as part of normal development, the person will be exposed to critical incidents as part of the normal life process. The person will interpret and react to the critical incidents. The resulting reaction will be based on the basic and conditional beliefs that the person has developed and incorporated into his or her schema.

The literature suggests that people develop different styles or patterns of information processing based on their life experiences; these schemas may influence a person's reaction (for example, resulting in cognitive distortion) when he or she interprets a current situation or event (Beck, Rush, Shaw, & Emery, 1979; Burns, 1980). Beck et al. (1979) listed the types of systematic errors that can lead to emotional distress as

- *Arbitrary inferences*—Conclusions are not based on accurate supporting evidence.
- *Selective abstractions*—One or more details in a situation are taken out of context, and the more pronounced features of the incident or situation are ignored.
- *Overgeneralization*—A global generalization is drawn from a single and possibly isolated incident.
- *Magnification and minimization*—What has happened is distorted, inappropriately representing the magnitude of what has actually transpired.
- *Personalization*—A person relates external events to himself or herself without any basis for doing so.
- *Absolutist, dichotomous thinking*—Experiences are perceived in an intense and possibly polarized manner.

In Beckian CBT, treatment involves four stages: (1) establishing a therapeutic alliance and rationale, (2) teaching the client how to self-monitor dysfunctional thoughts, (3) teaching the client to test automatic thoughts and silent assumptions, and (4) involving the client in homework assignments related to tracking and disputing dysfunctional thoughts. Typically Beck's CBT is a short-term (less than 20 sessions) program, initially held weekly and then less often. In a comprehensive overview of dozens controlled clinical trials of this short-term treatment, Jarrett and Rush (1989) concluded that "Beck's cognitive therapy is more effective than no treatment and is *at least* as effective as antidepressant medication in the treatment of nonpsychotic, nonbipolar depressed outpatients. While some patients preferentially benefit from a combination of medication plus cognitive therapy, this combination is not always more effective than cognitive therapy alone" (p. 1845).

CBTs based on Beck's model were among the earliest psychosocial treatments subjected to rigorous randomized, controlled clinical trials in the treatment of depression. Beck's approach also has been extended with favorable results to the treatment of clients with anxiety disorders, personality disorders, and substance abuse problems (Beck, 1993; Beck, Emery, & Greenberg, 1985; Beck & Freeman, 1990; Beck, Wright, Newman, & Leise, 1993), suggesting that this particular variant of CBT may have wide applicability for clinical social work in mental health.

## Ellis's Contributions to CBT

Albert Ellis is a clinical psychologist, also traditionally trained, who in the 1950s developed a form of brief therapy he called Rational Emotive Therapy (RET, recently retitled Rational Emotive Behavior Therapy (REBT), in recognition of its historic roots as a behavioral therapy (Ellis, 1993). Based on the extensive research literature, Ellis (1996) concluded that REBT results in lasting emotional and behavioral change in clients. A large number of controlled studies evaluating REBT have been published (reviewed in Lyons & Woods, 1991). The approach has developed into an institution in psychotherapy, with its own training institute, certification programs, and journal. REBT has been effectively and popularly applied to school and behavior problems in children. Several self-help books also have been published that use

REBT to assist the person in self-treatment of depression and dysfunctional relationships, among other problems. Although the REBT approach enjoys considerable evidence of effectiveness for selected disorders, the record is spotty. For example, cognitive therapies alone seem to be ineffective in the treatment of agoraphobia or specific phobias, have not been tested with generalized anxiety disorder, and have yielded mixed results with sexual disorders (Emmelkamp, 1994).

Overall, however, REBT is well worth exploring for use with a wide range of clients and client problems. Although RET has been discussed in the social work literature for more than 30 years (Werner, 1965, 1982), there do not appear to be any outcome studies conducted by social workers themselves that apply REBT as a single STT for clients experiencing serious psychosocial problems.

There can be some difficulty in discriminating between the theory and practice of Beckian CBT and of Ellis's REBT. Such distinctions have eluded some of the finest thinkers in psychotherapeutic theory. For practical purposes, both possess a substantial theoretical foundation, have produced well-proceduralized treatments, and seem to be effective for a number of serious problems. Time and empirical research will sort out any meaningful commonalities and differences.

## Other Short-term CBTs

Exposure therapy (ET) is among the more "behavioral" short-term CBTs, and it has been widely and effectively applied to a variety of serious behavioral and affective disorders. First developed as a treatment for specific and social phobias, ET has been shown to be an important element in therapy for people with panic disorder, agoraphobia, obsessive–compulsive disorder, posttraumatic stress disorder, morbid grief, and pathological jealousy. ET may be a useful treatment if a client experiences dysfunctional avoidance behavior, upsetting thoughts, or disturbed affect when exposed to situations that are in themselves harmless but may have been associated with pain, injury, or anxiety in the past. The social worker attempts to recreate the anxiety-evoking stimuli that upset the client and arrange for graduated exposure to these situations, thoughts, or circumstances, maintaining a balance between boredom and intolerable terror. Because there are concerns with maintaining and generalizing treatment gains, ET is preferably conducted in real-life contexts, with exposure in imagination reserved for circumstances that are impractical or impossible to reproduce in actuality. Detailed treatment protocols are available to help therapists assess clients for the suitability of ET and to design, conduct, and evaluate treatment (Marks, 1987; Thyer, 1987). Figure 10-1 lists selected disorders and corresponding citations of one or more well-controlled outcome studies pertaining to ET's effectiveness. Although the results of ET can vary considerably, it is usually a highly reliable technique that yields substantial improvements in a large number of clients. Dramatic effects in just one treatment session have been well documented. In one study of such exceedingly brief treatment, 20 patients received a single session of real-life ET (lasting about two hours) for the treatment of a specific phobia. At four-year follow-up, 90 percent remained much improved or were completely recovered (Ost, 1989).

A related, fairly new STT is Eye Movement Desensitization and Reprocessing (EMDR) therapy. Since its inception about 10 years ago (Shapiro, 1989), EMDR has been subjected to an impressive amount of controlled research on its effectiveness as a treatment for selected anxiety-related problems such as posttraumatic stress disorder (reviewed in Colosetti & Bordnick, 1997). EMDR seems like a

FIGURE **10-1**

### Selected Disorders for Which Exposure Therapy Can Be an Effective Short-term Treatment

| DISORDER | CITATION |
|---|---|
| Specific phobia | Marks (1987), Ost (1989) |
| Social phobia | Marks (1987) |
| Panic disorder | Barlow & Cerny (1988) |
| Agoraphobia | Jansson & Ost (1982) |
| Obsessive–compulsive disorder | Steketee, Foa, & Grayson (1982) |
| Posttraumatic stress disorder | Foa, Riggs, Danev, & Rothbaum (1991) |
| Morbid grief | Artelt & Thyer (1998) |
| Pathological jealousy | Cobb & Marks (1979) |

variant of exposure therapy—in imagination—to anxiety-evoking stimuli. There are some procedural differences and added elements, however, such as the distinctive waving of the therapist's finger back and forth at the client, who tracks it with his or her eyes (Shapiro, 1989, 1995). Several conclusions can be drawn from the literature to date (Acierno, Hersen, Van Hasselt, Tremont, & Mueser, 1994; Lohr, Kleinknecht, Tolin, & Barrett, 1995):

- Clients receiving EMDR report considerable therapeutic benefits that people not in treatment do not experience.
- The theory that EMDR is based on seems completely erroneous.
- The use of techniques to track external stimuli (such as finger waving and finger tapping) considered crucial to the procedure has been shown to be irrelevant to its success.
- EMDR has not been shown to be superior to credible placebo treatments.
- EMDR has not been shown to be superior to conventional exposure therapy.

Otherwise, more recent studies also have indicated that EMDR is not superior to placebo treatments (Colosetti & Thyer, 1997; Dunn, Schwartz, Hatfield, & Wiegele, 1996). The EMDR approach is mentioned here only because it has received an immense amount of publicity in the popular media and has generated a large number of outcome studies. These outcome studies have been improving in methodological rigor, and it is possible that EMDR will emerge as a superior version of ET. At present, however, this conclusion would be premature. The authors *do not* recommend that social workers undertake the substantial costs in time and money required to become an "approved" EMDR therapist until empirical research supports such efforts.

## TASK-CENTERED PRACTICE

Task-centered practice (TCP) is a relatively short-term treatment developed by social workers and is unusual in that it has been empirically tested in seven controlled studies, numerous additional uncontrolled trials, single-case studies, and demonstration projects (reviewed in Reid, 1997). The focus in TCP is helping the client operationally define problems and the steps necessary to overcome or cope with them.

The social worker assists the client with developing ways to work on specified extra-therapeutic tasks, which are the critical area of change (instead of intrapsychic maturation occurring during treatment sessions). Largely originated by William Reid, working with a number of social work colleagues and students over the past two decades, TCP is a highly empirically based approach to brief treatment—that is, it incorporates therapies with credible scientific evidence of efficacy as well as advocates for the systematic collection of valid data to help evaluate the outcomes of treatment with both individual and larger groups of clients. As described by Reid (1975), TCP is

> a short-term, time-limited form of practice designed to help individuals and families with specific psycho-social problems. The practitioner and client are expected to reach an explicit agreement on the particular problems to be dealt with and the probable duration of service (generally from 8 to 12 sessions within a two to four month period). (p. 3)

Figure 10-2 presents selected client problems and the controlled studies documenting the effectiveness of TCP in resolving them. As a disciplinary endeavor, TCP is a model of practice in which social workers can take some pride, and Reid and coworkers deserve much credit for persevering in this line of research for more than two decades. Moreover, TCP is constantly expanding in its applications to more types of problems (Naleppa & Reid, 1998). As an eclectic approach, it enjoys the benefit of a broad array of empirically supported intervention, but at the expense of theoretical consistency. Some social work professionals consider TCP to be simply an attenuated form of behaviorism, a view endorsed, with qualifications, by Gambrill (1994) but repudiated by Reid (1995). Certainly it is clear that TCP relies heavily on behavioral therapies and principles. Isolating the critical components of this model will be challenging because of the plethora of interventions and theoretical approaches it incorporates. Regardless, TCP is a social work–derived approach to brief treatment that is widely used and has at least a modest degree of empirical support.

FIGURE **10-2**

| **Selected Client Problems That Have Been Effectively Addressed by Task-Centered Practice** | |
|---|---|
| **PROBLEM** | **CITATION** |
| Parasuicide | Gibbons, Bow, & Butler (1985) <br> Gibbons, Butler, Urwin, & Gibbons (1978) |
| Delinquency | Larsen & Mitchell (1980) |
| Chronic mental illness | Newcome (1985) |
| Problems in school | Reid (1975, 1978) <br> Reid, Epstein, Brown, Tolson, & Rooney (1980) |
| Problems of adult mental health clients | Reid (1975, 1978) |
| Poor grades | Reid & Bailey-Dempsey (1995) <br> Reid, Bailey-Dempsey, Cain, Cook, & Burchard (1994) |
| Truancy | Reid & Bailey-Dempsey (1995) <br> Reid, Bailey-Dempsey, Cain, Cook, & Burchard (1994) |

SOURCE: Derived from Reid, W. (1997). Research on task-centered practice. *Social Work Research, 21,* 132–137.

## SOLUTION-FOCUSED THERAPY

In solution-focused therapy, it is assumed that clients already have the skills they need to address their problems and are capable of change (deShazer, 1985). Finding possible solutions to a problem rather than specifically solving it is emphasized. Little emphasis is placed on recognizing or establishing the cause or actual function of the problem, because change can occur without this link (O'Hanlon & Weiner-Davis, 1989). Pathology is not stressed, and as Fanger (1995) stated, "Learning to be the person you want to be is quite different—and often less time consuming—than learning why you are the way you are" (p. 88).

The therapist is active in helping the client find and identify strengths and existing functional patterns of behavior. A dialogue of "change talk" rather than "problem talk" is created (Walter & Peller, 1992). The problem is viewed positively, emphasizing patterns of change that may be successful for the client. Positive aspects of and exceptions to the problem are explored, a process that allows alternate views of the problem to develop. Once the small changes have been achieved, the client becomes empowered to elicit larger ones (O'Hanlon & Weiner-Davis, 1989; Walter & Peller, 1992). To adapt a solution-based approach to short-term practice, the social worker should consider these steps:

1. Create a hopeful atmosphere while eliciting the client's definition of the problem.
2. Establish what the client's desired outcome is.
3. Analyze and develop solutions.
4. Develop and implement a plan of action.
5. Assist with termination and follow-up issues, if needed.

Few published studies empirically validate solution-focused therapy. Scientifically credible evidence from controlled, single-system research designs and, ultimately, randomized, controlled clinical trials are required to demonstrate the effectiveness of solution-focused brief treatments in ameliorating mental disorders of clients seen by social workers (Araoz & Carrese, 1996).

## CONSTRUCTIVIST THERAPY

The development of solution-focused therapy and the introduction of constructivist models of treatment are part of a paradigm shift in psychotherapy in general (Franklin & Jordan, 1997; Neimeyer, 1993). Some constructivist theorists have suggested that traditional methods of scientific research and evaluation are not compatible with the postmodern ontological and epistemological views of constructivism, and they have been reluctant to undertake conventionally designed outcome studies of this approach to treatment. Proponents of the method readily acknowledge that no well-controlled studies have demonstrated any evidence of treatment effectiveness of the constructivist therapies (Neimeyer, 1993; Neimeyer & Mahoney, 1995), despite some promising preliminary information gathered from case studies (Durrant, 1990; Gallant, 1994; White, 1986).

Some researchers, however, have attempted to bridge this philosophical divide between the traditional scientists and the postmodernists by using single-subject experimental designs to examine clinical outcomes. For example, Besa (1994) published a multiple-baseline evaluation of narrative therapy provided to several families. More studies of this type are needed to provide the empirical justification necessary to subject constructivist methods to larger-scale controlled evaluations. If these approaches can produce meaningful improvements in clients lives, then such effects are potentially measurable and amenable to quantitative research.

## BIBLIOTHERAPY AND ITS VARIATIONS

To the extent that psychotherapies are grounded in scientific principles that can be effectively communicated to others, the potential exists to format treatment techniques in such an intelligible manner that clients themselves can, through their own reading, undertake at least some elements of effective treatment themselves. This is the guiding principle behind the development of so-called bibliotherapies (BTs) (self-help books) (Rosen, 1987). Contemporary self-help books constructed along these lines differ sharply from their popular predecessors in that they are grounded in previous empirical research and have been empirically evaluated in terms of their effectiveness at helping clients help themselves.

Many mental health problems are addressed by current self-help books, and one by Clum (1990) will illustrate the genre. *Coping with Panic: A Drug-Free Approach to Dealing with Anxiety Attacks* describes contemporary cognitive–behavioral practice techniques for clients who meet the criteria for panic disorder. Much of the book is psychoeducational in nature, telling the reader what is known about panic disorder and how they can overcome it. Among the treatment elements taught are client self-exposure to anxiety-evoking situations, training in proper breathing and relaxation skills, and instruction in coping by use of effective self-talk. This work goes beyond the realm of a general-interest publication, however, because the author has empirically tested the outcomes of using it. Gould, Clum, and Shapiro (1993) randomly assigned 31 clients to a waiting list (WL); to bibliotherapy (BT) with Clum's self-help book; or to individual, office-based behavior therapy (OBBT). Therapist contact (for assessment only) was 2.5 hours for WL clients, 3.0 hours for BT clients, and more than 10 hours for OBBT clients. On average, WL clients did not improve, but BT and OBBT clients improved statistically and clinically. Moreover, BT and OBBT clients showed about the same results. These results were replicated in Gould and Clum (1995). This finding suggests that depending on the outcome of clinical assessment, many clients with panic disorder may benefit greatly from Clum's short-term BT. Barlow and Cerny's *Psychological Treatment of Panic* (1988) also has been shown in clinical trials to help such clients (Barlow, Craske, Cerny, & Klosko, 1989). In addition, Marks's *Living with Fear* (1978) was found to be effective with a mixed sample of clients with panic disorder, specific phobias, and obsessive–compulsive disorder (Greist, Marks, Berlin, Gournay, & Noshirvani, 1980).

Self-help books based on empirically substantiated treatment methods and written by social workers include *When Once Is Not Enough* (Steketee & White, 1990) for obsessive–compulsive disorder and Seagrave and Covington's *Free from Fears* (1987) for panic disorder and agoraphobia. Seagrave and Covington also have produced a commercially available STT program on audiotapes called CHAANGE (Center for Help for Agoraphobia/Anxiety through New Growth Experiences). The CHAANGE program has yet been subjected to a systematic evaluation of clinical efficacy, which would be a promising line of research.

Steketee and White's (1990) self-help book has recently been tested by Fritzler, Hecker, and Losee (1997). Treatment involved readings from *When Once Is Not Enough* and five meetings with therapists over 12 weeks. Posttreatment assessment

FIGURE **10-3**

| **Examples of Self-help Resources with Demonstrated Efficacy in Short-term Treatment of Selected Mental Health Problems** | |
|---|---|
| **DISORDER** | **CITATION** |
| Heavy drinking | Barber & Gilbertson (in press) |
| | Miller & Munoz (1982) |
| | Hester & Delaney (1997) |
| Obsessive–compulsive disorder | Fritzler, Hecker, & Losee (1997) |
| | Steketee & White (1990) |
| Panic disorder and agoraphobia | Barlow & Cerny (1988) |
| | Clum (1990) |
| | Ghosh, Marks, & Carr (1984) |
| | Gould & Clum (1995) |
| | Gould, Clum, & Shapiro (1993) |
| Specific and social phobias | Marks (1978) |
| Depression | Selmi, Klein, & Greist (1982) |
| | Selmi, Klein, Greist, Sorrell, & Erdman (1990) |
| Smoking cessation | Schneider (1986) |
| | Schneider, Walter, & O'Donnell (1990) |
| Child noncompliance | Dangel & Polster (1984) |
| Weight loss | Stuart (1978) |

took place three weeks after the fifth session. Twelve clients were assigned to delayed or immediate treatment. Delayed clients showed no improvement, although the treated clients did. Delayed clients who were later treated improved similarly to those who received immediate treatment. In social work practice this self-help manual could be used as a primary treatment, or at least as a useful adjunct treatment, for some clients suffering from obsessive–compulsive disorder.

Selected examples of self-help STTs for some specific mental disorders are presented in Figure 10-3. This is by no means a comprehensive listing, but it serves to illustrate the growing empirical foundations for the provision of STT by self-help.

## *STTs AND TECHNOLOGY*

Developments in computer and audiovisual technology brought about a number of interesting variations of STT. Computers, virtual-reality (VR) devices, and videotaped instructional methods are all affecting the delivery of brief therapies. For example, Ghosh, Marks, and Carr (1984) randomly assigned 71 patients with agoraphobia to receive either bibliotherapy (BT) using Marks's self-help book (1978), similar content delivered by computer (CT), or therapist-guided exposure therapy (ET). Blind assessments were used at the conclusion of treatment and at six-month follow-up. Nearly all patients showed considerable improvement at the end of the study, and these gains were maintained at six months. The number of dropouts was low and equivalent across treatment groups. The average amount of therapist time spent with each client was 40 minutes for the BT group, 4.2 hours for the CT condition, and 3.2 hours in ET. CT and ET patients had from three to 10 treatment sessions of an hour or less in duration.

Hester and Delaney (1997) evaluated a computerized version of a self-help manual (Miller & Munoz, 1982) for heavy drinkers. Forty clients assigned to immediate or delayed treatment received pre- and posttreatment assessments of their drinking (by use of reliable and valid measures). People who received the computer-based brief treatment (eight sessions of 15 to 45 minutes each over 10 weeks) significantly reduced their drinking, but the delayed group did not. After they began STT, however, the delayed group showed similar substantial reductions in alcohol consumption.

The relative advantages of brief treatment mediated through reading a book, compared with interacting with a computer, remain to be determined. However, the observation that substantial therapist contact is not essential to successful clinical outcomes supports the hypothesis that it is the psychosocial principles underlying the treatments, rather than nonspecific interpersonal factors, that are responsible for the results.

VR refers to software that depicts real or fantasy environments in which the viewer (using a headset that covers the eyes) can partially interact. For example, turning one's head causes the scene to shift in the direction of the turn. VR makes possible the recreation of anxiety-evoking stimuli that are difficult to arrange in real life. Rothbaum and colleagues (1995b) reported a case study, with credible pre- and posttreatment outcome measures, of one client with severe acrophobia. The study described an ET procedure that used VR technology to convey the sense of standing at a great height. Treatments were twice weekly for three weeks, for a total of five sessions. Meaningful clinical improvements were found on the outcome measures as well as on measures of the client's ability to ascend previously avoided high places in real life.

Rothbaum and collaborators (1995a) also reported on a controlled trial of this technique, which involved 17 clients with acrophobia who were randomly assigned to immediate treatment (graduated exposure by use of VR technology) or to a waiting list. With seven sessions of 35 to 45 minutes each over eight weeks, the treated clients improved, but the clients on the waiting list did not, as shown by several valid outcome measures. Before treatment, the two groups had been equivalent.

More prosaic perhaps, but very effective, is the parent-training video program WINNING!, which was developed by two social workers. Designed with the help of extensive consumer input, the 22-lesson program teaches parents effective child management skills that are generalizable across a wide array of problem areas, including those found in the conditions of oppositional defiant disorder and conduct disorder. Thousands of families from diverse backgrounds and socioeconomic levels have participated in the WINNING! program. Multiple outcome studies conducted by the developers of the program (Dangel & Polster, 1984) have demonstrated that this video training program is effective in teaching parents effective child management skills and reducing inappropriate child behavior. The program is favorably rated by parents themselves, dropouts have been low, and cost-effectiveness is high. It has been adopted by social services agencies in 40 states, and it represents an outstanding example of an effective, social work–designed STT with preventive elements as well as ameliorative ones.

Contemporary technology will have an increasing impact on the delivery of mental health services and will augment the effectiveness of existing brief treatments. Computer software developed by social workers and others is available to assist in the assessment process (see, for example, the Computer Assisted Social

Services software included in Bloom, Fischer, & Orme, 1995), treatment planning (Polk, 1997), and the conduct of STT (Bloom, 1992a; Hester & Delaney, 1997).

## Conclusion

Therapists' interest in STT has greatly increased and will probably continue to increase over the years (Bolter, Levenson, & Alverez, 1990). A planned STT format for treatment appears to be both a viable and an essential practice modality for social workers in today's managed care environment. Health maintenance organizations and employee assistance programs generally favor highly structured, brief forms of therapy, and as these organizations and programs continue to grow, so will use of the short-term models they support (Wells, 1994).

The existing research base for STTs is large, but a number of critical lacunae remain. Randomized controlled clinical trials of SSTs have typically been conducted under some form of sponsored research support, with clear inclusionary and exclusionary patient criteria; well-trained therapists who are carefully supervised; and fairly homogeneous, mostly white clients. The generalizability of such outcome studies to practice in the real worlds of private practice, managed care, and agency-based services, which involve clients with multiple diagnoses and members of all racial and ethnic minority groups, remains largely unknown. Replications and extensions of effectiveness trials under more naturalistic practice settings are urgently needed to augment the evidentiary foundations of brief treatments.

Meanwhile, the need for STTs has been clearly established. Models with demonstrated effectiveness, such as some of those presented in this chapter, appear to be both the present and future of social work practice in the managed care environment. The use of long-term psychotherapies in our current practice environment is coming to a close (Thyer, 1994). Apart from the external contingencies imposed by managed care, ethical standards pertaining to a client's right to effective treatment are evolving (Myers & Thyer, 1997). When empirical research indicates that a given psychosocial treatment is effective in helping clients with particular problems, the view that social workers and other clinicians should be obligated to provide these supported treatments as first-choice interventions is becoming more widely accepted. Take, as a practical example, nonpsychotic depression. CBT has been shown to be an effective psychosocial treatment for this problem, but solution-focused treatment has not. Therefore, social workers treating depressed clients should learn and apply CBT and provide other, less supported interventions only if the first-choice treatments do not work (after a legitimate trial of their efficacy). This view was recently codified by the federal Agency for Health Care Policy and Research (Depression Guideline Panel, 1993): "Since it has not been established that all forms of psychotherapy are equally effective in major depressive disorder, if one is chosen as the sole treatment, it should have been studied in randomized controlled trials. . . . long-term therapies are not currently indicated as first-line acute phase treatments for patients with major depressive disorder" (p. 84).

In the field of psychiatry, Klerman (1990) asserted, "The psychiatrist has a responsibility to use effective treatment. The patient has a right to the proper treatment. Proper treatment involves those treatments for which there is substantial evidence" (p. 417). Social worker Leslie Tutty (1990) endorsed a similar view: "It is important to provide the most effective treatment available" (p. 13).

Providing empirically supported treatments does not guarantee that clients will be helped, but it would increase the likelihood of therapeutic benefits. The standard need not be inflexible: If a clinician can provide a plausible reason why an otherwise first-choice treatment should not be used, then alternative therapies may well be justifiable.

Many available STTs have shown scientific evidence of efficacy. The use of time-limited treatment, mutually negotiated goals and objectives, empirically based treatments, and careful clinical assessments taken before and during treatment are becoming part of responsible mental health practice. This is not only what managed care agencies expect, it also is what social work clients rightfully deserve.

# References

Acierno, R., Hersen, M., Van Hasselt, V., Tremont, G., & Mueser, K. (1994). Review of the validation and dissemination of eye movement desensitization and reprocessing: A scientific and ethical dilemma. *Clinical Psychology Review, 14,* 287–299.

Alter, C. L., Fleishman, S. B., Kornblith, A. B., Holland, J. C., Biano, D., Levenson, R., Vinciguerra, V., & Rai, K. R. (1996). Supportive telephone intervention for patients receiving chemotherapy: A pilot study. *Psychosomatics, 37,* 425–431.

Araoz, D. L., & Carrese, M. A. (1996). *Solution-oriented brief therapy for adjustment disorders.* New York: Brunner/Mazel.

Artelt, T., & Thyer, B. A. (1998). Treating chronic grief. In J. S. Wodarski & B. A. Thyer (Eds.), *Handbook of empirical social work* (Vol. 2, Psychosocial Problems, pp. 341–356). New York: John Wiley & Sons.

Barber, J. G., & Gilbertson, R. (in press). Evaluation of a self-help manual for the female partners of heavy drinkers. *Research on Social Work Practice.*

Barker, R. L. (1995). *The social work dictionary* (3rd ed.). Washington, DC: NASW Press.

Barlow, D. H., & Cerny, J. A. (1988). *Psychological treatment of panic.* New York: Guilford Press.

Barlow, D. H., Craske, M. G., Cerny, J. A., & Klosko, J. S. (1989). Behavioral treatment of panic disorder. *Behavior Therapy, 20,* 261–282.

Beck, A. T. (1993). Cognitive therapy: Past, present, and future. *Journal of Consulting and Clinical Psychology, 61,* 194–198.

Beck, A. T., Emery, G., & Greenberg, R. L. (1985). *Anxiety disorders and phobias: A cognitive perspective.* New York: Basic Books.

Beck, A. T., & Freeman, A. (1990). *Cognitive therapy of personality disorders.* New York: Guilford Press.

Beck, A. T., Rush, A. J., Shaw, B. F., & Emery, G. (1979). *Cognitive therapy of depression.* New York: Guilford Press.

Beck, A. T., Wright, F. D., Newman, C. F., & Leise, B. S. (1993). *Cognitive therapy of substance abuse.* New York: Guilford Press.

Besa, D. (1994). Evaluating narrative family therapy: Using single-system research designs. *Research on Social Work Practice, 4,* 309–325.

Bloom, B. L. (1992a). Computer-assisted psychological intervention: A review of the empirical literature. *Clinical Psychology Review, 12,* 169–197.

Bloom, B. L. (1992b). Planned short-term psychotherapy: Current status and future challenges. *Applied and Preventive Psychology, 1,* 157–164.

Bloom, M., Fischer, J., & Orme, J. (1995). *Evaluating practice: Guidelines for the accountable professional* (2nd ed.). Needham Heights, MA: Allyn & Bacon.

Bolter, K., Levenson, H., & Alverez, W. (1990). Differences in values between short-term and long-term therapists. *Professional Psychology, 21,* 285–290.

Budman, S., & Gurman, A. (1988). *Theory and practice of brief therapy.* New York: Guilford Press.

Burns, D. D. (1980). *Feeling good.* New York: William Morrow.

Clum, G. (1990). *Coping with panic: A drug-free approach to dealing with anxiety attacks.* Pacific Grove, CA: Brooks/Cole.

Cobb, J. P., & Marks, I. M. (1979). Morbid jealousy featuring as obsessive–compulsive neurosis: Treatment by behavioural psychotherapy. *British Journal of Psychiatry, 134,* 301–305.

Colosetti, S. D., & Bordnick, P. S. (1997). Should clinical social workers support "eye movement desensitization and reprocessing" (EMDR) therapy? In B. A. Thyer (Ed.), *Controversial issues in social work practice* (pp. 56–69). Needham Heights, MA: Allyn & Bacon.

Colosetti, S. D., & Thyer, B. A. (1997). *The relative effectiveness of EMDR versus relaxation training with battered women prisoners.* Unpublished manuscript.

Crits-Christoph, P., & Barber, J. P. (1991). *Handbook of short-term dynamic psychotherapy.* New York: Basic Books.

Dangel, R. F., & Polster, R. A. (1984). WINNING!: A systematic, empirical approach to parent training. In R. F. Dangel & R. A. Polster (Eds.), *Parent training* (pp. 162–201). New York: Guilford Press.

Depression Guideline Panel. (1993). *Clinical practice guideline number 5: Depression in primary care, 2: Treatment of major depression.* Rockville, MD: U.S. Department of Health and Human Services, Agency for Health Care Policy and Research.

deShazer, S. (1985). *Keys to solution in brief therapy.* New York: W. W. Norton.

Dunn, T. M., Schwartz, M., Hatfield, R. W., & Wiegele, M. (1996). Measuring effectiveness of eye movement desensitization and reprocessing (EMDR) in non-clinical anxiety: A multi-subject, yoked control design. *Journal of Behavior Therapy and Experimental Psychiatry, 27,* 231–239.

Durrant, M. (1990). Saying "Boo" to Mr. Scary: Writing a book provides a solution. *Family Therapy Case Studies, 5,* 39–44.

Dziegielewski, S. F. (1996). Managed care principles: The need for social work in the health care environment. *Crisis Intervention and Time-Limited Treatment, 3,* 97–110.

Elkin, I. (1994). The NIMH treatment of depression collaborative research program: Where we began and where we are. In A. E. Bergin & S. L. Garfield (Eds.), *Handbook of psychotherapy and behavior change* (4th ed., pp. 114–139). New York: John Wiley & Sons.

Ellis, A. (1993). Changing Rational Emotive Therapy (RET) to Rational Emotive Behavior Therapy (REBT). *Behavior Therapist, 16*(10), 1–2.

Ellis, A. (1996). *Better, deeper, and more enduring brief therapy: The rational emotive behavior therapy approach.* New York: Brunner/Mazel.

Emmelkamp, P.M.G. (1994). Behavior therapy with adults. In A. E. Bergin & S. L. Garfield (Eds.), *Handbook of psychotherapy and behavior change* (4th ed., pp. 379–427). New York: John Wiley & Sons.

Epstein, L. (1995). Brief task-centered practice. In R. L. Edwards (Ed.-in-Chief), *Encyclopedia of social work* (19th ed., Vol. 1, pp. 313–323). Washington, DC: NASW Press.

Fanger, M. T. (1995). Brief therapies. In R. L. Edwards (Ed.-in-Chief), *Encyclopedia of social work* (19th ed., Vol. 1, pp. 323–334). Washington, DC: NASW Press.

Fischer, J. (1973). Is casework effective? A review. *Social Work, 18,* 5–20.

Fischer, J. (1976). *The effectiveness of social casework.* Springfield, IL: Charles C. Thomas.

Foa, E. B., Riggs, D. S., Danev, C. V., & Rothbaum, B. O. (1991). Treatment of post-traumatic stress disorder in rape victims: Comparison between cognitive–behavioral approaches and counseling. *Journal of Consulting and Clinical Psychology, 59,* 715–723.

Frank, E. (1991). Interpersonal psychotherapy as a maintenance treatment for patients with recurrent depression. *Psychotherapy, 28,* 259–266.

Franklin, C., & Jordan, C. (1997). Does constructivist therapy offer anything new to social work practice? In B. A. Thyer (Ed.), *Controversial issues in social work practice* (pp. 16–28). Needham Heights, MA: Allyn & Bacon.

Friedlander, M. L. (1993). Does complimentarity promote or hinder client change in brief therapy: A review of the evidence from two theoretical perspectives. *Counseling Psychologist, 21,* 457–486.

Fritzler, B. K., Hecker, J. E., & Losee, M. C. (1997). Self-directed treatment with minimal therapist contact: Preliminary findings for obsessive–compulsive disorder. *Behaviour Research and Therapy, 35,* 627–631.

Gallant, J. P. (1994). New ideas for the school social worker in the counseling of children and families. *Social Work in Education, 15,* 119–128.

Gambrill, E. (1994). What's in a name? Task-centered, empirical, and behavioral practice. *Social Service Review, 68,* 578–599.

Ghosh, A., Marks, I. M., & Carr, A. C. (1984). Controlled study of self-exposure treatment for phobics: Preliminary communication. *Journal of the Royal Society of Medicine, 77,* 483–487.

Gibbons, J., Bow, I., & Butler, J. (1985). Task-centered social work after parasuicide. In E. Goldberg, J. Gibbons, & I. Sinclair (Eds.), *Problems, tasks and outcomes: The evaluation of task-centered casework in three settings* (pp. 169–257). Boston: Allen & Unwin.

Gibbons, J. S., Butler, J., Urwin, P., & Gibbons, J. L. (1978). Evaluation of a social work service for self-poisoning parents. *British Journal of Psychiatry, 133,* 111–118.

Gorey, K. M. (1996). Effectiveness of social work intervention research: Internal versus external evaluations. *Social Work Research, 20,* 119–128.

Gorey, K. M., Thyer, B. A., & Pawluck, D. E. (in press). Differential effectiveness of prevalent social work practice models. *Social Work.*

Gould, R. A., & Clum, G. A. (1995). Self-help plus minimal therapist contact in the treatment of panic disorder: A replication and extension. *Behavior Therapy, 26,* 533–546.

Gould, R. A., Clum, G. A., & Shapiro, D. (1993). The use of bibliotherapy in the treatment of panic. *Behavior Therapy, 24,* 241–252.

Greist, J. H., Marks, I. M., Berlin, F., Gournay, K., & Noshirvani, H. (1980). Avoidance versus confrontation of fear. *Behavior Therapy, 11,* 1–14.

Hepworth, D. H., & Larsen, J. (1993). *Direct social work practice.* Pacific Grove, CA: Brooks/Cole.

Hester, R. K., & Delaney, H. S. (1997). Behavioral self-control program for Windows: Results of a controlled clinical trial. *Journal of Consulting and Clinical Psychology, 65,* 686–693.

Jansson, L., & Ost, L-G. (1982). Behavioral methods for agoraphobia: An evaluative review. *Clinical Psychology Review, 2,* 311–336.

Jarrett, R. B., & Rush, A. J. (1989). Cognitive–behavioral psychotherapy for depression. In American Psychiatric Association (Ed.), *Treatments for psychiatric disorders* (pp. 1834–1846). Washington, DC: American Psychiatric Association.

Klerman, G. L. (1990). The psychiatric patient's right to effective treatment: Implications of *Osheroff v. Chestnut Lodge. American Journal of Psychiatry, 147,* 409–418.

Klerman, G. L., Budman, S., Berwick, D., Weissman, M. M., Damico-White, J., Demby, A., & Feldstein, M. (1987). Efficacy of a brief psychosocial intervention for symptoms of stress and distress among patients in primary care. *Medical Care, 25,* 1078–1088.

Klerman, G. L., Weissman, M. M., Rounsaville, B. J., & Chevron, E. S. (1984). *Interpersonal psychotherapy for depression.* New York: Basic Books.

Koss, M. P., & Shiang, J. (1994). Research on brief therapy. In A. E Bergin & S. L. Garfield (Eds.), *Handbook of psychotherapy and behavior change* (4th ed., pp. 664–700). New York: John Wiley & Sons.

Larsen, J., & Mitchell, C. (1980). Task-centered strength-oriented group work with delinquents. *Social Casework, 61,* 154–163.

Levenson, H. (1995). *Time-limited dynamic psychotherapy.* New York: Basic Books.

Lohr, J., Kleinknecht, R. A., Tolin, D. F., & Barrett, R. H. (1995). The empirical status of the clinical application of Eye Movement Desensitization and Reprocessing. *Journal of Behavior Therapy and Experimental Psychiatry, 26,* 285–302.

Lyons, L. C., & Woods, P. J. (1991). The efficacy of rational–emotive therapy: A quantitative review of the outcome research. *Clinical Psychology Review, 11,* 357–370.

Marks, I. M. (1978). *Living with fear.* New York: McGraw-Hill.

Marks, I. M. (1987). *Fears, phobias, and rituals.* New York: Oxford University Press.

Messer, S. B., & Warren, C. S. (1995). *Models of brief psychodynamic therapy: A comparative approach.* New York: Guilford Press.

Miller, M. D., Frank, E., Cornes, C., Imber, S., Anderson, B., Ehrenpreis, L., Malloy, J., Silberman, R., Wolfson, L., Zaltman, J., & Reynolds, C. F. (1994). Applying interpersonal psychotherapy to bereavement-related depression following loss of a spouse in late life. *Journal of Psychotherapy Practice and Research, 3,* 149–162.

Miller, W. R., & Munoz, R. F. (1982). *How to control your drinking* (rev. ed.). (Available from CASAA Research Division, Department of Psychology, University of New Mexico, Albuquerque, NM 87131.)

Molnos, A. (1995). *A question of time: Essentials of brief dynamic psychotherapy.* London: Karnac Books.

Mossey, J. M., Knott, K. A., Higgins, M., & Talericao, K. (1996). Effectiveness of a psychosocial intervention, interpersonal counseling, for subdysthymic depression in medically ill elderly. *Journal of Gerontology, 51*(Suppl. A.), M172–M178.

Myers, L. L., & Thyer, B. A. (1997). Should social work clients have the right to effective treatment? *Social Work, 42,* 288–298.

Naleppa, M., & Reid, W. (1998). Task-centered case management for the elderly: Developing a practice model. *Research on Social Work Practice, 8,* 63–85

Neimeyer, R. A. (1993). An appraisal of the constructivist psychotherapies. *Journal of Consulting and Clinical Psychology, 61,* 221–234.

Neimeyer, R. A., & Mahoney, M. J. (1995). *Constructivism in psychotherapy.* Washington, DC: American Psychological Association.

Newcome, K. (1985). Task-centered group work with the chronically mentally ill in day treatment. In A. E. Fortune (Ed.), *Task-centered practice with families and groups* (pp. 78–91). New York: Springer.

O'Hanlon, W. H., & Weiner-Davis, M. (1989). *In search of solutions: A new direction in psychotherapy*. New York: W. W. Norton.

Ost, L-G. (1989). One-session treatment for specific phobias. *Behaviour Research and Therapy, 27,* 1–7.

Persons, J. B. (1993). Outcome of psychotherapy for unipolar depression. In T. R. Giles (Ed.), *Handbook of effective psychotherapy* (pp. 305–323). New York: Plenum Press.

Persons, J. B., Thase, M. E., & Crits-Christoph, P. (1996). The role of psychotherapy in the treatment of depression: Review of two practice guidelines. *Archives of General Psychiatry, 53,* 283–290.

Polk, G. W. (1997). *Development and testing of an automated treatment planning system for persistently and severely mentally ill consumers of mental health services.* Unpublished doctoral dissertation, School of Social Work, University of Georgia, Athens.

Reid, W. (1975). An experimental test of a task-centered approach. *Social Work, 20,* 3–9.

Reid, W. (1978). *The task-centered system.* New York: Columbia University Press.

Reid, W. (1995). Eclecticism, empiricism, minimalism, and task-centered practice: A response to Gambrill. *Social Service Review, 69,* 157–163.

Reid, W. (1997). Research on task-centered practice. *Social Work Research, 21,* 132–137.

Reid, W., & Bailey-Dempsey, C. (1995). The effects of monetary incentives on school performance. *Families in Society, 76,* 331–340.

Reid, W., Bailey-Dempsey, C., Cain, E., Cook, T., & Burchard, J. D. (1994). Cash incentives versus case management: Can money replace services in preventing school failure? *Social Work Research & Abstracts, 18,* 227–238.

Reid, W., Epstein, L., Brown, L. B., Tolson, E. R., & Rooney, R. H. (1980). Task-centered school social work. *Social Work in Education, 2,* 7–24.

Reid, W., & Shyne, A. (1969). *Brief and extended casework.* New York: Columbia University Press.

Reynolds, C. F., Frank, E., Houck, P. R., Mazumdar, S., Dew, M. A., Cornes, C., Buysse, D. J., Begley, A., & Kupfer, D. J. (1997). Which elderly patients with remitted depression will remain well with continued interpersonal psychotherapy after discontinuation of antidepressant medication? *American Journal of Psychiatry, 154,* 958–962.

Reynolds, S., Stiles, W. B., Barkham, M., Shapiro, D. A., Hardy, G. E., & Rees, A. (1996). Acceleration of changes in impact during contrasting time-limited psychotherapies. *Journal of Consulting and Clinical Psychology, 64,* 577–586.

Roberts, A., & Dziegielewski, S. F. (1995). Foundation skills and applications of crisis intervention and cognitive therapy. In A. Roberts (Ed.), *Crisis intervention and time-limited cognitive treatment* (pp. 3–27). Thousand Oaks, CA: Sage Publications.

Rosen, G. M. (1987). Self-help treatment books and the commercialization of psychotherapy. *American Psychologist, 42,* 46–51.

Rothbaum, B. O., Hodges, L. F., Kooper, R., Opdyke, D., Williford, J. S., & North, M. (1995a). Effectiveness of computer-generated (virtual reality) graded exposure in the treatment of acrophobia. *American Journal of Psychiatry, 152,* 626–628.

Rothbaum, B. O., Hodges, L. F., Kooper, R., Opdyke, D., Williford, J. S., & North, M. (1995b). Virtual reality graded exposure in the treatment of acrophobia: A case report. *Behavior Therapy, 26,* 547–554.

Rounsaville, B. J., Chevron, E. S., Prusoff, B. A., Elkin, I., Imber, S., Sotsky, S., & Watkins, J. (1987). The relation between specific and general dimensions of the psychotherapy process in interpersonal psychotherapy of depression. *Journal of Consulting and Clinical Psychology, 55,* 379–384.

Rounsaville, B. J., Gawin, F., & Kebler, H. (1985). Interpersonal psychotherapy adapted for ambulatory cocaine abusers. *American Journal of Drug and Alcohol Abuse, 11*, 171–191.

Schneider, S. J. (1986). Trial of an on-line behavioral smoking cessation program. *Computers in Human Behavior, 2*, 277–286.

Schneider, S. J., Walter, R., & O'Donnell, R. (1990). Computerized communication as a medium for behavioral smoking cessation treatment: Controlled evaluation. *Computers in Human Behavior, 6*, 141–151.

Seagrave, A., & Covington, F. (1987). *Free from fears.* New York: Poseidon.

Segal, S. P. (1972). Research on the outcome of social work therapeutic interventions: A review of the literature. *Journal of Health and Social Behavior, 13*, 3–17.

Selmi, P., Klein, M. H., & Greist, J. H. (1982). An investigation of computer-assisted cognitive–behavior therapy in the treatment of depression. *Behavior Research Methods and Instrumentation, 14*, 181–185.

Selmi, P. M., Klein, M. H., Greist, J. H., Sorrell, S. P., & Erdman, H. P. (1990). Computer-assisted cognitive–behavioral therapy for depression. *American Journal of Psychiatry, 147*, 51–56.

Shapiro, F. (1989). Efficacy of the eye movement desensitization procedure in the treatment of traumatic memories. *Journal of Traumatic Stress, 2*, 199–223.

Shapiro, F. (1995). *Eye movement desensitization and reprocessing: Basic principles, protocols and procedures.* New York: Guilford Press.

Sholomskas, A. J., Chevron, E. S., Prusoff, B. A., & Berry, C. (1983). Short-term interpersonal therapy (IPT) with the depressed elderly: Case reports and discussion. *American Journal of Psychotherapy, 38*, 552–566.

Spinelli, M. G. (1997). Interpersonal psychotherapy for depressed antepartum women: A pilot study. *American Journal of Psychiatry, 154*, 1028–1030.

Steketee, G. S., Foa, E. B., & Grayson, J. (1982). Recent advances in the behavioral treatment of obsessive–compulsives. *Archives of General Psychiatry, 39*, 1365–1371.

Steketee, G. S., & White, K. (1990). *When once is not enough.* Oakland, CA: New Harbinger.

Stuart, R. B. (1970). *Trick or treatment: How and when psychotherapy fails.* Champaign, IL: Research Press.

Stuart, R. B. (1978). *Act thin, stay thin.* New York: W. W. Norton.

Taft, J. (1933). The time element in mental hygiene therapy as applied to social case work. In H. R. Knight (Ed.), *Proceedings of the National Conference of Social Work* (pp. 368–381). Chicago: University of Chicago Press.

Thyer, B. A. (1987). *Treating anxiety disorders.* Newbury Park, CA: Sage Publications.

Thyer, B. A. (1992). The term "cognitive-behavior therapy" is redundant [Letter]. *Behavior Therapist, 15*(5), 112, 128.

Thyer, B. A. (1994). Is psychoanalytic therapy relevant for public mental health programs? No! In S. A. Kirk & S. D. Einbinder (Eds.), *Controversial issues in mental health* (pp. 123–128). Needham Heights, MA: Allyn & Bacon.

Thyer, B. A., & Myers, L. L. (1997). Behavioral and cognitive theories. In J. R. Brandell (Ed.), *Theory and practice in clinical social work* (pp. 18–37). New York: Free Press.

Thyer, B. A., & Myers, L. L. (1998). Social learning theory: An empirically-based approach to understanding human behavior in the social environment. *Journal of Human Behavior in the Social Environment, 1*, 33–52.

Tutty, L. (1990). The response of community mental health professionals to client's rights: A review and suggestions. *Canadian Journal of Community Mental Health, 9*, 1–24.

Walter, J. L., & Peller, J. E. (1992). *Becoming solution-focused in brief therapy.* New York: Brunner/Mazel.

Wattie, B. (1973). Evaluating short-term casework in a family agency. *Social Casework, 54,* 609–616.

Weissman, M. M. (1984). The psychological treatment of depression: An update of clinical trials. In R. L. Spitzer & J. Williams (Eds.), *Psychotherapy research: Where are we and where should we go?* (pp. 89–105). New York: Guilford Press.

Weissman, M. M. (1994). Psychotherapy in the maintenance treatment of depression. *British Journal of Psychiatry, 26*(December Suppl.), 42–50.

Weissman, M. M., & Akiskal, H. A. (1984). The role of psychotherapy in chronic depressions: A proposal. *Comprehensive Psychiatry, 25,* 23–31.

Weissman, M. M., Jarrett, R. B., & Rush, A. J. (1987). Psychotherapy and its relevance to the pharmacotherapy of major depression: A decade later (1976–1985). In H. Y. Meltzer (Ed.), *Psychopharmacology: The third generation of progress* (pp. 1059–1069). New York: Raven.

Weissman, M. M., & Klerman, G. L. (1989). Interpersonal psychotherapy. In American Psychiatric Association (Ed.), *Treatments for psychiatric disorders* (pp. 1863–1872). Washington, DC: American Psychiatric Association.

Weissman, M. M., Klerman, G. L., Prusoff, B. A., Sholomskas, D., & Padian, N. (1981). Depressed outpatients: Results one year after treatment with drugs and/or interpersonal psychotherapy. *Archives of General Psychiatry, 38,* 51–55.

Wells, R. A. (1994). *Planned short-term treatment* (2nd ed.). New York: Free Press.

Werner, H. D. (1965). *A rational approach to social casework.* New York: Association Press.

Werner, H. D. (1982). *Cognitive therapy.* New York: Free Press.

White, M. (1986). Family escape from trouble. *Family Therapy Case Studies, 1,* 29–33.

# Advances in Psychopharmacology and Psychosocial Aspects of Medication Management: A Review for Social Workers

Kia J. Bentley and Joseph Walsh

Psychopharmacology, a specialized field within pharmacology, is the study of drugs that affect thinking, emotions, and behavior. It is an exciting field because a tremendous amount of hope and expectation is associated with psychiatric medications today. During the past few years, in almost every class of medication there have been dramatic or important developments that have translated into impressive improvements in the quality of people's lives. In addition, the uses and possible misuses of psychiatric drugs in society have been widely discussed in both the scholarly literature and the public media.

In 1992 Keshavan and Kennedy devoted an entire volume to such topics as overdosing and abuse of psychotropics, drug-induced syndromes, and problematic interactions. In social work, Cohen (1988; Cohen & McCubbin, 1990) has been a critical but intelligent voice for prudence with respect to psychiatric drugs. Most professionals and many members of the public are familiar with the controversy associated with Prozac, the first new selective serotonin reuptake inhibitor (SSRI) to be widely available. Critics described it as an expensive placebo, or worse, an invasive agent that causes aggression. Breggin is perhaps the best-known critic of psychiatric medications today (although he echoes the earlier criticisms of Thomas Szasz and others). He popularized his strong objections to the biological model of human dysfunction and concomitant "chemical lobotomies," as he called them, in *Psychiatric Drugs: Hazards to the Brain* (1987) and *Toxic Psychiatry* (1991). Likewise, there is the debate regarding the use of methylphenidate, whose well-known brand name Ritalin causes considerable unease among many people. The dramatic increase in the use of stimulants with children have some claiming that such use hides the "true" origins of problems and leads to stunted growth and underuse of effective psychosocial interventions. These criticisms persist even in the face of disconfirming evidence (as in the case of prolonged stunted growth and Ritalin) or unsuccessful legal challenges (as in the case of violence and Prozac). At best, they serve as an important check on the use of powerful pharmacologic agents that profoundly affect thoughts, actions, and emotions. At worst, they perpetuate myths and stereotypes and serve as barriers to the accessibility and acceptability of an effective tool in mental health care.

For social workers in mental health and other related fields, there is an increased mandate to know and appreciate all these developments, both those that are positive and exciting and those that are negative or foreboding. Social work is the largest provider of mental health care in the United States, and psychiatric medications are a frequent component of care. Social workers must have the knowledge, values, and skills to work more closely with and be more responsive to clients on medications, their families and, especially, prescribing physicians. With clients and families, social workers must be able to translate complex information into understandable, useful knowledge for living. Social workers should be able to dispel myths but provide realistic cautions and should be able to offer both concrete help and empathetic understanding in decision making concerning medication-related issues. With prescribing physicians, social workers should be able to freely and competently consult on treatment and rehabilitation plans as well as collaborate on specific issues related to medication management and adherence. To do all this with confidence, social workers need an up-to-date knowledge base on the basics of psychopharmacology, the classes of medications, and common drugs and their effectiveness with diverse populations. Social workers need to know about ongoing outcome research related to the additive or interactive effects of various psychosocial interventions and medication. Social workers need theory and skills to work with clients, families, and physicians on improving adherence to medications. As social workers—who often claim to more fully appreciate the environmental context of behavior, whether individual or societal—we also need up-to-date knowledge about managing parallel relationships with other mental health providers and about the social and personal meaning of psychiatric medication use for the consumer and others.

A basic premise of *Advances in Mental Health Research* is that there has been an explosion of knowledge in the mental health field during the past two decades and that social workers and schools of social work have been too slow to incorporate this new knowledge into practice or teaching. It is essential to close the gap between what is known and what social workers use. This chapter summarizes the literature on these topics and discusses their meaning for both social work practice and social work research.

## Effectiveness Research in Psychopharmacology

This section reviews five classes of psychotropic medication (antipsychotic, antidepressant, mood stabilizing, antianxiety, and psychostimulant drugs) to provide information about their evolution, current status, and promise for improved effectiveness. The primary references used to prepare the descriptive information include Bentley and Walsh (1996); Bernstein (1995); Grob (1983, 1991); Hyman, Arana, and Rosenbaum (1995); Janicak, Davis, Preskorn, and Ayd (1993); Parmelee (1996); and Schatzberg and Nemeroff (1995). (Figure 11-1 summarizes the specific medications discussed in this chapter.)

### *NEUROTRANSMITTERS AND PSYCHOTROPIC MEDICATION*

All human thoughts, emotions, and behaviors are associated with the activity of nerve cells—neurons—in the brain and spinal cord. Molecules or ions pass through the neuron membrane to enter or leave a cell through special channels governed by chemical activities within the cell. Impulse transmissions occur through the cell's long axon, through which one cell sends signals to neighboring cells, and the numerous dendrites, which receive signals sent by other neurons.

FIGURE **11-1**

## Trade and Generic Names for Psychiatric Medications

| TRADE NAME | GENERIC NAME | TRADE NAME | GENERIC NAME |
|---|---|---|---|
| **Antipsychotic Medications** | | **Mood-Stabilizing Medications** | |
| Clorazine, Promapar, Thorazine | chlorpromazine | Calan, Covera-HS, Isoptin, Verelan | verapamil |
| Clozaril | clozapine | Depakene, Depakote | valproate, valproic acid |
| Haldol | haloperidol | | |
| Mellaril, SK-thioridazine | thioridazine | Eskalith, Lithium, LITHOBID, Cibalith-S | lithium carbonate |
| Orap | pimozide | Tegretol | carbamazepine |
| Risperdal | risperidone | **Antianxiety Medications** | |
| Serlect | sertindole | Ambien | zolpidem |
| Stelazine, Suprazine | trifluoperazine | Ativan | lorazepam |
| Zyprex | olanzapine | BuSpar | buspirone |
| **Antidepressant Medications** | | Equanil, Meprospan, Miltown | meprobamate |
| Amitril, Elavil, Endep | amitriptyline | | |
| Anafranil | clomipramine | Klonopin | clonazepam |
| Asendin | amoxapine | Librium, Libritabs, Limbritol, Librax | chlordiazepoxide |
| Desyrel | trazodone | | |
| Janimine, SK-pramine, Tofranil | imipramine | Dizac, Valium, Val-release, Vazepam | diazepam |
| LUVOX | fluvoxamine | Xanax | alprazolam |
| Nardil | phenelzine | | zopiclone *(not available in the United States)* |
| Norpramin, Pertofrane | desipramine | | |
| Parnate | tranylcypromine | **Psychostimulant Medications** | |
| Prozac | fluoxetine | Catapres | clonidine |
| Serzone | nefazodone | Cylert | pemoline |
| Wellbutrin | bupropion | Dexampex, Dexedrine, Ferndex | dextroamphetamine |
| | moclobemide *(not available in the United States)* | Ritalin | methylphenidate |

Neurons maintain a negative electrical charge when at rest, but an impulse gives them a temporary positive charge. The transmission of signals through the nervous system begins when a cell generates an impulse, which is a momentary change in the electrical charge within the membrane. The transmission of an impulse to a receiving cell is accomplished by a chemical neurotransmitter, which is released into the synapse from the axon and then attaches to receptors in the dendrite of the neighboring cell (referred to as the postsynaptic receptors). A receptor usually responds to only one type of neurotransmitter, but there are often different types of receptors for a given neurotransmitter, which are characterized by molecular structure, location, the medications that bind to them, and their role in cell function. Information is passed from cell to cell along a pathway—or series of interconnecting neurons working for some coordinated purpose. Psychotropic medications act on these pathways. An agonist drug binds to a receptor and stimulates the same cellular activity as the neurotransmitter. An antagonist drug binds to a receptor but fails to stimulate cellular activity, thereby inhibiting the effect of the neurotransmitter.

Psychotropic drugs work by modifying natural events that occur in the synapses of nerve cell pathways in specific areas of the brain and subsequently affect brain function by

- altering presynaptic activity to prompt neurotransmitter release
- altering postsynaptic activity to affect receptor binding
- interfering with normal reuptake processes
- altering the manufacture of receptors.

More than 40 chemical neurotransmitters have been discovered, but the intended benefits of psychotropic drugs are generally attributed to the influence of only five of these, including acetylcholine, norepinephrine, dopamine, serotonin, and gamma-aminobutyric acid (GABA). Together these account for transmissions at fewer than half of the brain's synapses (glutamate, not discussed in this chapter, is the most common neurotransmitter). Although all these substances are crucial in regions of the nervous system concerned with emotional behavior, it is likely that medications act on neurons in other ways that are not yet fully understood.

Much of the current research on psychotropic medication is focused on learning more about neurotransmitters and their subtypes, discovering the possible role of additional neurotransmitters in producing symptoms of metal illnesses, and targeting new medications as specifically as possible to only those neurotransmitter subtypes believed to have a role in the production of symptoms. At present, any of the psychotropic medications are effective, with a few exceptions, for only 60 percent to 70 percent of those patients for whom they are prescribed. The social worker, therefore, should be active in prescribing processes with the physician, client, and the client's family to ensure a positive outcome for the patient.

## Antipsychotic Medications

The field of psychopharmacology was practically nonexistent until after World War II. Drugs were used only for the sedative control of the symptoms of mental illness and emotional distress. Medications such as opiates, morphine, bromide derivatives, chloral hydrate, and other barbiturate compounds were used in state hospital settings starting at the beginning of the 19th century. After World War II, however, the great successes of the new antibiotic drugs led to a strong faith in the power of medications to treat diseases of all types. It was in this context that the first antipsychotic medications were introduced.

The story of the development of chlorpromazine is a fascinating example of how science and serendipity governed the early days of psychopharmacology. In 1900 research began on antihistamines as potentially effective drugs for treating shock in medical patients. In Germany and France, research on synthetic antihistamines was underway in earnest during the 1930s because of the demands of treating World War I casualties, and as early as the 1940s, these drugs were used in some settings for the sedation of manic patients. In the populous "laboratories" of the state hospitals, it had previously been observed that people in acute psychotic states did not seem to suffer from allergic diseases and had a decreased histamine sensitivity. Through a curious reverse logic, this led to the experimental use of antihistamines as a means of reducing the symptoms of schizophrenia.

By 1950 the antihistamine chlorpromazine had been developed and was used in medicine as an anesthetic and analgesic. It also had hypnotic effects and its primary use was for the treatment of shock. Observations during earlier testing had shown that chlorpromazine lowered the body temperatures of animals; so, because cold water and cold packs had long been used as a means of sedating patients with mental illness, it was hypothesized that the new drug might have the same effect. It failed to lower body temperatures but was effective in controlling behavior. By 1952 a series of articles had appeared in the medical literature that noted the positive impact of chlorpromazine on a range of mental disorders (Swazey, 1974).

Between 1952 and 1954, chlorpromazine was formally tested as an antipsychotic drug and showed positive results (Kinross-Wright, 1954; Winkelman, 1954). However, its American manufacturers, Smith, Kline, and French, had difficulty marketing it in the United States because of psychiatry's adherence to the psychodynamic model of treatment and the problem of public financing of the drug for state hospital use. Through aggressive lobbying, the company was able to persuade state legislatures to invest money in the drug by arguing that the resulting deinstitutionalization would lower the total cost of public mental health care. Eventually chlorpromazine became widely used and proclaimed in many quarters as psychiatry's first "wonder drug."

At issue, though, after the introduction of chlorpromazine, was evidence of its long-term effectiveness and safety with regard to adverse effects. There was a strong demand among psychiatrists for its systematic evaluation, but this was difficult to organize on a national scale because the research methodologies available during the 1950s were limited. Formal evaluation of the drug was not initiated until 1961, and the results of the national study were not published for three years (Cole, 1964). Although the outcomes were positive, the episode provides an example of how enthusiasm for a drug can sometimes obscure safety concerns. Since 1964, potentially serious long-term effects of using chlorpromazine and other neuroleptics, such as tardive dyskinesia (involuntary smooth muscle movements of the face and limbs), have been well documented (Jeste & Caligiuri, 1993).

More than a dozen antipsychotic drugs were developed in the 10 years after chlorpromazine was evaluated to find effective medicines that would not feature anticholinergic side effects (sedation, photosensitivity, blurred vision, dry mouth, constipation, and weight gain). Effectiveness research on these first-generation antipsychotic drugs was summarized by Klein and Davis (1969). First, each drug was compared to placebo, and all but one (pimozide) were highly effective in these trials. Other studies compared the medications with either chlorpromazine, thioridazine, or trifluoperazine, all considered early standards, with regard to symptom reduction. In more than 100 studies of this type, the drugs were found to be equally effective but not superior to one another (Schooler & Keith, 1993). However, in the case of clozapine, a newer drug, differences in effectiveness have been found (Safferman, Lieberman, Kane, Szymanski, & Kinon, 1991). Clozapine is equal to chlorpromazine for general populations of people with schizophrenia, but it also is 30 percent to 40 percent effective with people who have not responded to the standard drugs. Risperidone, another new antipsychotic, was found in a series of trials in the United States, Canada, and Europe to be equally effective as haloperidol and to demonstrate a less problematic side effects profile (Kane & Marder, 1993). In two multicenter studies, risperidone was found to be superior to haloperidol in moderate doses on measures of positive and negative symptoms (Borison, Pathiraja, Diamond, & Meibach, 1992; Chouinard et al., 1993).

It is widely accepted, but still hypothetical, that people with schizophrenia have a relatively high concentration of the neurotransmitter dopamine, or a high sensitivity at its receptor sites, in pathways extending into the cerebral cortex and limbic system (Lieberman & Koreen, 1993). Firm evidence exists that antipsychotic drugs are dopamine antagonists—that is, they act on postsynaptic receptors to bind to dopamine receptors and block dopamine transmission. The medications differ primarily in their side effects and the milligram amounts required for equivalent doses. Most of the first generation of antipsychotic medications (those introduced from the 1950s through the 1970s) are more effective at reducing the positive symptoms of psychosis (an excess or bizarre distortion of normal functions such as delusions and hallucinations) than the negative symptoms (loss or reduction of normal functions, withdrawal, poverty of speech and thought, and lack of motivation). Several newer drugs, such as risperidone and clozapine, may be more effective in treating both types of symptoms.

Most antipsychotic medications act on all dopamine sites in the brain, but only those in the forebrain are sites of symptom-producing neuron activity. The other pathways extend from the midbrain to the basal ganglia area, which governs motor activity through the peripheral nervous system. A reduction in dopamine in these other areas, which are not critical for psychotic symptoms, causes adverse effects. Clients may experience muscle spasms, tremors, or stiffness, as dopamine is needed in normal amounts in the midbrain and basal ganglia for muscle activity. Symptoms of parkinsonism (muscle stiffness and tremor) and tardive dyskinesia are caused by dopamine reduction in the lower brain.

It was once assumed that there was a single type of dopamine receptor in the brain, but researchers have now identified five subtypes, named simply by the order in which they were described (Wilson & Claussen, 1993). During the 1970s and 1980s, research on postmortem brain samples and positron emission tomography of living persons with schizophrenia indicated that they tend to possess an abnormally high amount of dopamine subtype 2 ($D_2$) receptors. As new medications are developed to act differentially on these receptors, more is being learned about the actions of the drugs and their appropriate, increasingly specific targets. The first generation of antipsychotic medications are now known to affect $D_2$ receptors.

Two new antipsychotic medications have been introduced in the American market that act differently from the drugs used throughout the 1970s. Clozapine, available in Europe since 1960 and introduced in the United States in 1990, is a relatively weak $D_2$ antagonist but has a high affinity for $D_4$ receptors as well as interactions with $D_1$, $D_3$, serotonin, and other receptors (Meltzer, 1991). Its sites of action are hypothesized as being limited to the limbic forebrain and the frontal cortex, and thus it does not carry the risk of side effects in the muscular system. This blocking of receptors for serotonin raises the possibility that this neurotransmitter has a role in the development of psychotic symptoms for some people. The U.S. Food and Drug Administration (FDA) mandates that physicians prescribe clozapine only if the client does not first respond to more traditional antipsychotic drugs, because of its rare but serious adverse effect of agranulocytosis (white blood cell depletion). The more recently introduced (1994) drug risperidone, which also has fewer adverse effects than the first-generation drugs, has a high affinity for both $D_2$ and serotonin receptors, which supports the hypothesis that the serotonin antagonist effects diminish extrapyramidal effects (restlessness, spasms, rigidity, and tremors). The actions of the newer drugs make it difficult to argue that any single effect is responsible for their clinical activity. Furthermore, the new compounds' alleviation of the negative symptoms of schizophrenia suggests that serotonin antagonist activity is important in this regard. Clozapine also seems to suppress the potential for tardive dyskinesia.

Several other drugs have been or soon will be introduced in the United States for the treatment of schizophrenia (Tamminga, 1996). The first, olanzapine, was approved for use in the autumn of 1996. It is an antagonist of all dopamine receptors; some serotonin receptors; and also noradrenergic, cholinergic, and histamine receptors. It has a regionally selective effect on dopamine, affecting those tracts that go to the limbic and frontal cortex. In multicenter clinical trials olanzapine is equivalent to traditional neuroleptics for positive symptoms. However, it produces 50 percent fewer motor side effects and results in fewer negative symptoms. Quetiapine fumarate, a strong serotonin blocker, was approved in September 1997. It has fewer motor side effects because it is thought to affect dopaminergic pathways that are most associated with psychosis (Malhotra, Pinsky, & Breier, 1996). Sertindole is more specifically targeted than olanzapine, interacting predominantly with $D_2$ receptors but without attaching to receptors that produce sedative and anticholinergic effects. Like olanzapine, it is equal in effectiveness to traditional antipsychotic drugs for positive symptoms and has a greater therapeutic effect on negative symptoms, as well as a milder side effects. Like clozapine and olanzapine, sertindole selectively affects dopamine receptors in the limbic and frontal cortex. Approval of sertindole is expected soon. Clinical trials continue on a number of other antipsychotic medications in development (see Bentley, in press).

Despite advances in the pharmacologic treatment of schizophrenia, the importance of the psychosocial therapies must not be de-emphasized. Although a variety of studies in the 1960s showed no additional improvements in mental status for people being treated with psychotherapy in addition to medication, the methods in use then were more analytic than what is typically used today with this population (Klein & Davis, 1969). More recent studies of interactions between medications and individual, group, and family behavioral and educational interventions suggest substantially enhanced outcomes for clients on measures of rehospitalization and symptom relapse (Schooler & Keith, 1993). The most impressive outcomes related to functional level result from family-based interventions. The social worker has a clear role in the provision of these services in addition to the medication roles discussed elsewhere in this chapter.

## Antidepressant Medications

Until the early 1980s it was believed that clinical depression resulted from a deficiency of either norepinephrine or serotonin neurotransmitters in the limbic area of the brain. These are naturally regulated by breaking down in the synapse or through reuptake. The antidepressants developed in the 1950s and 1960s were thought to work by increasing the prevalence of norepinephrine in the nervous system. The newer antidepressants are known to act differently, and it is suspected that all antidepressants have additional effects on pre- and postsynaptic receptors and perhaps other neurotransmitter systems. Interactive hypotheses about the etiology of depressive symptoms are now emerging. The various endogenous mood disorders are believed to result from combinations of effects of norepinephrine, serotonin, and other neurotransmitters including GABA, dopamine, and the opioids.

The first specific antidepressant medications, the monoamine oxidase (MAO) inhibitors, were introduced in the mid-1950s after it was observed that one such drug, iproniazid, used in the treatment of tuberculosis, energized many of those patients. After this discovery, several drugs from the MAO chemical class were developed for use as antidepressants. They continue to be effective medications. Klein and Davis (1969) and Frank, Karp, and Rush (1993) have summarized research from the drugs' first decade of use, which demonstrated a 52 percent to 70 percent rate of effectiveness in relieving symptoms of depression. At present, two MAO medications are marketed in the United States, phenelzine and tranylcypromine. Phenelzine has been studied more extensively, and in addition to its antidepressant effect, it is useful in treating panic and other anxiety disorders (Ballenger, 1993). Tranylcypromine is structurally related to amphetamine and has a stimulant effect on some people (Himmelhoch, Thase, Mallinger, & Houck, 1991). The antidepressant effects of both drugs result from the inhibition of enzymes within cells that metabolize norepinephrine and serotonin. The medications also have an inhibitory effect on dopamine. MAO inhibitors are effective with some clients who do not respond to the other antidepressant medications, and they are sometimes the drug of choice for older adults, who tend to have an excess of MAO in the nervous system. Nevertheless, these drugs are not frequently prescribed today because of the rather extensive dietary restrictions that must be followed for the prevention of serious adverse effects. The amino acid tyramine, which is found in many foods, must not be ingested by the consumer of an MAO inhibitor because the combination of substances may produce serious hypertension. Many popular foods, including cheeses, wines, and some meats, contain tyramine.

During the 1980s it was learned that there are two types of MAO—A and B—and that medications that selectively affect type A will not produce the side effect of tyramine deamination (Lecrubier & Guelfi, 1990). Several new selective MAO inhibitors that have less interaction with tyramine are in development. One of these is moclobemide, which is available in much of the world but not yet in the United States. This medication has been found to be equal in effectiveness to both the cyclic (described below) and SSRI antidepressant medications (Bakish et al., 1992; Williams et al., 1993). Although these new medications will not be completely free of dietary restrictions, they may be an attractive alternative to consumers because of their absence of anticholinergic effects.

The cyclic drugs, so named because of the number of rings in their chemical structures, were the most commonly prescribed antidepressants from the late 1950s through the 1980s. The first antidepressant of this class was imipramine. This drug is closely related in structure to chlorpromazine (both are antihistamines), and it was first tested in 1948 for the treatment of psychotic agitation. The cyclic drugs are believed to work by blocking the reuptake of norepinephrine and serotonin, and their metabolites also have antidepressant action. Klein and Davis (1969) summarized the first 10 years of research on cyclic drugs, which indicated a 60 percent to 70 percent rate of effectiveness. Davis, Janicak, Wang, Gibbons, and Sharma (1992) summarized more than 100 studies conducted since then that support the earlier findings. The medications vary in their side effects, although many of the cyclic drugs include anticholinergic effects. For many patients, tolerance does develop to certain side effects but not to the therapeutic effects. Also, cyclic drugs can be taken only once per day.

Despite uncertainties about their specific actions in alleviating depression, some general characteristics of the above two classes of drugs can be described. They must usually be taken for several weeks before the patient experiences beneficial effects, because their actions are initially resisted by cells at the sites of action. They have a low therapeutic index, which means that there is not a great difference between the amounts required for therapeutic effect and overdose. This is a particular problem because the drugs are often prescribed for clients with self-destructive tendencies.

As with all psychotropic drug classes, researchers look for antidepressant drugs that affect specific neurotransmitters and sites to maximize therapeutic effects and minimize adverse effects. Clomipramine is one antidepressant drug that often has been much used for treating obsessive–compulsive disorder, but not as an antidepressant, because of its side effects. It is effective in serotonin reuptake inhibition, but its potent effects on norepinephrine, histamines, and acetylcholine neurotransmitters make it extremely discomforting to many people.

Beginning in 1987, various other SSRIs were introduced in the United States; fluoxetine (Prozac) was the first of these. The selectivity of these drugs for serotonin only adds to the uncertainty about the relevant actions of antidepressant drugs on the neurotransmitters that correlate with depression. The actions of SSRIs may include the stimulation of certain neurotransmitter building blocks in the cell body in ways that are not yet understood. These medications are more potent than the cyclic drugs, and they have a long half-life. Two of their major attractions is their reduced overdose potential and fewer adverse effects than other antidepressant groups. Fluvoxamine is an SSRI used exclusively to treat obsessive–compulsive disorder, generally with far fewer side effects than clomipramine. The SSRIs demonstrate an effectiveness rate of 60 percent to 70 percent across studies (Janicak et al., 1993).

Other atypical drugs that do not fit neatly into the above classes of antidepressant medication include trazodone, bupropion, amoxapine, and nefazodone. These are considered part of the "second generation" of psychoactive drugs but are atypical in that their chemical structures are unique. However, they act on the same transmitter systems. These drugs are equal to standard antidepressants in effectiveness (55 percent to 75 percent), and they tend to differ in side effects from each other and from other drugs (Frank et al., 1993; Janicak et al., 1993).

Important advances made in the past few years with these medications include some indications about which drugs work best with which mood disorders. It also has been learned that some antidepressants are effective with anxiety disorders, particularly panic disorder. A recent review by Charney, Miller, Licinio, and Salomon (1995) suggested that all antidepressant medications work with comparable effectiveness in treating major depression. There is some evidence, however, that atypical depressions (those characterized by mood reactivity with transient remissions) may be responsive to the MAO inhibitors (Liebowitz et al., 1988). Delusional depression requires a combination of antipsychotic and antidepressant medication. For treatment of refractory patients, lithium carbonate may potentiate the antidepressant effect of a medication (Austin, Souza, & Goodwin, 1991; Stein & Bernadt, 1993), although it is not generally effective as a maintenance drug (41 percent relapse rates, compared with 23 percent for other antidepressant drugs). Also, it may initiate a manic episode for people with bipolar disorder.

In the treatment of depression, the importance of the psychosocial therapies is clear. Several studies have compared psychotherapy, cyclic medication therapy, and control groups (Klerman, Weissman, Rounsaville, & Chevron, 1984; Kupfer et al., 1989). Most research has focused on cognitive interventions, although behavioral and interpersonal techniques also have been studied (Frank et al., 1993). The combined interventions demonstrate better client outcomes on various measures of social functioning.

## Mood-Stabilizing Medications

Lithium carbonate is the oldest and most widely prescribed medication for the treatment of bipolar disorder. Discovered as an element in 1817, lithium carbonate was first used medically in 1859 as a treatment for gout. By 1900 a variety of lithium products (waters, salts, tablets, and even beer) were marketed for the treatment of gout and other physical ailments, as well as, in one case, "nervous disorders in all their forms" (Bernstein, 1995, p. 197). These products fell out of public favor by 1910, after the cardiac side effects of lithium carbonate were noted, but in the 1920s a lithium bromide was developed as a sedative. The first specific reference to carbonate lithium (from certain water wells) as a treatment for mental illness was made in 1944, but it was not until 1949 that Australian scientist John Cade serendipitously discovered its role in stabilizing people who had agitation. He had been studying the urine toxicity of manic patients and noticed that guinea pigs developed lethargy after ingesting the lithium urate used as a solvent in his experiments. After Cade's successful trials with 10 human subjects, physicians in Europe began using lithium carbonate for treating bipolar disorder. It was not approved for use in the United States until 1969, partly because some people who used lithium carbonate as a salt substitute during the 1940s and 1950s experienced hypertension and death.

Lithium is the lightest of the solid elements, and it circulates through the body as a small ion with a positive electrical charge. Several theories of how lithium carbonate achieves its therapeutic effect have been considered. One hypothesis asserted that the drug's action is characterized by a high rate of passage through cell membrane ion channels, which results in a stabilization of electrolyte imbalances in the cell membrane and the impediment of naturally occurring impulses that contribute to mania. Another hypothesis differentiated the antidepressant and antimanic effects of the drug. The antidepressant effect of lithium carbonate may result from its reduction of the sensitivity of postsynaptic receptors for serotonin, which increases the amount of that transmitter in the nervous system. The antimanic effect may be related to a reduction in dopamine receptor sensitivity and an inhibition of cellular enzymes that produce dopamine. Lithium carbonate is more effective at stabilizing manic than depressive episodes (Gelenberg & Hopkins, 1993). It also is the most extensively studied of the mood-stabilizing drugs with regard to maintenance therapy. Patients experience 50 percent fewer recurrences of mania with the drug, compared with placebo (Scou, 1989).

Lithium carbonate circulates freely through the body and does not bind with plasma proteins. It must be taken two to three times daily, except in the time-release form. At steady states an equilibrium is reached: plasma lithium reflects total body lithium, thus the drug can be efficiently monitored by measuring its blood levels. Lithium carbonate has a relatively low therapeutic index, thus adverse effects (such as muscle tremor and kidney damage) can occur at blood levels only slightly higher than a therapeutic level. Therapeutic effects begin several weeks after initiation, and the drug sometimes is given, at least temporarily, with an antipsychotic drug to stabilize a manic person.

Despite its dramatic positive effects for many patients, lithium carbonate is only 70 percent to 80 percent effective (Gelenberg & Hopkins, 1993). Two other medications, both anticonvulsants, emerged in the late 1970s as alternative drugs for treatment of bipolar disorders. The antimanic effect of carbamazepine was discovered in the 1960s, when it was observed that the drug improved mood in many people who used it for seizure control. It was approved by the FDA, but only for anticonvulsant use, in 1974. At least one study has shown that carbamazepine is equally effective to lithium carbonate in both the acute (Small et al., 1991) and maintenance treatment of bipolar disorder; both limit relapse rates to 50 percent (Coxhead, Silverstone, & Cookson, 1992). Some studies have shown carbamazepine to be more effective with rapid cycling bipolar disorder (Goodwin & Jamison, 1990). Valproate was approved as an anticonvulsant medication in 1978, although its antimanic effects were discovered in the 1960s. It is comparable in effectiveness to lithium carbonate, with 60 percent to 70 percent of patients responding to its antimanic actions (Bowden et al., 1994; Gelenberg & Hopkins, 1993). Although the overall response rates for all three mood stabilizers are similar, a patient who does not respond to one may respond to another. Furthermore, all three are more effective at controlling mania than depression. There is some evidence that carbamazepine has an antidepressant effect, and it is occasionally used as an adjunct with traditional antidepressant drugs (Charney et al., 1995).

Carbamazepine, a potent blocker of norepinephrine reuptake, inhibits the repetitive firing of sodium channel impulses by binding to them. It also may function as an inhibitor of enzymes in the central nervous system that break down GABA. The GABA neurotransmitter may have antimanic properties, thus its increased prevalence in the nervous system may enhance mood stability. Valproate also has pre- and postsynaptic GABA receptor effects. It increases levels of GABA by blocking the convulsive effects of GABA antagonists. These medications are generally not prescribed unless lithium carbonate is first ruled out, because they have not been subjected to the same amount of study as the primary drug.

Like those of lithium carbonate, the alternative drugs' mechanisms of action in controlling mania are not clear. One theory holds that they control a "kindling" process in limbic system neuron tracts that contributes to the development of manic states and cycles. This theory was first introduced to explain the phenomenon of epilepsy, which helps explain how two anticonvulsant medications came to be used for the treatment of bipolar disorder. Researchers have speculated that in mania, as well as epilepsy, a repetitive application of low-grade electrical or chemical stimuli gradually rewires the brain by changing the composition of the affected brain cells. The altered cells become sensitive to more subtle stimuli and eventually respond with activity that produces a manic episode. As the stimulus continues, neighboring cells may be altered as well. Kindling theory also helps explain why, in some forms of mania, the cycle may quicken or become more severe. This process may imply that drugs that are effective early in the treatment of bipolar disorder may be less effective later. The anticonvulsant drugs are more effective in treating episodes of acute mania, rapid-cycling bipolar disorder (more than three cycles per year), and dysphoric mania (Calabreze & Delucchi, 1990). However, it is not clear how well these two drugs work in the maintenance of mood stability over the long term, and some research has suggested that their effectiveness may not persist (Janicak et al., 1993).

Other drugs, more fully summarized by Walsh (in press), appear to have some potential as antimanic agents, either as adjuncts to the major drugs or as sole interventions. Several drugs in the benzodiazepine class, which are primarily used as antianxiety medications, have been tested for antimanic qualities. Clonazepam has received the most attention as an adjunctive drug for use with lithium carbonate, particularly in acute mania, because of the rapid onset of its effects, its long duration of action, and its anticonvulsant effects, which may impede the kindling process (Chouinard, 1987). Lorazepam has demonstrated a possible effect in this way. These drugs have been shown in limited studies to be equally effective to haloperidol in adjunctive treatment of bipolar disorder (Bradwejn, Shriqui, Koszycki, & Meterissian, 1990; Sachs, Weilburg, & Rosebaum, 1990). They may provide an alternative to adjunctive use of antipsychotic drugs in stabilizing people in a manic state because the adverse effects of the antipsychotic drugs discourage some patients from adherence. The calcium channel blockers (verapamil is the best known of these), primarily used in the treatment of cardiovascular disorders, also are under investigation as antimanic drugs. They have effects on intracellular calcium ion concentrations similar to those of lithium carbonate and thus are hypothesized to have antimanic effects. A number of studies have shown effects comparable with those of lithium carbonate, whereas others have shown a poor response (Dubovsky, 1993; Hoschl & Kozeny, 1989). These drugs merit further study but are not yet warranted as antimanic agents. If effective, their relatively mild side effects, including safety during pregnancy, will make them attractive alternatives.

## Antianxiety Medications

Through the centuries people have relied on a variety of substances to control their anxiety and insomnia. Alcohol has always been a popular drug for these purposes, and during the late 19th century, bromide drugs were used to control anxiety and agitation in people with mental illness. In 1903 the barbiturate compounds came into use as central nervous system depressants, and they were widely prescribed through the 1940s and 1950s. A major problem with all of these substances has been their potential for abuse and addiction. A purportedly safer sedative and muscle relaxant, meprobamate, was introduced in 1955 but eventually was found to have serious addiction potential.

With the introduction of the benzodiazepines, barbiturates have become almost obsolete as antianxiety agents. The name derives from their chemical structure, in which benzene and diazepine rings are fused. Compared with their predecessors, these drugs have lower abuse potential, a lower potential for dependence and tolerance, a higher therapeutic index, and a higher dose margin between antianxiety and sedation effects. Chlordiazepoxide (Librium), introduced in 1960, was the first benzodiazepine. The second, diazepam (Valium), was for a time the most prescribed medication in the world, and between 1964 and 1973, antianxiety drug prescription worldwide rose to heights not seen since.

There may be natural benzodiazepine chemicals in the brain that are potentiated by the inhibitory GABA neurotransmitter. The benzodiazepine medications achieve their therapeutic effect by increasing the efficiency with which the GABA neurotransmitter binds to its receptor sites. They affect neurons in the limbic system, where receptors are known to decrease anxiety. GABA receptors in various regions of the brain mediate the antianxiety, sedative, and anticonvulsant effects of the benzodiazepines. In this way the medications block central nervous system stimulation and diminish activity in areas associated with emotion. They also raise the patient's seizure threshold because antiseizure activity is located in the cerebral cortex and limbic areas. The benzodiazepine drugs bind to specific sites on GABA receptors, but it is not clear how they achieve specificity as antianxiety agents. The benzodiazepines reduce anxiety in lower doses and are sedative in higher doses.

Benzodiazepines are highly effective medications. They achieve therapeutic effect within one week in treating most anxiety disorders (Downing & Rickels, 1985), and 75 percent of patients demonstrate moderate to marked improvement with them (Meibach, Dunner, Wilson, Ishiki, & Dager, 1987; Rickels, 1982). Their therapeutic benefit appears to peak after four to six weeks of use (Rickels, 1987), but many patients use these medications for months or years without developing a tolerance to them.

Benzodiazepines are quickly absorbed in the gastrointestinal tract and have a rapid effect, usually within 30 minutes. They have a high therapeutic index and do not present a risk for overdose, but they are physically addictive at some dosages with continuous use. Long-term use (four to six weeks or longer) can cause production of the body's natural benzodiazepine compounds to shut down. Thus, if the drug is abruptly withdrawn, no natural production will occur in the system for a certain period. Patients must gradually decrease these medications to prevent the effects of physical withdrawal. For these reasons, the benzodiazepines are intended for comparatively short-term use. American investigators recommend no more than four months of continuous use, and British guidelines published by the Committee on the Review of Medications call for two- to four-week regimens (as cited in Taylor, 1995).

During the past 20 years, research has focused on the therapeutic indications for the four types of benzodiazepine drugs. The high-potency drugs, which may be short- or long-acting (alprazolam and clonazepam, among others), have the highest relative withdrawal potential but are well suited for the treatment of particularly disabling anxiety states such as panic attacks (Ballenger et al., 1988). The antidepressants imipramine (cyclic) and phenelzine (MAO inhibitor) also are effective treatments for this disorder, but they are not fast acting. One study shows that alprazolam is 20 percent to 25 percent more effective than placebo in eliminating panic attacks (Ballenger, 1993). Tesar et al. (1991) studied both drugs and found similar effectiveness in them (approximately 50 percent). The low-potency benzodiazepines, which also may be short- or long-acting, are indicated for the control of milder anxiety states as well as for muscle relaxation and as preoperative drugs. The short-acting drugs are appropriate for treating insomnia and anticipatory anxiety.

Several other classes of medications are used for the control of anxiety. These include the beta-blockers, so named because they compete with norepinephrine at beta-adrenergic (a type of receptor) sites in the brain and peripheral nervous system that regulate cardiac and muscular functions. These medications are effective in treating anticipatory anxiety by reducing the visceral symptoms of rapid heartbeat, muscle tension, and dry mouth. Because patients do not experience these physiological indicators, their subjective experience of anxiety is diminished. Liebowitz et al. (1991) have shown the effectiveness of beta-blockers in treating social phobia.

Another type of antianxiety medication, buspirone (originally developed in 1968 as an antipsychotic medication), is a partial agonist of serotonin receptors. Serotonin is believed to be anxiolytic in the hippocampus and limbic areas, although its role in anxiety is not yet understood. Unlike the benzodiazepines, buspirone must be taken regularly to reach and maintain effectiveness. It is quickly absorbed and must be taken three times per day, but it is not potentially addictive. Clinicians treating patients who have taken benzodiazepines for an extended time often will change their prescription to buspirone. It seems to be particularly effective in treating generalized anxiety disorder (Sussman, 1993). Furthermore, in one study (Rickels & Schweizer, 1990), participants taking either type of medication were functioning at the same level after 40 months, but although none of the buspirone users were still taking the drug, 65 percent of the benzodiazepine users were doing so.

The antihistamines are still occasionally used as antianxiety agents. These drugs block histamine receptors in the central and peripheral nervous systems that are associated with anxiety and agitation. They are rapidly absorbed and maintain a therapeutic effect for at least 24 hours. The antihistamines tend to be sedating, however, and are effective as antianxiety agents for only a few months. They are not addictive, but neither are they as effective as the benzodiazepines. These drugs are most frequently used as relatively safe sleep-inducing agents.

The newest antianxiety drug available in the United States is zolpidem. Like buspirone, it is an atypical drug, and it affects a smaller subset of GABA than do the benzodiazepines. Zolpidem has been shown to be effective in the short-term treatment of insomnia but reports of discomforting side effects may delay its broad adoption. Another atypical drug, zopiclone, is available in Canada and some other countries and is prescribed as an antianxiety medication with anticonvulsant properties.

Obsessive–compulsive disorder is classified as an anxiety disorder, but medications from this class are not useful in its treatment. Clomipramine, an SSRI, has been the drug of choice for more than 10 years. Nine large-scale studies have demonstrated that it alleviates the symptoms for 35 percent to 42 percent of people with obsessive–compulsive disorder (Clomipramine Collaborative Study Group, 1991; Jenike, 1993). Research consistently bears out the effectiveness of SSRI for this disorder.

There also is research evidence that psychosocial intervention with panic disorder enhances the long-range outcome, compared with the use of medications alone (Ballenger, 1993; Jenike, 1993). Cognitive restructuring, breathing retraining, relaxation, exposure, and panic control treatments demonstrate 60 percent or greater levels of effectiveness, rates that are comparable with the medications. Once again, this result indicates that medications alone are not sufficient to maximize the social functioning of clients, and that the social work roles are essential in client intervention.

## Psychostimulant Medications

Psychostimulants produce states of wakefulness, mood elevation, alertness, and initiative, as well as the sense of competence. The first known stimulant, cocaine, was isolated in the mid-19th century and used by Bavarian soldiers as early as 1884 to decrease fatigue. The prototype of the current psychostimulant drugs is amphetamine, which has been a topic of medical interest and controversy since it was synthesized in 1887. Amphetamines were first used with children in the 1920s by a Rhode Island physician named Bradley in a successful effort to help survivors of an influenza epidemic with neurologic and mental impairments become more teachable and less agitated. They also were used in the 1930s as bronchial dilators, respiratory stimulants, and analeptics as well as for treating parkinsonism. Amphetamines were widely used by Japanese and American soldiers during World War II, after which they became well-known drugs of abuse. Until the development of the MAO inhibitors, they were used in the treatment of various conditions such as obesity and depression. Eventually, because of their abuse potential, the amphetamines were reclassified in 1972 as Schedule II drugs by the U.S. Drug Enforcement Agency. This is the most restrictive classification for prescription drugs; it indicates their high abuse potential and ensures that they cannot be prescribed by telephone or with refills. The amphetamines are currently approved only for the treatment of attention-deficit hyperactivity disorder (ADHD) and narcolepsy.

ADHD, which is among the most common psychiatric disorders seen in children and adolescents, begins in childhood but may persist into adolescence and even continue in modified form into adult life. Three percent to 5 percent of children are estimated to have the disorder, with boys having it two to three times as often as girls. The severity of the disorder is variable and likely to worsen in situations that demand sustained effort or high levels of structure. The decision to medicate is based on symptoms of inattention, impulsivity, and hyperactivity that are sufficiently persistent to cause functional impairment at school, at home, and with peers.

Stimulants have been used in the treatment of ADHD since 1936, when amphetamine drugs were found to be effective in controlling hyperactivity. The drugs release norepinephrine, dopamine, and serotonin from presynaptic terminals in the frontal portion of the brain, where attention and impulsivity are regulated. They also inhibit norepinephrine and dopamine reuptake. The mechanism of action of the psychostimulants in treating ADHD is not known. Between 70 percent and 90 percent of children respond positively to the major psychostimulant drugs currently available, which include dextroamphetamine, methylphenidate, and pemoline (Jacobvitz, 1990). Twenty percent of children who do not respond to one of these drugs will respond to another of the three, and true nonresponders are rare (Mercugliano, 1993). Moderate doses appear to improve attention, concentration, and cognitive functioning in adults as well, although ADHD in adults remains a somewhat controversial and less thoroughly studied condition.

Methylphenidate, the most widely used and studied psychostimulant, was introduced in 1958 as a treatment for children with hyperactivity (Jacobvitz, 1990). Since 1990 the number of children taking the drug in the United States has multiplied by two and one-half (Hancock, 1996). Although it must be taken two to four times daily, methylphenidate has a short half-life, which is advantageous because it does not impair sleep. It requires only 30 to 60 minutes to take effect but is associated with symptom aggravation 10 to 20 hours after a dose. A time-release form of the drug is available. Another psychostimulant, Pemoline, has a longer half-life: It is taken only once daily and thus may be easier for children and families to manage. Pemoline's lesser stimulant effect also may lessen its abuse potential. However, it has not been researched as extensively as methylphenidate and may require several weeks to demonstrate a therapeutic effect. Dextroamphetamine remains an alternative medication. It acts quickly and is taken only twice per day. However, it has a high potential for abuse and diversion to the illicit drug trade.

The common transient adverse effects of the stimulants include anorexia, weight loss, irritability, insomnia, and abdominal pain. Occasional but more serious adverse effects include increased blood pressure, tachycardia, nightmares, rash, and liver toxicity. When these drugs are used to treat children, the possibility of stunted growth is a valid concern, but there is a rebound growth spurt to normal height during drug holidays or if the drug is discontinued (Sylvester, 1993). However, further research is needed to study this effect on children who take psychostimulants continuously through adolescence. In most cases, patients are given drug holidays for at least two weeks to assess the status of their condition. These are practical during times of the year when children are out of school and have fewer persistent demands on their attention. Children with ADHD can remain symptomatic through adolescence and early adulthood, but there are few studies of drug effectiveness beyond puberty.

There is evidence, however, that treatment in childhood leads to better outcomes in adulthood. Hechtman, Weiss, and Perlman (1984) found that children using psychostimulants for three years or longer had better outcomes relative to further psychiatric treatment, levels of education, independent living, and aggression. Wender, Remherr, and Wood (1985) found a positive response rate of 57 percent in adults using methylphenidate for the first time.

Evidence of the effectiveness of other medications in treatment of ADHD is emerging. These drugs have not been extensively evaluated, but isolated clinical studies have demonstrated their promise for some people who do not respond to the primary drugs or cannot tolerate their adverse effects (Janicak et al., 1993). The cyclic antidepressants, including imipramine, desipramine, and amitriptyline, have been effective with ADHD and are particularly useful for patients who have a family history of depression or anxiety. These drugs demonstrate the same efficacy as the psychostimulants but also have more adverse effects, which many children cannot tolerate. Clonidine, an antihypertensive agent also used in the treatment of Tourette syndrome, has been effective with children who have severe problems with mood, activity level, cooperation, and frustration tolerance. It is often prescribed with a stimulant, for a combined effect. One positive feature of this medication is that it can be dispensed by use of a five-day transcutaneous patch. Finally, bupropion and fluoxetine, atypical antidepressants, may be therapeutic in some cases of ADHD.

All researchers emphasize, for children more than any others, that psychostimulant treatment must never take place in a vacuum. ADHD is a disorder with quality-of-life implications for the entire family, and psychosocial interventions have a major role in affecting the course of the disorder. Further, Gadow (1991) noted that children who take medication for ADHD may come to attribute their adjustment problems to factors outside their control, fail to acquire adaptive behaviors once symptoms are suppressed, and learn that taking medicine is an effective means of coping with all stresses. Satterfield, Satterfield, and Shell (1987) conducted a study that provides evidence of the benefits of multimodal interventions over medication alone. For these reasons, the social worker has much to contribute to the family of a child with ADHD.

## DIFFERENTIAL IMPACT OF MEDICATIONS ON SPECIAL POPULATIONS

A major strength of the social work profession is its appreciation of human diversity. Social workers understand that all people are unique, but members of different genders, age groups, and racial and ethnic populations tend to experience certain biological as well as social differences. This appreciation of diversity influences psychopharmacology as much as any other aspect of social work intervention. Although discussion of these differences is beyond the scope of this chapter, it should be emphasized that along with the well-known general actions of medications, distinct reactions to them also can occur in some special populations. Knowledge of these differences in therapeutic effects, side effects, and dosage is only beginning to emerge in the treatment of women, elderly people, members of several racial and ethnic populations, and people diagnosed with both mental illness and substance abuse problems. Because few other professions are educated about issues of diversity, social workers have an important responsibility to understand these differences and communicate them to both client and physician as well as to others involved in client care. With this professional strength and the partnership perspective, social workers can contribute important insights into the client's experience of taking medication, in both the social and physical senses.

# Research on Psychosocial Aspects of Medication Management and Use

Social workers need a knowledge base in psychopharmacology that extends beyond neurotransmission, pharmacokinetics, pharmacodynamics and drug classes, names, and typical dosages. They also need to understand how medications can be used most effectively in conjunction with psychosocial interventions, such as the various psychotherapies, support groups, education, skills training, case management, and other forms of rehabilitation. There is extensive information about how to improve adherence to medications that is important to social workers as they assume expanded roles as partners in psychopharmacologic treatment of their clients. However, much less research exists on managing relationships with prescribing physicians and how social workers can better appreciate and respond to the meaning that taking psychiatric medications has for their clients. This section examines the information available that can help social workers understand these important issues.

## EFFECTS OF COMBINED PSYCHOSOCIAL INTERVENTIONS AND PSYCHIATRIC MEDICATION

Outcome research in mental health that specifically examines the interactive or additive effects of psychosocial interventions with medications is particularly relevant for the social work profession. For example, Gerard Hogarty, MSW, has spent his career looking for the optimal combinations of different psychosocial treatments and certain dosages of antipsychotic medications for people with schizophrenia and other serious mental illnesses. In recent articles he described a complex series of clinical trials that attempted to either lower the dose of subjects' regular neuroleptic medication or find the appropriate dose of an adjunctive medication for people with schizophrenia who still have lingering negative symptoms, anxiety, and depression (Hogarty et al., 1995b). Another article described the impact of personal therapy combined with medication on patients with schizophrenia (Hogarty et al., 1995a). Personal therapy is a psychosocial intervention concerned with building internal awareness of feelings and enhancing coping strategies. Too often, social workers rely on colleagues in related disciplines to lead or conduct this kind of research. As Beitman and Klerman (1991) stated, both solid empirical research and decades of clinical experience support the belief that a combination of medication and psychosocial interventions will likely lead to the best client outcomes across a range of populations and problems, such as various affective, thought, and anxiety disorders as well as selected personality disorders.

In 1993, a special issue of the journal *Psychopharmacology Bulletin,* published by the National Institute of Mental Health, presented articles by leading psychiatrists, psychologists, and pharmacologists that catalogued the rich database on psychosocial treatment efficacy in mental health care, countering the general disparagement of psychiatric treatments. Keith and Matthews (1993) pointed out in their introduction to that volume that psychiatric treatment of mental disorders, which optimally almost always includes a combination of pharmacologic and nonpharmacologic interventions, compares favorably with traditional physical health treatments both in efficacy and effect size.

Obviously, there is considerable variation in the specific psychosocial intervention strategies used with respective symptoms, disorders, and populations, in combination with the various types of psychoactive medications. The ultimate clinical research question is, What works best for whom and under what conditions? Research continues, but many empirically based generalizations can be made right now. For example, effective psychosocial interventions commonly used with people with schizophrenia include skills training, psychoeducation, and family treatment; for people with depression—interpersonal psychotherapy, cognitive–behavioral interventions, and electroconvulsive therapy; for people with bipolar disorder—short-term individual treatment and group and family therapy; for people with panic disorder—cognitive restructuring, relaxation training, exposure and breathing training; and for people with obsessive–compulsive disorder—exposure and response prevention. Researchers have published promising results on studies of additive effects of participation in other treatment programs or models, including peer-run or employment programs, support groups, and case management (Wallace, 1993; Yank, Bentley, & Hargrove, 1993).

A survey of psychodynamically oriented group therapists summarized some of the identified benefits and challenges of integrating psychosocial and pharmacologic treatments. Rodenhauser and Stone (1993) analyzed the survey responses of 143 therapists across disciplines (social workers, psychiatrists, psychologists, nurses, and others) regarding their opinions, attitudes, and practices related to treatment integration, especially for group therapy. The respondents noted that prescribing and transference issues sometimes became confused and that they worried about splitting the therapeutic alliance and coordinating the actual arrangements for medication. They expressed concern about the overreliance on medications and whether clients on medication feel more shame or feel more "sick" than those in their groups not on medication. They worried about misinformation about medications being shared in the group context and its impact on the group process in general. On the other hand, the respondents recognized the positive effect of medication in reducing symptoms and helping clients be more accessible and amenable to group treatment. They noted that group members taking medication increase the heterogeneity of their groups, which may contribute to destigmatization. They recognized that medication can reflect nurturing and reassurance and give the message that each gets individualized care. Finally, they acknowledged that collaboration with physicians yields a better and more comprehensive treatment plan.

## *IMPROVING ADHERENCE TO PSYCHIATRIC MEDICATIONS*

Nonadherence to a medication regime can be anything from not filling the prescription to not taking all of it to stopping before a therapeutic effect can be achieved to self-adjusting the dose or timetable—or anything in between. Numerous authors (Buckalew & Sallis, 1986; Kane, 1984; Weiden et al., 1994) have pointed out that adherence to psychotropic medication is not usually an all-or-nothing proposition. In general, about half the time there is some degree of nonadherence, or as Jamison and Akiskal (1983) put it, "intermittent compliance" can be expected. Outright refusal is rare and is usually found in the context of inpatient care of people with psychosis.

In an earlier work (Bentley & Walsh, 1996), we presented a model for understanding medication adherence as a precursor to intervention. The model suggested that people do not take psychiatric medications in a "thoughtless vacuum" (Stimson,

1974) but rather in a unique biopsychosocial and cultural context. We agree with others who have pointed out that whether or not someone actually takes medication as prescribed should be seen in light of that person's view of his or her illness, treatment, life experiences, and expectations. Current theory and research suggest that social workers can look to four contextual dimensions to gain a full appreciation of the complexity of this issue for clients:

1. *Characteristics of the client.* This includes clients' "health beliefs"—how they see the medication as being related to some personally important desired outcome (not necessarily a medical or health outcome). However, Aspler and Rothman (1984) found that adherence was inversely related to perceived degree of health; the healthier clients think they are, the less likely they are to take their medication. In all the research examining hundreds of factors associated with adherence and nonadherence, few studies have found consistent, statistically significant relationships with demographic variables such as gender, age, socioeconomic status, education level, diagnosis, or length of symptoms (Frank, Perel, Mallinger, Thase, & Kupfer, 1992; Jamison & Akiskal, 1983). There are, however, few notable exceptions: Draine and Solomon (1994) found that older patients with fewer symptoms and a wider array of daily activities had better attitudes toward adherence. However, impairments in the senses, dexterity, or memory and greater complexity of drug regimens, according to these authors, may put elderly patients at greater risk of nonadherence. A study by Seltzer, Roncari, and Garfinkel (1980) found that living alone also puts people at greater risk of nonadherence. Another study found that a higher locus of control was associated with better compliance (Kucera-Bozarth, Beck, & Lyss, 1982). New areas of research include investigation into the role of visual memory and cognitive function as a factor in adherence (Isaac, Tamblyn, & McGill–Calgary Drug Research Team, 1993) and differential perceptions of toxicity and addictiveness across racial and ethnic groups.

2. *Aspects of treatment and the treatment environment.* Probably the most important factor related to nonadherence that is associated with treatment itself is negative physical side effects. It is certainly what clients themselves report is the most important. The most bothersome side effects, however, are not necessarily the most common or the most severe. Side effects such as akathesia (internal restlessness and agitation), mental slowness, confusion, weight gain, and tremors were all found to be the most problematic in terms of effect on compliance (Gitlin, Cochran, & Jamison, 1989; VanPutten, 1974). There are numerous other factors related to the medication itself that are associated with nonadherence. For example, research has shown that problems with adherence are more frequent when the medication regimen is more complex, when long-term maintenance medication is needed, and when there is higher cost or inaccessibility (Blackwell, 1979; Diamond, 1983). Morris and Schulz (1993) also found, however, that clients are less compliant when they receive free medications, perhaps because they do not value them as much as those for which they have to pay. It has been speculated that even the shape, color, size, and taste of medications influence adherence (Buckalew & Sallis, 1986). Another study examined factors associated with compliance rather than nonadherence. In a project that examined adherence to imipramine

among 53 patients with depression, Frank et al. (1992) found effective prophylaxis (prevention of symptoms) to be the factor most often associated with
compliance.

Social workers' person-in-environment perspective requires assessing aspects of the larger treatment environment, as well, for information on adherence. For example, many researchers have speculated that the attitudes
and beliefs of clinicians play an important role in adherence (Bentley,
Rosenson, & Zito, 1990; Jamison & Akiskal, 1983; Weissman, 1972). One
study (Jamison, Gerner, & Goodwin, 1979) showed that physicians' attitudes
were strongly associated with compliance. Others have found that clear
communication and quality provider–client relationships play an important
role in adherence (Hays & DiMatteo, 1987; Kane, 1984; Weiden et al.,
1994). Kupfer and Siegal's (1995) important research supported what others
have argued for decades—that a strong treatment alliance is perhaps the
best intervention (or prevention) of all. Their research showed that a solid
treatment alliance, characterized by continuous education and mutual sharing in which the patient is seen as "expert," was associated with a less than
10 percent dropout rate and high rates of adherence to medication (85 percent) over several years. Similarly, in a study of 90 people with serious mental illness and their case managers, Solomon, Draine, and Delaney (1995)
found a positive relationship between the pairs' working alliance and a
range of outcome measures, including quality of life and attitudes toward
medication compliance.

3. *Aspects of the social environment.* Few, if any, studies have systematically examined the impact of societal or familial mores and values on medication compliance by clients. However, it seems likely that the social culture of medication, cues and contingencies in the environment, and extent of family and
   social support play a role. As Leventhal, Diefenbach, and Leventhal (1992)
   pointed out, "social myth can dominate the interpretive process" of mental
   health clients and their families and thus substantially influence the decision-
   making process (p. 152).

4. *Aspects of the mental illness (symptoms).* Little research, especially in recent years,
   has examined the degree to which client symptoms negatively influence adherence. A number of studies done in the 1960s, reviewed by VanPutten
   (1974), related noncompliance to intrapsychic conflict. More recently, a
   study by Rodenhauser, Schwenker, and Khamis (1987) of 378 forensic patients in a maximum-security facility concluded that patient denial was the
   primary factor in noncompliance. However, the conclusions were reached
   by interpreting the chart recordings of nurses. As noted by Bentley (1993),
   because neither the nurses' nor the researchers' preconceived beliefs and attitudes were reported, the potential for bias or self-fulfilling prophesy has to
   be considered. Although there is not much research support, many mental
   health providers can point to years of clinical experience that suggests that
   some symptoms, such as denial, paranoia, lack of energy, or mania, have
   gotten in the way of proper administration of psychotropic drugs at some
   point.

Research on the effectiveness of interventions to improve adherence also is important for social workers. Perhaps the most widely examined intervention to improve adherence is patient education. For example, many of the comprehensive

psychoeducational and skills-training programs for families of people with schizophrenia include information about medication. Although it is difficult to isolate specific causal effects of any aspect of treatment packages, reports of increased medication compliance, among numerous other positive outcomes, are common (Anderson, Reiss, & Hogarty, 1986; Eckman, Liberman, Phipps, & Blair, 1990; Falloon, Boyd, & McGill, 1984). Other controlled and uncontrolled studies support a position of cautious optimism. Batey and Ledbetter (1982) found that medication education was associated with increased compliance as well as greater client involvement in treatment and increased levels of staff comfort with clients. Using a controlled experimental design, Youssef (1984) evaluated a group education program's impact on both compliance with medication and compliance with aftercare appointments. Results for subjects in the two-session intervention, compared with the no-education control subjects, were significantly associated with better outcomes on both of those variables.

Other studies have tried to ascertain the types of education that may have the greatest impact on compliance or other client outcomes. Robinson, Gilbertson, and Litwak (1986), for example, compared three types of structured drug education strategies that involve different combinations of written instructions, an information sheet, and individual consultation with a nursing or psychology student. Not surprisingly, an individual meeting paired with written materials was superior to the usual brief explanations given to clients. A study by Brown, Wright, and Christenson (1987), however, was not able to replicate the relationship between the acquisition of medication knowledge and increased adherence. This study had only a small number of subjects in the sample and used unvalidated measures, but other studies also have found equivocal results. Kelly, Scott, and Mamon (1990) found that psychiatric patients receiving individualized medication instruction in a Veterans Administration clinic had better adherence than did a comparison group (a home-based family consultation), but adherence actually worsened over time for both the experimental group and the comparison group.

Several other strategies have been suggested to improve medication adherence, including use of traditional behavioral strategies, reinforcement, prompts, and contracting (Bentley et al., 1990; Dunbar, Marshall, & Hovell, 1979) as well as cognitive strategies such as guided imagery, thought stopping, or self-instruction (DiMatteo & DiNicola, 1982; Turk, Salovey, & Litt, 1986). In addition, teaching clients how to communicate and negotiate with mental health providers and make decisions in a systematic way may contribute to adherence (Bentley & Walsh, 1996; Collins-Colon, 1990; Liberman, Kane, Vaccaro, & Wirshing, 1987). These strategies are suggested based on their proven success in applications to other problems, not because of results from direct and purposeful inquiry into their effectiveness with improving medication adherence.

The model of adherence calls for social workers to first fully assess clients' health beliefs—their desired outcomes and expectations with respect to medication. Assessment should include the medication's accessibility and affordability, degree of family support and, especially, the social worker's own attitudes and behaviors about psychiatric medication use. Perhaps the most overlooked strategy for improving adherence is open, honest reflection and discussion to clarify assumptions and beliefs. All in all, "achieving adherence and dealing productively with refusal over the long haul calls for using a number of combined strategies such as self-monitoring, education, and cognitive, behavioral, and other psychosocial strategies in the context of a caring relationship" (Bentley & Walsh, 1996, p. 151).

## *MANAGING INTERPROFESSIONAL RELATIONSHIPS AROUND MEDICATION ISSUES*

Given the data that support using an integrated or combined approach to the treatment of people with mental illness and serious emotional distress by both medication and psychosocial interventions, it is crucial for social workers to work toward open and productive collaborations with physicians. Only a few articles exist on the complex management of treatment and "turf issues" that can arise in these three-party or parallel relationships (client, prescribing physician, and social worker). Kelly's (1992) advice to work only with those whom you know and trust and both Busch and Gould's (1993) and Bradley's (1990) discussions of the positive and negative impact of transference and countertransference are an important part of that literature. But the question remains: Is there a research literature that can help social workers understand and then develop these cross-disciplinary relationships? Two distinct topics are useful in answering this broad question: (1) research on interdisciplinary collaboration and the role of social work in general and (2) studies that examined the referral processes involved in prescribing medication.

Toseland, Palmer-Ganeles, and Chapman (1986) published a classic and still useful study on social work and interdisciplinary teams in mental health. They surveyed 15 teams, involving more than 70 team members from eight disciplines, to ascertain their composition, structure, and roles. Social workers were perceived by the respondents to have the second-highest degree of influence (physicians had the highest) and were more likely to have served as coordinators of care, negotiators, conflict diffusers, and client advocates. Also, social workers were found to have a wider range of roles in general. Seventy-five percent of the respondents noted an overlap in roles among the disciplines. There was considerable disagreement as to whether team members should have equal power or whether there should be a clear differentiation of roles, and despite high rates of satisfaction with team functioning, the respondents reported confusion about supervisory responsibilities and accountability issues.

The issue of perceived roles in interdisciplinary contexts is an important one for social workers, especially as we consider expanded roles in medication management. Social workers' perceptions of their role often differ from those of others on interdisciplinary teams. For example, Pray (1991) found that physicians viewed hospital social workers basically as discharge planners who merely connect clients to concrete services. They also perceived social workers as having a limited perspective on patients' psychosocial problems. Another study in a medical setting suggested that physicians and nurses do not see social workers as competent to assess emotional difficulties or as having any particularly exclusive domain (Cowles & Lefcowitz, 1992). Such beliefs can lead professionals in other disciplines to subtly constrain social work functions and put social workers in a position of constantly trying to demonstrate their indispensability (Dane & Simon, 1991; Mailick & Jordan, 1977).

Social workers also may tend to stereotype other professionals. Although it is perhaps outdated now, a survey of 41 mental health professionals at three community mental health centers in Sacramento, California, in the early 1980s showed considerable stereotyping in the adjectives used to describe professionals in other fields (Folkins, Wieselberg, & Spensley, 1981). Respondents were asked to describe the "typical" social worker, psychologist, and psychiatrist (raising the possibility of problematic generalizations). The characterizations of others were largely positive, but the authors noted that issues of gender and power(lessness) seemed to be the major factors in the tendency to stereotype. However, a recent study by Sherer (1995) of mental health agencies in Israel found only minor differences among social workers, psychiatrists, and psychologists in role perceptions and functions. The author noted similar types of clients, problems, techniques, tasks, and workload among the three disciplines and little role ambiguity. However, the physician's status as an independent contractor to the agency, as well as education and gender issues, influenced perceptions of the physician as team leader.

The research of Mizrahi and Abramson (1985) on the training and socialization of physicians and social workers provides insight into the disparate views of appropriate social work roles in health and mental health as they relate to interdisciplinary collaboration. Specifically, physicians' training emphasizes hard science and offers little in terms of valuing the clinical relationship or sharing and expressing emotions. They are socialized to be more autonomous and authoritative. Social work, however, strongly emphasizes values, relationships, and self-awareness. Not surprisingly then, a more recent study by Abramson and Mizrahi (1996) that compared positive and negative accounts of collaboration by social workers and physicians found that physicians in general give lower priority to collaboration. These differences are likely to become apparent in the functioning of teams or in the management of collaborative relationships.

Vinokur-Kaplan (1993, 1995) suggested a theoretically and empirically based model for improving the effectiveness of interdisciplinary teams. Her model, based on a normative model of team effectiveness from organizational psychology, integrates data from her own research in psychiatric facilities in Michigan. According to Vinokur-Kaplan, the outcome of a team's work should be a high-quality product (for example, an individualized treatment plan), high team satisfaction and willingness to continue working together, and the participants' belief that each contributed to the well-being of the others. The extent to which these can be achieved comes from creating or establishing certain prerequisites, such as being clear about tasks and having a supportive physical and organizational environment, as well as establishing enabling (continuing process) conditions, such as sufficient effort to achieve the tasks and operating from an adequate knowledge and technical base. This kind of research is needed if interdisciplinary colleagues are to overcome the "separatist tendencies," "deep-rooted antagonisms," "parochialism," and "rigid cultism" that too often have characterized the relationship between the disciplines and become a stubborn barrier to treatment integration (Karuso, 1982).

It is important to restate the value of role clarity in interdisciplinary teams here. In another study in Israel, Rabin and Zelner (1992) started with the assertion that "the ability to attain job clarity without compromising professional standards may be crucial to solving status issues between different professions" (p. 19). They surveyed 87 social workers in a wide variety of mental health settings and found that a social worker's assertiveness (willingness to act) was directly linked to role clarity and job satisfaction.

Only a few empirical studies directly concern the referral process in psychiatric medication management. Goldberg, Riba, and Tasman (1991) surveyed psychiatrists regarding their attitudes toward and practices in working collaboratively with nonmedical psychotherapists. Of the 60 psychiatrists who worked in such an arrangement (medication backup), 73 percent said they worked with social workers who had master's degrees. Although two-thirds of the psychiatrists were satisfied with their level of involvement in cases (25 percent preferred more), they expressed a number of ethical concerns about three-party arrangements, including concerns about liability. It is interesting that medication was first suggested by the nonmedical psychotherapist in three-fourths of the cases. In a survey of social work field instructors, Littrell and Ashford (1994) found that the likelihood of referring to a prescribing physician was related to treatment setting and perceived severity of symptoms. For example, social workers in family services agencies were less likely to make a referral than are those in mental health centers or those working with clients whose symptoms were less severe. In cases of major depression, however, practice setting did not influence referrals.

## RESEARCH ON THE MEANING OF PSYCHIATRIC MEDICATION

We have stated elsewhere (Bentley & Walsh, 1996) that understanding the client's subjective experience with psychiatric medications, as well as the meaning that taking medication has for the individual, is crucial not only to relationship development but also to designing responsive and respectful intervention strategies around medication management. Social work's person-in-environment perspective, with its emphasis on the context of behavior, is helpful in this regard. It is interesting that psychoanalytic interpretations dominated the few early writings on the meaning of medication for clients in the 1950s and 1960s. For example, Sarwer-Foner (1975) emphasized the connection between the physiological effects of a drug and the patient's life experiences, internal conflicts, and drives. Hausner (1985–1986) built on some of these early formulations by suggesting that medication represented a "transitional object" that serves a soothing function, as protection from anxiety while the client is away from the therapist.

Encouraging discussions of the meaning of medication have emerged from anthropological, philosophical, and sociological perspectives. Jonsen (1988) described the symbolic meaning of medications as historically corresponding to one of three ancient Greek meanings for the word "drug": remedy (the power to cure), poison (risk–benefit ambiguities), and magical charm (the power of placebo). Similarly, Brody (1988) proposed a "meaning model" that connects the meaning of drug use to our faith in medicine and a personal physician and the concomitant placebo effect. In addition, Montagne (1988) stated, "the symbolic power of interpersonal interactions in health care might be more influential in structuring and guiding the healing process than the pharmacologic activity of specific substances" (p. 140).

A naturalistic study by a sociologist (Karp, 1992) was an exciting development in the study of the meaning of psychiatric medication. Over a period of several years, the researcher himself was a participant–observer in a case study of a support group for people with an affective disorder. According to Karp, the group's work "constituted a collective search for meaning" (p. 139). He noted that medication use was discussed at every meeting and that these conversations were most often characterized by confusion or ambiguity, with a tremendous variability in experience and opinion. Participants viewed medication as only a partial answer to their individual struggles with depression or bipolar disorder.

Powerful personal accounts can help social workers better appreciate the various meanings that medication can have for clients. Major journals, such as *Schizophrenia Bulletin* and *Psychiatric Services,* now regularly include columns written by mental health services consumers or their family members. Dozens of books, both heartbreaking and heartwarming, describe the personal experiences of people with mental illness or those of their families. The authors invariably emphasize the meaning that medication has for them. Among the best known of these are *A Brilliant*

*Madness* (Duke & Hochman, 1992), *Nobody's Child* (Balter & Katz, 1992), *I Never Promised You a Rose Garden* (Greenberg, 1964), *The Eden Express* (Vonnegut, 1975), *Is There No Place Else on Earth for Me?* (Sheehan, 1982), and *Girl, Interrupted* (Kaysen, 1993). This literature, which can be both profoundly dramatic and positively life altering as well as unspeakably traumatic and disillusioning, is a powerful and engaging way to build empathy and appreciation for the physical and emotional experiences of clients (Davis & Bowker, 1988).

Brekke, Levin, Wolkon, Sobel, and Slade (1993) reviewed the limited but more quantitatively oriented scholarly literature on the subjective experience in mental illness. Although their research did not explicitly pursue meaning or medication issues per se, it suggested the importance of the relationship of subjective, first-hand experiences and attributed meanings to everyday social functioning. Awad (1993), on the other hand, did expressly study the subjective experiences of select groups of consumers with their medications. He presented and tested a conceptual model for understanding the impact of medications and concluded: "subjective interpretation of the physiological changes that accompany the medicated state can influence the behavioral outcome of pharmacological therapy, including the experience of side effects" (pp. 609–610). Other research by Awad and others has noted the connection between a negative subjective experience with neuroleptics and poor adherence among a group of people diagnosed with schizophrenia.

Perhaps the best known scholar making a plea for more study of the subjective experience in mental illness is Yale's John Strauss (1989). His basic argument is that ignoring the subjective experience causes one to miss the interaction between the person and the disorder. If the two are separated, according to a recent profile of the famous psychiatrist, "you end up with a sort of rag bag of symptoms and signs and a label" (Strauss, quoted in Davidson, 1996, p. 1). The renewed recognition of this line of inquiry is welcome and will be useful in understanding the meaning of medications in clients' lives.

## Implications for Social Work Roles in Practice and Research

In our text on social work practice and psychotropic medication (Bentley & Walsh, 1996), we suggested a number of contemporary roles for social workers in medication management that can be carried out in the context of a partnership model of practice. The social worker can be a collaborator or consultant, educator, monitor, and advocate. Specifically, knowledge of the basics of psychopharmacology and research on the effectiveness of psychotropic medications prepare social workers to converse articulately with both clients and physicians and build state-of-the-science treatment plans. Social workers can describe the rationale for drug or combined treatment and make appropriate referrals when needed. This knowledge puts social work practitioners in a much better position to fully assess and then prepare clients for such a referral. Information about drug action, typical therapeutic indexes, and dosing can be shared, and clients' expectations, doubts, fears, and meanings can be elicited. Social workers also are equipped to help clients, families, and physicians in monitoring medications' effects over time, better explaining and empathizing with frustrations about lag time and bothersome side effects as well as about the ambiguities of less than full adherence to medication regimens. Social workers can and should use professional problem-solving processes and models of skills training to help clients and families with the range of medication-related issues and concerns.

Social workers also have an important potential role as educators. Knowledge of psychopharmacology, combined with good data on medication education's positive effects and social work's interpersonal and change-oriented skills, prepares us to design and deliver, ideally in collaboration with other providers, the education for which clients and their families are asking. This knowledge of both psychopharmacology and the psychosocial aspects of medication management helps social workers competently manage the parallel relationships that may exist and to advocate for clients when needed. One part of the advocate's role may be to assist individual clients with negotiations with their physician, facility, agency, or insurance company (Bentley, 1993; Cohen, 1988). Higgins (1995) also noted the role of social workers in political advocacy, especially in trying to improve the availability and affordability of certain expensive psychiatric medications for all classes of clients.

The role of the social worker as researcher is increasingly recognized. Mental health researchers from various fields have called for more studies by social workers in the area of psychopharmacology. The need continues for outcome research on the combined or interactive effects of interventions with a range of populations and problems. Cohen (1988) has urged practitioners to publish case studies about both the positive and the negative effects of medications. Clearly, there is more to discover about side effects and adherence and about successfully managing interprofessional issues and collaborative relationships in the mental health field. Finally, a more sophisticated and client-centered understanding of the meaning of medication in the lives of the children and adults we social workers serve would certainly make us more responsive, compassionate professionals.

# References

Abramson, J. S., & Mizrahi, T. (1996). When social workers and physicians collaborate: Positive and negative interdisciplinary experiences. *Social Work, 41,* 270–281.

Anderson, C., Reiss, D., & Hogarty, G. (1986). The survival skills workshop. In C. Anderson, D. Reiss, & G. Hogarty (Eds.), *Schizophrenia and the family: A practitioner's guide to psychoeducation and management* (pp. 71–131). New York: Guilford Press.

Aspler, R., & Rothman, E. (1984). Correlates of compliance with psychoactive prescriptions. *Journal of Psychoactive Drugs, 16,* 193–199.

Austin, M. P., Souza, F. G., & Goodwin, G. M. (1991). Lithium augmentation in antidepressant-resistant patients: A quantitative analysis. *British Journal of Psychiatry, 159,* 510–514.

Awad, A. G. (1993). Subjective response to neuroleptics in schizophrenia. *Schizophrenia Bulletin, 19,* 609–618.

Bakish, D., Bradwejn, J., Nair, N., McClure, J., Remick, R., & Bulger, L. (1992). A comparison of moclobemide, amitriptyline, and placebo in depression: A Canadian multicenter study. *Psychopharmacology, 106*(Suppl.), 98–101.

Ballenger, J. C. (1993). Panic disorder: Efficacy of current treatments. *Psychopharmacology Bulletin, 29,* 477–486.

Ballenger, J. C., Burrows, G., DuPont, R., Lesser, I. M., Pecknold, J. C., Noyes, R., Rifkin, A., & Swinson, R. P. (1988). Alprazolam in panic disorder and agoraphobia—Results from a multicenter trial. I. Efficacy in short-term treatment. *Archives of General Psychiatry, 45,* 413–422.

Balter, M., & Katz, R. (1992). *Nobody's child.* Reading, MA: Addison-Wesley.

Batey, S. R., & Ledbetter, L. E. (1982). Medication education for patients in a partial hospitalization program. *Journal of Psychosocial Nursing and Mental Health Services, 20*(7), 7–15.

Beitman, B. D., & Klerman, G. L. (Eds.). (1991). *Integrating pharmacotherapy and psychotherapy.* Washington, DC: American Psychiatric Press.

Bentley, K. J. (1993). The right of psychiatric patients to refuse medications: Where should social workers stand? [Points & Viewpoints]. *Social Work, 38,* 101–106.

Bentley, K. J. (in press). Psychopharmacological treatment of schizophrenia: What social workers need to know. *Research on Social Work Practice.*

Bentley, K. J., Rosenson, M., & Zito, J. (1990). Promoting medication compliance: Strategies for working with families of mentally ill people. *Social Work, 35,* 274–277.

Bentley, K. J., & Walsh, J. (1996). *The social worker and psychotropic medications: Toward effective collaboration with mental health consumers, families and providers.* Pacific Grove, CA: Brooks/Cole.

Bernstein, J. G. (1995). *Handbook of drug therapy in psychiatry* (3rd ed.). St. Louis: C. V. Mosby.

Blackwell, B. (1979). The drug regimen and treatment compliance. In R. B. Haynes, D. W. Taylor, & D. L. Sackett (Eds.), *Compliance in health care* (pp. 144–156). Baltimore: Johns Hopkins University Press.

Borison, R. L., Pathiraja, A. P., Diamond, B. I., & Meibach, R. C. (1992). Risperidone: Clinical safety and efficacy in schizophrenia. *Psychopharmacology Bulletin, 28,* 213–218.

Bowden, C. L., Brugger, A. M., Swann, A. C., Calabreze, J. R., Janicak, P. G., Petty, F., Dilsaver, S. C., Davis, J. M., Rush, A. J., & Small, J. G. (1994). Efficacy of divalproex vs. lithium and placebo in the treatment of mania. *JAMA, 271,* 918–924.

Bradley, S. (1990). Non-physician psychotherapist—physician pharmacotherapist: A new model for concurrent treatment. *Psychiatric Clinics of North America, 13,* 307–322.

Bradwejn, J., Shriqui, C., Koszycki, D., & Meterissian, G. (1990). Double-blind comparison of the effects of clonazepam and lorazepam in acute mania. *Journal of Clinical Psychopharmacology, 10,* 403–408.

Breggin, P. R. (1987). *Psychiatric drugs: Hazards to the brain.* New York: Springer.

Breggin, P. R. (1991). *Toxic psychiatry.* New York: St. Martin's Press.

Brekke, J. S., Levin, S., Wolkon, G. H., Sobel, E., & Slade, E. (1993). Psychosocial functioning and subjective experience in schizophrenia. *Schizophrenia Bulletin, 19,* 599–608.

Brody, H. (1988). The symbolic power of the modern personal physician: The placebo response under challenge. *Journal of Drug Issues, 18,* 149–161.

Brown, C. S., Wright, R. G., & Christenson, O. B. (1987). Association between type of medication, instruction and patient's knowledge, side effects and compliance. *Hospital and Community Psychiatry, 38,* 55–60.

Buckalew, L., & Sallis, R. (1986). Patient compliance and medication perception. *Journal of Clinical Psychology, 42,* 49–53.

Busch, F. N., & Gould, E. (1993). Treatment by a psychotherapist and a psychopharmacologist: Transference and countertransference issues. *Hospital and Community Psychiatry, 44,* 772–774.

Calabreze, J. R., & Delucchi, G. A. (1990). Spectrum of efficacy of valproate in 55 patients with rapid cycling bipolar disorder. *American Journal of Psychiatry, 147,* 431–434.

Charney, D. S., Miller, H. L., Licinio, J., & Salomon, R. (1995). Treatment of depression. In A. F. Schatzberg & C. B. Nemeroff (Eds.), *The American Psychiatric Press textbook of psychopharmacology* (pp. 575–601). Washington, DC: American Psychiatric Press.

Chouinard, G. (1987). Clonazepam in the acute and maintenance treatment of bipolar disorder. *Journal of Clinical Psychiatry, 48*(10), 29–36.

Chouinard, G., Jones, B., Remington, G., Bloom, D., Addington, P., MacEwan, G. W., Labelle, A., Beauclair, L., & Arnott, W. (1993). A Canadian multicenter placebo-controlled study of fixed doses of risperidone and haloperidol in the treatment of chronic schizophrenia patients. *Journal of Clinical Psychopharmacology, 13*, 25–40.

Clomipramine Collaborative Study Group. (1991). Clomipramine in the treatment of patients with obsessive–compulsive disorder. *Archives of General Psychiatry, 48*, 730–738.

Cohen, D. (1988). Social work and psychotropic drug treatments. *Social Service Review, 62*, 576–599.

Cohen, D., & McCubbin, M. (1990). The political economy of tardive dyskinesia: Asymmetries in power and responsibility. *Journal of Mind and Behavior, 11*, 465–488.

Cole, J. O. (1964). Phenothiazine treatment in acute schizophrenia. *Archives of General Psychiatry, 10*, 246–261.

Collins-Colon, T. (1990). Do it yourself: Medication management for community-based clients. *Journal of Psychosocial Nursing and Mental Health Services, 28*(6), 25–29.

Cowles, L. A., & Lefcowitz, M. (1992). Interdisciplinary expectations of the medical social worker in the hospital setting. *Health & Social Work, 17*, 57–65.

Coxhead, N., Silverstone, T., & Cookson, J. (1992). Carbamazepine versus lithium in the prophylaxis of bipolar affective disorder. *Acta Psychiatrica Scandinavica, 85*, 114–118.

Dane, B. O., & Simon, B. L. (1991). Resident guests: Social workers in host settings. *Social Work, 36*, 208–213.

Davidson, L. (1996, Spring). Mental illness and the person: A profile of John Strauss, M. D. *NARSAD Research Newsletter*, p. 1.

Davis, J. M., Janicak, P. G., Wang, Z., Gibbons, R., & Sharma, R. (1992). The efficacy of psychotropic drugs. *Psychopharmacology Bulletin, 28*, 151–155.

Davis, L. F., & Bowker, J. P. (1988). Living with mental illness: Examining personal experience. In J. Bowker (Ed.), *Services for the chronically mentally ill* (pp. 1–17). Washington, DC: Council on Social Work Education.

Diamond, R. (1983). Enhancing medication use in schizophrenic patients. *Journal of Clinical Psychiatry, 44*(6, Part 2), 7–14.

DiMatteo, M. R., & DiNicola, D. D. (1982). *Achieving patient compliance: The psychology of the medical practitioner's role.* Tarrytown, NY: Pergamon Press.

Downing, R. W., & Rickels, K. (1985). Early treatment response in anxious outpatients treated with diazepam. *Acta Psychiatrica Scandinavica, 72*, 522–528.

Draine, J., & Solomon, P. (1994). Explaining attitudes toward medication compliance among a seriously mentally ill population. *Journal of Nervous and Mental Disease, 182*, 50–54.

Dubovsky, S. L. (1993). Calcium antagonists in manic–depressive illness. *Neuropsychobiology, 13*, 224–228.

Duke, P., & Hochman, G. (1992). *A brilliant madness: Living with manic–depressive illness.* New York: Bantam Books.

Dunbar, J., Marshall, G., & Hovell, M. (1979). Behavioral strategies for improving compliance. In R. B. Haynes, D. W. Taylor, & D. Sackett (Eds.), *Compliance in health care* (pp. 174–190). Baltimore: Johns Hopkins University Press.

Eckman, T. A., Liberman, R. P., Phipps, C. C., & Blair, K. E. (1990). Teaching medication management skills to schizophrenic patients. *Journal of Clinical Psychopharmacology, 10*(1), 33–38.

Falloon, I., Boyd, J., & McGill, C. (1984). *Family care of schizophrenia: A problem-solving approach to the treatment of mental illness.* New York: Guilford Press.

Folkins, C., Wieselberg, N., & Spensley, J. (1981). Discipline stereotyping and evaluative attitudes among community mental health center staff. *American Journal of Orthopsychiatry, 51,* 15–28.

Frank, E., Karp, J. F., & Rush, A. J. (1993). Efficacy of treatments for major depression. *Psychopharmacology Bulletin, 29,* 457–475.

Frank, E., Perel, J. M., Mallinger, A. G., Thase, M. E., & Kupfer, D. J. (1992). Relationship of pharmacologic compliance to long-term prophylaxis in recurrent depression. *Psychopharmacology Bulletin, 28,* 231–235.

Gadow, K. D. (1991). Clinical issues in child and adolescent psychopharmacology. *Journal of Counseling and Clinical Psychology, 59,* 842–852.

Gelenberg, A. J., & Hopkins, H. S. (1993). Reports on efficacy of treatments for bipolar disorder. *Psychopharmacology Bulletin, 29,* 447–456.

Gitlin, M. J., Cochran, S. D., & Jamison, K. R. (1989). Maintenance lithium treatment: Side effects and compliance. *Journal of Clinical Psychiatry, 50,* 127–131.

Goldberg, R. S., Riba, M., & Tasman, A. (1991). Psychiatrists' attitudes toward prescribing medication for patients treated by nonmedical psychotherapists. *Hospital and Community Psychiatry, 42,* 276–280.

Goodwin, F. K., & Jamison, K. R. (1990). *Manic–depressive illness.* New York: Oxford University Press.

Greenberg, H. (Hannah Green). (1964). *I never promised you a rose garden.* New York: Holt, Rinehart and Winston.

Grob, G. (1983). *Mental illness and American society: 1875–1940.* Princeton, NJ: Princeton University Press.

Grob, G. (1991). *From asylum to community: Mental health policy in modern America.* Princeton, NJ: Princeton University Press.

Hancock, L. (1996, March 18). Mother's little helper. *Newsweek,* pp. 51–56.

Hausner, R. (1985–1986). Medication and transitional phenomena. *International Journal of Psychoanalytic Psychotherapy, 11,* 375–407.

Hays, R. D., & DiMatteo, M. R. (1987). Key issues and suggestions for patient compliance assessment: Sources of information, focus of measures, and nature of response option. *Journal of Compliance in Health Care, 2,* 37–53.

Hechtman, L., Weiss, G., & Perlman, T. (1984). Young adult outcome of hyperactive children who received long-term stimulant treatment. *Journal of the American Academy of Child Psychiatry, 23,* 261–269.

Higgins, P. B. (1995). Clozapine and the treatment of schizophrenia: Implications for social work practice. *Health & Social Work, 20,* 124–132.

Himmelhoch, J. M., Thase, M. E., Mallinger, A. G., & Houck, P. (1991). Tranylcypromine versus imipramine in anergic bipolar depression. *American Journal of Psychiatry, 148,* 910–916.

Hogarty, G. E., Kornblith, S. J., Greenwald, D., & DiBarry, A. L., Cooley, S., Flesher, S., Reiss, D., Carter, M., & Ulrich, R. (1995a). Personal therapy: A disorder-relevant psychotherapy for schizophrenia. *Schizophrenia Bulletin, 21,* 379–393.

Hogarty, G. E., McEvoy, J. P., Ulrich, R. F., DiBarry, A. L., Bartone, P., Cooley, S., Hammill, K., Carter, M., Munetz, M. R., & Perel, J. (1995b). Pharmacotherapy of impaired affect in recovering schizophrenia patients. *Archives of General Psychiatry, 52,* 29–41.

Hoschl, C., & Kozeny, J. (1989). Verapamil in affective disorders: A controlled, double-blind study. *Biological Psychiatry, 25,* 128–140.

Hyman, S. E., Arana, G. W., & Rosenbaum, J. F. (1995). *Handbook of psychiatric drug therapy* (3rd ed.). Boston: Little, Brown.

Isaac, L. M., Tamblyn, R. M., & McGill–Calgary Drug Research Team. (1993). Compliance and cognitive function: A methodological approach to measuring unintentional errors in medication compliance in the elderly. *Gerontologist, 33,* 772–781.

Jacobvitz, D. (1990). Treatment of attentional and hyperactivity problems in children with sympathomimetic drugs: A comprehensive review. *Journal of the American Academy of Child and Adolescent Psychiatry, 29,* 677–688.

Jamison, K. R., & Akiskal, H. S. (1983). Medication compliance in patients with bipolar disorder. *Psychiatric Clinics of North America, 6,* 175–192.

Jamison, K., Gerner, R., & Goodwin, F. (1979). Patient and physician attitudes toward lithium. *Archives of General Psychiatry, 36,* 866–869.

Janicak, P. G., Davis, J. M., Preskorn, S. H., & Ayd, F. J. (1993). *Principles and practice of psychopharmacotherapy.* Baltimore: Williams & Wilkins.

Jenike, M. A. (1993). Obsessive–compulsive disorder: Efficacy of specific treatments as assessed by controlled trials. *Psychopharmacology Bulletin, 29,* 487–499.

Jeste, D. V., & Caligiuri, M. P. (1993). Tardive dyskinesia. *Schizophrenia Bulletin, 19,* 303–312.

Jonsen, A. R. (1988). Ethics of drug giving and drug taking. *Journal of Drug Issues, 18,* 195–200.

Kane, J. M. (Ed.). (1984). *Drug maintenance strategies in schizophrenia.* Washington, DC: American Psychiatric Press.

Kane, J. M., & Marder, S. R. (1993). Psychopharmacologic treatment of schizophrenia. *Schizophrenia Bulletin, 19,* 113–128.

Karp, D. A. (1992). Illness and ambiguity and the search for meaning: A case study of a self-help group for affective disorders. *Journal of Contemporary Ethnography, 21,* 139–170.

Karuso, T. (1982). Psychotherapy and pharmacotherapy: Toward an integrated model. *American Journal of Psychiatry, 139,* 1102–1113.

Kaysen, S. (1993). *Girl, interrupted.* New York: Turtle Bay Books.

Keith, S. J., & Matthews, S. M. (1993). The value of psychiatric treatment: Its efficacy in severe mental disorders. *Psychopharmacology Bulletin, 29,* 427–430.

Kelly, G. R., Scott, J. E., & Mamon, J. (1990). Medication compliance and health education among outpatients with chronic mental disorders. *Medical Care, 28,* 1181–1197.

Kelly, K. V. (1992). Parallel treatment: Therapy with one clinician and medication with another. *Hospital and Community Psychiatry, 43,* 778–780.

Keshavan, M. S., & Kennedy, J. S. (1992). *Drug-induced dysfunction in psychiatry.* New York: Hemisphere.

Kinross-Wright, V. (1954). Chlorpromazine—A major advance in psychiatric treatment. *Postgraduate Medicine, 16,* 297–299.

Klein, D., & Davis, J. M. (1969). *Diagnosis and drug treatment of psychiatric disorders.* Baltimore: Williams & Wilkins.

Klerman, G. L., Weissman, M. M., Rounsaville, B. J., & Chevron, E. S. (1984). *Interpersonal psychotherapy of depression*. New York: Basic Books.

Kucera-Bozarth, K., Beck, N. C., & Lyss, L. (1982). Compliance with lithium regimens. *Journal of Psychosocial Nursing and Mental Health Services, 20*(7), 11–15.

Kupfer, D. J., Frank, E., Perel, J. M., Cornes, C., Mallinger, A. G., Thase, M. E., McEachran, A. B., & Grochocinski, V. J. (1989). Five-year outcome for maintenance therapies in recurrent depression. *Archives of General Psychiatry, 49*, 769–773.

Kupfer, D. J., & Siegal, C. R. (1995). Alliance not compliance: A philosophy of outpatient care. *Journal of Clinical Psychiatry, 56*(Suppl. 1), 11–16.

Lecrubier, Y., & Guelfi, J. D. (1990). Efficacy of reversible inhibitors of monoamine oxidase-A in various forms of depression. *Acta Psychiatrica Scandinavica, 360*, 18–23.

Leventhal, H., Diefenbach, M., & Leventhal, E. A. (1992). Illness cognition: Using common sense to understand treatment adherence and affect cognition interactions. *Cognitive Therapy and Research, 16*, 143–163.

Liberman, R., Kane, J., Vaccaro, J., & Wirshing, W. (1987, October). *Negotiating medication issues with schizophrenic patients*. Workshop conducted at the Institute on Hospital and Community Psychiatry, Boston.

Lieberman, J. A., & Koreen, A. R. (1993). Neurochemistry and neuroendocrinology of schizophrenia: A selective review. *Schizophrenia Bulletin, 19*, 197–255.

Liebowitz, M. R., Quitkin, M., Stewart, J. W., McGrath, P. J., Harrison, W. M., Markowitz, J. S., Rabkin, J. G., Trichamo, E., Goetz, D. M., & Klein, D. F. (1988). Antidepressant specificity in major depression. *Archives of General Psychiatry, 45*, 129–137.

Liebowitz, M. R., Schneier, F. R., Hollander, E., Welcowitz, L., Saouno, J. B., Feerick, J., Camperas, R., Fallon, B. A., Street, L., & Gitow, A. (1991). Treatment of social phobia with drugs other than benzodiazepines. *Journal of Clinical Psychiatry, 52*(11, Suppl.), 10–15.

Littrell, J., & Ashford, J. B. (1994). The duty of social workers to refer for medications: A study of field instructors. *Social Work Research, 18*, 123–128.

Mailick, M. D., & Jordan, D. (1977). A multimodel approach to collaborative practice in health care settings. *Social Work in Health Care, 2*, 445–457.

Malhotra, A. K., Pinsky, D. A., & Breier, A. (1996). Future antipsychotic agents: Clinical implications. In A. Breier (Ed.), *The new psychopharmacology of schizophrenia* (pp. 41–56). Washington, DC: American Psychiatric Press.

Meibach, R. C., Dunner, D., Wilson, L. G., Ishiki, D., & Dager, S. R. (1987). Comparative efficacy of propranolol, chlordiazepoxide, and placebo in the treatment of anxiety: A double blind trial. *Journal of Clinical Psychiatry, 48*, 355–358.

Meltzer, H. Y. (1991). The mechanism and action of novel antipsychotic drugs. *Schizophrenia Bulletin, 17*, 71–95.

Mercugliano, M. (1993). Psychopharmacology in children with developmental disabilities. *Pediatric Clinics of North America, 40*, 593–614.

Mizrahi, T., & Abramson, J. (1985). Sources of strain between physicians and social workers. Implications for social workers in health care settings. *Social Work in Health Care, 10*(3), 33–51.

Montagne, M. (1988). Philosophies of drug giving and drug taking. *Journal of Drug Issues, 18*, 139–148.

Morris, L. S., & Schulz, P. M. (1993). Medication compliance: The patient's perspective. *Clinical Therapeutics, 15*, 593–606.

Parmelee, D. X. (1996). *Pediatric psychopharmacology*. Richmond, VA: Commonwealth Institute for Child and Family Studies.

Pray, J. E. (1991). Responding to psychosocial needs: Physician perceptions of their referral practices for hospitalized patients. *Health & Social Work, 16,* 184–192.

Rabin, C., & Zelner, D. (1992). The role of assertiveness in clarifying roles and strengthening job satisfaction of social workers in multidisciplinary mental health settings. *British Journal of Social Work, 22,* 17–32.

Rickels, K. (1982). Benzodiazepines in the treatment of anxiety. In E. Usdin, P. Skolnick, J. F. Tallman, D. Greenblatt, & S. M. Paul (Eds.), *Pharmacology of benzodiazepines* (pp. 37–44). London: Macmillan.

Rickels, K. (1987). Antianxiety therapy: Potential value of long-term treatment. *Journal of Clinical Psychiatry, 48,* 7–11.

Rickels, K., & Schweizer, S. (1990). The clinical course and long-term management of generalized anxiety disorder. *Journal of Clinical Psychopharmacology, 10,* 101–110.

Robinson, G., Gilbertson, A., & Litwak, L. (1986). The effects of psychiatric patient education to medication program on post-discharge compliance. *Psychiatric Quarterly, 58,* 113–118.

Rodenhauser, P., Schwenker, C. E., & Khamis, H. J. (1987). Factors related to drug treatment refusal in a forensic hospital. *Hospital and Community Psychiatry, 38,* 631–637.

Rodenhauser, P., & Stone, W. N. (1993). Combining psychopharmacotherapy and group psychotherapy: Problems and advantages. *International Journal of Group Psychotherapy, 43,* 11–28.

Sachs, G. S., Weilburg, J. B., & Rosebaum J. F. (1990). Clonazepam vs. neuroleptics as adjuncts to lithium maintenance. *Psychopharmacology Bulletin, 26,* 137–143.

Safferman, A., Lieberman, J. A., Kane, J. M., Szymanski, S., & Kinon, B. (1991). Update on the clinical efficacy and side effects of clozapine. *Schizophrenia Bulletin, 17,* 55–70.

Sarwer-Foner, G. J. (1975). Psychiatric symptomatology: Its meaning and function in relation to the psychodynamic action of drugs. In H.C.B. Denbar (Ed.), *Psychopharmacological treatment: Theory and practice* (pp. 201–224). New York: Marcel Dekker.

Satterfield, J. H., Satterfield, B. T., & Shell, A. M. (1987). Therapeutic interventions to prevent delinquency in hyperactive boys. *Journal of the American Academy of Child and Adolescent Psychiatry, 26,* 56–64.

Schatzberg, A. F., & Nemeroff, C. B. (Eds.). (1995). *The American Psychiatric Press textbook of psychiatry.* Washington, DC: American Psychiatric Press.

Schooler, N. R., & Keith, S. J. (1993). The clinical research base for the treatment of schizophrenia. *Psychopharmacology Bulletin, 29,* 431–446.

Scou, M. (1989). Lithium prophylaxis: Myths and realities. *American Journal of Psychiatry, 146,* 573–576.

Seltzer, A., Roncari, I., & Garfinkel, P. (1980). Effect of patient education on medical compliance. *Canadian Journal of Psychiatry, 25,* 638–645.

Sheehan, S. (1982). *Is there no place else on earth for me?* New York: Random House.

Sherer, M. (1995). Division of work among mental health professionals in Israel. *Administration and Policy in Mental Health, 22,* 447–456.

Small, J. G., Klapper, M. H., Milstein, V., Kellams, J. J., Miller, M. J., Marhenke, J. D., & Small, I. F. (1991). Carbamazepine compared to lithium in the treatment of mania. *Archives of General Psychiatry, 48,* 915–921.

Solomon, P., Draine, J., & Delaney, M. A. (1995). The working alliance and consumer case management. *Journal of Mental Health Administration, 22,* 126–134.

Stein, G., & Bernadt, M. (1993). Lithium augmentation therapy in tricyclic-resistant depression: A controlled trial using lithium in low and normal doses. *British Journal of Psychiatry, 162,* 634–640.

Stimson, G. V. (1974). Obeying doctor's orders: A view from the other side. *Social Science and Medicine, 8,* 97–104.

Strauss, J. S. (1989). Subjective experiences of schizophrenia: Toward a new dynamic psychiatry—II. *Schizophrenia Bulletin, 15,* 179–187.

Sussman, N. (1993). Treating anxiety while minimizing abuse and dependence. *Journal of Clinical Psychiatry, 54*(Suppl. 5), 44–51.

Swazey, J. P. (1974). *Chlorpromazine in psychiatry: A study of therapeutic innovation.* Cambridge, MA: MIT Press.

Sylvester, C. (1993). Psychopharmacology of disorders in children. *Psychiatric Clinics of North America, 16,* 779–788.

Tamminga, C. T. (1996, Winter). The new generation of antipsychotic drugs. *NARSAD Research Newsletter,* pp. 4–6.

Taylor, C. B. (1995). Treatment of anxiety disorders. In A. F. Schatzberg & C. B. Nemeroff (Eds.), *The American Psychiatric Press textbook of psychopharmacology* (pp. 641–656). Washington, DC: American Psychiatric Press.

Tesar, G. E., Rosenbaum, J. F., Pollack, M. H., Otta, M. W., Sachs, G. S., Herman, J. B., Cohen, L. S., & Spier, S. A. (1991). Double-blind, placebo-controlled comparison of clonazepam and alprazolam for panic disorder. *Journal of Clinical Psychiatry, 52,* 69–76.

Toseland, R., Palmer-Ganeles, J., & Chapman, D. (1986). Teamwork in psychiatric settings. *Social Work, 31,* 46–52.

Turk, D., Salovey, P., & Litt, M. (1986). Adherence: A cognitive–behavioral perspective. In K. Gerber & A. Nehemkis (Eds.), *Compliance: The dilemma of the chronically ill* (pp. 44–72). New York: Springer.

VanPutten, T. (1974). Why do schizophrenic patients refuse to take their drugs? *Archives of General Psychiatry, 31,* 67–72.

Vinokur-Kaplan, D. (1993, February). *Integrating team effectiveness into social work practice: Some responses to disciplinary diversity.* Paper presented at the Annual Program Meeting of the Council on Social Work Education, New York.

Vinokur-Kaplan, D. (1995). Enhancing the effectiveness of interdisciplinary mental health treatment teams. *Administration and Policy in Mental Health, 22,* 521–530.

Vonnegut, M. (1975). *The Eden Express: A personal account of schizophrenia.* New York: Praeger.

Wallace, C. J. (1993). Psychiatric rehabilitation. *Psychopharmacology Bulletin, 29,* 537–548.

Walsh, J. (in press). The psychopharmacological treatment of bipolar disorder: What social workers need to know. *Research on Social Work Practice.*

Weiden, P., Rapkin, B., Mott, T., Zygmut, A., Goldman, D., Horvitz-Lennon, M., & Frances, A. (1994). Rating of medication influences (ROMI) scale in schizophrenia. *Schizophrenia Bulletin, 20,* 297–307.

Weissman, M. (1972). Casework and pharmacotherapy in the treatment of depression. *Social Casework, 53,* 38–44.

Wender, P. H., Remherr, F. W., & Wood, D. (1985). A controlled study of methylphenidate in the treatment of attention deficit disorder, residual type, in adults. *American Journal of Psychiatry, 142,* 547–552.

Williams, R., Edwards, R. A., Newburn, G. M., Mullen, R., Menkes, D. B., & Segkar, C. (1993). A double-blind comparison of moclobemide and fluoxetine in the treatment of depressive disorders. *International Clinical Psychopharmacology, 7,* 155–158.

Wilson, W. H., & Claussen, A. M. (1993). New antipsychotic medications: Hope for the future. *Innovations & Research, 2*(1), 3–12.

Winkelman, N. W. (1954). Chlorpromazine in the treatment of neuropsychiatric disorders. *JAMA, 155,* 18–21.

Yank, G. R., Bentley, K. J., & Hargrove, D. S. (1993). The vulnerability-stress model of schizophrenia: Advances in psychosocial treatment. *American Journal of Orthopsychiatry, 63,* 55–69.

Youssef, F. (1984). Adherence to therapy in psychiatric patients: An empirical investigation of the impact of patient education. *International Journal of Nursing Studies, 21,* 51–57.

# Psychoeducation and Severe Mental Illness: Implications for Social Work Practice and Research

Ellen P. Lukens and Helle Thorning

Psychoeducation is increasingly valued as a critical component in the treatment of severe mental illness, particularly schizophrenia. During the past 20 years, a range of psychoeducational models have been developed and tested to address the needs of people with schizophrenia and their family members. Some of these models are strictly educational in design; others include a treatment or therapy component, hence the term "psychoeducation." The models are generally designed to impart information about the illness to family members and other primary caregivers.

This chapter reviews the literature on psychoeducation and severe mental illness in a way that is relevant to social work. The objectives are to

- reflect on the critical components of psychoeducation by describing the evolution and history of the models
- review the research literature on psychoeducational interventions
- discuss the implications of psychoeducation for the person with illness and his or her family, as well as for the clinician
- examine psychoeducation as a key component in treatment from the perspective of both practice and research.

The research described in this chapter is focused on schizophrenia because the psychoeducational models evolved in response to observations of this illness. Schizophrenia is a severe brain disease characterized by symptoms that can include delusions, hallucinations, disorganized thinking and speech, and disorganized behavior as well as restricted affect and speech, loss of volition, and social withdrawal (American Psychiatric Association [APA], 1994). It is well documented that schizophrenia also is associated with denial or unawareness of illness and poor compliance with treatment (Amador, Strauss, Yale, & Gorman, 1991).

## Social Work, Education, and Empowerment

Social workers traditionally have placed a strong emphasis on education as an important means of empowering and enabling clients to assume mastery and control over their lives (Germain & Gitterman, 1996; Simon, 1994). Advocates for an empowerment-based practice consider teaching, training, and education to be central to the social work process (Cochran, 1993; Parsons, Jorgenson, & Hernandez, 1994;

Simon, 1994). Thus, psychoeducational models have important implications for treatment, research, and training in social work.

According to Kieffer (1984), the process of empowerment generally proceeds through several stages, including

1. the individual's personal growth, with implications for larger social change
2. increased sense of self-esteem, self-efficacy, and control, combined with an ability to critically assess the situation and cultivate and use resources
3. a social movement that begins with the education and politicization of powerless people who collectively work to gain power and change oppressive structures.

As disempowered people gain knowledge, they are increasingly prepared to make informed decisions regarding their own lives and the lives of those for whom they are responsible and to adequately advocate for themselves and their needs, both individually and collectively. Such a process of education has been central in the evolution of powerful self-help movements such as the Alliance for the Mentally Ill (AMI) (Sommer, 1990). In turn, demands from such well-organized groups for research and new approaches to rehabilitation have increased interest and awareness among social workers and other mental health professionals regarding education, policy, and treatment for severe mental illness.

## What Is Psychoeducation?

Psychoeducation has not been consistently defined, either in terms of what it is or how it is presented. Although common themes have emerged in the literature, models vary considerably in terms of content, breadth and length of presentation, how and when information is presented, who is included in the process, and how education is combined with other forms of intervention.

Some discussion can be found in the literature about the differences between education per se and psychoeducation. Although the terms are often used interchangeably, some distinction can be made as to how information is imparted and processed. "Education" implies a presentation of facts and information regarding the illness in question and could be taught by either a layperson or a professional. "Psychoeducation" suggests an additional treatment component, usually facilitated by a mental health professional who has been trained in clinical intervention (Hatfield, 1990; Lam, 1991).

Educational models generally include information on the epidemiology and nature of illness, diagnosis and symptoms, etiology, course and outcome, and medication (Anderson, Reiss, & Hogarty, 1986; Lam, 1991; Lukens & Thorning, 1996; McFarlane et al., 1995; Mueser & Gingerich, 1994). Additional topics include stress management, street drugs, side effects of medication, and community resources (Falloon, Boyd, & McGill, 1984; Smith & Birchwood, 1987). Depending on the intervention, the educational material might be covered in one or two condensed sessions (Barrowclough & Tarrier, 1987; Berkowitz, Eberlein-Fries, Kuipers, & Leff, 1984; Falloon et al., 1984), in a one-day workshop that serves as an introduction to an on-going intervention (Anderson et al., 1986; McFarlane et al., 1995), or in a series of sessions over time (Thorning & Lukens, in press; Tunnel, Albert, Jacobs, & Osiasom, 1988).

The psychoeducational interventions extend the education to include a range of psychotherapeutic approaches using cognitive, behavioral and psychosocial techniques (Anderson et al., 1986; Falloon et al., 1984; Köttgen, Sönnichsen, Mollenhauer, & Jurth, 1984; McFarlane et al., 1995). Models have been designed for the person with the illness alone as well as for individual family sessions with or without the presence of the person with the illness (Barrowclough & Tarrier, 1987; Berkowitz et al., 1984; McGill, Falloon, Boyd, & Wood-Siverio, 1983). Other programs have been designed for a group of families meeting together, hence the term "multiple-family groups" (Abramowitz & Coursey, 1989; Cozolino, Nuechterlein, West, & Snyder, 1988; McFarlane et al., 1995, Smith & Birchwood, 1987). Proponents of the multiple-family group approach describe the important role the group plays in enhancing the educational process through the expansion of the social network as well as community and professional supports (McFarlane et al., 1995). In some cases, the person with the illness is invited to attend the sessions, both to gain knowledge and to serve as an expert witness; in others, emphasis has been placed on work with only relatives (Leff et al., 1989; Thorning & Lukens, in press). Often the decision whether to include the person with the illness depends on readiness for treatment.

## Changing Attitudes toward Family Involvement in Treatment

Any chronic illness has a devastating impact on both the person with the illness and the family, regardless of where the person with the illness resides. In the United States, an estimated 50 percent to 75 percent of adults who currently have schizophrenia reside with their families (Kuipers & Bebbington, 1988). Family members are often the primary caregivers, so questions about the relationship between the clinical characteristics of the person with illness and the effects of those characteristics on other family members are important to consider.

Over the past 10 years, the relationship between families and mental health professionals has become more collaborative, building on the strengths and expertise of all parties to establish mutual goals for treatment and rehabilitation (Lukens & Thorning, 1996; Marsh, 1994). However, such attitudes have changed relatively slowly over the course of the 20th century.

At the turn of the century, early researchers, led by Kraepelin (1971) and Bleuler (1950), postulated that schizophrenia was the result of a central nervous system defect that differed from other neurological conditions. However, no clear pathology was found at postmortem examination, a discovery that incited debate among early theoreticians, so emphasis was placed instead on the impact of environmental factors on the illness.

A series of case studies on family dynamics and schizophrenia, influenced by the psychoanalytic movement, were published during the first half of the 20th century. Findings negatively portrayed the family, and particularly the mother, in relation to onset and course of illness (Fromm-Reichmann, 1948; Kasanin, Knight, & Sage, 1934; Levy, 1931; Tietz, 1949). Fromm-Reichmann coined the term "schizophrenogenic" mother, characterizing both parent and child as defective. This work provided the syntax for later research on expressed emotion, clarity of communication, and affect among family members.

The family therapy movement that evolved in the 1950s also was influenced by this early research. The early family therapists focused on the impact of family dynamics on the mental status of individual family members (Nichols & Schwartz, 1995) and how illnesses such as schizophrenia should be treated. Arguing that the problems and symptoms associated with severe mental illness arose from unhealthy relationships with family members and could best be alleviated by treatment through a private relationship between therapist and client (Mishne, 1993), family clinicians tended to discourage contact between people labeled as patients and their relatives. Thus, families were often separated from the person with the illness during hospitalization and either directly or indirectly excluded from treatment.

Those attitudes toward families were reinforced by the nature of the paternalistic relationship between families and professionals that emerged in many areas of medicine during the 1950s, 1960s, and 1970s. As Starr (1982) emphasized in the introduction to his important work on the rising power and sovereignty of the medical profession in the 20th century, "When professionals claim to be authoritative about the nature of reality, whether it is the structure of the atom, the ego, or the universe, we generally defer to their judgment" (p. 4). Given this deference, medical or mental health professionals would have had to yield some of their power if the perspective of the family were to be accepted as even remotely valid.

In their work on childhood disabilities, Gliedman and Roth (1980) argued that the paternalistic nature of this relationship encouraged professionals to see *both* parents and the person with illness or disability as the patient. Family members were expected to take on a classic sick role, to be passive and agree with the experts. If they disagreed, they were treated as uncooperative children. This combination of blaming the victim, professional dominance, and underlying societal stigma regarding disabilities put the family in a classic double bind: "either submit to professional dominance (and be operationally defined as a patient) or stand up for one's rights and risk being labeled emotionally maladjusted (and therefore patientlike)" (p. 150).

## Psychoeducation as an Intervention for Expressed Emotion

The use of neuroleptic medications in treatment for schizophrenia also became widespread in the 1950s, leading to deinstitutionalization—the discharge into the community of large numbers of people with chronic mental illness. With such a change in locus of care from hospital to community, and hence to the family, the emphasis on how family attitudes and behavior might be related to the cause of illness received renewed attention from research.

Thus, an interest in what came to be called "expressed emotion" among family members of people with schizophrenia developed during this period. The early research in this area focused on the clinical observation that the family atmosphere of people with schizophrenia was characterized by overstimulation, dominance, overprotection, rejection, criticism, and contradictory messages (Brown, Monck, Carstairs, & Wing, 1958; Brown & Rutter, 1966). This phenomenon was usually measured by a dichotomous variable that reflected either high or low expressed emotion (that is, presence or absence of criticism and overinvolvement) expressed by parents in regard to a family member with schizophrenia.

Initial findings and subsequent replication studies suggested that such high levels of emotion were strongly associated with the exacerbation or relapse of symptoms, particularly among men suffering from schizophrenia (Brown, Birley, & Wing, 1972; Leff & Vaughn, 1981; Vaughn & Leff, 1976; Vaughn, Snyder, Jones, Freeman, & Falloon, 1984). As a result, specific educational interventions were designed to teach families how to provide a low-key and less stressful environment in the home to protect the person with illness from relapse. Such interventions included emphasis on education in combination with improved communication skills, problem solving, coping effectiveness, and development of realistic expectations and symptom monitoring, particularly among family members.

Leff and colleagues (Leff et al., 1989; Leff, Kuipers, Berkowitz, Eberlein-Fries, & Sturgeon, 1982; Leff & Vaughn, 1985) conducted two small studies of educational interventions to lower expressed emotion among family members. In the earlier study, 24 people with schizophrenia who had relatives described as high in expressed emotion were randomly assigned to two treatment groups. The experimental treatment included education of the relatives, a relatives' group, and individual family therapy in the relatives' home. The control group included regular hospital follow-up of the person with illness, but with little family contact. Over two years of follow-up, only two of the 10 subjects who received the experimental treatment relapsed, but seven of nine control subjects relapsed. The relatives in the treatment group were described as statistically significantly less critical toward the person with schizophrenia at two-year follow-up, but there was no change in the relatives in the control group. The treated relatives also showed an increase in optimism over time.

In the second study 24 families classified as high in expressed emotion were assigned to either education along with ongoing family therapy in the home or education along with a relatives' support group. In both treatments, people with illness were excluded from the process. Compliance with treatment was low in the relatives' support group, with only five of the 11 families attending even once. Among families who attended the support group, the nine-month relapse rate of people with illness was 17 percent, comparable with that of people with illness in the family therapy group. Both groups showed decreased criticism and increased warmth toward the person with illness over the course of treatment.

Hogarty and collaborators (1986) conducted a large trial ($N = 90$) of social treatment and medication aimed only at those families labeled as high in expressed emotion. The study included four groups: (1) family treatment and medication ($N = 21$), (2) social skills training and medication ($N = 20$), (3) family treatment combined with social skills and medication ($N = 20$), and (4) drugs alone ($N = 29$). The family treatment included a one-day educational workshop followed by additional sessions at home that focused on application of educational principles, reduction of isolation, and help in coping with problems. The social skills training was designed to reduce the vulnerability of a person with illness to family stress and improve his or her assertiveness during family interactions by enhancing verbal and nonverbal social behaviors and increasing the accuracy of social perceptions and judgment.

The researchers found that people treated with drugs alone had a relapse rate of 42 percent during the year-long follow-up. In both the family education group and the social skills training group, the people with illness had a continued high risk of relapse when expressed emotion was high at follow-up, even when contact between the person and his or her family remained low (33 percent). However, when family education and social skills training were combined, relapse rates were zero, even when expressed emotion at follow-up remained high (Hogarty et al., 1986).

Falloon and colleagues (1982, 1985) obtained similar results when they compared 18 subjects who received standard treatment with an experimental group also composed of 18 subjects. The experimental group received a series of educational sessions and family interventions in the home over nine months, with emphasis on problem solving in the context of an educational format (Falloon et al., 1982, 1984;

McGill et al., 1983). The goal was to lower expressed emotion by promoting clear communication and the direct expression of thoughts and feeling among family members: "The therapist functions as a model of these effective communication skills while prompting, coaching, and reinforcing the efforts and competence performance of each family member. During family problem-solving discussions, he or she continuously monitors the communication process to assess specific assets and deficits that enhance or detract from effective problem resolution" (Falloon et al., 1984, p. 260). Both groups consisted primarily of families who were described as high in expressed emotion. During the nine-month period of the study, the control group had a relapse rate of 44 percent and the experimental group had a 6 percent relapse rate. At two years 83 percent of the control subjects had relapsed, in contrast to 17 percent in the experimental group.

Tarrier and colleagues (1988) found strong associations between expressed emotion among family members and relapse of the positive (that is, psychotic) symptoms among people with illness. The investigators randomly assigned 64 families described as high in expressed emotion to one of four intervention groups—two groups that focused on variations in behavioral intervention in combination with a brief educational piece, one group described as "education only" and one group described as "routine" treatment. An additional 19 families described as low in expressed emotion were assigned to either "education only" or "routine" treatment. Two findings were particularly important and consistent with the other studies on expressed emotion and relapse. First, the subjects in the two behavioral intervention cells combined had significantly lower relapse rates over the nine-month period after discharge (12 percent) compared with the "education only" group (43 percent) and the "routine" treatment group (53 percent). Second, the people returning to live with relatives described as high in expressed emotion following either "education only" or "routine" treatment interventions had significantly higher relapse rates than did those returning to low expressed emotion homes following treatment described as "education only" (22 percent) or "routine" treatment (20 percent).

The work of Glick and colleagues (Glick et al., 1985; Haas et al., 1988) was different from the other studies in that it was conducted in a hospital and was designed to educate families of 84 people diagnosed with schizophrenia and 60 with major affective disorders. The families received between six and eight educational sessions focusing on education and support during the inpatient stay. At short-term follow-up, the psychiatric symptoms had decreased significantly among the female inpatients, and the families rated themselves as more open to support as well as more positive regarding treatment and less negative toward the family member with the illness.

In an earlier study of psychoeducation, Goldstein, Rodnick, Evans, May, and Steinberg (1978) assigned 96 people with schizophrenia to family therapy or no family therapy. Subjects were first stratified as to good and poor premorbid functioning and then randomly assigned to treatment. The six family therapy sessions concentrated on education, crisis management, acceptance of illness, and long-term planning. Although lowering expressed emotion was not a stated goal, negative symptoms, such as social withdrawal and blunted affect, significantly decreased among subjects in the family therapy group after six weeks, but this outcome was not sustained at six-month follow-up.

Based on these studies, it is difficult to draw firm conclusions about the role that education and psychoeducation play in outcome, primarily because the educational components were imprecisely and inconsistently defined and had little impact alone. In those studies in which education alone was compared with education along with an additional intervention, outcomes in the combined intervention were more impressive, at least at short-term follow-up.

Nonetheless, these studies did fuel the idea that expressed emotion among family members is a causal factor in relapse of the psychotic symptoms of schizophrenia. Not surprisingly, this emphasis on family variables and causality triggered anger and criticism from family advocates. In the 1970s and 1980s, as families became more politically active through national self-help groups, such as AMI, family members became increasingly willing to challenge professional authority, including that based on the work on family variables such as expressed emotion. AMI members interpreted such studies as a distraction from more biologically oriented research into the causes of such severe illness and as yet another way to divert money and time from the critical need of people with illness for housing and rehabilitation (Hatfield, 1987, 1988; Kanter, Lamb, & Loeper, 1987; Leff, 1989; Lefley, 1992; Mintz, Mintz, & Goldstein, 1987).

The literature on expressed emotion has been criticized for additional reasons, including the ambiguity, narrowness, and rigidity of the construct itself; inconsistent definition of relapse in the intervention studies; the emphasis on relapse as the outcome variable to the exclusion of other phases and aspects of symptomatology (Birchwood & Smith, 1987; Gottschalk et al., 1988; MacMillan, Gold, Crow, Johnson, & Johnstone, 1986); the implication that families are to blame for outcomes among people suffering from illness (Hatfield, 1987; Lefley, 1987); and the emphasis on labeling instead of describing family situations as well as the focus on illness instead of strengths (Hatfield, 1988). As the families and their advocates have argued, high levels of involvement ("overinvolvement") may serve a self-protective function, particularly given the hostile and exclusionary attitudes toward the family that have been described (Terkelsen, 1983). Little emphasis has been placed on the positive aspects of family involvement and how they might serve both the family and the person with illness (Kanter et al., 1987; Terkelsen, 1983), nor have researchers focused on the possible negative consequences of low expressed emotion for both the family and the person with the illness (Hogarty et al., 1995; Kanter et al., 1987; Lefley, 1992). Critics have suggested that low expressed emotion is poorly understood, and lack of involvement or criticism could reflect rejection or neglect as well as acceptance (Koenigsberg & Handley, 1986; Kanter et al., 1987). Such absence of positive conditions (such as lack of support and stimulation) also might serve as a source of stress (Cassell, 1976; Link & Phelan, 1995).

The conclusion that the relationship between expressed emotion and relapse is truly causal also has been challenged (Hogarty et al., 1986; Kuipers, 1987; Kuipers & Bebbington, 1988; MacMillan et al., 1986). In its place a more complex reciprocal model has been proposed, which combines both internal and external stressors, coping mechanisms and other personality variables, and external supports and resources (Hyde & Goldman, 1992; Leff, 1989; Lukens, 1993). Strachan, Feingold, Goldstein, Miklowitz, and Nuechterlein (1989) provided preliminary evidence that expressed emotion among key relatives may reflect transactional processes between the person with illness and his or her family. In a sample of 36 subjects with schizophrenia during both an acute hospitalization and the aftercare period, these authors compared the coping styles of the patients with high and low expressed emotion within the family. In a family assessment session, they found that patients interacting with relatives with low expressed emotion made significantly less critical and more autonomous statements than those interacting with relatives described as high in expressed emotion. In addition, when the dominant coping style of the patient was described as negative, the level of expressed emotion within the family was high. The authors concluded that the quality of behavior for both the families and the patients may predict subsequent functioning for the person with illness.

Expressed emotion and, by association, psychoeducation became a source of controversy in the mental health field. Unfortunately, the potential impact, relevance, and value of educational interventions were overshadowed by the fact that they were designed specifically to decrease expressed emotion. As Mintz and colleagues (1987) observed, "parents of schizophrenic patients have resisted what appears to be a new attempt to blame them for the illness, through the concept of stress as a cause of breakdown, while professionals who view the basis of schizophrenic illness as biological have argued against the allocation of resources to the study of psychosocial factors" (p. 314).

## Stress–Diathesis Models

Despite the debate over expressed emotion, it is generally well established that course, outcome, and symptoms of the severe mental illnesses are worsened by stress. The Stress–Diathesis Model (also known as the Vulnerability Stress Model) forms the basis for understanding schizophrenia and other severe mental illnesses from the perspective of genetic, biological, and environmental (psychosocial) factors. It posits a multifactorial relationship among provoking agents (stressors), vulnerability and symptom formation (diathesis), and outcome (Zubin & Spring, 1977). In applying this model, Heinrichs and Carpenter (1983) noted that either excessive arousal or low levels of arousal can interfere with individual functioning on many levels: "Most individuals have learned that excessive levels of anxiety (excessive arousal) interfere with their functioning but, if they lack the fine edge that moderate anxiety provides and are too apathetic (insufficient arousal), their performance, again, is less that optimal" (p. 269).

They further observed that any form of treatment will vary in specificity of effect for a particular person at any given point in time. They suggested that treatment should therefore depend on a person's mix of symptoms and where he or she is in the course of the illness. Ideally, this approach would mean that stimuli in the environment could be identified, adjusted, and "titrated" in much the same way that medicine is titrated. From this perspective, it would follow that a delicate balance would have to be achieved if both the family and the person with illness were to function at an optimal level at any given time. In this context the relationship between the environment and symptoms and behaviors associated with illness could be considered interactive or reciprocal.

It is assumed that the creation of a healthy environment for the person with illness is important for the long-term prognosis of schizophrenia, that people with schizophrenia respond to stress, and that dysfunction within a family can contribute to a stressful environment for any person, whether or not he or she has a mental disorder. Therefore, educating families about the range of stressors that contribute to outcome should serve as a protective function. Marsh (1994) identified these potential stressors as family life events, such as the occurrence of the illness itself, and both concurrent and previous life events; family resources, such as family process, socioeconomic status, coping strategies, and both professional and personal supports; and family appraisal, including a family's understanding, perspective, and knowledge of mental illness. As family members begin to identify stressors in their own lives and to work with the person with the illness to identify stressors, they can begin to recognize patterns and cycles of illness and how these may be exacerbated by stress. Recognizing these patterns is critical to the educational process and to weathering the fluctuation of symptoms that frequently characterizes schizophrenia and other severe mental illnesses. The psychoeductional models provide an opportunity to gain this perspective.

## RECENT APPLICATIONS OF THE PSYCHOEDUCATIONAL MODELS

Treatment provides the client with a place to step away from the onslaught and challenges of everyday life, reflect on this reality, and achieve increased mastery and acceptance of his or her situation (Saari, 1991). Because of the nature of schizophrenia, the environment serves as an important frame of reference for the person with illness, a setting where symptoms and behaviors can be grounded or "cued" through external structures and events (Scheflen, 1981; Weinberger, 1987). Psychoeducation can offer valuable opportunities for families and professionals to use such knowledge to calm the impact of severe mental illness on the family and on the person with illness and to learn how to assess and titrate levels of stress both at home and in other environments. If conducted in a group setting, psychoeducation effectively combines the strengths of both self-help and psychotherapeutic models (McFarlane et al., 1995).

## A RESEARCH-BASED PSYCHOEDUCATIONAL MODEL

Much of the work reported to date concerned the development of educational models in combination with behavioral interventions aimed directly at the family, the person with illness, or both. During the past 20 years, multiple-family groups have come to be perceived as an effective and practical means of enabling the family to cope with severe mental illness by helping group members support each other and share and address issues of managing the illness. They serve as an educational forum and typically include six or seven families meeting together with two or more mental health professionals (McFarlane, 1983; McFarlane et al., 1995).

Research by McFarlane and colleagues (1995) found that the modality is strongly associated with decreased relapse among people with illness when the group is conducted on an outpatient basis with both families and people with illness attending the same group for at least two years. In this study, 172 recently hospitalized people diagnosed with schizophrenia were randomly assigned to psychoeducational single- or multiple-family groups in six hospitals across the state of New York. Over two years of treatment, the subjects in the multiple-family groups had significantly lower cumulative relapse rates than did those in the single-family groups. Subjects in both groups showed increased compliance with medication regimens and significantly fewer hospitalizations.

The model of McFarlane and colleagues, which was adapted from the work of Anderson and colleagues (1986), consists of four treatment stages: (1) joining, (2) education and skills training, (3) re-entry, and (4) social and vocational rehabilitation. *Joining* is the process of establishing a relationship between the clinician and the family that is characterized by a spirit of collaboration rather than "treatment." The objectives for this phase are to establish a working alliance, identify and assess the needs of the family in a collaborative manner, identify the family's strengths and resources both in general and in dealing with the illness, and create a contract with mutual and realistic goals.

Thus, the joining relationship serves a pivotal function: It provides a safe forum and refuge for the family, a bridge between the family's perspective and the clinician's professional world. It also is the preliminary step toward empowering families through the educational process. Throughout their work together, the clinician functions as a "point person," an available resource and advocate for the family who can mediate or negotiate with any part of the mental health or social services system that may be required by the illness of their relative (Anderson et al., 1986).

After the clinician has formed an alliance with the family, family members are invited to an educational and skills training workshop conducted by the clinician and other relevant professionals. The workshop provides information to families about the complexities of the illness and is another key step in the implementation of the psychoeducational model. The workshop is specifically for family members and friends of the people with illness. The person with illness is invited only if he or she is particularly well compensated and not delusional or denying illness. The clinicians working with the family conduct the workshop, assisted by the psychiatrist treating the person with illness.

After the workshop, the clinician begins meeting twice monthly with the families and the people with illness in either multiple- or single-family groups. The goal during this phase is to design and test strategies for coping and helping the person as he or she recovers from an acute episode of schizophrenia. Major content areas include education regarding adherence to treatment regimens, medication compliance, helping the person with illness understand the importance of avoiding the use of street drugs and alcohol, and setting realistic goals for the initial period of recovery. Formal problem-solving and communication skills training drawn from the work of Falloon and colleagues (1984) characterizes each session and is used to amplify and reinforce the education and skills training presented during the earlier workshop. Each session follows a prescribed format, which enhances coping effectiveness and strengthens the alliance among the families, the people with illness, and the clinicians. A brief period of socialization also is included in each session to encourage and normalize social interaction among participants on topics unrelated to illness.

It is in this context that the multiple-family group process is particularly important and effective in helping families and people with illness increase their understanding of the problems associated with schizophrenia. As the professional and nonprofessional group members work together, they provide each other with insights and observations that are critical to compliance with treatment and bringing about change.

In the second year of treatment in the multiple-family group, emphasis is placed on the rehabilitative needs of the person with illness, addressing social skills and the ability to obtain and maintain employment in particular. Sessions are usually conducted once a month, although this frequency may vary depending on the needs of the group. The sessions are used to role-play situations likely to cause stress for both the person with the illness and the family. Family members actively assist in various aspects of this training. They also are encouraged to rebuild their network of family and friends, which has usually been weakened as a consequence of having a family member with schizophrenia.

At this stage, insight into the realities and limitations of the illness begins to emerge, and the illness is reconsidered as a relative rather than an absolute disability (McFarlane & Lukens, 1998). Group leaders, relatives, and other group members can help the person with illness understand his or her strengths and limitations and increase insight by providing a supportive, nonstigmatizing environment. The goal is to focus on strengths and progress, along with some degree of acceptance of limitations and continuing treatment compliance.

In the cases treated during the two-year period of the study by McFarlane and colleagues, the people with illness increasingly cooperated with treatment, as suggested by high rates of medication compliance. If they remained stable for at least six months during the second year in treatment, they were offered an abbreviated version of an educational videotape that had been shown to their families during the initial educational workshop. This information enabled them to help other group members with illness reflect on the connections between symptoms and environmental stress and begin to acknowledge the fact that they were living with an illness.

## AN EXPLORATORY CLINICAL APPLICATION

The psychoeducational models described in the research literature provide important guidelines for further investigation. Drawing on these applications, we developed two clinical models for psychoeducational multiple-family groups to explore the efficacy of this treatment modality on an inpatient service with intermediate length of stay (five to six months). This work, which was conducted between 1990 and 1995, compared two ongoing groups, one in which both people with illness and families were present, the other in which the people with illness were not present. For both inpatient groups, *family* was loosely defined to include not only immediate family but also significant others such as close friends, church members, and in one case, the owner of an apartment where a person with illness lived.

In these models, as in the model of McFarlane and colleagues, the joining relationship was critical in providing the link between the inpatient treatment team and the family. Although an initial educational workshop was tried in accordance with the work of McFarlane et al., the presentation was eventually modularized to accommodate the rotating membership characteristic of an inpatient unit, based on the impression that families would more easily grasp and use information presented over time (Tunnel et al., 1988). Educational materials were presented through rotating modules (Mueser & Gingerich, 1994) over a period of five to six months. Each session lasted approximately two hours. The first hour of each session focused on a didactic presentation that covered such topics as symptoms of schizophrenia and schizoaffective illness, the epidemiology of schizophrenia, stress management, crisis interventions, community resources, and medication and side effects. As we worked with the families over time, it became clear that the groups needed time to assimilate the knowledge presented. They also needed time to address issues in their lives that seemed to interfere with the integration and application of information. Thus, in the second hour of each session, application of the didactic presentation was discussed in relation to both the long-term and immediate needs of the group members. During this hour the co-leaders drew on the behavioral techniques delineated by Anderson and colleagues (1986) and McFarlane and colleagues (1995) as well as on life cycle and narrative models of treatment.

The following vignette illustrates this process:

> In the group including people with illness, Mary began to discuss some difficulties she was having on the unit. She was distraught because she experienced the male nurses as abusing her. In a voice that grew increasingly more agitated, she told how she worried they would hurt her: "At night they stare through the door. I think they want to rape me." As the group members listened to this, a sense of alarm began to spread through the group; members were fearful that her accusations were true. After all, abuse and sexual abuse of inpatients had been reported in the media; were they putting their daughters in an unsafe environment at the time when they were most vulnerable? The group leaders tried to address this by providing the following educational intervention designed to influence the group process.
>
> "Mary," one of the leaders said, "I know from what you are saying that you have been very frightened on the unit, and that you are worried that the staff will hurt you. You have not known the staff for very long. When one has been hurt in the past, it is very hard to trust people and know that you will not be hurt again." The group listened intensely to this. The leader continued, "I am now going to say something that may be difficult to hear, but important for me to tell both you and the group." Mary nodded her head. "Mary is talking about how frightened she is, and that she worries that she may be hurt by the staff. But, Mary, you feel this way in many situations, and sometimes these feelings get blown way out of proportion to the situation. When the staff thinks about this and how schizophrenia can affect people, we say that you have paranoid feelings. This doesn't mean that we shouldn't listen to what you have to say, but we have to understand this in the context of your illness. I will talk to the staff about the fact that at this time you may need some special sensitivity with regard to regaining a sense of privacy and control, and to help you with this particular fear."
>
> The tension in the group abated as they began to comprehend the meaning of paranoia, and how this symptom affected the situation. In addition, group members expressed an increased understanding of the difficulties of Mary's predicament. In subsequent groups, several parent members expressed more warmth and understanding toward both her and their own daughters.

## LIFE CYCLE MODELS

Family systems theory suggests that individual family members interact in such a way that change in one member directly or indirectly affects other members, in what becomes a circular chain of influence. This is the basis of the family life cycle model, which evaluates symptoms and functioning in relationship to normal functioning over time (Carter & McGoldrick, 1989). Rolland (1994a) drew on this perspective in his Family Systems-Illness model, which provides a paradigm for psychoeducation, assessment, and intervention with families based on prevention. Rolland's typology examined illness in relationship to onset (acute or gradual), course (progressive, constant, or relapsing), and expectation as to outcome (nonfatal, shortened life span or sudden death, progressive and usually fatal) and incapacitation (none to severe); it also can include an overarching category of degree of uncertainty or unpredictability. Encouraging families to reflect on illness in this context enables them to identify and understand the kinds of stressors and challenges they may face over time. The role of the mental health professional is to work with the family and the person with illness to re-establish a normal momentum and equilibrium in the face of major disruption in the life cycle (Carter & McGoldrick, 1989). Such preparation can help families weather the often variable course that characterizes schizophrenia.

In confronting the severe mental illness or disability of a child of any age, the family must undergo a complete reorganization of lifestyle, self-perception, roles, economic security, and belief system. These processes all involve loss, which may be exacerbated by the cultural and personal stigma attached to the illness (Fox, 1992; Link, Cullen, Struening, Shrout, & Dohrenwend, 1989; White, 1989). MacGregor (1994) proposed that grief is experienced as both an external loss of normal and predictable family atmosphere, privacy, financial resources, and independence and an internal loss of self-esteem, positive memories of the family's past life, pride, dreams, and pleasure in the anticipated success of what a child might have been. This sense of internal loss can contribute to sadness, guilt, shame, and stigma. It may be exacerbated by anger directed toward the family, the person with illness, and the limitations of the mental health system (Thorning & Lukens, in press).

In her pioneering work on death, Kübler-Ross (1969) suggested that terminally ill people and their families experience five stages of bereavement: denial and isolation, anger, bargaining, depression, and acceptance. After her work, several models sequencing the phases of emotions evoked in the process of mourning associated with severe mental illness were formulated (MacGregor, 1994; Tessler, Killian, & Gubman, 1987). Common to these models is an end stage in which there is no resolution or acceptance but rather a prevailing sense of worry about the future. The intensity of the feelings of sadness can fluctuate as they are triggered by changes in the life cycle, medical or psychiatric crises, and other stressors (Rolland, 1994b; Thorning & Lukens, 1996). This sense of loss is illustrated by the following example:

> The group without patients present was often able to reflect more directly on the impact that the illness has on their lives, and profound sadness frequently permeated the mood of the group. The mother of a 33-year-old son who was hospitalized with schizophrenia talked about her healthy daughter's upcoming wedding. As she discussed her reservations about having her ill son attend the wedding, another mother became tearful. This mother said how upsetting it was for her to hear how the family was planning a wedding for their well daughter: "I only have one daughter, and she is so ill. She will probably never have a wedding." The room was thick with sadness. A general discussion emerged among the group members as each of them offered their unique sadness in having a mentally ill adult child. A father remarked that his sadness is reawakened whenever a son or daughter of a friend successfully goes though yet another developmental milestone: graduating from high school or college, getting married, having children. "The wound is reopened," he said, "and I cry again as I fall asleep."

Recognizing and coming to terms with severe mental illness in a family member are important steps toward re-establishing a bond with that person, and they increase the possibility of a restoration of some semblance of equilibrium both for the individual family member and for the family as a whole. Such coming to terms does not imply passive acceptance of the status quo. Rather it focuses on the importance of identifying options and opportunities for change given the constraints of the situation. For some family members this process may mean joining a self-help group or becoming involved in other forms of advocacy; for others it may mean attending to neglected aspects of their own lives. In this process, the sense of hope that emerges helps family members maintain and strengthen existing relationships and establish new ones.

## NARRATIVE AND STRENGTHS MODELS

Loss of hope has detrimental effects on both the person with illness and family members. Severe mental illnesses such as schizophrenia attack a person's sense of self (Hatfield, 1989; Thorning & Lukens, 1996). The negative symptoms that frequently characterize schizophrenia may serve a protective role in that they moderate stimulation existing in the environment. Yet these symptoms, which include apathy, resignation, submissiveness, and withdrawal, also characterize learned helplessness, described by Deegan (1992) as a "cycle of despair and disempowerment." Breaking into this cycle—that is, instilling hope—can be critical in successful management and coping with the illness. For example, when we gave a presentation on mourning and loss during a local chapter meeting of AMI, we were struck by the response of one parent. He felt that pride in what his son *had* accomplished, given the son's longstanding struggles with mental illness, far outweighed any feelings of loss that the family had experienced. Acceptance of the person as worthwhile in the face of such chronic illness is a critical component of hope (Deegan, 1988; Woodside et al., 1994).

Helping family members and people with illness assume such a hopeful stance is an important component of the psychoeducational models. The narrative approaches to treatment provide important paradigms for enhancing psychoeducation and are critical in encouraging hope. Based on constructivist theory, which emphasizes strengths, and on social constructionism, with its emphasis on personal history, cultural perspectives, and diversity, narrative models can provide an important forum for education, empowerment, and change (Cowger, 1994). The narrative model emphasizes a working parity between the mental health professional and the family in which a mutual effort is made to identify strengths among all family members, including the person with illness. From this perspective, clinicians are not so much preoccupied with what causes a problem but with how the effects of the problem cause stress in individuals and families and are played out over time (Nichols & Schwartz, 1995). The clinician takes the role of participant–facilitator, working with the family to elicit, contextualize, mirror, and amplify the situation so that reasonable alternative solutions to old problems can be reached (Greene, Jensen, & Harper Jones, 1996; Real, 1990). Through this process, family members can begin to confront and come to terms with the illness by describing and reflecting on the situation and by telling, elaborating on, and retelling their story. Through such externalization and re-examination of the problems, events, and challenges they have faced, they confront the continuing stress of the illness and the disruption it has caused in their lives. Both mental health professionals and family group members also can begin to value the strengths and personality of the person with illness separately from the symptoms of the illness. This is particularly important with an illness such as schizophrenia, in which the illness attacks a person's sense of self (Hatfield, 1989; Thorning & Lukens, 1996). As Saari (1991) stated, "by relating to the client as more than that person currently experiences himself or herself to be, the client does, in fact, gradually become more than he or she initially was" (p. 162). This approach enables the families and clinicians to focus on assessment rather than diagnosis and develop a realistic and comprehensive treatment plan. It is this mobilization of competence, emphasis on strengths, and capacity to build connections with others that contributes to self-confidence and stimulates hope (Cowger, 1994; Real, 1990). Thus, a critical function of the psychoeducational multiple-family group modality is that families, people with illness, and clinicians working together are able to educate themselves and each other, confront loss, recognize strengths, and identify possibilities for hope, as facilitated and witnessed by the presence of others. The following vignette illustrates this process.

> During an educational session focused on the symptoms of schizophrenia, Peter launched into a description of the voices he hears constantly. The group members, both people with illness and their family members, listened carefully as he shared how he was being tortured by voices that were constantly commenting negatively about anything he did: "Clean your room. You forgot to wash your hands, you dope. You are nothing but a filthy liar and a no-good son of a bitch." One mother sat quietly listening to Peter, tears streaming down her cheeks. "My daughter has never been able to tell me what goes on with her," she said. "I see her looking over her shoulders all the time. I know that she must be listening to something, but I may have been afraid to really ask her. You have given me a little window into her world, a world I was not able to understand before."

## Discussion

In response to the long-standing implication that families contribute to the onset and outcome of mental illness and disability, family advocates have debated the value of psychoeducation and the power differential it implies. They argue that family members do not want or need treatment but are critically in need of information and knowledge—education—if they are to stay abreast of current research and approaches to care (Hatfield, 1990). Because of the tendency of some health care providers to disempower and foster dependence among people with illness, the history of blaming the family, and the social stigma attached to disability, it is not surprising that families have responded in this fashion. Therefore, mental health professionals must carefully examine their own perspectives on illness and blame, both in training and in practice, to provide families with what is now known about biological and environmental factors in the onset and course of severe mental illness. As Tunnel et al. (1988) stated, this "allows professionals to work with families without holding them responsible. In fact taking an interactional view can decrease the family's sense of hopelessness and lack of control over the illness" (p. 80).

To even begin to struggle with schizophrenia or other severe mental illness, both family members and clinicians must have information and facts about and insight into the illness itself; coping skills specific to the particular psychiatric disorder; and tremendous patience. Families develop methods of dealing with the problems and disabilities associated with severe mental illness, but these methods may be productive or nonproductive depending on the circumstances. Expecting families or other caregivers to intuitively know how to handle such conditions is unrealistic (McFarlane & Lukens, 1998). The goal, then, for the psychoeducational approaches should be to help families regain some sense of control, mastery, and equilibrium in their lives in the face of the ongoing and overwhelming stress and pervasive sadness associated with the severe mental illness of a family member.

Increasing understanding of the origins of the illness, in association with a non-stigmatizing, tolerant, and accepting environment, is central in this process for the family caregiver, the person with illness, and the clinician. Psychoeducation should be viewed as a collaborative effort among family, clinician, and person with illness—a dynamic and interactive relationship in which the health care professional serves as consultant, facilitator, advocate, and also educator and student. The traditional, hierarchical relationship, in which the clinician provides structure and topics to be discussed, is replaced by a mutual collaborative effort in which the mental health professional and family members work together to develop increased understanding (Marsh, 1994). Ideally, the clinician can provide the broad picture, based on wide experience with many people struggling with similar kinds of symptoms; family members and people with illness can provide perspectives on individual strengths, day-to-day occurrences, subtle changes in individual symptoms, and patterns in the illness over time. Families who are involved provide a continuity of interest, knowledge, and caring that is impossible for mental health professionals to replicate, particularly given current trends toward managed care and short-term hospitalization. Moving from this interactive or reciprocal model, family members and mental health professionals can acknowledge gaps in knowledge on both sides and achieve respect for both each other and what is known. This combined effort creates a rich opportunity for enhanced care for the person with illness as well as support for the family. Borkman (1976) referred to this as the value of combining both "experiential" and "professional" knowledge. As Rolland (1994a) observed, such approaches "respect the limits of scientific knowledge, affirm basic competency and promote the flexible use of multiple biological and psychosocial healing strategies" (p. 466).

Thus, for psychoeducation to work effectively, medical jargon and euphemism must be demystified and the family involved in the treatment planning and process. Stotland (1984), referring to an interaction with a medical professional that concerned his own disabled child, observed that "by involving us in the process and by giving us his professional opinion as an opinion, he returned to us our parental rights of making the important decision that would affect our child's life. We were in control, but we were no longer alone" (p. 72). Other authors have noted that simple inclusion and the style of interaction are critical to the involvement of families. For professionals to show some humility, to appropriately acknowledge ambiguity and lack of clarity in the current state of knowledge—whether in mental illness in general or the subtleties of an individual treatment plan—is an important part of forming an inclusionary relationship (Lee, 1996; Rolland, 1994a).

The psychoeducational multiple-family group is an ideal forum for such a paradigm. Critical information about an illness and its management is usually provided by co-leaders, as is an opportunity for group members to share experiences, make connections, decrease isolation, and develop new ideas. The presence of several families moderates the intensity that would be characteristic of individual family sessions and normalizes the families' experiences. This is reinforced by the presence of co-leaders who work together to provide a range of information and perspectives. The clinicians, in turn, serve as a link between the families and other resources within the mental health and social services system. Thus, a broad-based safety net—a "community of care"—is created to enhance the families and the clinicians' recognition of and responsiveness to the needs of both the family and the person with illness (Pescosolido, Wright, & Sullivan, 1995). Families can provide new perspectives to members of another family (sometimes called "cross-parenting"). People with illness who are in different stages of recovery or who have different strengths may serve as models or consultants for each other or for the parents or relatives of another group member with illness. Problem-solving skills can be introduced, modeled, practiced, and applied. Both clinicians and family group members can "witness" the experiences of other group participants, an important step in re-establishing equilibrium and moving toward empowerment (Simon, 1994; Thorning & Lukens, in press). In this way, educational principles are explicated, tested, and reinforced.

## Implications for Further Research

The current literature on psychoeducation leaves many questions unanswered. There are many areas for future research, particularly in topics relevant to the field of social work. These include

- work with families to identify and describe the critical factors that should be included in a well-defined educational program
- examination of factors that enhance or inhibit the educational process
- applications of educational and psychoeducational models in a range of field settings, with both inpatients and outpatients
- comparison of the impact of educationally based models of intervention (that is, self-help models) with professionally led psychoeducational models
- evaluation of the impact of educational and psychoeducational interventions on outcomes over time
- expanding the definition of outcome to include variables relevant to the quality of life for all family members, such as stigma, mourning and loss, hope, self-efficacy, and burden
- broad-based evaluation over time of the impact of such models on the person with illness, including measures of social and vocational function and other quality-of-life variables as well as relapse
- research that addresses cost-effectiveness, length, and intensity of intervention relative to outcome, given the current trend in managed care toward intermittent and short-term treatment
- additional research on the interaction between the illness's impact on the family and the availability and quality of external care and resources for the person with the illness
- assessment and research regarding the differential needs of and impact on those from a range of cultural and ethnic backgrounds.

Readily available treatment manuals to assist training, testing, and replication for both clinicians and researchers also are needed.

Social workers and other mental health professionals must broaden our goals to include educating the larger community, including both health care professionals and laypeople, about the severe mental illnesses. This approach is particularly important because people with mental illness rely heavily on many resources outside the family for care and rehabilitation, and an unknown percentage have little or no contact with their families. In addition, psychoeducation has tremendous potential for applications to treatment of other illnesses, both medical and psychiatric. These possibilities also need to be explored.

# References

Abramowitz, I. A., & Coursey, R. C. (1989). Impact of an educational support group on family participants who take care of their schizophrenic relatives. *Journal of Consulting and Clinical Psychology, 57,* 232–236.

Amador, X., Strauss, D., Yale, S., & Gorman, J. (1991). Awareness of illness in schizophrenia. *Schizophrenia Bulletin, 17,* 113–132.

American Psychiatric Association. (1994). *Diagnostic and statistical manual of mental disorders* (4th ed.). Washington, DC: Author.

Anderson, C., Reiss, D., & Hogarty, G. (1986). *Schizophrenia and the family: A practitioner's guide to psychoeducation and management.* New York: Guilford Press.

Barrowclough, C., & Tarrier, N. (1987). A behavioural family intervention with a schizophrenic patient: A case study. *Behavioural Psychotherapy, 15,* 252–271.

Berkowitz, R., Eberlein-Fries, R., Kuipers, L., & Leff, J. (1984). Educating relatives about schizophrenia. *Schizophrenia Bulletin, 1,* 418–429.

Birchwood, M., & Smith, J. (1987). Expressed emotion and first episodes of schizophrenia. *British Journal of Psychiatry, 152,* 859–860.

Bleuler, E. (1950). *Dementia praecox or the group of schizophrenias* (Translated by J. Zinkin, Ed.). New York: International University Press. Originally published in 1911.

Borkman, T. (1976). Experiential knowledge: A new concept for the analysis of self-help groups. *Social Service Review, 50,* 445–456.

Brown, G. W., Birley, J.L.T., & Wing, J. K. (1972). Influence of family life on the course of schizophrenic disorders: A replication. *British Journal of Psychiatry, 121,* 241–258.

Brown, G. W., Monck, E. M., Carstairs, G. M., & Wing, J. K. (1958). Influence of family life on the course of schizophrenic illness. *British Journal of Social Medicine, 16,* 55–68.

Brown, G. W., & Rutter, M. (1966). The measurement of family activities and relationships. *Human Relations, 19,* 241–263.

Carter, B., & McGoldrick, M. (1989). *The changing family life cycle: A framework for family therapy.* Needham Heights, MA: Allyn & Bacon.

Cassell, J. (1976). The contribution of the social environment to host resistance. *American Journal of Epidemiology, 104,* 107–123.

Cochran, M. (1993). Parent empowerment: Developing a conceptual framework. *Family Science Review, 5,* 81–92.

Cowger, C. (1994). Assessing client's strengths: Clinical assessment for client empowerment. *Social Work, 39,* 262–268.

Cozolino, L., Nuechterlein, K., West, K., & Synder, K. (1988). The impact of education about schizophrenia on relatives varying in expressed emotion. *Schizophrenia Bulletin, 14,* 675–687.

Deegan, P. (1988). Recovery: The lived experience of rehabilitation. *Psychosocial Rehabilitation Journal, 11*(4), 11–19.

Deegan, P. (1992). The independent living movement and people with psychiatric disabilities: Taking back control over our own lives. *Psychosocial Rehabilitation Journal, 15*(3), 3–19.

Falloon, I., Boyd, J., & McGill, C. (1984). *Family care of schizophrenia.* New York: Guilford Press.

Falloon, I., Boyd, J., McGill, C., Williamson, M., Razani, J., Moss, H., Gilderman, A., & Simpson, G. (1985). Family management in the prevention of morbidity of schizophrenia. *Archives of General Psychiatry, 42,* 887–896.

Falloon, I., Jeffrey, M., Boyd, L., McGill, C., Razani, J., Moss, H., & Gilderman, A. (1982). Family management in the prevention of exacerbations of schizophrenia. A controlled study. *New England Journal of Medicine, 306,* 1438–1439.

Fox, P. (1992). Implications for expressed emotion therapy within a family therapeutic context. *Health & Social Work, 17,* 207–213.

Fromm-Reichmann, F. (1948). Notes on the development of treatment of schizophrenics by psychoanalytic psychotherapy. *Psychiatry, 2,* 263–273.

Germain, C., & Gitterman, A. (1996). *The life model of social work practice.* New York: Columbia University Press.

Glick, I., Clarkin, J., Spencer, J., Haas, G., Lewis, A., Peyser, J., DeMane, N., Good-Ellis, M., Harris, E., & Lestelle, V. (1985). A controlled evaluation of inpatient family intervention. *Archives of General Psychiatry, 42,* 882–896.

Gliedman, J., & Roth, W. (1980). *The unexpected minority: Handicapped children in America.* New York: Harcourt Brace Jovanovich.

Goldstein, M., Rodnick, E., Evans, J., May, P., & Steinberg, M. (1978). Drug and family therapy in the aftercare treatment of acute schizophrenia. *Archives of General Psychiatry, 35,* 1169–1177.

Gottschalk, L., Falloon, I., Marder, S., Lebell, M., Gift, T., & Wynne, L. (1988). The prediction of relapse of schizophrenic patients using emotional data obtained from their relatives. *Psychiatry Research, 25,* 261–276.

Greene, G., Jensen, C., & Harper Jones, D. (1996). A constructivist perspective on clinical social work practice with ethnically diverse clients. *Social Work, 41,* 172–180.

Haas, G., Glick, I., Clarkin, J., Spencer, J., Louis, A., Peyser, J., Demane, N., Good-Ellis, M., Harris, E., & Lestelle, V. (1988). Inpatient family intervention: A randomized clinical trial. *Archives of General Psychiatry, 45,* 84–94.

Hatfield, A. (1987). Taking issue: The expressed emotion theory: Why families object. *Hospital and Community Psychiatry, 38,* 341.

Hatfield, A. (1988). Issues in psychoeducation for families of the mentally ill. *International Journal of Mental Health, 17*(1), 48–64.

Hatfield, A. (1989). Patients' accounts of stress and coping in schizophrenia. *Hospital and Community Psychiatry, 40,* 1141–1144.

Hatfield, A. (1990). *Family education in mental illness.* New York: Guilford Press.

Heinrichs, D., & Carpenter, W. (1983). The coordination of family therapy with other treatment modalities. In W. R. McFarlane (Ed.), *Family therapy in schizophrenia* (pp. 267–287). New York: Guilford Press.

Hogarty, G., Anderson, C., Reiss, D., Kornblith, S., Greenwald, D., Javna, C., & Madonia, M. (1986). Family psychoeducation, social skills training, and maintenance chemotherapy in the aftercare treatment of schizophrenia. *Archives of General Psychiatry, 43,* 633–642.

Hogarty, G., Kornblith, S., Greenwald, D., DiBarry, A., Cooley, S., Flesher, S., Reiss, D., Carter, M., & Ulrich, R. (1995). Personal therapy: A disorder-relevant psychotherapy for schizophrenia. *Schizophrenia Bulletin, 21,* 379–393.

Hyde, A., & Goldman, C. (1992). Use of a multi-modal multiple family group in the comprehensive treatment and rehabilitation of people with schizophrenia. *Psychosocial Rehabilitation Journal, 15*(4), 77–86.

Kanter, J., Lamb, H., & Loeper, C. (1987). Expressed emotion in families: A critical review. *Hospital and Community Psychiatry, 38,* 374–380.

Kasanin, J., Knight, E., & Sage, P. (1934). The parent–child relationship in schizophrenia. *Journal of Nervous and Mental Disease, 79,* 249–263.

Kieffer, C. (1984). Citizen empowerment: A developmental perspective. *Prevention in Human Services, 3*(3), 9–36.

Koenigsberg, H., & Handley, R. (1986). Expressed emotion: From predictive index to clinical construct. *American Journal of Psychiatry, 43,* 1361–1373.

Köttgen, C., Sönnichsen, I., Mollenhauer, K., & Jurth, R. (1984). Group therapy with families of schizophrenic patients: Results of the Hamburg Camberwell Family Interview Study III. *International Journal of Family Psychiatry, 5,* 83–94.

Kraepelin, E. (1971). *Dementia praecox and paraphrenia* (R. Barclay & G. Robertson, Eds. & Trans.). New York: Robert E. Krieger. Originally published in 1919.

Kübler-Ross, E. (1969). *On death and dying.* New York: Macmillan.

Kuipers, L. (1987). Research in expressed emotion. *Social Psychiatry, 22,* 216–220.

Kuipers, L., & Bebbington, P. (1988). Expressed emotion research in schizophrenia: Theoretical and clinical implications. *Psychological Medicine, 18,* 893–909.

Lam, D. (1991). Psychosocial family intervention in schizophrenia: A review of empirical studies. *Psychological Medicine, 21,* 423–441.

Lee, M. (1996). A constructivist approach to the help-seeking process of clients: A response to cultural diversity. *Clinical Social Work Journal, 24,* 187–202.

Leff, J. (1989). Review article: Controversial issues and growing points in research on relatives' expressed emotion. *International Journal of Social Psychiatry, 35,* 133–145.

Leff, J., Berkowitz, R., Shavit, N., Strachan, A., Glass, I., & Vaughn, C. (1989). A trial of family therapy v. a relatives' group for schizophrenia. *British Journal of Psychiatry, 154,* 58–66.

Leff, J., Kuipers, L., Berkowitz, R., Eberlein-Fries, R., & Sturgeon, D. (1982). A controlled trial of social intervention in the families of schizophrenic patients. *British Journal of Psychiatry, 141,* 121–134.

Leff, J., & Vaughn, C. (1981). The role of maintenance therapy and relatives' expressed emotion in the relapse of schizophrenia: A two-year follow-up. *British Journal of Psychiatry, 139,* 102–104.

Leff, J., & Vaughn, C. (1985). *Expressed emotion in families: Its significance for mental illness.* New York: Guilford Press.

Lefley, H. (1987). Families of the mentally ill: Meeting the challenges. In A. B. Hatfield (Ed.), *New directions for mental health services* (pp. 3–21). San Francisco: Jossey-Bass.

Lefley, H. (1992). Expressed emotion: Conceptual, clinical, and social policy issues. *Hospital and Community Psychiatry, 43,* 591–598.

Levy, D. M. (1931). Maternal overprotection and rejection. *Archives of Neurology and Psychiatry, 25,* 886–889.

Link, B., Cullen, E., Struening, E., Shrout, P., & Dohrenwend, B. (1989). A modified labeling theory approach to mental disorders: An empirical assessment. *American Sociological Review, 54,* 400–423.

Link, B., & Phelan, J. (1995). Social conditions as fundamental causes of disease. *Journal of Health and Social Behavior, 36*(Suppl.), 80–94.

Lukens, E. (1993). *The relationship among family variables and symptom groupings of patients with schizophrenia in a prospective study of family intervention.* Unpublished doctoral dissertation, Columbia University, New York.

Lukens, E., & Thorning, H. (1996). Schizophrenia and the family. In C. Kaufman & J. Gorman (Eds.), *Schizophrenia: New directions for clinical research and treatment* (pp. 197–206). New York: M. A. Liebert.

Marsh, D. T. (1994). The psychodynamic model and services for families: Issues and strategies. In H. Lefley & M. Wasow (Eds.), *Helping families cope with mental illness* (pp. 105–128). Chur, Switzerland: Harwood.

MacGregor, P. (1994). Grief: The unrecognized parental response to mental illness in a child. *Social Work, 39*, 160–166.

MacMillan, J., Gold, A., Crow, T., Johnson, A., & Johnstone, E. (1986). Expressed emotion and relapse. *British Journal of Psychiatry, 148*, 133–143.

McFarlane, W. (1983). Multiple family therapy in schizophrenia. In W. McFarlane (Ed.), *Family therapy in schizophrenia* (pp. 141–172). New York: Guilford Press.

McFarlane, W., & Lukens, E. (1998). Insight, families and education: An exploration of the role of attribution in clinical outcome. In X. Amador & A. David (Eds.), *Insight and psychosis* (pp. 317–331). New York: Oxford University Press.

McFarlane, W., Lukens, E., Link, B., Dushay, R., Deakins, S., Newmark, M., Dunne, E., Horen, B., & Toran, J. (1995). Multiple family groups and psychoeducation in the treatment of schizophrenia. *Archives of General Psychiatry, 52*, 679–687.

McGill, C., Falloon, R., Boyd, J., & Wood-Siverio, C. (1983). Family educational intervention in the treatment of schizophrenia. *Hospital and Community Psychiatry, 34*, 934–938.

Mintz, J., Mintz, L., & Goldstein, M. (1987). Expressed emotion in relapse of first episodes of schizophrenia. *British Journal of Psychiatry, 151*, 314–320.

Mishne, J. (1993). *The evolution and application of clinical theory.* New York: Free Press.

Mueser, K., & Gingerich, S. (1994). *Coping with schizophrenia: A guide for families.* Oakland, CA: New Harbinger.

Nichols, M., & Schwartz, R. (1995). *Family therapy: Concepts and methods.* Needham Heights, MA: Allyn & Bacon.

Parsons, R., Jorgensen, J., & Hernandez, S. (1994). *The integration of social work practice.* Pacific Grove, CA: Brooks/Cole.

Pescosolido, B., Wright, E., & Sullivan, W. (1995). Communities of care: A theoretical perspective on case management models in mental health. *Advances in Medical Sociology, 6*, 37–79.

Real, T. (1990). Therapeutic use of self in constructivist/systemic therapy. *Family Process, 29*, 255–272.

Rolland, J. S. (1994a). *Families, illness and disability.* New York: Basic Books.

Rolland, J. S. (1994b). Working with illness: Clinicians' personal and interface issues. *Family Systems Medicine, 12*, 149–169.

Saari, C. (1991). *The creation of meaning in clinical social work.* New York: Guilford Press.

Scheflen, A. (1981). *Levels of schizophrenia.* New York: Brunner/Mazel.

Simon, B. (1994). *The empowerment tradition in American social work: A history.* New York: Columbia University Press.

Smith, J., & Birchwood, M. (1987). Specific and non-specific effects of educational intervention with families living with schizophrenic relative. *British Journal of Psychiatry, 150*, 645–652.

Sommer, R. (1990). Family advocacy and the mental health system: The recent rise of the Alliance for the Mentally Ill. *Psychiatric Quarterly, 61*, 205–221.

Starr, P. (1982). *The social transformation of American medicine.* New York: Basic Books.

Stotland, J. (1984). Relationship of parents to professionals: A challenge to professionals. *Journal of Visual Impairment and Blindness, 2*, 69–74.

Strachan, A., Feingold, D., Goldstein, M., Miklowitz, D., & Neuchterlein, K. (1989). Is expressed emotion an index of a transactional process? II. Patient's coping style. *Family Process, 28,* 169–181.

Tarrier, N., Barrowclough, C., Vaughn, C., Bamrah, J., Porceddu, K., Watts, S., & Freeman, H. (1988). The community management of schizophrenia: A controlled trial of a behavioural intervention with families to reduce relapse. *British Journal of Psychiatry, 153,* 532–542.

Terkelsen, K. (1983). Schizophrenia and the family: II. Adverse effects of family therapy. *Family Process, 22,* 191–200.

Tessler, R. C., Killian, L. M., & Gubman, G. D. (1987). Stages in family response to mental illness. *Psychosocial Rehabilitation Journal, 10*(4), 3–16.

Thorning, H., & Lukens, E. P. (1996). Schizophrenia and the self. In C. Kaufman & J. Gorman (Eds.), *Schizophrenia: New directions for clinical research and treatment* (pp. 177–187). New York: M. A. Liebert.

Thorning, H., & Lukens, E. (in press). Clinical social work in psychiatry. In B. Fallon & J. Gorman (Eds.), *The New York State Psychiatric Institute—American psychiatry at the centennial, 1896–1996.* New York: New York State Psychiatric Institute.

Tietz, T. (1949). A study of mothers of schizophrenic patients. *Psychiatry, 12,* 55–65.

Tunnel, G., Albert, M., Jacobs, J., & Osiasom, J. (1988). Designing a family psychoeducation program to meet community needs: The NYU–Bellevue Project. *International Journal of Mental Health, 17,* 75–98.

Vaughn, C., & Leff, J. (1976). The influence of family and social factors on the course of psychiatric illness: A comparison of schizophrenic and depressed neurotic patients. *British Journal of Psychiatry, 129,* 125–137.

Vaughn, C. E., Snyder, K. S., Jones, S., Freeman, W. B., & Falloon, I. R. (1984). Family factors in schizophrenia relapse: A replication in California of British research on expressed emotion. *Archives of General Psychiatry, 42,* 1169–1177.

Weinberger, D. (1987). Implications of normal brain development for the pathogenesis of schizophrenia. *Archives of General Psychiatry, 44,* 660–669.

White, M. (1989). *Selected papers.* Adelaide, Australia: Dulwich Centre Publications.

Woodside, H., Landeen, J., Kirkpatrick, H., Byrne, C., Bernardo, A., & Pawlick, J. (1994). Hope and schizophrenia: Exploring attitudes of clinicians. *Psychosocial Rehabilitation Journal, 18,* 140–141.

Zubin, J., & Spring, B. (1977). Vulnerability: A new view of schizophrenia. *Journal of Abnormal Psychology, 86,* 103–126.

# Cancer Support Groups and Group Therapies

Pat Fobair

> But the greatest thing that turned me back towards my feelings was what I learned in the Survivors' Group. One night when I was feeling bad, a young Latin woman entered the group. She had recently completed her therapy for lymphoma. She cried every time she attempted to talk about her pain. Finally, she spoke about not being able to feel good about anything, about not feeling lovable. For the first time, I heard someone talking about experiencing what I had experienced and suddenly, I realized that I was not the problem, but instead that I had a problem.
>
> —Robert Watts, Jr. (1998)

**M**oments of clarity, identification, and connection that come with storytelling are part of the emotional healing process that group therapies offer cancer patients, a process that helps return patients to a sense of inner control. Just as illness has biochemical and emotional components, healing requires emotional as well as physical assistance (Emonds, 1995).

This review of support groups and group therapies offers a perspective on research-based cancer groups as they occur along a continuum, moving from open-ended, drop-in groups that provide supportive, educational, or self-help experiences to time-limited or closed groups that use principles of existential group psychotherapy, such as the supportive–expressive group therapy (Spiegel & Spira, 1991). This chapter reviews the history and theoretical background of groups; describes the breakthroughs in mental health research that have shown how support groups and group therapies reduce psychological distress and enhance quality of life; discusses the continuum of group format, group organization, and leadership issues; reviews the possible negative experiences and problems that challenge group leaders; and discusses the special aspects of group therapy for cancer patients. Psychotherapeutic groups for cancer patients have been rigorously studied and provide an important example of research-based clinical practice (Spiegel et al., 1996).

## History

### THEORETICAL PERSPECTIVE

The theoretical base of cancer support groups comes from both historical roots and current trends in therapy. The historical origins began with the development of social work and group psychotherapy at the beginning of the 20th century. Group work began in settlement houses and in the early days of hospital social work.

## EARLY MODELS

In the 1880s and 1890s, in response to the challenge of large waves of European immigration to the United States, there was a burst of American social innovations that blossomed into such social services as the settlement house movement and hospital social work. The origins of today's hospital-based support group lie in social work pioneer Jane Addams's work at Hull House in Chicago, where social group work began, and in the development of hospital social work with group services for chronically ill people by Ida Cannon (1923) at Massachusetts General Hospital in Boston.

Jane Addams (1860–1935) was called the "conscience of America" because of the importance of her innovative work. Hull House opened in 1889 to address the needs of poor and unemployed people by forming educational groups and community action programs to help people deal with social, economic, and personal problems. Such settlement house groups provided information, education, and support for and encouraged self-help among the new Americans (Galinsky & Schopler, 1989). In 1931, Addams shared the Nobel peace prize with educator Nicholas Murray Butler, and she was elected president of the Woman's International League for Peace. Social work historians credit the settlement house movement and the work of Hull House as an important forerunner of today's support groups (Bruno, 1964a; Friedlander, 1968; Shaffer & Galinsky, 1989).

Medical social work began in 1905 in four places at nearly the same time (Friedlander, 1968). Richard Cabot introduced social work as an important factor in hospital treatment at Massachusetts General Hospital in Boston. His concept was that the social worker would help achieve a more accurate diagnosis and effective treatment program. Cannon worked with Cabot to demonstrate the utility of the social treatment of sick people (Bruno, 1964a). In 1923, she dedicated her book *Social Work in Hospitals: A Contribution to Progressive Medicine* to Cabot, "whose insight, constructive imagination, and fearless pioneer spirit have been the chief factors in starting and bringing to its present status in this country, organized hospital social service" (p. iii). She defined the *hospital social worker* as "one who sees the patient not merely as an isolated, unfortunate person occupying a hospital bed, but as a member belonging to a family or community group that is altered because of his ill health. The social worker seeks to remove obstacles either in the patient's surroundings or in his mental attitude that interfere with successful treatment, thus freeing the patient to aid in his own recovery" (pp. 14–15). During the same period, medical social work also began at Bellevue Hospital in New York, Johns Hopkins Hospital in Baltimore, and the Berkeley Infirmary in Boston (Friedlander, 1968).

Cannon, working with physicians and other social workers, created the early models of group treatment. She described the social worker's role in group treatment of chronically ill people and encouraged her staff to participate in groups for heart disease, diabetes, infantile paralysis (polio), scoliosis, and nutrition. According to Cannon (1923), "The group treatment helps to develop a loyalty and cooperation which bring patients back to the clinic more ready to follow advice. It gives a sense of comradeship which is of great value. New patients soon lose their shyness, those consumed with self-pity seldom fail to find others making less of greater handicaps, and the discouraged man or woman hears how someone else gained when conditions seemed quite as hopeless" (p. 77). She anticipated the future when she wrote, "careful social case work may thus not only serve the patient but also contribute to medical–social research" (p. 77).

Social group work was first described by early social worker Helen Hart. As head social worker at Kingsley House in Pittsburgh, she spoke about the changing functions of settlements in the settlement house movement: "The central objective for settlement programs is the [development of] personality through group relations" (cited in Bruno, 1964b). Social group work was influenced by the views from progressive education, and it later became part of the program of child guidance centers and family agencies. In 1935, Grace Coyle defined *social group work* as an educational process aiming at the development and social adjustment of people through voluntary group association (cited in Bruno, 1964b). Support groups for cancer patients were first reported in the 1970s (Krupnick, Rowland, Goldberg, & Daniel, 1993). Today's open-ended hospital support groups continue in the spirit of their origins.

The early model for group psychotherapy in medicine began in 1905 at Massachusetts General Hospital when Joseph Pratt, a Boston internist, developed the "tuberculosis class" for chronically ill patients there. Pratt understood the need to treat the psychological health of a person as well as his or her disease. In 1923 Cannon, who worked with Pratt, described the weekly group meetings with the doctor and social worker and noted that the patient was encouraged to keep up his spirits "in order that he may persist in the regimen prescribed, live within his physical limitations, and preserve or develop his sense of responsibility in carrying his share of the treatment" (p. 76). Pratt designed a treatment regimen that included physician home visits and diary keeping by the patients as well as the weekly meetings at the hospital. Cohesiveness and mutual support were created in the classes as a result of the mutual reporting of progress in weight gain and testimonials by successful patients (Cannon, 1923; Pratt, 1922; Yalom, 1985). Although physicians usually did not continue to lead the groups for chronically ill people, psychiatrists did begin to experiment with group methods with psychotic patients during the 1920s and 1930s (Lonergan, 1985; Yalom, 1985). J. L. Moreno, best known for the development of psychodrama, first coined the term "group therapy" in the 1920s (Yalom, 1980). Freudian-inspired group psychotherapy for interpersonal and intrapsychic conflicts began in the United States in the 1930s. During World War II the use of group therapy expanded considerably because of the need to treat large numbers of servicemen. During the 1950s a number of innovations in group therapy developed, including the existential–humanist model. Viktor Frankl, Rollo May, and Carl Rogers were popular exponents of the existential approach (Shaffer & Galinsky, 1989; Yalom, 1980).

## CURRENT THEORY

Integrating theory from models such as cognitive–behavioral therapy, group work has drawn on systems theory and small-group theories as well as psychological and sociological perspectives (Galinsky & Schopler, 1989). Most recently, theories from postmodernist and narrative therapy perspectives are being integrated into group therapies (Pardeck, Murphy, & Choi, 1994; White & Epston, 1990).

A key concept in social work group theory is the "open systems" model, which is based on an ecological perspective that stresses the reciprocal nature of relationships among people and systems. The concept of "person-in-environment" is particularly relevant for social workers in a hospital setting, where the group leader acknowledges the organizational influence of the larger system, including its influence on the patient (Perlman, 1957). The group is seen as a system with a defined boundary and interrelated parts. Support group conditions are viewed as an adaptation to external conditions and participant characteristics that confront each group system (Schopler & Galinsky, 1993). The impact between the group leaders and the group members is reciprocal, that is, interactions affect each person and reverberate through the system.

The social worker recognizes how forces in the small group promote two kinds of internal group leadership—task-oriented and social–emotional—which are both important to the development and maintenance of the ongoing group (Shulman, 1992). The activities of peer support and mutual aid are encouraged by group leaders. A positive outcome is group cohesion—that is, the attractiveness of the group (or "we-ness" value) described by group members as they discuss their reasons for group participation. When a group is cohesive, participants feel accepted by the other members. They perceive a similarity among themselves and others and they are willing to talk without defensiveness about themselves and share feelings for other group members. Discovering that one's feelings are shared by others is a curative element of groups. Group members help each other learn that each member is not the only one with a particular problem. The effect of this mutual sharing is bolstered by the feeling of being accepted—of not being alone with a problem (Yalom, 1985).

The ideas of postmodernism—a linguistic theory that proposes that the social world is more than a tangible, objective system—have penetrated social work practice and are useful for group leaders working with cancer patients (Pardeck et al., 1994). Postmodernism developed as a response to both scientific positivism and the humanistic ideas expressed in existentialism (Miller, 1993). Postmodernism posits a view of the self as responsive to the culture's use of language and power. How we know and what we believe to be true is connected to language, and truth is a product of language rather than something that is objective and universal. Social reality is a matter of the way we conceive and define it. As individuals, we create our own culture as we interact with each other in groups. Each person confirms his or her own reality by constructing and interpreting personal values, beliefs, and commitments through developing a personal narrative. Social groups invent their own community identity much as a person creates his or her own personal identity (Pardeck et al., 1994). Group members create a culture, with a starting point of the profound shift in their lives caused by, for example, the threat to their survival posed by a diagnosis of cancer. As they continue to participate, group members retell their life stories to each other; they explain the meaning that the intrusion of the illness has had in their lives. In open-ended cancer groups, participants are allowed to join, say what they need, and decide when their needs are met. Group members are encouraged to determine what they want to achieve and decide when they have achieved a successful outcome (Pardeck et al., 1994).

Social work values practical experience and historically has recognized the friction between scientific knowledge and real-life experience. As Gowdy (1994) said, "Much of human knowing is intuitive, subtle and sensory" (p. 364). It is important for members of marginalized groups to see themselves as their own authorities. Life is for growth of the human spirit and one's expanding consciousness (Reynolds, 1939). A common practice in group work is the "naming" of the experience. As Pozatek (1994) put it, "giving voice to something previously unacknowledged can be incredibly empowering for clients. Providing an opportunity for this new awareness can be a transformative moment for both patient and worker" (p. 400). The ideas of postmodernism have made important contributions to the theory and goals of client-centered group work by social workers in hospitals.

## EXISTENTIAL GROUP THERAPY

A second source of theory for support groups and group therapies comes from the application of existential philosophy to group therapy. Originating with Kierke-gaard in Sweden in the 1830s, the philosophy of existentialism was expanded and popularized in Europe through the work of Heidegger and Jaspers in the 1920s. In the United States, existentialism penetrated the fields of psychology, psychiatry, and the social sciences during the late 1940s and the 1950s, largely as the result of the popular book *Existence: A New Dimension in Psychiatry and Psychology* (May, Angel, & El-lenberger, 1958). This was a major development in American psychotherapy, a third force after Freudian psychoanalysis and Watsonian behaviorism (Yalom, 1980). As response to the positivist tradition that valued empirical research, existentialists took a new look at the nature of knowledge. The existential therapists repudiated Freudi-an psychology's emphasis on the role of biological drives in human development, yet they absorbed rather than abandoned the major Freudian concepts of unaware-ness, anxiety, and resistance (Yalom, 1985).

The term "existentialism" comes from the concept in this school of philosophy that existence and essence are the same—that the essence of the human being is to exist. The emerging self evolves, taking responsibility for potentiality and self-actual-ization. Existentialists believe that the most important issue is the cognitive need to give meaning to one's life. In existential psychotherapy, therapists take a nonjudg-mental attitude toward clients' previous decision making, and they act as role models of openness, sharing more of themselves than Freudian therapists do (Shaffer & Galinsky, 1989). Existentialism serves as a reminder that beneath the elaborate struc-ture of the knowable world remains the fact of biological existence. Our awareness of the limits of our own existence can inspire both terror and a sense of awe, which encourage us to evaluate the meaning in life. We realize that we are vulnerable, our relationship to the world is contingent, and the world we each experience will die with us. The more we face the ultimate aloneness, the more we sense that life's meaningfulness can be confirmed or refuted on the most personal level (Yalom, 1980).

Four important themes appear in reviews of existentialism: death, freedom, iso-lation, and meaning. Yalom (1980), writing about life, death, and anxiety in *Existen-tial Psychotherapy*, noted that avoidance of the thought of one's own death can lead to greater anxiety and defenses, such as the irrational belief in our own "specialness" or belief in the ultimate rescuer. Specialness might take the form of workaholism or a drive for power and money, narcissism that interferes in interpersonal relations by distancing a person from others. Wishing to be rescued is another escape from facing one's death. The desire to be rescued from the edge of the abyss by an omnipotent presence is pervasive in human culture. Either form is an effort to gain control over one's death anxiety.

In existentialist thought, freedom is the absence of external structure. Each per-son is responsible for creating his or her own world, life design, choices, and actions. One's responsibility is to discover the choices to further one's potential and create meaning in life. Existentialist isolation is the fact of entering and existing in life

FIGURE **13-1**

**Types of Support Groups**

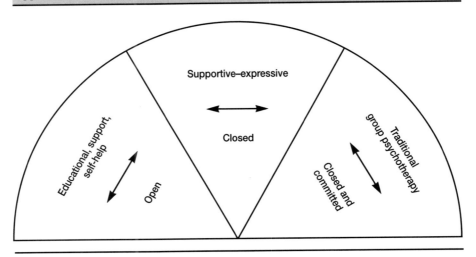

alone, no matter how close we become to one another. There is a tension between the wish to be part of a larger whole—to have intimate contact with others—and the awareness that each person is, ultimately, alone. Why do we live? How will we live? Each person must construct his or her own meaning in life in a universe that has no meaning (Yalom, 1980).

The supportive–expressive group therapy model bridges the gap between tradition-al group psychotherapy and the educational and support groups (see Figure 13-1). It draws on the philosophy of existential group therapy and meets a need arising from the cancer patient's relationship to a world that is finite. Supportive–expressive groups build social support and help members express emotions, thereby helping them come to terms with their personal circumstances, revise and strengthen rela-tionships, and re-examine meaning in their lives. For example, in a group for women with metastatic breast cancer, group members can experience special moments of closeness through participating in the daily life of a group member who is dying. In-stead of avoiding an unpleasant reality, they extend their friendship into the dying group member's home and spend time with her and her family. Group meetings may be held even in the dying patient's home. After the death, group leaders and members attend the funeral or memorial service. Thus, group members become important to each other despite the emotional pain of grieving a loss: They become a new support system for one another.

In supportive–expressive therapy, group members are encouraged to examine their personal choices, increase their emotional expressiveness, and work on im-proving doctor–patient relationships and social and family support. Other themes include working through grief as group members die and group survivors face the possibility of their own death. Group leaders create an atmosphere of empathy and unconditional positive regard. They strive to be genuine and share their own expe-riences using transparency of self as a way of modeling desired behaviors for the group member. As group members discuss their uncertainty about the future and their feelings of vulnerability, they begin to focus on the issues facing them, such as their treatment-related concerns, the effect of the illness on their family, and the implications for their personal choices and goals. In supportive–expressive groups, the more a group member faces the ultimate aloneness provoked by the possibility of death, the more the personal meaning of life becomes vivid. Therapists use this model to help patients focus on the issues and feelings they are facing in the moment and to encourage group members to move from emotion-focused coping to active coping (Classen et al., 1993).

Existential therapy and the supportive–expressive group therapy model derive from the idea that our biological survival precedes all other issues in life. When it was adopted into the medical model in the late 1940s, existential philosophy provided a major shift toward focusing on the individual as a cognitive person with choices in self-development and in reappraising life goals. The supportive–expressive model is concerned with the importance of facing one's finite relationship with the world and redefining the meaning in one's life when threatened by a diagnosis of cancer or other serious illness.

Although existential humanism and postmodernism share certain philosophies, there also are essential differences in their views of the self. Both schools are responses to reductionist thinking in scientific positivism. Both drew on the philosophical thoughts of Nietzsche, Heidegger, and Wittgenstein. Postmodernist ideas were a reaction to existential humanism (Miller, 1993). Frustrated with existentialists' failure to address the issues of language and power, Foucault broke with existentialism and developed many concepts important to postmodernism. When existentialists think of "the self," they think of the innate potentiality of each person, personal freedom and responsibility, and the opportunities in life to examine personal meaning (Yalom, 1980). Postmodernists come to their view of the self from their understanding of language and power—that is, reality is defined by language (Pardeck et al., 1994). According to the postmodernists, it is through the institutions of power that truth is delivered to us (Saleebey, 1994). People are encouraged to examine how they have collaborated in the control of their own lives as they adhere to the truths learned during their lives. They are seen as essentially blameless in creating their own problems, and each person is viewed as an expert in her own experience. Instead of concentrating on defining problems, clients are encouraged to picture solutions. Possibility and narrative therapies are two therapeutic descendants of postmodernism; both encourage therapists to invite the person not to blame himself or herself (White & Epston, 1990). The tasks of the possibility therapist are to validate the person and his or her experience, and to change the view of the problem (O'Hanlon, 1993). In narrative therapy, a new narrative is coauthored, distinct from the problem-saturated story, to assist clients in redefining their lives (Chang & Phillips, 1993).

Existentialism examines individual issues of death, freedom, isolation, responsibility, and meaninglessness, and postmodernists are concerned with power, truth, making meaning, responsibility, and uncertainty. Both hold that the consciousness within a person is an important area of study (White, 1993; Yalom, 1980). For example, the concept of power in existentialism can be seen as a deception in one's view of the self as special (Yalom, 1980), but a postmodernist views power as part of the culture's use of language and control of others (Saleebey, 1994).

The role of the leader in support groups or group therapies also is viewed differently. Existential therapists are encouraged to be open, expressive, and less judgmental in their work with clients. Postmodernist therapists are encouraged to see clients as their own authorities, honor what has evolved within the person, and help clients create scenarios of possibility as they retell the story of their personal journeys

(Gowdy, 1994; Pardeck et al., 1994; Saleebey, 1994). Both postmodern and existential therapists acknowledge the client's experience, validate the client's point of view, encourage his or her thoughts and actions, and incorporate their own experience into the conversation as they move toward solutions (O'Hanlon, 1993; Yalom, 1980).

## Research on the Effectiveness of Group Work

One of the breakthroughs in mental health research during the past 20 years has been demonstration of the effectiveness of support groups and group therapies in improving the quality of life and life expectancy for cancer patients. The two most dramatic studies by Spiegel, Bloom, Kraemer, and Gottheil (1989) and Fawzy et al. (1990) found reductions in emotional distress and mortality among the cancer patients randomly assigned to the experimental arm of the group therapy research. Improvements in emotional distress were found in eight additional group therapy studies when cancer patient group members were compared with cancer patient control subjects (Cella, Sarafian, Snider, Yellen, & Winicour, 1993; Evans & Connis, 1995; Jacobs, Ross, Walker, & Stockdale, 1983; Johnson, 1982; Kelly et al., 1993; Telch & Telch, 1986; Toro, Rappaport, & Seidman, 1987; Weisman, Worden, & Sobel (1980).

The expanding professional literature indicates that group psychotherapy is effective in helping cancer patients cope better with their disease. In a review of psychosocial interventions, Fawzy, Fawzy, Arndt, and Pasnau (1995) found evidence that several forms of group intervention were effective in improving patient mood. This section reviews the research for open-ended, educational, cognitive–behavioral, self-help and supportive–expressive groups, and cognitive education or emotionally expressive group discussion.

### OPEN-ENDED GROUPS

Open-ended groups have been popular with social work practitioners working in hospital settings, but there has been little research to review their effectiveness. In an early study, Wood, Milligan, Christ, and Liff (1978) reported on a pilot study with 15 cancer patients who attended eight weekly 90-minute meetings. They found that the patients had wanted the group experience; 11 of 13 patients felt that the group experience was helpful, eight thought it helped them face anxieties and fears, and six found it easier to speak in the group about feelings and concerns related to their illness. Getting factual information from the group was helpful for nine patients, nine felt less isolated, 11 felt support and warmth from the leaders, and 12 said they would recommend the group experience to other cancer patients. Both social workers and psychiatrists have reported open-ended support groups to be useful in their work with inpatients who have chronic and psychiatric illness (Cannon, 1923). Lonergan (1985), who described social work groups, and Beeber (1988) and Yalom (1983), who described inpatient psychiatry groups, found that open-ended support groups were helpful for patients particularly because they offered a flexibility that closed, time-limited groups could not.

### EDUCATIONAL GROUPS

Two comparative studies of patient education groups were carried out by Johnson (1982) and Jacobs et al. (1983). Johnson developed a structured educational program for cancer patients randomly selected from a group of adults who had been diagnosed with cancer within the past year and were receiving treatment in a hospital outpatient care setting. The patients were paired after being matched by age, gender, and their scores from three pretest dependent variables (that is, the State–Trait Anxiety Inventory—Spielberger, Gorsuch, & Lushene, 1968; the Purpose in Life Test—Crumbaugh, 1973; and the Course Inquiry—Johnson & Flaherty, 1980), indicators of anxiety, meaning in life, and knowledge about cancer. Each of the 26 pairs was then randomly assigned to either the treatment or control group. Treatment included eight educational counseling sessions, titled "I Can Cope," which were conducted over four weeks and covered learning about the disease, coping with daily health problems, communication, liking oneself, living with limits, and identifying helpful resources. At the end of the eight weeks, the treatment group had lower anxiety scores (Spielberger et al., 1968) and reported better knowledge of their illness and an increased sense of meaning in life (Johnson & Flaherty, 1980), compared with the control group.

Jacobs and colleagues (1983) conducted two prospective controlled studies to determine if psychological and social functioning could be enhanced in patients with Hodgkin's disease by either education or participation in a peer support therapy group. A total of 81 patients were evaluated in the two studies by use of the Cancer Patient Behavior Scale before and after the intervention. Among the 47 patients in the education study, the 21 experimental patients experienced significant reduction in the frequency of anxiety, treatment problems, depression, and disruption in life, compared with the 26 patients in the control group. However, in the second study of 34 patients using peer group support, the 16 patients in the experimental arm showed no improvement in any of the areas studied when compared with the 18 control patients.

## COGNITIVE–BEHAVIORAL GROUPS

In the 1980s, two studies pioneered the use of cognitive–behavioral techniques in work with cancer patients. The Omega Project (Weisman et al., 1980) used a structured intervention that addressed common questions and concerns of cancer patients, provided education, and taught relaxation techniques. The program used four audiotapes and 10 sets of illustrated "problem" cards to focus discussions. Fifty-nine subjects participated in four group sessions over a six-week period. All patients, including 58 control subjects, were screened for variables such as religion, socioeconomic status, race, and other demographic data. They were assessed by the Profile of Mood States (POMS) (McNair, Lorr, & Drappelman, 1971), the Index of Vulnerability, Therapist Rating Form, Patient Evaluation of Psychosocial Intervention, and Inventory of Current Concerns. Patients randomly assigned to group intervention reported increased communication and coping skills and a positive psychological outcome, as measured by the POMS, the Index of Vulnerability, and the Inventory of Current Concerns, when compared with patients in the control group.

Telch and Telch (1986) compared group coping-skills instruction with supportive group therapy for cancer patients and found the cognitive–behavioral and affective coping strategies to be more effective in the patients' psychosocial adjustment to their illness. Forty-one patients were randomly assigned to one of three conditions for six weeks: 13 patients to group coping-skills instruction, 14 patients to support group therapy, and 14 patients to no treatment (control). Coping-skills training included instruction in relaxation and stress management, assertive communication, cognitive restructuring and problem solving, feelings management, and pleasant activity planning. Pretests and posttests using the POMS and the Cancer Inventory of Problem Situations were the primary instruments used to assess affective states. Results demonstrated that patients who received the coping-skills training had a greater benefit in mood outcome than did the other two groups. The patients who received supportive group therapy exhibited little improvement, and the untreated patients showed a decline in their psychological adjustment between the pre- and posttest six weeks later.

Important efforts have taken place systematically to examine immune system changes among cancer patients attending group therapies and later to observe the survival of the cancer patients involved. Fawzy and colleagues (1990) studied components of several therapy programs that resulted in positive effects. They combined specific parts of the Omega Project (Weisman et al., 1980) and studies by other researchers (Jacobs et al., 1983; Spiegel, Bloom, & Yalom, 1981; Telch & Telch, 1986) to create a six-week structured group intervention to encompass health education, stress management, coping skills, and supportive group psychotherapy. Sixty-eight patients who had already received the standard surgical treatment for their illness were randomly assigned to the control or the experimental group. The groups received the same routine medical care, but the 34 patients assigned to the experimental group received the intervention. Although all the patients reported moderate to high levels of psychological distress at baseline, as measured by the POMS, at the end of the six weeks the experimental subjects exhibited significantly lower levels of distress than did the control subjects. Six months later, the group differences were even more pronounced. The patients who had received the intervention reported better mood, less confusion and fatigue, greater use of active coping techniques, and healthier immune systems. Six years later, they reported having experienced fewer recurrences of cancer and fewer deaths (Fawzy et al., 1995).

## SELF-HELP GROUPS

Over a three-year period, Cella and colleagues (1993) studied the effects of a self-help group intervention on quality of life for 77 patients with cancer in one of seven groups participating in an eight-week program. The study was based on the premise that mutual support provided by group members is the essential helpful factor in the group experience. As expected, self-reported quality-of-life scores, as measured by the Functional Living Index–Cancer (FLIC) improved statistically significantly ($p < 0.05$) by the final session, compared with reports completed at the start of the intervention. Although the study subjects positively rated the leaders, they described peer support as the most helpful component of the intervention.

Perhaps the most important research on self-help groups was reported by Toro and colleagues (1987), who studied the implementation of 33 self-help groups affiliated with GROW International, an organization that sponsors weekly group meetings for former patients of psychiatric hospitals who are adjusting to living in the community. The 33 GROW groups, with a total of 170 members, were compared with 25 psychotherapy groups ($N = 180$ patients) to examine the self-help groups' development of the necessary therapeutic social climate. Both groups were assessed by use of the Group Environment Scale (Moos, 1981, 1986). The mean differences between the two groups showed significant differences in the nature of the self-help groups in nine of 10 dimensions. The self-help groups were found to be more cohesive and had more active leadership than the psychotherapy groups. They were more task oriented and better organized, and they scored somewhat higher on the "independence" variable. The psychotherapy groups, which included both inpatients and outpatients and were led by professionals with a psychodynamic orientation, were found to be directed toward the open expression of anger, and they showed more flexibility and innovation (Moos, Finney, & Maude-Griffin, 1993).

## SUPPORTIVE–EXPRESSIVE GROUP THERAPY

Pioneering work in this area has been done by Spiegel and his colleagues (1981, 1989, 1991). They compared 50 patients with metastatic breast cancer receiving group therapy and regular medical care with a control group of 36 closely matched patients receiving only regular medical care. Patients receiving the intervention met in weekly 90-minute therapy groups for one year. The families of these group members met once a month for one year. The intervention included providing an environment in which patients were encouraged to express thoughts and feelings about their illness and its effects on their lives. Group members also were encouraged to develop close personal ties with each other in and out of the group. Group cohesion, sharing of mutual fears, and emotional self-disclosure were emphasized. Self-hypnosis was taught for pain management, stress reduction, and facing difficult fears. The POMS was the principal outcome measure used in the study (McNair et al., 1971). Group members and control patients were assessed at three-month intervals. At 12 months, the patients in the experimental group showed statistically significantly ($p < 0.01$) less tension, fatigue, and confusion and more vigor than the control group as well as much less pain. At 10-year follow-up, three of the 86 patients were still alive. Review of medical records and death certificates showed that survival was significantly ($p < 0.0001$) different, with a mean of 36.6 months in the intervention group compared with 18.9 months in the control group. Lower mood disturbance and higher ratings of vigor on the POMS at the end of the intervention were significantly associated with greater longevity (Fawsy et al., 1995; Spiegel, 1993; Spiegel et al., 1981; Spiegel et al., 1989).

## COGNITIVE EDUCATION OR EMOTIONALLY EXPRESSIVE GROUP DISCUSSION

Some clinicians have wondered whether cognitive exercises or emotionally expressive group discussion have greater value for therapeutic group treatment outcome. Studies by Evans and Connis (1995) and Kelly and colleagues (1993) supported the conclusion that support group therapies, modeled on expressive–supportive groups that focus on the expression of emotion by group members, are more successful than cognitive–behavioral group therapies in helping patients experience fewer psychiatric symptoms and maladaptive interpersonal sensitivity, anxiety, and behavior patterns. Kelly and collaborators (1993) randomly assigned 68 men diagnosed with HIV infection and depression to one of three study conditions: an eight-session cognitive–behavioral group, an eight-session social support group, or a comparison condition. Data were collected at three time points: before and after the intervention and three months later. All participants were assessed individually using the Center for Epidemiologic Studies Depression Scale (CES-D). Substance abuse and sexual practices were self-reported and a single index was created. The results showed that relative to the comparison group, both the cognitive–behavioral and the social support group therapies produced reductions in depression, hostility, and somatization. The social support intervention also produced reductions in overall psychiatric symptoms and tended to reduce maladaptive interpersonal sensitivity, anxiety, and frequency of unprotected receptive anal intercourse; cognitive–behavioral intervention resulted in less-frequent illicit drug use during the follow-up period. At postintervention and three-month follow-up, participants in the social support group intervention continued to show greater reduction in depression scores compared with participants in the other two arms of the study.

Evans and Connis (1995) also were interested in comparing outcomes of counseling techniques among emotionally distressed men going through cancer treatment. They randomly assigned 72 cancer patients with depression who were undergoing radiation therapy to one of three conditions: cognitive–behavioral treatment, social support, or no-treatment control. Before and after intervention and at six-month follow-up, study participants were individually assessed using CES-D. Both the cognitive–behavioral and social support therapies resulted in less depression, hostility, and somatization when compared with the no-treatment group. The social support intervention, compared with the cognitive–behavior treatment, also resulted in fewer psychiatric symptoms, reduced maladaptive interpersonal sensitivity and anxiety, and demonstrated more changes that were evident at six-month follow-up. These two studies supported the theory that when patients focus on the expression of emotion, they can shift from emotion-focused coping to more effective, problem-solving coping (Spiegel, 1995b).

## SUMMARY OF RESEARCH ON GROUPS

At least 10 studies have found that group interventions improve patient mood, provide information, encourage active coping skills, and increase the number of health-enhancing behaviors. Positive outcomes were found across the board in educational, cognitive–educational, self-help, and supportive–expressive groups. Fawzy et al. (1995) noted that "the need for a variety of psychosocial interventions is enhanced as increasing numbers of patients with cancer have longer survival" (p. 100).

# Group Process

A support group for patients with cancer provides both emotional and social support for those who participate. Goals include helping participants learn about themselves in relation to the illness; buffering the experience of stress by offering a safe, confidential atmosphere in which patients can discuss making difficult decisions; and talking with others who are experiencing similar life changes. The group provides a place to talk about emotions and assists patients in recognizing and accepting the uncertainty of the future. It ensures organization for crisis intervention when critical moments occur for the person with cancer, aids communication, encourages assertive behavior, provides for reality testing and relief from a sense of guilt, and assists patients and survivors with grief and bereavement (Cordoba, Shear, Fobair, & Hall, 1984; Fobair, Cordoba, Pluth, & Bloom, 1982).

The first task of the group leader is to decide the goals of the group (Bernard, 1979). In an environment where patients are facing a life-threatening situation, the group leader encourages group members to re-examine their values and personal goals and establish priorities that are congruent with their situation at the moment. The goals in open-ended groups are to support treatment-related discussion that allows patients to determine that they are in harmony with their medical plans; talk about patients' concerns and feelings; encourage psychological movement from emotion-focused coping to action-oriented coping; and provide a network of patients who can offer each other regular, frequent acceptance and nurturance.

As the group evolves, the group leader might be asked to advocate for a group member—for example, intervening in a community agency when a patient needs assistance. The patients' right to determine their own needs is affirmed. Challenging bureaucratic rules or discriminatory practices that interfere with a group member's rights or opportunities is a frequent task for group leaders (Fobair & Wax, 1995).

The style and content of social work groups varies among counseling support, educational, or self-help groups. Groups might include teaching materials from cognitive skills development or an action-oriented component such as process art or spontaneous writing. Process art and spontaneous writing encourage group members to experience themselves in the moment, letting go of thoughts of end results and paying attention to their own process. In addition to verbal exchanges, process art and sometimes journal writing are used to encourage personal expression (Fobair & Wax, 1995). Group leaders encourage the open expression of both positive and negative feelings by offering supportive responses to member concerns and by accepting differences among group members. As the group develops, members may share in the performance of leadership functions (Galinsky & Schopler, 1989).

Essential resources for support groups include a cancer patient population of sufficient size to enroll in a group eight to 12 people who want or need such services; leaders with time available; a group plan; materials such as notebooks; and a location, date, and time. The assistance needed to start a group has been well described by others (Cordoba et al., 1984; Lonergan, 1985; Yalom, 1985).

## GROUP FORMAT

### Open-Ended Groups

Open-ended groups can take the form of counseling and support or education and discussion. They may be led by a professional or may be self-help and peer support in nature. In a hospital setting an open-ended group may be available to everyone on a given medical service or may have a focused membership by diagnosis or age group. Group preparation may be as simple as a verbal invitation to join or involve a short screening interview. Patients and their families may attend for one session or more. Membership depends on patient availability and enthusiasm for the group. Shifts in participation should be expected (Lonergan, 1985). Leaders in counseling support groups have described their task as facilitating, enabling, validating, and mirroring the patients' discourse on their experiences since the cancer diagnosis, although educational groups are more tutorial in style (Cordoba et al., 1984). The leader in supportive group interventions builds patients' self-esteem and reduces anxiety and regression to more childish behavior. The result is that group members feel better about themselves after each meeting. New members experience an immediate feeling of relief (Lonergan, 1985). In educationally oriented groups, the leader helps patients understand and master the practical and emotional aspects of their situation so they will be confident in participating in the medical environment.

Open-ended counseling, support, and information groups are often used in hospitals with numerous cancer patients and easy access to group meetings. The impetus for starting a counseling information group may come from the social worker's knowledge of patients' emotional suffering. The open-ended support group begins when patients with a pressing concern get together to share their personal experiences and engage in the development of a cohesive, supportive system (Schopler & Galinsky, 1993). Open-ended groups can provide a forum for patients to talk about their cancer treatment experience, share emotional release, find validation of their concerns, reduce social isolation, learn new information, experience group support and cohesion, and heal the psychic wound from having experienced a threat to one's life. Open-ended groups are inclusive and recognize that some patients may come for one session only (Fobair et al., 1981; Lonergan, 1985; Schopler & Galinsky, 1993).

Group members may experience a variety of situations in their disease course while they are participating. Any subject may come up in an open-ended group (Christ, 1991; Cordoba et al., 1984). The group members' feelings and concerns guide the content of each group meeting and will evolve as the group coalesces and becomes more intimate. Some of the themes that participants raise frequently are

- the impact of the cancer diagnosis
- threat to their survival
- overwhelming emotional reaction (why me?)
- wish to deny the reality of the disease
- need for further information
- need to make decisions about appropriate treatment and understand the treatment plan
- reorganization of the family to incorporate the demands of treatment and offer support to the patient
- restoration of self-esteem when there is hair loss, weight loss, and fatigue
- ambivalence about treatment caused by its disturbing side effects
- relationships with physicians
- loss of control
- loneliness and isolation
- fear of being dependent
- problems with practical resources related to medical needs and daily life (for example, financial security, housing, transportation, and insurance).

These themes reflect the adaptive tasks patients face during diagnosis and treatment (Christ, 1991; Cordoba et al., 1984). At the end of treatment and during early survivorship, patients experience new worries, such as

- fears of having less medical surveillance or of recurrence
- continuation of some problems that predated the diagnosis
- physical losses
- communication problems with family and friends
- resuming work and family tasks with a changed sense of body and life expectancy
- confronting social stigma and barriers to normalization
- new interest in nutrition and activity patterns
- turf issues at work and home
- death and the process of dying
- new values and goals
- changes in priorities
- negative feelings and thoughts
- active coping techniques.

Should illness recur, the patient will need to talk about his or her understanding of the new situation, express disappointment and negative feelings, alleviate a sense of guilt or self-blame, reconceive perspective, and make decisions about the new treatment.

## Educational Groups

Educational and discussion groups are based on the premise that the more people know about how to cope with their situation, the greater their chances of achieving their maximum level of well-being (Krumm, Vanetta, & Sanders, 1979). Patients and family members are comfortable with educational groups because such groups convey respect for their ability to take responsibility for their own care. The educational group provides a forum for those who want to learn more but are not ready to talk about their feelings (Cordoba et al., 1984; Fobair et al., 1982).

The process in educational and discussion groups embraces the concept of behavior change through the learning experience. As in a classroom or seminar, the objectives and goals are arranged in advance of the group meeting. Set times and dates, even a printed schedule, may announce the class. The group can be larger than in counseling and therapy groups. The group leaders present materials or introduce speakers and encourage group members to discuss the presentation, integrating it through discussion with others and, when possible, using the ideas presented and discussed to anticipate new situations.

Education and discussion groups are especially helpful for patients with newly diagnosed cancer who are flooded with negative feelings and the stress of an overwhelming situation. Such patients need to learn more about their medical condition and treatment options at the same time that their coping techniques are being challenged. Information helps reduce patients' anxiety (Lonergan, 1985). One of the challenges for group leaders is to manage the group's communication when they are ready to talk about feelings or personal concerns. The group leader may have to choose between covering educational content or allowing patient spontaneity (Cordoba et al., 1984; Fobair et al., 1982).

## Cognitive–Behavioral Groups

One of the most useful materials in educational programs involves teaching such coping skills as assertive communication, constructive thinking, feelings management, and relaxation techniques. Developed in the fields of education and psychology, cognitive–behavioral interventions assist patients in gaining the skill needed to manage and reduce stress, alter thoughts that increase depression, and develop adaptive behavioral coping strategies (Evans & Connis, 1995). Cognitive–behavioral techniques can help patients gain control over negative thoughts and feelings, begin the process of reframing the cancer experience, and help in choosing active coping techniques (Telch & Telch, 1986; Worden & Weisman, 1984). Behavioral therapies encourage patients to develop specific coping skills for specific problems. Group leaders teach these active coping skills to augment the patients' current resources and improve their life and coping strategies (Spiegel & Spira, 1991).

Group members frequently will describe moments when they experienced loss of control and a flood of difficult feelings, such as shock, fear, isolation, anxiety, anger, sadness, depression, uncertainty, low self-esteem, demoralization, guilt, panic, and disappointment (see Figure 13-2). When these feelings become overwhelming, negative thoughts, such as blaming oneself or others, become repetitious and painful. Additional negative thoughts and feelings might include defiance, partial denial or dissociation, magical thinking, "black-and-white" thinking, "awfulizing" or "catastrophizing," or helplessness and hopelessness (Matano & Yalom, 1991). Group leaders encourage patients to learn about these normal coping processes (defense mechanisms) and recognize their own thoughts and feelings so that they can progress to more active coping or problem solving as soon as they understand what they are doing mentally. The active coping techniques include giving oneself permission to feel, identifying feelings, giving feelings a name, recognizing feeling through body tensions, accepting situations that are beyond personal control, and changing what is possible by use of constructive thinking and problem solving. Allowing for relaxation, communicating with others, using humor, and forgiving oneself and others whenever possible also are important tasks (Telch & Telch, 1986).

When I use the teaching tool shown in Figure 13-2, I sometimes find it useful to tell group members about my personal experience with breast cancer. Sharing these experiences with group members helps normalize some of the issues and feelings that group members find hard to talk about. My early-stage breast cancer was diagnosed in 1986, and I remember the shock and fear I felt when I found the skin puckering on my left shoulder. I was struck by the sense of personal isolation, feeling as though a glass shield covered my head and shoulders. "Oh, this is how I am going to die," I first thought. Then, "No, this is how I am going to have to live—UGH!" When my negative feelings were too high, I found myself having "blaming" thoughts and reverting to denial and dissociation. Although I was able to make medical plans and move life forward, it was months before I could accept the full impact of the diagnosis. I had to learn to soothe myself, prepare for the events to come, give myself permission to feel all the feelings and tolerate the tears. Gradually, I learned to identify the negative feelings more rapidly, give them a name, and focus on what to do. Moments of helplessness were reduced to brief times when I understood that as soon as I took one small step toward an active choice, I would feel better. As quickly as I could, I learned not to delay in moving toward personal problem solving, because that was the quickest way for me to calm down and stop "awfulizing and catastrophizing." Although, they were more difficult to talk about at first, there were brief moments of suicidal thoughts that were usually related to low energy because of my earlier treatment. I also experienced helpless and hopeless feelings of "being in a prison."

## Self-Help Groups

Self-help and mutual-aid groups are an important resource in modern society (Moos et al., 1993). They provide support systems aimed at helping fellow patients and family members overcome their sense of being victims of a disease (Cole, O'Connor, & Bennett, 1979) and assist group members by providing a forum in which to learn coping skills and share with others. Self-help groups are often leaderless or run by the group as a whole. They comfort group members who previously felt isolated by helping them identify common patterns resulting from previous stress or behavior patterns. Such groups flourish in situations in which patients have found that the hardships and stigma of their illness have prevented their full participation in the normal course of events or when professional help has been unresponsive or unavailable (Adams, 1979). Self-help groups create a support system through their membership structure, group commitment to goals, and member identification with the group. Older members help newer ones by convincing them of the importance of participating. Self-help groups are effective because they destigmatize the role of patient,

FIGURE **13-2**

## Coping with Loss of Control

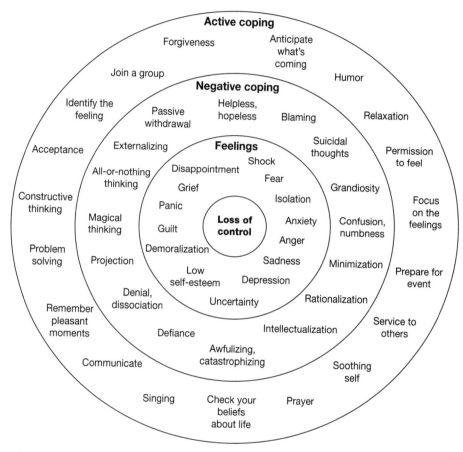

### Using the Coping Circles
- Having cancer can make us feel out of control and bring up strong feelings.
- When you feel "out of control" and do not know why, try this.
- Trace back your thoughts and review feelings that have been recently disturbing for you.
- Negative feelings can be overwhelming and bring up defensive thoughts.
- Regaining a sense of control involves our identifying the negative feelings, discovering the source, recognizing defensive coping, accepting what cannot be changed, changing what we can, problem solving, practicing relaxation, using assertive behavior, examining old beliefs about life that may not fit today's problems, forgiving ourselves and others, and sharing and communicating with others.
- Using the coping circles involves catching yourself in that passive, helpless, hopeless, defensive place, figuring out one thing you can do for yourself and then moving on to problem solving.

SOURCE: Adapted from Bob Matano, PhD, Department of Psychiatry, Stanford University, 1995. Used with permission.

reduce social isolation, and provide social and emotional support (Cole et al., 1979; Spiegel & Spira, 1991; Wax, 1991).

Self-help groups have been described as antielitist and democratic in nature (Fobair et al., 1982; Katz & Binder, 1976). Their leadership comes from peers who have experienced the same problems as all the others in the group. Members can be active, judgmental, critical, or supportive. They divulge their experiences to each other and provide a level of acceptance that other kinds of groups may not. Emphasis in the group may be placed on self-control, will power, or faith. The group urges appropriate behavior and celebrates day-to-day victories (Ascheim, Horman, Queisser, & Silverman, 1978). Group members' self-disclosure can be enormously helpful to new members.

Problems in self-help groups may occur if the flow of new patients dwindles or the group members become stuck in one or two ways of doing things. When a new member's needs exceed the knowledge of the group, there can be a breakdown in role modeling as an effective helping technique. Recognizing the limits of group options for members and encouraging appropriate referrals may be additional limits to self-help groups (Fobair et al., 1982).

A debate exists among professional and patient-oriented organizations over the virtues of professionally led groups versus self-help groups, especially concerning group members' expression of boundaries in relating to each other. When leaders have not experienced serious illness, they may not as easily bridge the gap between health care providers and patients. They may not share compassion or understanding with patients in the group as much as the patients desire. Self-help groups, on the other hand, may overexpress an antiprofessional bias or become overidentified with helping individual members rather than looking to the needs of the group as a whole.

## Closed-Format Groups

Time-limited, closed, or continuously committed groups provide the opportunity for group members to get to know each other well and explore important issues in depth. The supportive–expressive therapy group can offer an excellent model for achieving these goals in group therapy.

### Supportive–Expressive Group Therapy

The goals of supportive–expressive group therapy for cancer patients are to help patients normalize the cancer experience, feel less alone, integrate a changed self-image, increase emotional expressiveness, improve coping skills, and improve doctor–patient communication and social and family support. For example, as members of a group for patients with metastatic breast cancer confront their mortality, it is the therapist's goal to help them reduce their fear and anxiety and "detoxify" the death and dying process by working through their experiences of grief. The therapist helps patients think about how they want to use their time well, possibly by developing a life project, and enhance their quality of life.

In supportive–expressive group therapy, leaders encourage group members to discuss current issues and feelings, keeping the group focused on the here and now. Group members, distressed by the cancer experience, focus on coping with the illness. Contact outside the group is encouraged by the leaders. Empathy, genuineness, and nonjudgmental, positive regard are values the group leaders try to model.

Leaders create a group culture by encouraging interaction, spontaneity, and self-disclosure. Like social work groups, supportive–expressive groups include educational information as well as coping-skills training and cognitive restructuring, but the major goal of the leader in a supportive–expressive group is to encourage group members to talk about their feelings (Classen et al., 1993; Spiegel & Spira, 1991).

Coleading a supportive–expressive group for metastatic breast cancer patients with David Spiegel at Stanford University Medical Center in California, has allowed me to see how patients benefit from this group model. We have met continuously since 1990 with a group of women who are participants in a research project. Most have been involved in the group for at least one year. Sandy, a successful journalist, has used the group to get closer to her feelings, improving and becoming more authentic in her communication with her husband and daughters. She started and maintains a life project, a student scholarship encouraging women in journalism. Marianne, a former therapist and nurse, has used the group to continue her process of seeking options in life while she prepares for her death. Sheila has role modeled assertiveness with doctors and compassion for dying members, contributing to the group's cohesiveness. Sally received validation for finding her assertive voice with physicians and family members. Victoria found new hope and personal control in her medical care as she defined what she wanted with her physicians. Group members move along at their own pace and benefit from the group caring and cohesion.

## TRADITIONAL GROUP THERAPY

Traditional group psychotherapy has both a different focus and a different task for leaders and patients. Group members attend to deal with a psychological difficulty, and the therapist encourages them not to contact each other outside the group. The leader's purpose is to help group members achieve the personal or character change over time by exploring long-standing patterns of behavior. The therapist may facilitate regression within the group or may use a periodic instillation of anxiety and frustration to encourage movement (Lonergan, 1985; Spiegel & Spira, 1991). Shaffer and Galinsky (1989) noted that the analytic group therapist

- sets limits
- encourages group interaction by helping establish an open and accepting atmosphere
- offers support to a group member when he or she is in need of it but is not getting it from the group
- is alert to manifestations of resistance and transference in the various participants, as well as to countertransference reactions within himself or herself
- points out resistance and transference to group members when they are at a point of sufficient awareness to accept and integrate such an intervention
- interprets at an appropriate time some of the meanings of these various resistances and transferences, including, if possible, their relationship to crucial childhood events and patterns.

Although the first three responsibilities are similar to those of leaders in cancer support groups, several areas of difference exist—the psychological purpose, the leader's use of regression techniques, and interpretation of resistance or transference issues to group members.

## GROUP ORGANIZATION AND LEADERSHIP ISSUES

How well any group will do is influenced by environmental as well as participant and group conditions. In the open-systems model of support group organization, Schopler and Galinsky (1993) described the characteristics of group structure that lead to positive or negative outcomes. The environmental conditions include such resources as the sponsoring organization, funding, staff, and potential group members. Potential constraints, such as availability of transportation to meetings and conflicting demands on staff, also are part of the environmental conditions. Important participant characteristics include the number of group leaders, their knowledge and experience, and their skill and interventive approach. The number of group members, their descriptive and behavioral attributes, and the group's history and continuity also are important. Group conditions include members' and leaders' goals, the group structure, the roles and bonds of group members and leaders, the culture in the group, operating procedures, and meeting format. The group outcomes—positive or negative effects, group problems, or ethical and legal issues—are created in large part by these conditions.

## MANAGING GROUP MEETINGS

Yalom (1983) suggested that it is important for group leaders to provide structure and a consistent, coherent group procedure for patients. He outlined four points for group leaders:

1. During the first few minutes, launch the meeting, orient new members, and introduce them to each other.
2. Define and select the most profitable direction for the group to move in its work.
3. Guide the group as they address the issues and feelings expressed.
4. End the meeting—in the last few minutes, allow for review of the work accomplished and seek feedback from new members and those who did not participate.

An open-ended group can be launched in one of several ways.

- The group leader can describe the purpose of the group and invite each participant to join as part of a discussion of the patients' thoughts or feelings about their medical issues.
- The group leader can offer an opening question, group members answer, and conversation flows from that point.
- Group members ask questions and tell stories, and the group leader makes verbal interventions as indicated.

Each method enhances different circumstances. When patients have not yet met, it is important for them to learn each other's names and diagnoses and, early in the session, describe themselves by telling what brings them to the group and sharing something about their current lives. This encourages discussion of each patient's personal cancer story, treatment, and other medical issues. It provides the group leader with a perspective from which to decide which are the greatest patient needs. When all the group members know each other, the leader may begin less formally with a question such as "What's been important for you this week?" or "Has anyone brought issues to be discussed today?" Group members may seize the opening initiative with their own questions and personal stories. Picking out what can be described as the "point of urgency" is one of the leader's central tasks.

Group interaction may flow from introductions. Sometimes it is helpful for the leader to summarize the issues and feelings heard so far and ask the group what questions they have for each other. Sometimes group members are drawn to a person's dilemma with the greatest universal interest or to a situation in which they feel great commonality and compassion with the other. After a problem has been explored for a while, the leader can ask if others have had similar feelings. Spontaneity of responses is encouraged. As long as cancer-related issues or pertinent feelings remain central to the group's agenda, the group leader serves best by staying out of the way (Spiegel & Spira, 1991; Yalom, 1980).

All groups that continue meetings, even open-ended groups, will have stages of development. Beeber (1988) described a systems model of short-term, open-ended group therapy with four stages:

1. *Re-beginning.* Ongoing groups experience destabilization of external boundaries when group members or leaders change. Signs of destabilization can be late-arriving group members or seasoned group members acting like new arrivals. Group leaders can restabilize the group by identifying and clarifying the source of the disruption, reviewing who has left the group, restating the purpose, orienting new members, or acknowledging changes in therapists. The therapist's own lateness or failure to keep track of patient turnover may be examples of his or her own reaction to changes in the group.

2. *Subgrouping.* Patient–therapist subgroups include newly arrived patients who tend to direct their remarks to the therapist as if they were in consultation and the other group members were not there. Usually leadership from the senior group members helps a newly arrived member move on to concerns about boundaries among subgroups of patients. Subgroups of patients tend to define themselves by sitting together. Group members frequently use identification of similarities and differences or projection as major coping mechanisms in the group. Part of feeling better after participating in a group has to do with having talked with "people just like me" or with having realized that there are people who are less well off. Upward or downward comparisons are powerful therapeutic tools that each member brings to the group (Taylor, Falke, Shoptaw, & Lichtman, 1986).

3. *Work Phase.* Group members now concern themselves with boundaries within themselves as well as their link to the others. They are more introspective and more open to recognizing denied parts of the self. There is a surge of group cohesion. At this stage scapegoating of the most fragile member can take place as group members act out their fear of closeness. The leader should interpret the underlying anxieties to the group members because these identifications and projections mirror concerns of the members.

4. *Termination.* Group members begin to realize that group experience is finite, and those left behind as well as those leaving have feelings of sadness and loss. Ongoing groups are forever ending and forever beginning, and boundary issues are reconsidered as needed.

## GROUP PROBLEMS AND NEGATIVE EXPERIENCES

In a review of the literature, Galinsky and Schopler (1994) concluded that negative group experiences can result from any interaction, and it is difficult to learn about negative aspects of social relationships. When they asked 20 group leaders to report on the problems in their current groups, irregular attendance and membership at different stages of involvement were the two most frequently mentioned. "Finding open communication threatening" was first on the list of leaders' reports of negative effects among currently participating group members.

Group members have complained that sometimes they feel pressure to conform or feel stress related to group obligations. Sometimes group experiences leave them feeling overwhelmed and less adequate (Shumaker & Brownell, 1984). Lack of group direction and being bothered by disruptive or controlling members are additional complaints (Galinsky & Schopler, 1994). A person's anxiety and personal defenses can be stirred by group participation. Fears of seeming stupid, that one's problems are worse than others, or that one will not be liked are felt by many group members when they begin. "Is this group for me?" is a question often in patients' minds. The answer will be yes, if before the end of the first meeting they are able to find a sympathetic ear with the leader or another group member who understands their dilemmas or has a similar problem.

Group members also are vulnerable to the defensive behaviors provoked and expressed in groups. The difficult group member, the one who monopolizes or cannot quit talking, the moralizer, the competitive group member, the help-rejecting complainer, and the silent member are all behaving in their defensive modes, provoked by fears of dependency, emotional blocks, or the need to control (Yalom, 1985). In response, leaders can reframe the situation and address the underlying feelings of fear, anger, or sadness that the difficult group member may be unable to disclose directly. A helpful technique in reframing and redirection is to summarize what the difficult group member just said, then follow with a question to the patient or other group members. The leader's redirection will allow the other group members to continue their exploration of issues and feelings. The leader also may thank the monopolizer for sharing important experiences and then add, "Now, let's see how others in the group experienced that situation."

Occasionally, in a closed group, a group member will scapegoat another group member. When this happens, the attacking group member is usually projecting the most disliked aspect of himself or herself. As Shulman (1992) pointed out, this process is a form of communicating to the leader the group members' feelings about themselves. The group leader helps first by using identification with the member under attack and asks "How was it for you to hear that?" The leader then validates how it seemed to the scapegoated member: "It must have felt pretty strange, when you were anticipating a warmer welcome." Then turning to the speaker and the rest of the group, the leader can ask, "What are your feelings about what you've just heard?" The speaker may reply, for example, "Well, I realize I've missed her and seeing her reminds me how angry I feel when I don't know how people are doing. Sometimes its hard for me to attend meetings, and I resent it when others skip meetings." When the feelings have been identified and expressed, the group leader can reframe the attack as a worry or an unexamined turf issue that reflects a difference in priorities. The group leader defuses the tension by helping both sides express their feelings and by reframing the problem as a semantic misunderstanding or priority difference.

Getting directly to the negative feelings helps address the loss of inner control that difficult or defensive group members are frequently experiencing. Many members with problem behaviors are feeling vulnerable, needy, dependent, or angry. Finding a way to help them access their feelings may detoxify the negative coping their behavior embodies and open a deeper level of communication within the group. The leader can ask "How are you feeling now?" or interject "How did that feel to you?" when such questions are appropriate. As Spiegel (1995a) said, "You don't have to wait until the end of the story to intervene. If you are feeling uncomfortable, chances are other patients are too" (p. 253).

## TYPE AND MEETING SCHEDULE

Groups for patients with serious illness are begun during their treatment course and continue during the early months of recovery. Discussion over the years about what kind of group to plan—open-ended or closed group formats—has centered on educational, cognitive, and supportive group processes. Educational workshops may be the most acceptable for patients during the acute phase of treatment. Krupnick et al. (1993) suggested a three-tiered flow chart for group leaders planning support groups for cancer patients. Educational workshops could take place where treatment is provided, during the (treatment) workday, and last from six weeks to three months. Emotionally oriented groups could be offered in a closed-group format after treatment has been completed for members who are free of disease, at midday or in the evening, lasting for three to four months, or as an open-ended group lasting one year or more for patients receiving maintenance treatment for continued or recurrent illness. Emotionally focused groups could be held away from the hospital. Zampini and Ostroff (1993) described the need for educational supports for patients after treatment has ended. For all patients and interested family members, update workshops could be held periodically during the year, away from the hospital.

My experience supports and contrasts with the thoughtful review by Krupnick and colleagues (1993). Educational groups, such as our coping-skills classes, are successful in drawing patients who might not be attracted to a feelings-oriented group, and some of these patients will later join our open-ended groups. Our most popular groups in the hospital are an open-ended group for younger patients and a time-limited group for patients with breast cancer, both of which focus on personal issues and feelings. Roth and Covi (1984) noted that, in their experience, neither the open-format nor the time-limited group was preferable over the other, although absence of time constraints favored open-ended groups because they give both leaders and members greater flexibility. Lengths of participation in an open-ended group vary from a few weeks to many months, while group members reorganize their lives. Several patients treated for Hodgkin's disease have attended our young people's group at Stanford for one or two years as they worked out negative feelings and restabilized career plans. The issues of finding forgiveness, letting go of negative defenses, and moving toward active coping techniques are emotional shifts that are difficult for patients until they are physically and emotionally ready.

## Leadership Issues

Attentiveness, warmth, being respectful and humane, and a willingness to talk about oneself are characteristics of effective group leaders (Yalom, 1985). Effective group leaders establish a warm, accepting, understanding relationship with group members. Research has supported these characteristics as important to group members: Cella and colleagues (1993) asked 48 members of groups for patients with cancer to rate their group leaders on a postintervention assessment of 13 one-word descriptions of characteristics. The four top-rated characteristics were "care," "committed," "sensitive," and "understanding." Moos et al. (1993) found that the leader's willingness to openly discuss personal issues affects the group climate and the members' learning of helping skills. Group members can identify more easily with leaders who share some of their own thoughts and personal vulnerability.

A common dilemma for patients—seeing one's own situation as different from everyone else's—can be addressed in the first meeting of time-limited or closed groups with possible benefits for retention of group members. In many support groups for patients with cancer, there is a diversity of medical situations—from less serious illness to those that pose greater threat to life. Patients with minimal disease are frightened when they hear worst-case scenarios, and patients with greater medical problems worry that there will not be time for all their concerns to be heard. The group leader can address this naturally occurring discrepancy by saying "When you first begin a group, it is natural for you to see your personal differences from each other. This can be disappointing and may prompt you to consider dropping out of the group. We feel certain that over time you will see your similarities to each other and will feel more comfortable in participating."

Groups will advance and deepen as their leaders gain experience. A parallel process exists among leaders' wisdom and personal growth, the comments and group direction they provide, and the ability of the group to move in the same direction. Ringler, Whitman, Gustafson, and Coleman (1981) described the technical advances they made in leading a cancer support group. As Ringler and colleagues began to verbalize their feelings about the group to each other, they were able to express their feelings more honestly with the patients in the group. The countertransference issues (that is, overidentification or failure to understand a patient) of the leaders had interfered with their ability to help the patients face difficult ideas and feelings. "Under the guise of 'protecting the patients,' we were actually projecting our own terror of disfigurement, pain, loss of functioning, and death onto the group members and leaving them to face those issues alone" (p. 339).

## Patient Issues

### PARTICIPATING

The need for social support is a leading motivation for cancer patients to join groups. In three studies (Bauman, Gervey, & Siegel, 1992; Sutherland & Goldstein, 1992; Theil de Bocanegra, 1992), patients who felt that they had an inadequate social support network, such as a spouse or parent who did not understand their feelings, were more likely to join a support group. Other characteristics of group participants in the study by Bauman and colleagues were higher education; younger age; being unmarried, a joiner, or a help seeker wanting more information; or being more expressive of emotional feelings. In Theil de Bocanegra's study, time was a factor in patients wanting group support. Those diagnosed more recently (from zero to 14 weeks before) and those with less education were those most likely to want to join a group. Participants in Sutherland and Goldstein's study were physically healthier, more oriented to self-care, and less satisfied with their existing social support system. Patients chose not to participate because they felt alone in their feelings, could not relate to what others in the group were saying, felt that being with other people with cancer was too frightening or depressing, felt physically better off and wanted to put the cancer behind them, or were not "group people." According to Bauman and colleagues, a major motivation for attending a group was to compare individual emotional and physical progress with that of others, learn more about the illness, and share concerns with other patients.

The risk factors and timing of interventions was the focus of a recent analysis of a large study (948 women with breast cancer) reported by Bloom and Kessler (1994). Women older than 50 were found to be more depressed, as were divorced and widowed women. The overall burdens of treatment; health status; the number of changes in one's life as a result of having cancer; and poor self-esteem, social support, or family support were variables associated with negative mood and greater distress. Women who participated in the study during the early months after surgery (from zero to three months) were found to be more depressed than women who joined later (as measured by the Depression Scale and the Global Symptom Inventory), which suggests that early intervention can be important.

Gender differences have been considered a possible problem area in group participation. Harrison, Maguire, and Pitceathly (1995) examined patterns of confiding related to gender among patients with cancer and found that men were as likely as women to have confided their main concern to others. However, men were much more likely to have had only one confidant, and women confided in a wider circle of family, friends, and partners, overall. Although it is usually easier to interest women in attending a support group, men do attend when they feel a need for more information, when they feel misunderstood at home, or when they have experienced a loss of control (Fobair, 1989).

One participant, Robert, six years after his treatment ended, expressed his reason for joining our group at Stanford:

> Before I was diagnosed, I was a professional athlete. I was used to putting problems aside. I could not think about injuries when I was playing, or I would get injured, and instead I would picture myself doing what needed to be done, picture myself winning. That didn't work with having Hodgkin's disease, although I used it as my model for getting through treatment. But it was after treatment that problems began. I would find myself getting overwhelmingly anxious, feel tight in the chest. I remember working out in my gym at home and after 15 seconds with skipping rope, my chest tightened up, my muscles were tight from the radiation, and I didn't know how to deal with that. I was scared I was going to die. But I wasn't allowed to be scared. It got to where I found myself parked in my car on the Golden Gate Bridge thinking, well if death is going to get me, let's just get it over with. I can't live with this. I called Dr. Hancock, and he said, "Get down here." Sometime during treatment someone needs to lead you by the hand and take you to the group. I felt overwhelmed at the thought that I wasn't the same man I was when I walked in, that I couldn't solve things by just working out more. I couldn't accept being someone who was sick, who had the risk of dying. Since I have been to the group, I have cried. I feel better because I can accept better who I am now.

For a man like Robert, whose physical strength had been the symbol of well-being, it took feeling the emotional pain in his body before he could reach out to others for help.

## NEEDING TO HEAR ONE'S VOICE

Group leaders have noticed that there is a necessary repetition in patient story-telling over the weeks of group participation (Lonergan, 1985). It is beneficial for group members to hear their own voices (Pozatek, 1994). The psychic wound of experiencing the threat to life of cancer diagnosis and the need to grieve the loss of trust in one's body seem to be important in provoking this response. Many patients report a psychic numbing in their initial response to hearing their cancer diagnosis. Before patients can gain perspective on their grief, they need to talk together—as Freud said, "remembering, repeating, and working through" (cited in Spiegel et al., 1981, p. 35). When group members explore their experience, it helps them discover the meaning the situation has for them. As Pozatek (1994) observed, social workers can be useful to clients "by facilitating their naming of an experience" (p. 400). Sometimes patients spontaneously voice something previously unacknowledged. Providing an opportunity for new awareness is empowering for the client and transformative for both the group leader and the group member.

## EXAMINING OLD BELIEFS, FINDING MEANING IN THE NEW SITUATION

Serious illness threatens dreams, diminishes the illusion of autonomy and control over life, and causes the loss of the illusion that life is predictable. These are important themes for group discussion. The discrepancy between what one's view of life had been versus what life means now brings up many old beliefs, such as expecting life to be fair or believing that bad things do not happen to good people. The question "Why has this happened?" often means "How could this have happened to *me*?" There is a human need to find a positive purpose for a negative event. We attach meaning to what we perceive according to our worldview, our personal inner–outer perception. This influences our behavior and is influenced in turn by what we do. It is linked to our identity and is the basis for our sense of continuity between past and present. Meaning in our personal lives is predicated on our specific cognitive response to particular events, and it influences the coping strategies we use to deal with the stress we encounter (Fife, 1994).

Concentrating on meaning has a practical outcome for patients seeking the return of a sense of inner control. Using the Constructed Meaning Scale, Fife (1995) measured meaning in the lives of 422 patients with various types of cancer. The specific meaning that people gave to their situation was based on the amount of social support in their lives and their coping strategies, and that meaning was predictive of their personal sense of control, body image, and psychological adjustment. The greater the social support from friends, health care professionals, and family members, the more positive the meaning of the illness in their lives. Emotional defenses, such as denial, avoidance, and positive focusing, also were predicted by the nature of the meaning people developed about their illness. These results are consistent with the work of Bloom (1982), Spiegel and colleagues (1981, 1993, 1995b), Cella and Yellen (1993), and Yalom (1980), who found that participation in support groups brought about a positive perspective on the illness. Fife (1995) concluded that the meaning patients make in their lives after a cancer diagnosis might be viewed as a clinical marker of psychosocial vulnerability. The task for group leaders is to encourage patients to reconsider their old beliefs that are no longer helpful in their current situation and to discover the present meaning that cancer has in their lives.

### *DISCOVERING A NEW PERSPECTIVE IN DEALING WITH CONFLICT*

Group members bring their current and former conflicts with them into the room. Having a cancer diagnosis, recognizing that your life is threatened when you thought you were healthy, is *the* most powerful level of conflict. However, other issues, such as having conflicts in values at home or at work, being worried about financial and other resources, or having turf disputes with coworkers or family members, remain important. When patients express confusion over which issue to deal with (confusion in their priorities), I share with them a perspective adapted from the work of Wax (1991) and invite them to reorder their current problems. With the conflict chart shown in Figure 13-3 as a visual cue, patients can reconsider their concerns and begin focusing on the most pressing issue—that is, "What's the most important issue here?" We discuss how it can be helpful to escalate their communication with family or colleagues and use assertiveness techniques when they are not getting the necessary attention. When they want to defuse tension and feel more comfortable, they can be coached to locate the overlapping priorities they share with the other partner in tension and use reconciling communication techniques, such as negotiation, bargaining, and compromise. Although this concept in conflict management was originally designed for use with interdepartmental tensions in large work groups, it also is very useful when adapted for use with cancer patients (Fobair & Wax, 1995).

## Benefits of Groups

Group work with cancer patients helps both patients and group leaders (Yalom, 1985) and can provide an economic benefit for the hospital (Friedman, Sobel, Myers, Caudill, & Benson, 1995). Some of the curative factors (Yalom, 1985) have been mentioned here, such as the value that comes from belonging (group cohesiveness) and learning that you are not alone (universality), but patients also benefit from helping others (altruism), group member guidance, catharsis, identification

FIGURE **13-3**

**Levels of Conflict**

1. **Survival:** Hearing the diagnosis leads to a sense that one's life is threatened, to shock and feelings of isolation and fear (physical, professional, and financial). These feelings can lead to a high level of anxiety, aggression, and irrationality.
2. **Values:** Basic beliefs for which people will fight (such as respect, doctor–patient relationship, health, survival, conservation of body, sexuality, body image, quality of life).
3. **Resources:** Money, facilities, medical choices.
4. **Turf:** Whose job is it? (family roles, physician's role, patient's role).
5. **Priorities:** What is most important? Life, body conservation, sexual feelings, family life, or work and career?
6. **Communication:** Escalate or de-escalate by use of assertiveness, negotiation, bargaining, or reconciliation of viewpoints.
7. **Semantics:** "Let me say that a different way." Changing words that are offensive—for example, from anger to disappointment.

SOURCE: Adapted from the work of John Wax, LCSW, 1994. Used with permission.

with someone in the group who is better adjusted, self-understanding, finding inspiration and hope in seeing others get better, and existential factors such as recognizing that life is at times unfair and unjust and, ultimately, there is no escape from some of life's pain and death.

Results of a literature review suggest that group treatment was more effective than individual treatment in 25 percent of the studies. Toseland and Siporin (1986) located 74 studies comparing individual and group treatments. In 32 studies subjects were randomly assigned to individual or group treatments and independent and dependent variables were measured by one or more standardized instruments. Their results showed that group treatment was as effective as individual treatment in 75 percent of the studies and significantly more effective in the remaining 25 percent of the studies.

Cost-effectiveness can result from group interventions. Although the primary purpose of psychosocial interventions is to improve health outcomes, some studies have shown that patients had fewer clinic visits when they participated in behavioral medicine groups (Friedman et al., 1995). In a study of chronic pain, the patients who received the behavioral medicine intervention enjoyed the benefits of decreases in negative psychological symptoms such as anxiety, depression, and hostility, and their clinic use decreased by 36 percent, a decrease that is cost-effective for the medical setting (Caudill, Schnable, Zuttermeister, Benson, & Friedman, 1991). In teaching self-management skills to patients with arthritis, Lorig, Mazonson, and Holman (1993) noted that participants at four-year follow-up enjoyed a greater sense of self-efficacy, a 20 percent reduction in pain, and a 43 percent reduction in visits to physicians. There is a growing literature describing the efficacy of stress management in the treatment of cancer, including the work of Fawzy et al. (1993) and Spiegel and colleagues (1989). Although further systemic work needs to be done in this area, one sees examples in clinical practice that suggest groups can be cost-effective interventions.

The social support that flows from the group experience decreases isolation and provides information and opportunities for support in treatment decision making (Friedman et al., 1995). This support also reduces psychological distress (Spiegel, 1993), improves efficacy in stress management (Fawzy et al., 1993), provides impetus and validation for improving healthy habits and supporting behavior change (Ornish et al., 1990), reduces panic disorders that commonly accompany chest pain (Yingling, Wulsin, Arnold, & Rouan, 1993), and helps reduce pain when relaxation, self-hypnosis, and meditation techniques are taught along with the group interaction (Caudill et al., 1991).

For professionals who lead groups, group work is a pleasant, if challenging, innovation to introduce in the hospital setting. Viewed as an efficient use of the professional's time (Lonergan, 1985), it also can be the highlight of the week. The group leader's reward comes when patients rethink hardened positions, and those with negative thoughts and feelings find active coping choices—when he or she sees lives changing and improving over time. Ron, for example, expressed suicidal thoughts when he first came to the hospital for radiation treatment. A year after he had spent six weeks in the group, he commented, "It helped out at a bad time. It was broadening. I saw people and looked at reality. I am an orderly person. The illness caused me to look at the flaws in my life. This was upsetting. It was very helpful for me to see that I wasn't the worst off nor did I have the most unique situation."

Ron's cognitive shift from negative thoughts to more life-affirming, active coping choices continues today. The emotional shift he made came after he had interacted with other patients, some of whom had worse situations than his own.

Finally, a group leader benefits personally from knowing that he or she had a significant place in the group members' lives. For example, Paul, a Jungian psychiatrist, joined our group at Mount Zion Hospital in San Francisco after receiving a diagnosis of Hodgkin's disease. A husband and father of three young children, he had been driving his psychiatrist wife Sally "crazy" (her word) when he asked to attend our group. He needed more time to talk, to process his treatment experience. As a group we wrote poetry twice a month. Paul wrote

> Control, Control, know what it's all about,
> Where it came from, where it goes,
> What will happen, when will it happen,
> How will it turn out.
> Bull shit, there is no certainty
> All the above is a waste of time
> An energy drain,
> A mind fuck, a circle of nothingness.
> This is it here and now,
> The future doesn't add meaning
> To the present, just gives it more significance.
> Just flow with it
> Make choices even though you don't know the point
> Like all searches,
> You come back to where you are.

We kept in touch over the years. When Paul came for follow-up appointments, he and Sally shared their family news. When Paul wrote stories about paddling his kayak in the San Francisco Bay, we republished them in the *"Surviving!"* newsletter. Although his original disease went into remission, Paul had difficulty breathing and had coronary problems as a result of radiation. On what would be his last follow-up visit, I walked him out to the parking lot and gave him a warm hug. After that, he called me to say that things were getting worse. In late June 1996, I returned from vacation to find this message on my voice mail: "Hi Patricia, Paul. Just wanted to say hello and goodbye. I'm going downhill awfully fast since I last saw you. Call soon, you can still get me, perhaps. I appreciate all the years we've known each other. Thanks, you were great. I think I'm handling it okay. I can't go on much longer. Bye-Bye, Pat."

I saved that message for weeks before writing it down. Sally and I had lunch a few weeks later. She told me that as Paul was dying, his family around him, he asked his daughter to find my telephone number. Just as, years before, his comprehension of the existential issues had instructed me, Paul taught me in the 1990s by example, dying with a clear mind and open heart. As group leaders, we can enjoy the opportunity to be transformed by special moments in our groups and experience for ourselves how we are all connected.

# References

Adams, J. (1979). Mutual-help groups: Enhancing the coping ability of oncology clients. *Cancer Nursing, 2*, 95–98.

Ascheim, B., Horman, E., Queisser, T. D., & Silverman, P. (1978). *Development of special mental health technical assistance materials for self-help groups in particular populations* (Contract No. 278-77-0038-SM). Rockville, MD: National Institute of Mental Health.

Bauman, L. J., Gervey, R., & Siegel, K. (1992). Factors associated with cancer patients' participation in support groups. *Journal of Psychosocial Oncology, 10*(3), 1–20.

Beeber, A. R. (1988). A systems model of short-term, open-ended group therapy. *Hospital and Community Psychiatry, 39*, 537–542.

Bernard, M. (1979). *Some thoughts on groups and their organization.* (Available from the American Cancer Society, California Division, 1710 Webster, Oakland, CA 94617.)

Bloom, J. R. (1982). Social support, accommodation to stress, and adaptation to breast cancer. *Social Science and Medicine, 16*, 1329–1338.

Bloom, J. R., & Kessler, L. (1994). Risk and timing of counseling and support interventions for younger women with breast cancer. *Journal of the National Cancer Institute Monographs, 16*, 199–206.

Bruno, F. J. (1964a). The conscience of America. In F. J. Bruno (Ed.), *Trends in social work, 1874–1956* (pp. 112–119). New York: Columbia University Press.

Bruno, F. J. (1964b). Social group work. In F. J. Bruno (Ed.), *Trends in social work, 1874–1956* (pp. 270–277). New York: Columbia University Press.

Cannon, I. M. (1923). *Social work in hospitals: A contribution to progressive medicine.* New York: Russell Sage Foundation.

Caudill, M., Schnable, R., Zuttermeister, P., Benson, H., & Friedman, R. (1991). Decreased clinic use by chronic pain patients: Response to behavioral medicine interventions. *Clinical Journal of Pain, 7*, 305–310.

Cella, D. F., Sarafian, B., Snider, P. R., Yellen, S. B., & Winicour, P. (1993). Evaluation of a community-based cancer support group. *Psycho-Oncology, 2*, 123–132.

Cella, D. F., & Yellen, S. B. (1993). Cancer support groups: The state of the art. *Cancer Practice, 1*, 56–61.

Chang, J., & Phillips, M. (1993). Michael White and Steve deShafer: New directions in family therapy. In S. Gilligan & R. Price (Eds.), *Therapeutic conversations* (pp. 95–112). New York: W. W. Norton.

Christ, G. (1991). Principles of oncology social work. In A. Hollub, D. Fink, & G. Murphy (Eds.), *Textbook of clinical oncology* (pp. 594–605). Atlanta: American Cancer Society.

Classen, C., Diamond, S., Soleman, A., Fobair, P., Spira, J., & Spiegel, D. (1993). *Brief supportive–expressive group therapy for women with primary breast cancer: A treatment manual.* Stanford, CA: Stanford University, Breast Cancer Intervention Project.

Cole, S. A., O'Connor, S., & Bennett, L. (1979). Self-help groups for clinic patients with chronic illness, *Primary Care, 6*, 325–340.

Cordoba, C., Shear, M. B., Fobair, P., & Hall, J. (1984). *Cancer support groups practice handbook.* Oakland, CA: American Cancer Society.

Crumbaugh, J. C. (1973). *Purpose in Life Test, 1966: Everything to gain.* Chicago: Nelson-Hall.

Emonds, K. (1995). Environmental medicine: The hardware and software of psychoneuroimmunology. In R. Buczynski (Ed.), *The psychology of health, immunity and disease* (pp. 57–63). Mansfield, CT: National Institute of Clinical Application of Behavioral Medicine.

Evans, R. L., & Connis, R. T. (1995). Comparison of brief group therapies for depressed cancer patients receiving radiation treatment. *Public Health Reports, 110,* 306–311.

Fawzy, F. I., Cousins, N., Fawzy, N. W., Kennedy, M. E., Elashoff, R., & Morton, D. (1990). A structured psychiatric intervention for cancer patients: 1. Changes over time in methods of coping and affective disturbance. *Archives of General Psychiatry, 47,* 720–725.

Fawzy, F. I., Fawzy, N. W., Arndt, L. A., & Pasnau, R. O. (1995). Critical review of psychosocial interventions in cancer care. *Archives of General Psychiatry, 52,* 100–113.

Fawzy, F. I., Fawzy, N. W., Hyun, C. S., Elashoff, R., Guthrie, D., Fahey, J. L., & Morton, D. (1993). Malignant melanoma: Effects of an early structured psychiatric intervention coping, and affective state on recurrence and survival 6 years later. *Archives of General Psychiatry, 50,* 681–689.

Fife, B. L. (1994). The conceptualization of meaning in illness. *Social Science and Medicine, 38,* 309–316.

Fife, B. L. (1995). The measurement of meaning in illness. *Social Science and Medicine, 40,* 1021–1028.

Fobair, P. (1989, October). *Twelve clinical indicators of the level of distress among cancer patient survivors.* Paper presented at the 35th annual meeting of the National Association of Social Workers, Health and Mental Health Section, San Francisco.

Fobair, P., Cordoba, C., Pluth, C., & Bloom, J. (1982). Considerations for successful groups. In J. Cullen (Ed.), *Cancer rehabilitation: Proceedings of the Western States Conference on Cancer Rehabilitation* (pp. 105–128). Palo Alto, CA: Bull.

Fobair, P., & Wax, J. (1994). *Cognitive issues: Adapted teaching tool for use with cancer patients.* Stanford: University of California.

Fobair, P., & Wax, J. (1995, November). *Cognitive issues. Honing your group leadership skills.* Paper presented at Building Bridges to Hope, Leukemia Society of America, San Diego.

Fobair, P., Wolfson, A., Mages, N., Hall, J., Harrison, I., & Vose, J. (1981). Group work with cancer patients in radiation therapy. In P. Tretter, L. M. Leigner, A. H. Kutscher, R. J. Torpie, R. Bellis, & M. Tallmer (Eds.), *Psychosocial aspects of radiation therapy* (pp. 99–113). New York: Arno Press.

Friedlander, W. A. (1968). *Introduction to social welfare* (3rd ed.). Englewood Cliffs, NJ: Prentice Hall.

Friedman, R., Sobel, D., Myers, P., Caudill, M., & Benson, H. (1995). Behavioral medicine, clinical health, psychology, and cost offset. *Health Psychology, 14,* 509–518.

Galinsky, M. J., & Schopler, J. H. (1989). The social work group. In J.B.P. Shaffer & M. J. Galinsky (Eds.), *Models of group therapy* (pp. 18–40). Englewood Cliffs, NJ: Prentice Hall.

Galinsky, M. J., & Schopler, J. H. (1994). Negative experiences in support groups. *Social Work in Health Care, 20,* 77–95.

Gowdy, E. A. (1994). From technical rationality to participating consciousness. *Social Work, 39,* 362–370.

Harrison, J., Maguire, P., & Pitceathly, C. (1995). Confiding in crisis: Gender differences in pattern of confiding among cancer patients. *Social Science and Medicine, 4,* 1255–1260.

Jacobs, C., Ross, R. D., Walker, I. M., & Stockdale, F. E. (1983). Behavior of cancer patients: A randomized study of the effects of education and peer support groups. *American Journal of Clinical Oncology 6,* 347–350.

Johnson, J. (1982). The effects of a patient education course on persons with a chronic illness. *Cancer Nursing, 5,* 117–123.

Johnson, J., & Flaherty, M. (1980). The nurse and cancer patient education. *Seminars in Oncology, 7,* 63–70.

Katz, A. H., & Binder, E. I. (Eds.). (1976). *The strength in us: Self-help groups in the modern world.* New York: New Viewpoints.

Kelly, J. A., Murphy, D. A., Bahr, R., Kalicman, S. C., Morgan, B. A., Stevenson, Y., Koab, J. J., Brasfield, T. L., & Bernstein, B. M. (1993). Outcome of cognitive–behavioral and support group brief therapies for depressed, HIV-infected persons. *American Journal of Psychiatry 150,* 1679–1682.

Krumm, S., Vanetta, P., & Sanders, J. (1979). Group approaches for cancer patients: A group for teaching chemotherapy. *American Journal of Nursing, 79,* 916.

Krupnick, J. L., Rowland, J. H., Goldberg, R. L., & Daniel, U. V. (1993). Professionally-led support groups for cancer patients: An intervention in search of a model. *International Journal of Psychiatry in Medicine 23,* 275–294.

Lonergan, E. C. (1985). Mobilizing group members' coping devices. In E. C. Lonergan, (Ed.), *Group intervention: How to begin and maintain groups in medical and psychiatric settings* (pp. 145–170). New York: Aronson.

Lorig, K., Mazonson, P. D., & Holman, H. R. (1993). Evidence suggesting that health education for self-management in patients with chronic arthritis has sustained health benefits while reducing health care costs. *Arthritis and Rheumatism, 36,* 439–446.

Matano, R. A., & Yalom, I. D. (1991). Approaches to chemical dependence: Chemical dependency and interactive group therapy. A synthesis. *International Journal of Group Psychotherapy 41,* 269–293.

May, R., Angel, E., & Ellenberger, H. F. (Eds.). (1958). *Existence: A new dimension in psychiatry and psychology.* New York: Basic Books.

McNair, P. M., Lorr, M., & Drappelman, L. (1971). *POMS manual.* San Diego: Education and Industrial Testing Services.

Miller, J. (1993). *The passion of Michael Foucault.* New York: Simon & Schuster.

Moos, R. H. (1981). *Group Environment Scale manual.* Palo Alto: Consulting Psychologists Press.

Moos, R. H. (1986). *Group Environment Scale manual* (2nd ed.). Palo Alto: Consulting Psychologists Press.

Moos, R. H., Finney, J., & Maude-Griffin, P. (1993). The social climate of self-help and mutual support groups: Assessing group implementation, process, and outcome. In B. S. McCrady & W. R. Miller (Eds.), *Research on Alcoholics Anonymous: Opportunities and alternatives* (pp. 251–274). New Brunswick, NJ: Rutgers Center of Alcohol Studies.

O'Hanlon, W. H. (1993). Possibility therapy: From iatrogenic injury to iatrogenic healing. In S. Gilligan & R. Price (Eds.), *Therapeutic conversations* (pp. 3–17). New York: W. W. Norton.

Ornish, D., Brown, S. E., Scherwitz, L. W., Billings, J. H., Armstrong, W. T., Ports, T. A., McLanahan, S. M., Kirkeeide, R. L., Brand, R. J., & Gould, K. L. (1990). Can lifestyle changes reverse coronary heart disease? The Lifestyle Heart Trial. *Lancet, 1,* 129–132.

Pardeck, J. T., Murphy, J. W., & Choi, J. M. (1994). Some implications of postmodernism for social work practice. *Social Work, 39,* 343–346.

Perlman, H. (1957). *Social casework: A problem solving process.* Chicago: University of Chicago Press.

Pozatek, E. (1994). The problem of certainty: Clinical social work in the postmodern era. *Social Work, 39,* 396–404.

Pratt, J. H. (1922). Principles of class treatment and their application to various chronic diseases. *Hospital Social Service, 6,* 401.

Reynolds, B. C. (1939). Social case work: What is it? What is its place in the world today? In F. Lowry (Ed.), *Readings in social case work, 1920–1938* (pp. 136–147). New York: Columbia University Press.

Ringler, K. E., Whitman, H. H., Gustafson, J. P., & Coleman, F. W. (1981). Technical advances in leading a cancer patient group. *International Journal of Group Psychotherapy, 31,* 329–344.

Roth, D., & Covi, L. (1984). Cognitive group psychotherapy of depression: The open-ended group. *International Journal of Group Psychotherapy, 34,* 67–75.

Saleebey, D. (1994). Culture, theory, and narrative: The intersection of meanings in practice. *Social Work, 39,* 351–361.

Schopler, J. H., & Galinsky, M. J. (1993). Support groups as open systems: A model for practice and research. *Health & Social Work, 18,* 195–207.

Shaffer, J.B.P., & Galinsky, M. J. (1989). *Models of group therapy.* Englewood Cliffs, NJ: Prentice Hall.

Shulman, L. (1992). *The skills of helping: Individuals, families and groups* (3rd ed.). Itasca, IL: F. E. Peacock.

Shumaker, S. A., & Brownell, A. (1984). Toward a theory of social support: Closing conceptual gaps. *Journal of Social Issues, 40*(4), 11–36.

Spiegel, D. (1981). Vietnam grief work using hypnosis. *American Journal of Clinical Hypnosis, 24,* 33–40.

Spiegel, D. (1993). Psychosocial intervention in cancer. *Journal of the National Cancer Institute, 85,* 1198–1205.

Spiegel, D. (1995a). Essentials of psychotherapeutic intervention for cancer patients. *Supportive Care in Cancer, 3,* 252–256.

Spiegel, D. (1995b). How do you feel about cancer now? Survival and psychosocial support. *Public Health Reports, 110,* 298–300.

Spiegel, D., Bloom, J. R., Kraemer, H. C., & Gottheil, E. (1989). Effect of psychosocial treatment on survival of patients with metastatic breast cancer. *Lancet, 2,* 888–891.

Spiegel, D., Bloom, J. R., & Yalom, I. (1981). Group support for patients with metastatic cancer. A randomized prospective outcome study. *Archives of General Psychiatry, 38,* 527–533.

Spiegel, D., Morrow, G. R., Classen, C., Riggs, G., Stott, P. B., Mudaliar, N., Pierce, H. I., Flynn, P. J., & Heard, L. (1996). Effects of group therapy on women with primary breast cancer. *Breast Journal, 2,* 104–106.

Spiegel, D., & Spira, J. (1991). *Supportive–expressive group therapy: A treatment manual of psychosocial intervention for women with recurrent breast cancer.* Stanford, CA: Stanford University School of Medicine, Psychosocial Treatment Laboratory.

Spielberger, C. D., Gorsuch, R. L., & Lushene, R. (1968). *The State-Trait Anxiety Inventory (STAI).* Palo Alto, CA: Consulting Psychologists Press.

Sutherland, C. E., & Goldstein, M. S. (1992). Joining a healing community for cancer: Who and why? *Social Science and Medicine, 35,* 323–333.

Taylor, S. E., Falke, R. L., Shoptaw, S. J., & Lichtman, R. R. (1986). Social support groups and the cancer patient. *Journal of Consulting and Clinical Psychology, 54,* 608–615.

Telch, C. F., & Telch, M. J. (1986). Group coping skills instruction and supportive group therapy for cancer patients: A comparison of strategies. *Journal of Consulting and Clinical Psychology, 54,* 802–808.

Theil de Bocanegra, H. (1992). Cancer patients' interest in group support programs. *Cancer Nursing, 15,* 347–352.

Toro, P. A., Rappaport, J., & Seidman, E. (1987). Social climate comparison of mutual help and psychotherapy groups. *Journal of Consulting and Clinical Psychology, 55,* 430–431.

Toseland, R. W., & Siporin, M. (1986). When to recommend group treatment: A review of the clinical and the research literature. *International Journal of Group Psychotherapy, 36,* 171–201.

Watts, R., Jr. (1998). Cherish the goose bumps. In *People are never the problem* (pp. 1–30). Tulsa: Honor Books.

Wax, J. (1991). *Conflict management.* Unpublished manuscript.

Weisman, A. D., Worden, J. W., & Sobel, H. J. (1980). *Psychosocial screening and intervention with cancer patients* (the Omega Project, Grant No. CA-19797). Boston: Harvard Medical School, Massachusetts General Hospital.

White, M. (1993). Deconstruction and therapy. In S. Gilligan & R. Price (Eds.), *Therapeutic conversations* (pp. 18–30). New York: W. W. Norton.

White, M., & Epston, D. (1990). *Narrative means to therapeutic ends.* New York: W. W. Norton.

Wood, P. E., Milligan, M., Christ, D., & Liff, D. (1978). Group counseling for cancer patients in a community hospital [Abstract]. *Psychosomatics, 19,* 555–561.

Worden, J. W., & Weisman, A. D. (1984). Preventive psychosocial intervention with newly diagnosed cancer patients. *General Hospital Psychiatry, 6,* 243–249.

Yalom, I. D. (1980). *Existential psychotherapy.* New York: Basic Books.

Yalom, I. D. (1983). *Inpatient group psychotherapy.* New York: Basic Books.

Yalom, I. D. (1985). *The theory and practice of group psychotherapy.* New York: Basic Books.

Yingling, K. W., Wulsin, L. R., Arnold, L. M., & Rouan, G. W. (1993). Estimated prevalences of panic disorder and depression among consecutive patients seen in an emergency department with acute chest pain. *Journal of General Internal Medicine, 8,* 231–235.

Zampini, K., & Ostroff, J. S. (1993). The post-treatment resource program: Portrait of a program for cancer survivors. *Psycho-Oncology, 2,* 1–9.

# Mental Health Services for Children and Adolescents

Mary Carmel Ruffolo

Millions of children and adolescents suffer from serious emotional and behavioral problems. According to Cohen, Provet, and Jones (1996), during any given year, approximately 16 percent to 20 percent of children and adolescents have diagnosable emotional or behavior problems that cause at least temporary interference with function in family, school, or community settings. For children under age 18 with a mental disorder, prevalence rates, calculated by use of only clinical diagnosis measures, range from 17 percent to 22 percent (11 million to 14 million children) (National Institute of Mental Health [NIMH], 1990).

In defining serious emotional disturbance (SED) in children and adolescents, the Center for Mental Health Services (CMHS; Washington, DC), included guidelines that require a diagnosable mental, behavioral, or emotional disorder of sufficient duration to meet diagnostic criteria specified in the *Diagnostic and Statistical Manual of Mental Disorders,* 3rd edition, revised (DSM-III-R) (American Psychiatric Association, 1987). Children also must display functional impairment that substantially interferes with or limits their role or functioning in family, school, or community activities. Functional impairment is defined by CMHS as difficulties that substantially interfere with or limit a child or adolescent from achieving or maintaining one or more developmentally appropriate social, behavioral, cognitive, communicative, or adaptive skills (Brazelton Center for Mental Health Law, 1993).

Recent prevalence studies, such as the Methodological Epidemiological Catchment Area (MECA) study and the Great Smoky Mountains Study of Youth, assessed the presence of SED in children and adolescents by use of both clinical diagnostic measurements and functional impairment measurements. The studies found assessing functional impairment to be the most challenging aspect in estimating the prevalence of SED (Costello, Angold, Burns, Erkanli, et al., 1996; Costello, Angold, Burns, Stangl, et al., 1996; Lahey et al., 1996). The prevalence rates of SED in children and adolescents in these two studies varied considerably, depending on the measurements used to determine functional impairment. In a review of these studies and others (Bird et al., 1988; Jensen et al., 1995; Kashani, Ezpeleta, Dandoy, Doi, & Reid, 1991; Kessler et al., 1994) that included clinical diagnosis and functional impairment measures, Friedman, Kutash, and Duchnowski (1996) estimated that the prevalence of SED in children and adolescents is likely to be between 9 percent and 19 percent. A majority of the children and adolescents identified as having SED are not receiving professional help for their mental health needs. In the Great Smoky Mountains Study, when children and adolescents did receive mental health care, it was likely to be from a provider outside the specialty mental health sector (Burns et al., 1995). It has been estimated that between 70 percent and 80 percent of children with SED do not receive any mental health services (Costello, Burns, Angold, & Leaf, 1993; Tuma, 1989). When these children and adolescents receive mental health services, their families often encounter a disorganized, fragmented system of care.

Because of the serious discrepancy between the number of children and adolescents in need of mental health services and the number who actually receive services, many changes have been sought in the mental health services delivery system, especially for those with SED. This chapter reviews the history of mental health services for children and adolescents, presents the current philosophy and research base for mental health services for this population, examines major studies of the delivery of mental health services, explores the practical and clinical importance of the research findings, and discusses future challenges for research and social work practice in delivering mental health services to this population.

The "breakthroughs" in mental health research on children and adolescents with SED that are reviewed in this chapter are less definitive than those described elsewhere in this book. The major advances in this research have been the identification of child and adolescent mental health as a unique mental health problem, the prioritization of mental health research on children and adolescents, and greater emphasis on integrating clinical efficacy studies and service effectiveness studies.

## History of Mental Health Services for Children and Adolescents

There have been important changes in the delivery of mental health services for children and adolescents since the early 1980s. Before then, federal involvement in the provision of mental health services for children and adolescents was limited. According to Namir and Weinstein (1982), the role of the federal government before 1980 could be characterized as defining the needs of children and adolescents for services and delivery modalities, which are different from those of adults, and developing fragmented, noncomprehensive mental health services for specialized groups of children and adolescents. The major legislation that helped states fund mental health services for children and adolescents before the 1980s was the Community Mental Health Centers Act, Part F program (1972), which assisted local mental health programs in developing alternative mental health services for children and adolescents and in funding for staff (Myers, 1985).

In 1982, Knitzer published a landmark study, *Unclaimed Children: The Failure of Public Responsibility to Children and Adolescents in Need of Mental Health Services,* that focused on the inadequacies of the state-level systems across the United States in meeting the needs of children with SED. She reported that many state departments of mental health did not have even one full-time child mental health staff person. Knitzer and the Children's Defense Fund sought action from public agencies to "reclaim" responsibility for children with SED and for their families. This study served as a catalyst to focus national attention on the gaps in mental health services for youths. In 1984, the NIMH created the Child and Adolescent Service System Program (CASSP), the only program at the federal level concerned with providing mental health services to children with SED and their families. The CASSP initiative focused on expanding the capacity of the states to serve the children and adolescents with the gravest cases of SED and called for collaboration by multiple child-serving agencies to develop community-based systems of care. These agencies included such multiple services systems as mental health, child welfare, juvenile justice, developmental disability, and education agencies. The initial CASSP funds were used for system development activities at the state and community levels and not for direct services to children and adolescents. The program provided grants to states to improve services delivery to children and their families. During system development the target population was children and adolescents with SED. NIMH (1983) defined this target population as children ages 17 years or younger, who require not only mental health services but also services of at least one other human services agency (for example juvenile justice, child welfare, or special education) and who have a diagnosable mental health problem that has a disabling influence on functioning. In addition, problematic behaviors should be of at least one year's duration. Lourie, Katz-Leavy, and Jacobs (1986) reported that the initial CASSP goals were to

- improve the availability of continuums of care for children and adolescents with SED, thus improving availability and access to appropriate services across systems
- develop leadership and increase allocations of resources for child and adolescent mental health services
- establish coordination mechanisms among agencies and increase collaboration and efficiency of services delivery
- develop ways to include family input in planning and developing services systems, treatment options, and individual services planning
- develop the capacity for and provide technical assistance to child and adolescent services system development
- evaluate the principles and practices of CASSP.

A national technical assistance center was established at Georgetown University in Washington, DC, to support the CASSP development activities. Two research and training centers were funded by NIMH and the National Institute of Disability and Rehabilitation Research: the University of South Florida Mental Health Institute and the Regional Research Institute of Portland State University (Kutash, Duchnowski, & Sondheimer, 1994). These centers were established to develop a new model for providing mental health services with an emphasis on multiagency, community-based systems of care. The CASSP initiative was instrumental in the passage of the 1986 State Comprehensive Mental Health Services Plan Act, which requires that state departments of mental health include children and adolescent mental health services in their planning process.

Mental health reforms during the mid-1980s focused on expanding core services intended to keep children and adolescents in their own homes and communities. These included crisis intervention services, respite care for parents, day treatment programs, intensive case management services, and therapeutic foster care. In addition, cross-system collaboration in case planning and intervention was promoted.

A shift in the way mental health professionals viewed families began to emerge from this new CASSP initiative. The role assigned by mental health professionals to families in the treatment of children and adolescents with SED began to change from one of blame and cause to one of partnership and strength. This fostered the development of a national parent-run organization, the Federation of Families for

Children's Mental Health, in 1987. This organization provided strong advocacy for children's mental health and sought increased availability of appropriate services for children and adolescents with SED.

In 1989 the Institute of Medicine identified several gaps in the knowledge base that concerned the prevalence of mental disorders among children and adolescents, the services needs of this population, and their use of mental health services. This work sparked the development of the *National Plan for Research on Child and Adolescent Mental Disorders* (NIMH, 1990). This plan provided a coherent national strategy to address critical gaps in the knowledge base on mental disorders in children and adolescents and mental health services needs and use (Hoagwood & Hohmann, 1993). The plan was further operationalized into program announcements for Child and Adolescent Mental Health Service System research demonstration grants and research on child and adolescent mental disorders (NIMH, 1991a, 1991b). In addition, NIMH funded two Centers for Research on Mental Health Services for Children and Adolescents at Johns Hopkins University, Baltimore, and Children's Hospital, San Diego.

In 1992 the Comprehensive Community Mental Health Services Program for Children and Adolescents with Severe Emotional Disturbances was signed into law, bringing children's mental health services into a new era. This law, Section 119 of the Alcohol, Drug Abuse, and Mental Health Administration (ADAMHA) Reorganization Act (1992), P.L. 102-321, provided funding for the provision of services and their integration (Rog, 1995). The CASSP initiatives were moved to the newly created CMHS, and NIMH assumed the lead role in developing the services research component of the national plan. In 1994, $35 million was distributed under this program for systems of care in 38 localities (Rog, 1995). States also were required to restructure their services into an integrated, community-based system of care.

Currently the most important challenge facing mental health services for children and adolescents is the potential impact of health care reform and managed care. Maintenance of the "system of care" model as part of any reformed health care system for children and adolescents with SED is receiving considerable emphasis. Even after the changes initiated in the 1980s and early 1990s, there continues to be an enormous gap between the need for care and services system capability. Expenditures for child and adolescent mental health services still favor residential and hospital inpatient care. Burns (1991) estimated the cost of mental health care for adolescents (ages 10 to 18) in 1986 to be $3.5 billion, with more than 46 percent of that total spent for hospital inpatient care. The increase in the number of private psychiatric hospitals in the 1980s accounts for much of the increased inpatient care expenditures. Hoagwood and Rupp (1994) reported that 41 percent of the care provided in private psychiatric hospitals is to youths. This growth needs to be addressed as intermediate-level community-based interventions continue to evolve.

On November 8, 1993, a consortium of 16 national human services and advocacy organizations testified before the Labor and Human Resources Committee of the U.S. Senate that

> There currently is widespread consensus that community-based systems of care represent the state-of-the-art in treating children with serious emotional disorders, and the development of such systems has become a national goal. . . . it is especially important now . . . to ensure that the reformed health care system represents true reform—reform that encourages the provision of the most appropriate care for children and youth with mental and

emotional disorders in a flexible manner, based on clinical needs. (Testimony, 1993, pp. 3–4)

Friedman (1996) suggested that health care reform needs to involve the development of community-based systems of care in which

- Services are provided in a flexible, family-focused, comprehensive manner.
- Categorical barriers to comprehensive and flexible services are reduced, and integrated, holistic services are provided.
- Services are provided in individualized and culturally competent ways.
- Greater emphasis is placed on preventive and family support activities than on crisis and deep-end services (that is, services that require hospitalization or residential care).
- Financing policies support these approaches.
- Responsibility for planning and control of resources is decentralized so that greater control is exercised at the community and neighborhood levels.
- Accountability is defined in terms of client and system outcomes and is integrated into system operations.

## Current Philosophy and Research Base for Mental Health Services

The major philosophy underlying the current direction of development in the mental health services system emerged from the CASSP initiatives. The orientation that defined the work of states in designing their mental health services for children and adolescents is the system-of-care model. This model has influenced the development of family-centered and community-based innovations. Stroul and Friedman (1986) defined *system of care* as a comprehensive spectrum of mental health and other necessary services organized into a coordinated network to meet the multiple and changing needs of children and adolescents with SED. The system-of-care philosophy caused major changes in the delivery of mental health services to children, adolescents, and their families. The goal of mental health services for this population is to increase the accessibility, availability, and quality of services through a system of care that is organized to be flexible and meet the needs of children and adolescents with SED. According to Sondheimer and Evans (1995), the important elements of the CASSP system of care include

- early identification and intervention
- a comprehensive continuum of services
- development and monitoring of individualized treatment plans
- services provided in the least-restrictive environment
- involvement of families in treatment planning and delivery, and support for families as primary caregivers
- coordination of services across multiple providers and systems
- case management
- services that are responsive to cultural, racial, and ethnic diversity.

Another philosophical shift in the delivery of mental health services for children and adolescents has occurred in treatment interventions, with an emphasis on providing mental health services in the natural environment by "wrapping services around the child" (Kutash et al., 1994, p. 194). Traditionally, the intervention of choice for a child or adolescent with SED in need of intensive services was psychiatric hospitalization or a residential treatment center. The CASSP philosophy challenged the states to develop coordinated systems of care that extend beyond the boundaries of the mental health system to include all systems in which children are identified and served (Rog, 1995). In addition, partnership with parents and families has emerged as a major theme in the development of services delivery systems.

Greater cultural sensitivity and competence in the delivery of mental health services to this population have been recognized as essential. Eliminating barriers to services and access to care requires individualized, family-focused, and culturally competent interventions.

The National Plan for Research on Child and Adolescent Mental Disorders (NIMH, 1990) called for expanded support of research on services delivery and systems of care for children and adolescents, including clinical services research development. Hoagwood and Hohmann (1993) stressed the particular need for scientific study of epidemiology of childhood disorders, care and effectiveness of interventions for children, delivery of services to youths and their families, and services system organization and financing. They identified two major differences between child and adolescent services research and clinical research: the notions of extensionality and contextuality. Hoagwood and Hohmann reported that services research extends clinical research into everyday settings (extensionality) and examines the factors that affect the delivery of treatments and services in community settings (contextuality).

Burns and Friedman (1990) suggested that services systems research should ask two questions: (1) How should the system be organized to provide cost-effective services, and (2) how should it be financed? The answers to these simple questions are complex. Hoagwood and Rupp (1994) identified several problems that emerge in building a research base for services research: existing databases have diagnostic inconsistencies; responsibilities for services delivery to this population are shared by multiple, key systems; and estimates of the prevalence and incidence of children and adolescents with SED rely heavily on various community surveys that used different assessment instruments.

## Selected Research Studies on Mental Health Services for Children and Adolescents

As use of managed care increases, mental health services for children and adolescents need to be examined from the perspective of clinical and services system outcomes. A greater concentration on accountability, with emphasis on costs of care and services effectiveness, has emerged. Mental health services delivery systems must be modified to meet the specific clinical needs of children and adolescents with SED and to embrace efficacious treatments as they become available (Jensen, Hoagwood, & Petti, 1996). Hoagwood, Jensen, Petti, and Burns (1996) have proposed an inclusive model of outcomes that will promote, for both clinicians and researchers, a dynamic way to conceptualize outcomes broadly to include areas of impact for children and adolescents within their environmental contexts. The model proposed five outcome domains as important sources of evidence of impact: symptoms, functioning, consumer perspectives, environments, and systems. Symptoms in this model are defined as any of the emotional or behavioral symptoms a child may exhibit in one or more settings (for example, distractibility, impulsiveness, depression, anxiety, impatience, aggression). The functioning domain is the ability of children and adolescents to adapt to varying demands across systems (family, school, peer group, community). The consumer perspective domain encompasses the subjective experience of the family and the child as it relates to quality of life, satisfaction with care, and burden and family strain. The environmental domain addresses the child's or adolescent's functioning in such primary domains as school and home. The systems domain concerns the use, coordination, costs, type, and duration of services available to the child or adolescent and the family. According to Hoagwood et al. (1996), this model permits analysis of the relationships within and between children and their contexts, recognizing that these relationships change as the child develops. Minor variations in any of the domains can lead to radically different outcomes for children and adolescents with SED.

Current outcome research has focused on two main categories: (1) studies of clinical efficacy for children and adolescents with specific disorders and (2) studies of the impact of the services system on children and adolescents with heterogeneous symptoms. Jensen et al. (1996) examined previous research to determine the degree to which it addressed the five outcome domains proposed by Hoagwood and collaborators (1996) and found only 38 studies of children and adolescents with serious mental health disturbances that met minimal scientific criteria. The criteria used in these studies included the use of a control or comparison group, six months or more of follow-up, and having been conducted since 1988. Only two of the studies included outcome assessments across all five domains, and they focused primarily on services effectiveness outcomes. These two studies, the Fort Bragg Continuum of Care Study (Bickman et al., 1995) and the Robert Wood Johnson Foundation's Program for Youth (Saxe, Cross, Lovas, & Gardner, 1995), are discussed in detail later in this chapter. On the basis of their review of studies, Jensen and colleagues (1996) recommended that integrating research into clinical practice should become an increasingly important goal for researchers and clinicians.

For purposes of discussion here, studies that are beginning to address the gap between research and practice have been organized into two major categories. The first concerns services research that addresses systems of care for children and adolescents who have SED and services system effectiveness. The second concerns clinical services research and clinical efficacy studies for this population. The integration of clinical efficacy studies and services system effectiveness studies, as recommended by Jensen and colleagues (1996), is in the early stages of development.

## MENTAL HEALTH SERVICES SYSTEM RESEARCH STUDIES

Each of these major studies has provided important information about services system development and implementation of models for systems of care. Only the key features of these studies are noted in this review, but the studies are representative of much of the services system research currently being conducted. The landmark Fort Bragg Continuum of Care Study, completed in 1995, is discussed in the most detail because of its implications for future services system development.

### CHAMPUS Tidewater Demonstration Project

The Civilian Health and Medical Program for Uniformed Services (CHAMPUS) Tidewater Demonstration Project examined the level of care initially provided to children and adolescents receiving mental health services in Virginia under the CHAMPUS Contractor Provider Agreement capitation program (Burns, Thompson, & Goldman, 1993). Over a three-year period (1986–1989), it explored initial mental health services decisions for children and adolescents in the program, quality-of-care issues under this cost containment model, and criteria for placement decisions. This demonstration project was designed to evaluate shifts in use of different levels of care and the appropriateness of the initial disposition decisions under the capitated program model.

The population was children and adolescents ages 0 to 17 who presented for treatment during a 28-month period. The program regulated price and transferred financial risk and greater decision-making responsibility to independent health care contractors (Burns et al., 1993). The program required case management, services networking to give consumers a choice between contract or noncontract providers, partial hospitalization as an option, and independent quality-of-care monitoring. Data on demographic characteristics, beneficiary status, symptom and behavior problem ratings, functioning, diagnosis, and initial disposition were collected primarily from case manager records at point-of-services entry, and selected data were collected from treating clinicians. The levels of care for initial disposition in this study were outpatient, partial hospitalization, residential treatment center, and inpatient. The study population of children and adolescents for year 1 was 1,966, for year 2 was 2,298, and for year 3 was 3,648.

The major findings were

- The number of children and adolescents entering treatment increased during each year of the demonstration. Approximately 2 percent of the population received mental health services in year 1, and 3.8 percent received services in year 3.
- A dramatic rise in outpatient admissions was observed each year: 79.0 percent in year 1, 89.0 percent in year 2, and 95.5 percent in year 3.
- A major reduction of one-third each year occurred in inpatient admissions.
- Use of residential treatment centers was nearly eliminated; year 1, 3.5 percent; year 2, 0.3 percent; and year 3, 0.2 percent.
- The partial hospitalization option was rarely used (Burns et al., 1993).

These results suggest that under a capitated program, it is difficult to admit children and adolescents to more restrictive care, even when there is no indication of decreasing severity in their problems, diagnoses, and functioning levels.

### Robert Wood Johnson Foundation's Mental Health Services Program for Youth

Over a five-year period, this demonstration examined organization and financing mechanisms for child and adolescent mental health services. The research was funded by the Robert Wood Johnson Foundation in 1989.

The Mental Health Services Program for Youth (MHSPY) demonstration was implemented in California, Kentucky, North Carolina, Ohio, Oregon, Pennsylvania, Vermont, and Wisconsin. (Pennsylvania withdrew from the demonstration in the second year of the study.) The demonstration proposed that the provision of comprehensive and coordinated mental health care is more effective and efficient than the current fragmented systems of care for children and adolescents with SED (Saxe et al., 1995). The states that took part in the project developed interagency groups that cross systems of care for children and adolescents (for example, mental health, child welfare, education, and juvenile justice), and all the project sites used case management. The primary goal of the demonstration was to test the hypothesis that changes in the organization and financing of mental health care for children and adolescents can improve care. The secondary goal was to describe the diversity of forms that an effective services system can take as well as ways to implement these systems.

Three dimensions of services system operation were examined in this study: comprehensiveness, appropriateness, and coordination (Saxe et al., 1995). Comprehensiveness is the organization of services (range, capacity, and delivery), finances (resources, services costs, and innovations), and clients (profile, needs, and access to services). Appropriateness concerns the clinical model, treatment planning, and care. Coordination is the structure of the services system, interagency relationships, parent and community involvement, interagency financial cooperation, and innovations. The demonstration used a quasi-experimental design, and sites were assessed longitudinally, with data collected at three points in time. Three methods of data collection were developed for this demonstration: (1) organizational and financial data collection from document review, interviews, observations, and surveys; (2) case-specific data collection extracted from project management information systems; and (3) clinical assessment data collection based on diagnostic interviews, quality-of-care data, and clinical case conferences.

Baseline data were analyzed by Saxe et al. (1995). At baseline each project had

- developed or enhanced substantive collaborative relationships among participating agencies
- created or designated already existing interagency structures for planning and decision making
- incorporated parents, advocates, and community representatives in planning and policy making
- developed strong interagency case management programs
- implemented new or expanded community-based services as alternatives to inpatient care
- developed financial strategies to allow greater flexibility in the use of services funds.

At the midpoint in the data collection process, clinical evaluators at the demonstration sites reported that the MHSPY interventions demonstrated creativity, commitment, and enthusiasm of services providers from various fields and systems and involved parents effectively. All the project sites designed their services systems around the needs of children and adolescents, and at each site a needs-driven services system model was evolving and being implemented.

## Services Coordination for Children in State Custody in Tennessee

This study evaluated access to mental health services for children and adolescents who were at risk of being placed in state custody. Legislation was passed in Tennessee to implement a pilot project in 12 counties (two separate six-county areas) over a three-year period to study the effects of coordinating services from all state agencies that assume custody of children and adolescents (Glisson, 1994). These state agencies were concerned with child welfare, youth corrections, mental health, and mental disabilities. Autonomous six-person services coordination teams were created to assume responsibility for children and adolescents in state custody in each of the two pilot areas. These teams were responsible for assessment, residential placement, referral to appropriate services, and monitoring the child's progress while in state custody. A central intake procedure and uniform assessment tools were used.

A quasi-experimental design was used to compare placement decisions, the acquisition of mental health services, and the children's functioning in the pilot and the control areas (two six-county areas matched on key demographic variables to the pilot areas) (Glisson, 1994). More than 2,000 children and adolescents entered state custody each year in the areas studied. (Children up to age four were not included in the research sample.) The type of placement for each child or adolescent was indicated by three levels of restrictiveness: least restrictive, moderately restrictive, and most restrictive. The least-restrictive level involved such placements as living with relatives or foster families. At the moderately restrictive level were placements in nonsecure group homes and small residential programs. Placements at the most-restrictive level were in secure group homes, correctional institutions, or psychiatric hospitals.

No differences were found between the control and pilot areas in terms of the gender, age, ethnicity, and initial problem characteristics of the sample of children and adolescents placed in custody (Glisson, 1994). After six months, study subjects in the pilot areas were in less-restrictive and more-appropriate placements than were the children and adolescents in the control areas. Children and adolescents in the pilot areas were found to be more likely to receive mental health services. For those who entered state custody with higher levels of disturbance, more progress was made in the pilot areas than in the control areas. Seventy percent of the children and adolescents in both pilot and control areas who entered state custody scored in the 90th percentile clinical range on the Child Behavioral Checklist Total Problem Behavior Scale. Only 14 percent of all children and adolescents who entered state custody and required clinical intervention received services from the mental health system. Glisson concluded that the findings from this study support the value of autonomous interorganizational services coordination teams in meeting the mental health needs of children and adolescents in state custody.

## Fort Bragg Continuum of Care Study

The Fort Bragg Continuum of Care demonstration and evaluation project was the first comprehensive study of a managed behavioral health plan for children and adolescents. This five-year independent evaluation of an $80 million demonstration program, the Fort Bragg Child and Adolescent Mental Health Demonstration Project, funded by the U.S. Army, examined quality, cost, and effectiveness of a system of care model for children and adolescents with mental health and substance abuse problems. Cardinal Mental Health Group, Inc., a private, not-for-profit corporation in Fayetteville, North Carolina, received the contract to provide a continuum of care for the Fort Bragg catchment area. The demonstration project used a closed system, or an exclusive provider model, that required families who sought services for their children and adolescents to use the project's clinical services, which were free, or to choose to seek and pay for services on their own (Bickman et al., 1995). All children and adolescents who sought services received a comprehensive intake assessment to determine the appropriate level of services at the Rumbaugh Clinic, the facility used for the demonstration project. The range of services available under this exclusive provider model included traditional outpatient care, intensive outpatient care, inpatient hospitalization, in-home therapy, after-school group treatment, day treatment, therapeutic foster homes, specialized group homes, 24-hour crisis management teams, transportation, and wraparound services (Bickman et al., 1995). If a child or adolescent needed more than outpatient services, the clinical services were coordinated with the other child-serving agencies and practitioners in the community. Services within the continuum were linked through a case management component and interdisciplinary treatment teams led by a doctoral-level staff person. All services provided by the project were at no financial cost to the families, and no limits were placed on types of services offered. The philosophy of the demonstration project called for controlling costs by providing a continuum of services more appropriate for each child and adolescent.

The contract for independent evaluation of the demonstration project was awarded to the Center for Mental Health Policy of the Vanderbilt Institute for Public Policy Studies at Vanderbilt University, Nashville, Tennessee. The evaluation consisted of substudies of implementation, quality, mental health outcomes, and costs and use. The implementation substudy provided a comprehensive description of how the study was put into place. The quality substudy examined evidence of whether or not key components of service were of sufficient quality to warrant evaluation. A quasi-experimental longitudinal design was used in the mental health outcomes study. The cost and utilization substudy compared actual use of mental health services with the cost of providing those services for all children and adolescents. Two comparison sites at Fort Campbell, Kentucky, and Fort Steward, Georgia, that provided mental health services to children and adolescents were used to assess the relative impact of the demonstration project. Baseline data and two additional data waves (six months apart) were collected on a sample of children and adolescents at the demonstration site and the comparison sites.

Findings from the mental health outcome substudy and the cost and use substudy have direct implications for future services delivery development. The findings of the mental health outcomes study (Bickman et al., 1995) were

- The typical child or adolescent referred for services improved at each site.
- The level of mental health improvement was about the same at each site.
- Certain subgroups of children and adolescents (for example, those with high psychopathology and high functional impairment or those with multiple problems) who had been hypothesized to have better outcomes in the demonstration project showed similar improvement at the comparison sites.

The mental health outcomes study did not find support for the hypothesis that the demonstration project's system of care led to better mental health outcomes than did the traditional system of services at the comparison sites.

The cost and use substudy found that at the system level, instituting a continuum of care increased mental health expenditures. Services at the demonstration site were 3.29 times more expensive per child or adolescent than were services at the comparison sites (Bickman et al., 1995). The children and adolescents at the demonstration site also used more services and remained in treatment longer.

Thus, Bickman and collaborators (1995) concluded that

- The project increased access to services for children and adolescents, and these clients were the children and adolescents appropriate to treat.

- The project successfully treated children in less-restrictive environments.
- Parents and adolescents were more satisfied with services at the demonstration site.
- Cost control through appropriate care was not demonstrated to be effective.
- A continuum of care is not necessarily more expensive.
- Lack of clinical differences in outcomes leads to questions about current clinical practices.

According to Bickman and colleagues (1995),

> This evaluation brings to question currently held beliefs among experts concerning the necessity for a continuum of care and many of its features. It has been shown that the demonstration had a more systematic and comprehensive assessment and treatment planning approach, more parent involvement, better case management, more individualized services, fewer treatment dropouts, a greater range of services, enhanced continuity of care, increased length of treatment, and better match between treatment and needs as judged by parents. Still, there were no better outcomes reported. Thus commonly accepted wisdom about what is a better-quality system of care is called into question. A fragmented system of care, without these features, performed as well in this evaluation. (pp. 208–209)

An alternative explanation of these findings would consider the continuum of care model to be effective and challenge the assumption that clinical services provided in the community are effective, but this evaluation project was not designed to answer that question (Bickman et al., 1995). It is possible that the treatments provided to children and adolescents had a positive effect at both the demonstration project and the comparison sites.

In a review of the Fort Bragg experiment, Friedman and Burns (1996) raised several questions about the findings, including questioning the basic program theory used in the evaluation. They noted the lack of specificity in defining the population for which the program theory should apply, the failure of the program theory to specify the point in time at which changes should be found, and the differences in financing arrangements between the demonstration and the comparison sites. However, Friedman and Burns also noted that the evaluation study demonstrated the importance and complexity of assessing the level of implementation of a theory of change and the general issue of the adequacy of present measures of child and family functioning.

Henggeler, Schoenwald, and Munger (1996) stated that they did not find an absence of significant clinical outcomes to be surprising. In their view, positive effects of child psychotherapy demonstrated in studies conducted in university settings have rarely been observed in studies conducted in community settings. Henggeler and colleagues posited that if existing treatment models are not clinically effective, the provision of more treatment options to youths in a more coordinated and integrated fashion, as accomplished in the Fort Bragg experiment, would not necessarily lead to more positive clinical outcomes.

The Fort Bragg experiment did, however, demonstrate important differences in the area of family satisfaction with care and in services use patterns. For example, children and adolescents at the demonstration site used fewer residential treatment and inpatient care services.

In summary, the Fort Bragg experiment was not perfect, but it had many strengths, including reliable implementation analyses, low attrition, relatively strong measurement methods, appropriate data analyses, and adequate statistical power to detect minuscule effect sizes, if they existed (Henggeler et al., 1996).

## CLINICAL SERVICES RESEARCH STUDIES

The following clinical services studies addressed interventions to evaluate particular components of system-of-care models, such as case management, wraparound services, and multisystemic interventions for children with more serious mental health problems. They represent a sample of the work currently in progress across the United States.

### Multisystemic Family Preservation Services Project

Multisystemic family preservation (MFP) treatment is an innovative treatment and services strategy that has demonstrated long-term clinical efficacy in treating serious antisocial behavior in adolescents. It also is promising for the treatment of other serious clinical problems, such as substance abuse and severe emotional disturbance (Henggeler, Schoenwald, Pickrel, Rowland, & Santos, 1994).

The capacity of multisystemic therapy (MST) to reduce rates of antisocial behavior and institutionalization for violent and chronic juvenile offenders was examined in a research study in South Carolina funded by NIMH. Eighty-four serious juvenile offenders at imminent risk of incarceration were randomly assigned to MST or to services usually provided by the juvenile justice system—that is, incarceration (Henggeler, Melton, Smith, Schoenwald, & Hanley, 1993). MST intervention targets family, peers, and school and community systems and is child focused and family centered, with treatment goals and intervention strategies tailored to the needs, strengths, and goals of the youth and his or her family (Henggeler et al., 1994). Family treatment strategies are integrated from problem-focused treatment models such as structural family therapy, behavioral family treatment, and strategic family therapy. The primary goal of MST is to engage the youth and the family in systemic change. Scherer, Brondino, Henggeler, Melton, and Hanley (1994) identified the nine principles of multisystemic therapy:

1. The primary purpose of assessment is to understand the fit between the identified problems and their broader systemic context.
2. Interventions should be focused on the present and be action oriented, targeting specific and well-defined problems.
3. Interventions should concentrate on sequences of behavior within or between multiple systems.
4. Interventions should be developmentally appropriate.
5. Interventions should require daily or weekly effort by family members.
6. The therapist continuously evaluates intervention efficacy from multiple perspectives.
7. Interventions should promote treatment generalization and long-term maintenance of therapeutic change.
8. Therapeutic contacts should emphasize the positive and use systemic strengths as methods for change.

9.  Interventions should promote responsible behavior and decrease irresponsible behavior among family members.

Youths in this study averaged three to four previous arrests (59 percent had been arrested for violent crimes) and 8.2 weeks of previous incarceration, which attested to their high degree of antisocial behavior (Henggeler et al., 1994). MST was delivered by three full-time therapists, with an average duration of 13.4 weeks and 33.0 hours of face-to-face contact (Henggeler et al., 1993). At follow-up assessment, families in the MST condition of the study reported increased cohesion, decreased adolescent aggression with peers, and decreased criminal activity by the adolescent. At the 59-week follow-up, MST, compared with usual services, was found to be more effective at reducing recidivism rates (42 percent versus 62 percent), institutionalization (an average of 73 fewer days incarcerated), and cost ($3,000 per case versus $17,000 per case) (Henggeler et al., 1994). At the 2.4-year follow-up, adolescents in the MST condition continued to demonstrate reduced recidivism rates and institutionalization days.

### New York State Treatment Foster Care and Family-Centered Intensive Case Management Research Demonstration Project

This project compared the child, family, and services system outcomes of New York's treatment foster care program with those of a family-centered intensive case management program in three rural counties in that state. The New York State treatment foster care program, Family-Based Treatment (FBT), provides training, support, and respite treatment for foster families in the community (Armstrong & Evans, 1992). A family specialist in the program trains and provides support to a cluster of five treatment families and one respite family. The Family-Centered Intensive Case Management (FCICM) program provides intensive support and services through flexible funding, wraparound services, and interagency collaboration. The case manager and a parent advocate work as a team with eight families and two respite families in the FCICM program. The study used a positive, controlled, randomized design in which children ages six to 12, who had been referred to FBT by mental health professionals and human services workers, were assigned to either FBT or FCICM (Evans et al., 1994). The researchers collected data on functioning and symptoms at baseline and at six-month intervals, including six months after discharge from the program. Thirty-nine children in the three rural counties were randomly assigned to either FCICM ($N = 15$) or FBT ($N = 24$). Evans and colleagues (1994) found that when given intensive and individualized supports, children with SED can be cared for effectively in their own homes. The average length of stay in FCICM was 13.2 months.

### Seattle Homeless Adolescent Research Project

The goal of the Seattle Homeless Adolescent Research Project (Project Passage) was to implement and evaluate an intensive mental health case management program for adolescents. Project Passage was based on nine primary components: assessment, planning, linkage, monitoring or tracking, advocacy, counseling or the therapeutic relationship, treatment teams, crisis services, and flexible funds (Cauce et al., 1994). Caseload size was limited to no more than 12 homeless adolescents. The setting for the study was the Orion Multiservice Center in downtown Seattle, a drop-in center that provides homeless, runaway, and street-involved youths between ages 11 and 20 a safe place to stay during the day. The target population for Project Passage was homeless youths at risk for SED. To be eligible for Project Passage services, homeless youths had to be interested in receiving some type of services or treatment, willing to participate in the research, and have plans to stay in the Seattle area for at least six months. When the adolescents who met these criteria agreed to participate, they were assigned randomly to one of two treatment conditions: intensive case management (ICM) or regular case management. Regular case management was the control condition. The key differences between Project Passage ICM and regular case management were caseload size, availability of flexible funds, and educational qualifications; ICM involved a lower caseload size, had flexible funds available to meet the individual needs of the homeless youth, and required case managers to have a master's degree.

A pretest and posttest control group design model was used to evaluate the effectiveness of Project Passage ICM. Fifty-five subjects were assigned to ICM condition, and 60 subjects were assigned to regular case management. Data were collected during face-to-face interviews with study participants at baseline and then every three months. Results for the first 115 homeless youths in both conditions who had completed baseline assessment and the first three-month follow-up assessment showed improvement in mental health and social adjustment. There were no major differences between the two groups, except that the homeless youths in the Project Passage ICM reported a higher level of satisfaction with their quality of life and lower levels of self-reported aggression (Cauce et al., 1994).

## PRACTICAL AND CLINICAL IMPORTANCE OF THE RESEARCH FINDINGS

Research in mental health services system development and clinical interventions remains a national priority. The studies reviewed in this chapter have raised critical questions about traditional mental health interventions and the relative efficacy of continuum-of-care models. Studies of mental health services systems are needed to understand what types of organization and financing systems are effective and efficient in serving children and adolescents. The challenge will be to reach consensus on ways to operationalize concepts to measure the functioning of services systems, quality of care, positive outcomes, and effectiveness of services systems. The Fort Bragg study has raised serious concerns for policymakers and clinicians about the efficacy of continuum-of-care models and the overall effectiveness of clinical services delivered in the community. The services system research reviewed here demonstrated that access to care for children and adolescents improves with the development of system-of-care models and an interagency coordination effort using a case management model. They also have raised concerns about the major emphasis on community alternatives as more effective and appropriate for meeting the needs of children and adolescents. It appears that system-of-care models encourage clinicians and case managers to seek less-restrictive treatment intervention options for children and adolescents, which supports the CASSP philosophy.

The clinical services studies reviewed here bring to the forefront the real-world issues in the evaluation of innovative clinical interventions. Their small sample sizes and limited indications of positive outcomes, even in the MST intervention, demonstrate the difficulty of capturing the intervention effect in natural settings. The small sample sizes in these studies created problems in accurately assessing statistical power and treatment effect measures. Such studies are difficult to design and implement because changes in services delivery systems influence the effectiveness of many of the intervention outcomes. The MST intervention appears to be a particularly promising approach for working with children and adolescents with serious emotional and behavioral problems (Henggeler et al., 1994). Case management services that are designed to be intensive and require more skilled professionals have shown limited differences in outcomes for children and adolescents who use these services (Cauce et al., 1994; Evans et al., 1994).

These studies also raise questions about the sensitivity of the measures used to document outcomes and change. Horizontal diffusion can occur when random assignment is made within the same population at the same site. Burns and Friedman (1990) have recommended that more rigorous controlled studies (like the clinical services studies reviewed in this chapter) are needed to assess both the clinical and the cost outcomes of innovative services. Conceptualization of the research problems and the links to randomized clinical trials or comparison group models requires special attention from researchers working with children and adolescents. Attrition rates in small samples also may influence outcomes in services research.

Henggeler and colleagues (1996) suggested three primary sets of difficulties in achieving favorable clinical outcomes: (1) failure of most treatment approaches to attend to the multidetermined nature of serious clinical problems, (2) low ecological validity of many treatments, and (3) low accountability of mental health providers. Jensen et al. (1996) indicated that the gap between research and practice can be narrowed if studies of clinical efficacy and services effectiveness are integrated and linked to important public policy questions. They have identified three areas that are ripe for integrative research efforts: (1) studies that investigate the differential long-term effects of various treatment alternatives; (2) studies that package multifaceted treatments and export them into naturalistic settings, where they can be incorporated into routine practices; and (3) studies that examine and incorporate consumer perspectives with other outcome assessments.

## Challenges for Mental Health Services Research and Social Work Practice

Research on the effectiveness of services systems and specific service components in child and adolescent mental health is a relatively new endeavor. Social work professionals need to engage in this much-needed and difficult services research agenda. Clinical services innovations should be studied with rigor, by use of randomized clinical trials whenever possible. Measurement instruments are needed to capture the dynamic and ever-changing services system models and clinical interventions. Outcome studies should be a particular priority in this era of managed health care.

In work with children and adolescents, what do social workers do that is effective and demonstrates long-term positive outcomes for the children and their families? Are there particular models of services system organization and financing that contribute to more positive outcomes? What innovative clinical services work for whom—and when and for how long? Do different subgroups of children and adolescents need different levels of services interventions? These are just a few of the research questions that social workers need to address in their provision of mental health services to children and adolescents. Use of empirically based clinical services interventions should become an increasing part of social work's practice and training.

Rog (1995) stated,

> Often in service areas in which practice traditions have been in place long before research has been developed, it is difficult to change direction in the light of significant scientific evidence. There is often the danger that customary practice will prevail despite the lack of evidence to support its continuing or even in the face of contradictory findings. (p. 15)

Hoagwood and Hohmann (1993) identified a number of critical areas that have not been adequately investigated in child and adolescent services research:

- hospitalization and residential treatment of children and adolescents
- cultural appropriateness of mental health services (barriers and effectiveness)
- parental involvement
- school and mental health services interface
- legal and mental health services interface
- child welfare and mental health services interface
- innovative treatments or services approaches
- cost containment
- reimbursement mechanisms
- psychiatric emergency services.

The gaps in child and adolescent services research call for immediate attention from social workers, who can contribute to building the knowledge base for child and adolescent mental health services by engaging in critical studies of services and system responses.

# References

Alcohol, Drug Abuse, and Mental Health Administration Reorganization Act, P.L. 102-321, Title 42, U.S.C. 201 et seq., 106 Stat. 323 (1992).

American Psychiatric Association. (1987). *Diagnostic and statistical manual of mental disorders* (3rd ed., rev.). Washington, DC: Author.

Armstrong, M. I., & Evans, M. (1992). Three intensive community-based programs for children and youth with serious emotional disturbance and their families. *Journal of Child and Family Studies, 1,* 61–74.

Bickman, L., Guthrie, P. R., Foster, E. M., Lambert, E. W., Summerfelt, W. T., Breda, C. S., & Heflinger, C. A. (1995). *Evaluating managed mental health services: The Fort Bragg experiment.* New York: Plenum Press.

Bird, H. R., Canino, G., Rubio-Stipec, M., Gould, M. S., Ribera, J., Sesman, M., Woodbury, M., Huertas-Goldman, S., Pagan, A., Sanchez-Lacay, A., & Moscoso, M. (1988). Estimates of the prevalence of childhood maladjustment in a community survey in Puerto Rico. *Archives of General Psychiatry, 45,* 1120–1126.

Brazelton Center for Mental Health Law. (1993). *Federal definitions of children with serious emotional disturbance* (pp. 25–29). Washington, DC: Author.

Burns, B. J. (1991). Mental health service use by adolescents in the 1970s and 1980s. *Journal of the American Academy of Child and Adolescent Psychiatry, 30,* 144–149.

Burns, B. J., Costello, E. J., Angold, A., Tweed, D., Stangl, D., Farmer, E. M., & Erkanli, A. (1995). Children's mental health service use across service sectors. *Health Affairs, 14,* 147–159.

Burns, B. J., & Freidman, R. M. (1990). Examining the research base for child mental health services and policy. *Journal of Mental Health Administration, 17*, 87–98.

Burns, B. J., Thompson, J. W., & Goldman, H. H. (1993). Initial decisions by level of care for youth in the CHAMPUS Tidewater demonstration. *Administration and Policy in Mental Health, 20*, 231–246.

Cauce, A. M., Morgan, C. J., Wagner, V., Moore, E., Sy, J., Wurzbacher, K., Weeden, K., Tomlin, S., & Blanchard, T. (1994). Effectiveness of intensive case management for homeless adolescents: Results of a 3 month follow-up. *Journal of Emotional and Behavioral Disorders, 2*, 219–227.

Cohen, P., Provet, A. G., & Jones, M. (1996). Prevalence of emotional and behavioral disorders during childhood and adolescence. In B. L. Levin & J. Petrila (Eds.), *Mental health services: A public health perspective* (pp. 193–209). New York: Oxford University Press.

Community Mental Health Centers Act, P.L. 92-255, 86 Stat. 76, 77, 85 (1972).

Costello, E. J., Angold, A., Burns, B. J., Erkanli, A., Stangl, D. K., & Tweed, D. L. (1996). The Great Smoky Mountains Study of Youth. Functional impairment and serious emotional disturbance. *Archives of General Psychiatry, 53*, 1137–1143.

Costello, E. J., Angold, A., Burns, B. J., Stangl, D. K., Tweed, D. L., Erkanli, A., & Worthman, C. M. (1996). The Great Smoky Mountains Study of Youth. Goals, design, methods and the prevalence of DSM-III-R disorders. *Archives of General Psychiatry, 53*, 1129–1136.

Costello, E. J., Burns, B. J., Angold, A., & Leaf, P. J. (1993). How can epidemiology improve mental health services for children and adolescents? *Journal of the American Academy of Child and Adolescent Psychiatry, 32*, 1106–1114.

Evans, M., Armstrong, M. I., Dollard, N., Kuppinger, A., Huz, S., & Wood, V. (1994). Development and evaluation of treatment foster care and family-centered intensive case management in New York. *Journal of Emotional and Behavioral Disorders, 2*, 228–239.

Friedman, R. M. (1996). Mental health policy for children. In B. L. Levin & J. Petrila (Eds.), *Mental health services: A public health perspective* (pp. 234–248). New York: Oxford University Press.

Friedman, R. M., & Burns, B. J. (1996). The evaluation of the Fort Bragg Demonstration Project: An alternative interpretation of the findings. *Journal of Mental Health Administration, 23*, 128–136.

Friedman, R. M., Kutash, K., & Duchnowski, A. J. (1996). The population of concern: Defining the issues. In B. A. Stroul (Ed.), *Children's mental health: Creating systems of care in a changing society* (pp. 69–98). Baltimore: Paul H. Brookes.

Glisson, C. (1994). The effect of services coordination teams on outcomes for children in state custody. *Administration in Social Work, 18*(4), 1–23.

Henggeler, S. W., Melton, G. B., Smith, L., Schoenwald, S. K., & Hanley, J. H. (1993). Family preservation using multisystemic treatment: Long-term follow-up to a clinical trial with serious juvenile offenders. *Journal of Child and Family Studies, 2*, 283–293.

Henggeler, S. W., Schoenwald, S. K., & Munger, R. (1996). Families and therapists achieve clinical outcomes, systems of care mediate the process. *Journal of Child and Family Studies, 5*, 177–184.

Henggeler, S. W., Schoenwald, S. K., Pickrel, S. G., Rowland, M. D., & Santos, A. (1994). The contribution of treatment outcome research to the reform of children's mental health services: Multisystemic therapy as an example. *Journal of Mental Health Administration, 21*, 229–239.

Hoagwood, K., & Hohmann, A. A. (1993). Child and adolescent services research at the National Institute of Mental Health: Research opportunities in an emerging field. *Journal of Child and Family Studies, 2,* 259–268.

Hoagwood, K., Jensen, P. S., Petti, T., & Burns, B. J. (1996). Outcomes of mental health care for children and adolescents: I. A comprehensive conceptual model. *Journal of the American Academy of Child and Adolescent Psychiatry, 35,* 1055–1063.

Hoagwood, K., & Rupp, A. (1994). Mental health service needs, use and costs for children and adolescents with mental disorders and their families: Preliminary evidence. In R. W. Manderscheid & M. A. Sonnenshein (Eds.), *Mental health: United States 1994, Center for Mental Health Services* (DHHS Publication No. SMA 94-3000, pp. 52–64). Washington, DC: U.S. Government Printing Office.

Institute of Medicine. (1989). *Research on children and adolescents with mental, behavioral and developmental disorders.* Washington, DC: National Academy Press.

Jensen, P. S., Hoagwood, K., & Petti, T. (1996). Outcomes of mental health care for children and adolescents: II. Literature review and application of a comprehensive model. *Journal of the American Academy of Child and Adolescent Psychiatry, 35,* 1064–1077.

Jensen, P. S., Watanabe, H. K., Richters, J. E., Cortes, R., Roper, M., & Liu, S. (1995). Prevalence of mental disorder in military children and adolescents: Findings from a two stage community survey. *Journal of the American Academy of Child and Adolescent Psychiatry, 34,* 1514–1524.

Kashani, J. H., Ezpeleta, L., Dandoy, A. C., Doi, S., & Reid, J. C. (1991). Psychiatric disorders in children and adolescents. The contribution of the child's temperament and the parents' psychopathology and attitudes. *Canadian Journal of Psychiatry, 36,* 569–573.

Kessler, R. C., McGonagle, K. A., Zhao, S., Nelson, C. B., Hughes, M., Eshleman, S., Wittchen, H-U., & Kendler, K. S. (1994). Lifetime and 12-month prevalence of DSM-III-R psychiatric disorders in the United States: Results from the National Comorbidity Survey. *Archives of General Psychiatry, 51,* 8–19.

Knitzer, J. (1982). *Unclaimed children: The failure of public responsibility to children and adolescents in need of mental health services.* Washington, DC: Children's Defense Fund.

Kutash, K., Duchnowski, A., & Sondheimer, D. (1994). Building the research base for children's mental health services. *Journal of Emotional and Behavioral Disorders, 1,* 194–197.

Lahey, B. B., Flagg, E. W., Bird, H. R., Schwab-Stone, M., Canino, G., Dulcan, M. K., Leaf, P. J., Davies, M., Brogan, D., Bourdon, K., Horwitz, S. M., Rubio-Stipec, M., Freeman, D. H., Lichtman, J., Shaffer, D., Goodman, S. H., Narrow, W. E., Weissman, M. M., Kandel, D. B., Jensen, P. S., Richters, J. E., & Reiger, D. A. (1996). The NIMH methods for the epidemiology of child and adolescent mental disorders (MECA) study: Background and methodology. *Journal of the American Academy of Child and Adolescent Psychiatry, 35,* 855–864.

Lourie, I. S., Katz-Leavy, J., & Jacobs, J. H. (1986). *Division of Education and Service System Liaison (DESSL) Child and Adolescent Service System Program (CASSP): Fiscal year 1986 report.* Washington, DC: National Institute of Mental Health.

Myers, J. C. (1985). Federal efforts to improve mental health services for children: Breaking the cycle of failure. *Journal of Clinical Child Psychology, 14,* 182–187.

Namir, S., & Weinstein, R. S. (1982). Children: Facilitating new directions. In L. R. Snowdon (Ed.), *Reaching the underserved: Mental health needs of neglected populations: Vol. 3. Annual reviews of community mental health* (pp. 43–73). Beverly Hills, CA: Sage Publications.

National Institute of Mental Health. (1983). *Program announcement: Child and Adolescent Services System Program.* Washington, DC: Author.

National Institute of Mental Health. (1990). *National plan for research on child and adolescent mental disorders* (DHHS Publication No. ADM 90-1683). Rockville, MD: Author.

National Institute of Mental Health. (1991a). *Child and Adolescent Mental Health Service system research demonstration grants* (PA-91-40). Rockville, MD: Author.

National Institute of Mental Health. (1991b). *Implementation of the national plan for research on child and adolescent mental disorders* (PA-91-46). Rockville, MD: Author.

Rog, D. (1995). The status of children's mental health services: An overview. In L. Bickman & D. Rog (Eds.), *Children's mental health services: Research, policy and evaluation* (pp. 3–18). Thousand Oaks, CA: Sage Publications.

Saxe, L., Cross, T. P., Lovas, G., & Gardner, J. K. (1995). Evaluation of the Mental Health Services Program for Youth: Examining rhetoric in action. In L. Bickman & D. Rog (Eds.), *Children's mental health services: Research, policy and evaluation* (CMHS, Vol. 1, pp. 206–235). Thousand Oaks, CA: Sage Publications.

Scherer, D. G., Brondino, M. J., Henggeler, S. W., Melton, G. B., & Hanley, J. H. (1994). Multisystemic family preservation therapy: Preliminary findings from a study of rural and minority serious adolescent offenders. *Journal of Emotional and Behavioral Disorders, 2,* 198–206.

Sondheimer, D., & Evans, M. E. (1995). Developments in children's mental health services research: An overview of current and future demonstration directions. In L. Bickman & D. Rog (Eds.), *Children's mental health services: Research, policy and evaluation* (CMHS, Vol. 1, pp. 64–84). Thousand Oaks, CA: Sage Publications.

State Comprehensive Mental Health Services Plan Act, P.L. 99-660, Title 42, U.S.C. 300x et seq., 100 Stat. 3794–3797 (November 14, 1986).

Stroul, B. A., & Friedman, R. M. (1986). *A system of care for severely emotionally disturbed children and youth.* Washington, DC: Georgetown University, Child and Adolescent Service System Program, Technical Assistance Center.

Testimony submitted to Labor and Human Resources Committee, U.S. Senate, at hearings on mental health and substance abuse in health care reform. (1993, November 8). Washington, DC.

Tuma, J. M. (1989). Mental health services for children: The state of the art. *American Psychologist, 44,* 188–199.

## Suggested Reading

Attkisson, C. C., Dresser, K. L., & Rosenblatt, A. (1995). Service systems for youth with severe emotional disorder: System-of-care research in California. In L. Bickman & D. Rog (Eds.), *Children's mental health services: Research, policy and evaluation* (CMHS, Vol. 1, pp. 236–280). Thousand Oaks, CA: Sage Publications.

Bickman, L. (Ed.). (1996). The Fort Bragg Experiment [Special Issue]. *Journal of Mental Health Administration, 23.*

Catron, T., & Weiss, B. (1994). The Vanderbilt school-based counseling program: An interagency, primary care model of mental health services. *Journal of Emotional and Behavioral Disorders, 2,* 247–253.

Costello, E. J., Farmer, E. M., Angold, A., Burns, B. J., & Erkanli, A. (1997). Psychiatric disorders among American Indian and white youth in Appalachia: The Great Smoky Mountains Study. *American Journal of Public Health, 87,* 827–832.

Evans, M. E., Armstrong, M. I., & Kuppinger, A. D. (1996). Family-centered intensive case management: A step toward understanding individualized care. *Journal of Child and Family Studies, 5*, 55–66.

Evans, M. E., Armstrong, M. I., Thompson, F. T., & Lee, J. (1994). Assessing the outcomes of parent and provider-designed systems of care for children with emotional and behavioral disorders. *Psychiatric Quarterly, 65*, 257–272.

Henggeler, S. W., Pickrel, S. G., Brondino, M. J., & Crouch, J. L. (1996). Eliminating (almost) treatment dropout of substance abusing or depending delinquents through home-based multisystemic therapy. *American Journal of Psychiatry, 153*, 427–428.

Henggeler, S. W., Schoenwald, S. K., & Pickrel, S. G. (1995). Multisystemic therapy: Bridging the gap between university and community based treatment. *Journal of Consulting and Clinical Psychology, 63*, 709–717.

Hoagwood, K., & Cunningham, M. (1992). Outcomes of children with emotional disturbance in residential treatment for educational purposes. *Journal of Child and Family Studies, 1*, 129–140.

Hoagwood, K., Jensen, P. S., & Fisher, C. B. (1996). *Ethical issues in mental health research with children and adolescents.* Mahwah, NJ: Lawrence Erlbaum.

Koroloff, N. M., Elliott, D. J., Koren, P. E., & Friesen, B. (1994). Connecting low-income families to mental health services: The role of the family associate. *Journal of Emotional and Behavioral Disorders, 2*, 240–246.

Kutash, K., Rivera, V. R., Hall, K., & Friedman, R. M. (1994). Public sector financing of community-based services for children with serious emotional disabilities and their families: Results of a national survey. *Journal of Mental Health Administration, 21*, 262–270.

Rugs, D., & Kutash, K. (1994). Evaluating children's mental health service systems: An analysis of critical behaviors and events. *Journal of Child and Family Studies, 3*, 249–262.

Santos, A. B., Henggeler, S. W., Burns, B. J., Arana, G. W., & Meisler, N. (1995). Research on field-based services: Models of reform in the delivery of mental health care to populations with complex clinical problems. *American Journal of Psychiatry, 15*, 1111–1123.

Schlenger, W. E., Etheridge, R. M., Hansen, D. J., Fairbank, D. W., & Onken, J. (1992). Evaluation of state efforts to improve systems of care for children and adolescents with severe emotional disturbances: The CASSP initial cohort study. *Journal of Mental Health Administration, 19*, 131–142.

Schoenwald, S. K., Ward, D. M., Henggeler, S. W., Pickrel, S. G., & Patel, H. (1996). Multisystemic therapy treatment of substance abusing or dependent adolescent offenders: Costs of reducing incarceration, inpatient and residential placement. *Journal of Child and Family Studies, 5*, 431–444.

Silver, S. T., Duchnowski, A. J., Kutash, K., Friedman, R. M., Eisen, M., Prange, M. E., Brandenburg, N. A., & Greenbaum, P. E. (1992). A comparison of children with serious emotional disturbance served in residential and school settings. *Journal of Child and Family Studies, 1*, 43–59.

Yoe, J. T., Santarcangelo, S., Atkins, M., & Burchard, J. D. (1996). Wraparound care in Vermont: Program development, implementation and evaluation of a statewide system of individualized services. *Journal of Child and Family Studies, 5*, 23–38.

Young, S. C., Nicholson, J., & Davis, M. (1995). An overview of issues in research on consumer satisfaction with child and adolescent mental health services. *Journal of Child and Family Studies, 4*, 219–238.

# Community-Based Treatment Models for Adults with Severe and Persistent Mental Illness

Mary Ann Test

For more than 100 years in the United States, a system of large state and county hospitals was the primary site of treatment and care for adults with severe and persistent mental illnesses. Beginning in 1955 and accelerating in the late 1960s and the 1970s, this system changed dramatically as a result of the deinstitutionalization and community care movement—the release or transfer of former long-term inpatients and the treatment of people newly diagnosed with mental illnesses in the community (Mechanic & Rochefort, 1990).

The community care movement holds great promise because thousands of citizens with severe mental illnesses can potentially live in freedom among us rather than being isolated and segregated in distant institutions. Yet in most places this promise has not been realized because an effective community treatment system still does not exist. The tragic results are well known: Numerous people with severe mental illnesses revolve in and out of hospitals or suffer barren and empty lives in the community; many spend time in penal settings or are homeless.

One contributing factor to the failure to develop adequate community care systems has been a lack of knowledge about how to treat people with severe mental illnesses in community settings. Mental health services research has begun to reduce this gap—at least one well-defined, empirically validated, and widely replicated community treatment model now exists. Other promising approaches have been or are being developed but need further research. This chapter describes effective and promising models of community-based care and their research support. Knowledge of "what works" will contribute to more effective program development and practice with this population by social workers and other mental health professionals, and an introduction to promising approaches may stimulate the needed evaluative investigations.

Much of this chapter is devoted to a description of programs of assertive community treatment, the only full-services intervention that has been tested in multiple, randomized clinical trials (Burns & Santos, 1995). Drake and Burns (1995) stated, "No psychosocial intervention has influenced current community mental health care more than assertive community treatment" (p. 667). Two other promising models of community care, which share to a considerable extent the values and approaches of social work, also are presented. One—the psychosocial rehabilitation center or "clubhouse" model—has been used for many years, and information about its methods has been widely disseminated. The few controlled studies of this model revealed promising results, but much more evaluative work is needed. The other approach described—consumer-run programs—is relatively new and provides fertile ground for social work collaboration in its empirical evaluation.

# Programs of Assertive Community Treatment (PACT)

## BACKGROUND

My colleagues Arnold Marx, Leonard Stein, and I developed the community treatment model called "PACT" (also termed "Training in Community Living," or "TCL," in the earlier literature) in the early 1970s (Marx, Test, & Stein, 1973). We had come to realize that the comprehensive services provided by the hospital also were necessary if clients with severe and persistent mental illnesses were to survive and grow in the community. We were working on an inpatient ward of a state hospital in the late 1960s and had become discouraged because, after discharge, our clients almost invariably relapsed and rotated back to the hospital, although we believed they had been prepared for community living (Stein & Test, 1985). When we examined the community aftercare system available to our discharged clients, we noted that in several critical ways, it seemed a total mismatch with their characteristics and needs.

Many of the services and day-to-day supports that our clients needed were simply not available to them in the community. The community care system typically offered only supportive therapy and medications but, because of ongoing impairments from their illnesses and extreme vulnerabilities to stress, our clients often needed assistance in many other life domains, such as housing, daily living activities, general health care, economic support, friends and leisure activities, work rehabilitation, and crisis support. Even as some of these other services became available and we carefully linked our clients with them, dropout from services often happened rapidly. The various agencies required our clients to come to the center or program to receive their medications and other services, but the symptoms of severe mental illnesses, such as lack of motivation, poor social skills, cognitive impairments, and psychotic episodes, made this difficult for the clients to do. Then, as the services system became better developed, it also became complex and fragmented. For example, various services were provided under different roofs and diverse funding auspices. People with severe mental illnesses were not able to negotiate this system and often "fell through the cracks."

We developed the PACT model to ameliorate these problems and address specifically the characteristics and needs of people with severe and persistent mental illnesses. The basic tenets of the model were

- The community—not the hospital—should be the primary locus of care for these clients, because the community is where clients face daily, ongoing stressors.
- Treatments and supports in the community must be comprehensive, potentially addressing all areas of life.
- Treatment and care must be flexible and highly individualized to address the vast heterogeneity of this population as well as the changing needs of one client across time.

- These comprehensive and flexible treatments and supports must be organized and delivered to reach clients efficiently.

Pilot efforts of this new approach were implemented by hospital staff, who went into the community each day to help our newly discharged clients remain there (Marx et al., 1973). With experience, we came to believe that many people could avoid hospitalization altogether if they received comprehensive community care and supports instead. Thus, we moved our hospital staff to the community and used our new PACT model as an alternative to the mental hospital (Stein & Test, 1980). We are now implementing this community-based model to help young adult clients with severe mental illnesses remain in the community and improve their quality of life and functioning (Test, Knoedler, & Allness, 1985; Test et al., 1991). The PACT approach is now widely used in the United States (Deci, Santos, Hiott, Schoenwald, & Dias, 1995).

## DESCRIPTION OF THE MODEL

At the heart of the PACT model is the core services, or continuous treatment, team (Torrey, 1986). A core services team is a community-based, multidisciplinary team of mental health staff who serve as a fixed point of responsibility for a defined group of clients. The team is responsible for assisting the client with meeting needs in all areas of life. The size of the core team and the number of clients served vary considerably by geographic area. In our current long-term study in Madison, Wisconsin, for example, this interdisciplinary team consists of 14 staff who are responsible for 120 young adults with schizophrenia. The team provides coverage seven days a week, 24 hours a day, and operates out of an office in the community. Coverage during the night is provided by staff members who are on call through a beeper paging system.

There are three critical elements of the PACT core services team operation:

1. The core team is the primary provider of treatment, rehabilitation, and social services. The PACT model is a marked contrast to broker case management models in which a case manager links the client with other providers. The Madison PACT core team, for example, provides clients with medications; supportive and problem-solving therapy; crisis intervention; and assistance with housing, work rehabilitation, and daily living activities—whatever is needed to enable the client to remain and grow in the community with a decent quality of life. This minimizes the fragmentation and time-consuming (often unsuccessful) coordination that is needed in systems involving multiple agencies, each of which address only a part of the client's multiple and often rapidly changing needs. The PACT model ensures that someone always is responsible and available to provide the client with help in the many areas of spontaneous need that arise (for example, installing a lock on a door to make housing safe or assisting with budgeting). When the same team provides both treatment and rehabilitation services, the complex interaction of symptoms and psychosocial functioning can be efficiently and effectively addressed. Also, use of a core services team results in not only continuity of care across functional areas and across time, but also continuity of caregiver, because the client has to relate to only one set of staff.
2. The team is mobile—that is, team members use assertive outreach to provide most services where the client is, rather than in an office or agency setting.

Each morning the staff meet at the community-based office to receive assignments; they then spend their working day in the community, meeting clients in their places of residence, neighborhoods, or sites of work or leisure. Our data indicate that 78 percent of the time spent with clients takes place in their territory; only 22 percent is in our office (Brekke & Test, 1987). Such assertive outreach prevents the dropout of clients from services. In addition, the provision of services and skills training where the client uses them eliminates the need for the client to transfer training from an agency setting to his or her natural environment, something that people with severe mental illnesses often find difficult.

3. The services provided by the team are highly individualized. The great diversity of people with severe mental illness and the fact that both the person and the disorder are constantly changing over time require that services be personalized (Strauss, Hafez, Lieberman, & Harding, 1985). In PACT the treatment interventions are designed for the current needs and preferences of each client, and do not simply assign the client to a set of existing programs. The content, amount, timing, and kinds of treatment, rehabilitation, and supports provided vary enormously among clients, as well as for the same client across time.

The treatment process begins with a thorough clinical and functional assessment. Then the client and the team work together to devise an individualized treatment plan for symptoms and psychological functioning, housing and other environmental supports, activities of daily living (such as budgeting, cooking, or personal care), vocational skills, social relationships and leisure activities, relationships with family, and medical and general health. Assessment is ongoing, and treatment plans are regularly updated. Core team member interventions are based on the treatment plan.

In illness management, the core team provides medication, which is often delivered to clients. Also, staff have frequent one-to-one contacts with clients to help them solve problems and provide an abundance of emotional support. Over time and within the context of a long-term relationship, the team attempts to educate the client about his or her illness and, sometimes, helps the clients learn to self-manage symptoms. They also provide individualized psychoeducation to family and community members (such as landlords and employers). A team member is on call 24 hours a day to provide crisis intervention. Brief admission to a hospital is used as needed.

In the area of housing, staff primarily help clients find rooms or apartments in the community rather than use specialized residential settings. We have found that clients prefer these more integrated and normative settings, and support can be adjusted in such settings to the amount that the client needs at any given time. Team members spend much time helping clients meet their basic needs where they live. This work might involve teaching and assisting them with activities of daily living, such as grocery shopping, money management, laundry upkeep, and use of transportation. Staff also help clients establish friendships and find satisfying leisure activities in their own neighborhoods. Team members play the role of coach, teaching clients daily living skills as well as providing them with emotional support when something new or difficult is attempted.

Employment plays a central role in PACT and is the major means of establishing daily structure for clients (Frey, 1994; Frey & Godfrey, 1991; Russert & Frey, 1991). In the current PACT program in Madison, we use a supported employment model to assist each client with finding and keeping, in the community, a real job that matches her or his interests, skills, and current abilities. Some jobs are found by the client and the PACT vocational staff person by studying together the employment section of the newspaper and making formal applications for jobs that appear appropriate. Others are found by the staff person telephoning various employers to inquire about potential work opportunities that might be appropriate for the client. Most of these placements are part-time at first. We provide clients with active skills teaching and support in their jobs, which involves working with both the client and the employer to help them learn means of coping and structuring the environment so that clients are able to work despite what are often continuing psychotic symptoms. Our goal is that each client will be able to work at his or her optimal level.

The original PACT model was derived from our clinical experiences and sound knowledge of our clients and their illnesses rather than from theory. The model also fits comfortably within a vulnerability–stress theoretical framework of severe mental illnesses (Liberman, 1982; Nuechterlein & Dawson, 1984). Specifically, the PACT core services team provides clients with interventions to decrease their biological vulnerability; it helps them learn skills and provides social supports to strengthen protective factors; and it emphasizes helping clients meet basic needs and secure supportive work and living environments to weaken environmental stressors. Although we are constantly trying to help clients decrease the severity of their symptoms and illness and increase skills, it also is important to help them find environments in which they can function optimally, despite their continuing, often horrendous, illnesses.

## STAFFING AND IMPLICATIONS FOR SOCIAL WORK TRAINING

PACT core team members must have a wide range of aptitudes and professional skills. PACT teams are interdisciplinary and optimally include staff representing the various mental health professions of social work, psychiatric nursing, occupational therapy, psychology, rehabilitation counseling, and psychiatry. If possible, at least 75 percent of the members of a core team should have bachelor's or master's degrees in mental health–related fields, and no more than 25 percent of the total staff should be paraprofessionals.

Each team needs a clinical supervisor who is qualified in social work, nursing, rehabilitation counseling, or psychology, or who is a psychiatrist. The importance of competent clinical supervision cannot be overemphasized. If the team supervisor is someone other than a psychiatrist, it is essential that a psychiatrist be part of the team or provide routine and frequent psychiatric input.

A critical aspect of PACT is that staff work as a team rather than as a group of individual practitioners in the context of a case management program, with responsibility only for their own caseload. In the PACT model, all team members work with all clients. If a staff member is absent for any reason, clients and their family members can still rely on others with whom they have good working relationships. Having team members share responsibilities and create treatment plans together prevents the burnout that can occur when a single staff person is responsible for a caseload of clients, and it also is conducive to creative problem solving.

Although it is helpful to have the specialized skills and knowledge of each of the mental health professionals represented on the PACT team, team members operate interchangeably in the daily functioning of the program. All are constantly involved in the provision of treatment, rehabilitative, and social services because clients' biopsychosocial issues are intertwined, and each staff person needs to be able to respond appropriately and effectively to any situation that might arise. All team members need to be highly knowledgeable about severe mental illnesses and able to implement multiple methods of intervention.

Work by social workers in PACT models with people with severe mental illnesses requires training in both generalist social work methods and clinical social work as well as specific knowledge of and experience with people with severe mental illnesses. Much of the PACT model is founded on traditions of generalist social work practice that focus on the person in the environment and requires a constant use of systemic assessment and flexible problem-solving methods. Social workers have much to offer in the training of other team members in these methods. Good clinical skills also are essential and cannot be overemphasized. These skills include interviewing, assessment, treatment planning, and intervention. Finally, specific knowledge of severe mental illnesses is critical, including information about etiology, signs and symptoms, course, and specific treatment methods (medications and psychosocial). Although some training takes place on the job, as team members from each discipline learn the knowledge and skills of the others through exchanges at daily team meetings and working together, there is no substitute for quality generalized and specialized training in professional schools.

## RESEARCH ON THE EFFECTIVENESS OF THE PACT MODEL

Our initial study in the 1970s evaluated the use of PACT as an alternative to hospitalization (Stein & Test, 1980). The study subjects were an unselected group of diagnostically mixed clients (ages 18 to 62) who were seeking inpatient admission to the state mental hospital in Madison, Wisconsin, and who had any diagnosis other than severe organic brain syndrome, mental retardation, or primary alcoholism. These clients were randomly assigned to either PACT or a control group. Control subjects received the standard treatment used in that community, which was progressive for the time. Specifically, most were admitted to the hospital for a brief period of intensive inpatient treatment, then they were discharged to the community aftercare system. Subjects assigned to the experimental condition were usually not admitted to the hospital but instead were immediately involved in the community-based PACT model. In this study the experimental subjects received the PACT treatment for 14 months, after which they were discharged to the existing community programs in Dane County, Wisconsin. All study subjects were followed up and assessed by independent research analysts every four months, for a total of 28 months.

The within-treatment results were strikingly positive. During the 14 months that the experimental group was treated in the PACT model, they demonstrated markedly less time spent in psychiatric institutions, greater independent-living skills, less symptomatology, and higher satisfaction compared with the control group. They also showed advantages in the areas of work and social functioning: Compared with the control subjects, they spent more time in sheltered, although not competitive, employment and reported having more trusted friends and belonging to more social groups.

An additional part of the evaluation was a comprehensive economic benefit–cost analysis (Weisbrod, Test, & Stein, 1980). This analysis revealed that the new model was economically feasible, with the overall costs and benefits of the PACT model and the usual (traditional) model of care being similar. Meanwhile, an assessment of the relative social costs of PACT, compared with the traditional model, demonstrated that PACT resulted in no greater burden to family or community members, even though the clients in PACT were spending much more time in the community (Test & Stein, 1980).

The final part of the evaluation consisted of following clients for 14 months after they were discharged from PACT to ascertain if the within-treatment benefits held up. A critical finding was that for the most part, they did not; most of the positive effects were lost by the end of the 14-month follow-up period (Stein & Test, 1980). Similar results have been found with virtually all biological and psychosocial treatments studied to date (antipsychotic medications, day treatment, family psychoeducation, and so forth) (Bellack & Mueser, 1993; Hogarty et al., 1991; Test, 1981). These findings suggest that treatment programs for people with severe and persistent mental illnesses may need to be ongoing and long term rather than time limited.

After completion of the original PACT study, a number of other controlled studies of the model took place in various parts of the United States and abroad. These studies were needed to ascertain if the positive findings of the Madison project would generalize to other settings and client populations. Studies of early replications and adaptations of PACT took place in Kent County, Michigan (Mulder, 1985); Sydney, Australia (Hoult, Reynolds, Charbonneau-Powis, Weekes, & Briggs, 1983); Chicago (Bond et al., 1990); and three sites in Indiana (Bond, Miller, Krumwied, & Ward, 1988). The findings of these and other "first-generation" PACT studies were reviewed by Olfson (1990) and Test (1992). They showed consistent and marked effects of PACT in reducing the number of days spent in psychiatric hospitals. Some studies (Hoult et al., 1983; Stein & Test, 1980) found greater reductions in the symptoms of study subjects compared with control subjects. Clients in the PACT program expressed more satisfaction with life, compared with control subjects, in the majority of studies that measured this variable. Social and work functioning, when measured, revealed mixed results: The advantages of PACT, when found, were modest. Overall, studies suggested that the costs of PACT interventions were equal to or less than the control conditions (Hoult et al., 1983; Mulder, 1985; Weisbrod et al., 1980).

A second generation of controlled studies of PACT was completed between 1990 and 1994 and has recently been reviewed by Burns and Santos (1995). Some of these studies featured such methodological improvements as increased monitoring of the experimental and comparison interventions, larger sample sizes, and longer duration of treatment. They also involved a wider range of clients with severe mental illnesses, including veterans (Rosenheck, Neale, Leaf, Milstein, & Frisman, 1995), clients in Great Britain (Marks et al., 1994), young adults with recent-onset schizophrenia (Test et al., 1991), and homeless people with severe mental illnesses (Morse, Calsyn, Allen, Tempelhoff, & Smith, 1992). One study combined assertive community treatment with family psychoeducation (McFarlane, Stastny, & Deakins, 1992). After review of these studies, Burns and Santos (1995) concluded that there continues to be strong evidence for a powerful effect of PACT on reducing the number of days spent in psychiatric hospitals. In addition, they noted that several studies reported improvements in independent living and clinical status as well as high rates of client and family satisfaction associated with PACT. However, the impact on social and work functioning continued to be only modest, when found. The two studies that evaluated costs found them to be lower in PACT than the comparison condition (Knapp et al., 1994; Rosenheck et al., 1995).

More controlled studies of PACT are in progress. Among them are a comparison of PACT with a high-quality alternative model of community care (Essock &

Kontos, 1995), a study with homeless people in a large urban area (Dixon, Krauss, Kernan, Lehman, & DeForge, 1995), a study of mentally ill people with co-occurring substance abuse (Teague, Drake, & Ackerson, 1995), a rural study (Santos et al., 1993), and a study of long-term PACT treatment with a major emphasis on helping clients improve their work functioning (Test et al., 1991).

The completed trials have powerfully demonstrated the efficacy of the PACT model in reducing time spent in hospitals and increasing community tenure. Many studies have supported other benefits, such as increased independent living, reduced symptomatology, and greater client and family satisfaction. These findings have demonstrated generalizability for women and men (Test, Burke, & Wallisch, 1990), several ethnic groups (white people and African Americans have been studied most often), Americans and citizens of other countries, clients coming into the model from hospital or community settings, people living in large urban or smaller city settings, and homeless people. Thus, the PACT model is an effective approach to helping people with severe mental illnesses live in freedom among us with a decent quality of life, despite the presence of continuing illnesses for which we have not found a cure.

As a result of these positive research findings, the PACT model is being widely disseminated throughout the United States and elsewhere (Deci et al., 1995). Several states have adopted the model statewide, and some (for example, Rhode Island and Wisconsin) have developed clear program standards to define the PACT model. McGrew and colleagues (McGrew & Bond, 1995; McGrew, Bond, Dietzen, & Salyers, 1994) have developed a fidelity index of PACT program implementation in a study that used experts (that is, people who had done research on PACT or had been administrative–clinical leaders of PACT programs) to rate the critical components of the model. Brekke and Test (1992) also have presented and tested a model for measuring implementation of community support programs. These efforts to define and monitor program elements and implementation are critical to the valid replication of PACT, and they will enable empirical study of the aspects of the model that account for its positive outcomes.

# Psychosocial Rehabilitation Center Model

## BACKGROUND

An early community care model that has shown remarkable resilience and has some empirical support is the psychosocial rehabilitation center or "clubhouse" model. This well-defined approach evolved from Fountain House in New York City, which was begun in 1948 by a group of former psychiatric patients to provide mutual support and self-help. The philosophy and goals of the clubhouse approach were summarized by John Beard (1978), a clubhouse pioneer who was the director of Fountain House for many years:

> In brief, what we are trying to do in the daytime hours at Fountain House is to serve more adequately the increasing numbers of people leaving our mental institutions who are obviously not needed by the community to which they are returning. A contributing or participating role is simply not available to them. . . . In our day program at Fountain House, we are trying to create a community of people where the individual patient, as a club member, can make a genuine contribution, can be clearly needed, authentically appreciated

and recognized. We would like our environment to be one which expects individuals to arrive, and is aware of their absence. In many ways we are a
kind of family, a large extended family, where disappointments occur, aspira-
tions emerge, and opportunities of many kinds are available. Our relationships to each other reflect, we hope, a continuity and personal relevance to
whatever is happening in one's life, and the range of such experiences is indeed broad and diverse. (p. 203)

## DESCRIPTION OF THE MODEL

The site of this approach is a comfortable, community-based center to which clients
come during days and evenings—a kind of center of community life (Stroul, 1986).
Clubhouses are often open seven days a week, including evenings. Clients are called
"members," and the heart of the model is that the members themselves run the
clubhouse and its activities—it is *their* place. Thus, a strong consumer-centered, empowerment philosophy prevails.

Daily activities of running the clubhouse are work ordered. Members participate in one or more work units to greet visitors and answer the telephone, shop for
food, prepare and serve a lunch (most clubhouses serve at least a midday meal),
make hospital and home visits, or compose and issue a newsletter. Members participate in all decisions about clubhouse operation. As a result, clients are members of
a meaningful and supportive society to which they may belong without time limits
(Stroul, 1986). Staff have a nonhierarchical relationship with members, and it is often difficult to tell staff from clients. Illness issues are downplayed (clubhouses typically link members with providers of mental health services rather than providing
these themselves), and a focus on strengths prevails.

Most clubhouses now have extended programs that go beyond the center itself.
Social and recreational activities are available at the facility but typically extend to
allow members to use leisure opportunities in the community. Some clubhouses offer a range of residential options for members, ranging from highly supportive, supervised settings to more integrated settings, such as supervised apartments (which
are sometimes in an apartment complex operated by the center). The clubhouse
also provides general case management services, including helping with entitlements and advocacy.

Assistance with employment is a key aspect of the clubhouse approach. Clubhouses offer their own transitional employment programs (TEPs) (Macias, Kinney,
& Rodican, 1995). In the TEP model of work rehabilitation, the clubhouse finds
paid jobs that are available to its members who want to work. The clubhouse trains
and supervises its members in these jobs and assures the employer that the work will
be done—that is, if a member is not able to work on a given day, another member
might take his or her place, or a staff member might perform the job. Transitional
employment placements are part-time and time limited, usually 20 hours per week
and six months in duration. Members doing well in TEPs receive support and assistance from the clubhouse in securing and maintaining independent employment.

Grants from both the National Institute of Mental Health and private foundations have supported formal dissemination of the clubhouse model, and well over
200 clubhouses have been founded in the United States. In 1990, through a consen-
sual process, the clubhouse community created and adopted *Standards for Clubhouse
Programs* to define the clubhouse philosophy and the various aspects of the model
(Propst, 1992). Special issues of *Psychosocial Rehabilitation Journal* ("The Clubhouse

Model," 1992) and *New Directions for Mental Health Services* (Dincin, 1995) have provided further information about the clubhouse approach.

## RESEARCH ON THE EFFECTIVENESS OF THE CLUBHOUSE MODEL

The clubhouse model is widely used, so it is surprising and unfortunate that very few controlled studies have been conducted to examine its effectiveness. In an early study of Fountain House, Beard, Pitt, Fisher, and Goertzel (1963) followed relatively long-stay clients who had been discharged from hospitals to either Fountain House or a no-aftercare control group. Two years after admission to the clubhouse program, statistically significantly fewer of the Fountain House clients had been rehospitalized, compared with control subjects. There were no differences in employment rates. At nine-year follow-up the differences between the two groups had diminished (Beard, Malamud, & Rossman, 1978).

In a more comprehensive study Dincin and Witheridge (1982) evaluated Thresholds, a psychosocial rehabilitation center in Chicago. Clients (many were young adults with schizophrenic disorders) were randomly assigned to the comprehensive Thresholds program or the control condition, a part-time supportive treatment at a different location. Thresholds clients participated in the typical clubhouse activities (including prevocational and TEP work rehabilitation); received services from an individual caseworker; and were eligible to live in special, transitional residential facilities. After nine months there were statistically significant differences in the number of clients who had been rehospitalized (14 percent of Thresholds clients compared with 44 percent of control subjects). The results of the study also suggested that although clients of the psychosocial rehabilitation center developed stronger social networks, these networks did not result in greater employment, more participation in leisure activities, or less symptomatology, compared with control subjects.

Recent controlled evaluations of the full psychosocial rehabilitation center model have been lacking, but some clubhouses have conducted quasi-experimental research (Cook, 1995). Considerable attention is now being given to evaluations of different approaches to employment rehabilitation, a domain in which clubhouse methods pioneered. Reviews of this literature noted that although prevocational and TEP jobs enhance clients' work activities, they do not appear to have a meaningful effect on rates of competitive employment (Bond, 1992; Lehman, 1995). Nontransitional approaches, which involve direct placement and support in real jobs ("supported employment"), may hold more promise. As a result, some clubhouses are now beginning to incorporate employment approaches using direct placement and support into their work with members (Cook & Razzano, 1992).

## Consumer-Run Programs and Services

### BACKGROUND

The past decade has seen an enormous growth in consumer-run programs and services. Little research on their effectiveness has yet taken place, but this model of community-based services is discussed here because it is an important new direction in community care and one that may provide important opportunities for social work collaboration in research evaluation. Consumer-run programs can be loosely defined as services developed, controlled, and operated by their consumers—that is, the clients. They are usually organized so that responsibility, control, and decision making are shared among the consumer membership; participation is completely voluntary. These programs are an outgrowth of the psychiatric patients' movement that advocates self-determination (Zinman, 1986) and of the self-help movement and its philosophy that the best helpers may well be those who have experienced similar problems (Stroul, 1986).

Consumer-run programs are distinctive and powerful because consumers are in the dual roles of receiving services and, at the same time, providing services (Borkman, 1991). Both processes are hypothesized to be empowering and helpful because, in the former role, clients have access to needed resources and community, and in the latter role, they assume meaningful and responsible roles that are often denied to them in the larger society. Chamberlin, Rogers, and Sneed (1989) noted, "Empowerment within the group leads to a sense that members should have a say in mental health matters generally and to a rejection of the role of passive service recipient" (p. 101). Furthermore, over time gradual reductions in the stigma perceived by the general public may occur because those who are not mentally ill will see people with mental illnesses performing far more competently than earlier stereotypes allowed.

A wide range of services and programs are run by consumers with severe and persistent mental illnesses. These services vary in size, organization, type of activities, and linkages and relationships with the mental health system. They now go far beyond self-help and support groups to include consumer-run drop-in centers; social, recreational, and educational programs; advocacy and case management; and residential, crisis, and vocational services. Although they are often run by consumer volunteers, more and more such programs are now funded by local, state, and federal authorities. For example, from late 1988 through 1992, the National Institute of Mental Health's Community Support Program funded 13 three-year, consumer-operated demonstration projects (Brown & Parrish, 1995). These included drop-in centers, affordable housing, live-in companions, a program to feed homeless people, and consumer-provided linkage of inpatients to community supports to aid discharge and transition to community living.

## RESEARCH ON THE EFFECTIVENESS OF CONSUMER-RUN SERVICES

Little research has been conducted on the effectiveness of consumer-run services because implementation of these models is recent, and there are particular challenges involved in the study and evaluation of self-help efforts in general (Borkman, 1991). Methods and collaborative arrangements that preserve the integrity and autonomy of self-help groups and programs but allow scientifically valid conclusions to be drawn need to be developed. The October 1991 issue of the *American Journal of Community Psychology*, a special issue on self-help groups, published excellent articles describing these evaluation challenges and some innovative solutions to them (Borkman, 1991).

Most research on consumer-run services to date has been descriptive. Two relatively large studies examined who is served by self-help agencies or groups for mental health clients and why members joined (Segal, Silverman, & Temkin, 1995; Young & Williams, 1988). Other reports described specific programs and their operations (Lieberman, Gowdy, & Knutson, 1991; Mowbray, Chamberlain, Jennings, & Reed, 1988; Mowbray, Wellwood, & Chamberlain, 1988). Research on the self-help group GROW was among the most sophisticated and included theoretical examination (McFadden, Seidman, & Rappaport, 1992), but the focus was on process rather than outcome. Other reports have discussed or described how self-help groups relate to professionals (Emerick, 1990; Toro et al., 1988).

Three studies offered useful process evaluations of how consumer-run programs are implemented and the extent to which they carry out their proposed functions (Chamberlin, Rogers, & Ellison, 1996; Kaufmann, Ward-Colasante, & Farmer, 1993; Mowbray & Tan, 1993). These studies also included a soft "effectiveness" evaluation conducted by asking members about their satisfaction with the services. The work of Mowbray and Tan also asked consumers to evaluate retrospectively how the programs had affected their lives. All these studies found high satisfaction with services, and results of the Mowbray and Tan survey suggested positive influences on clients' lives. As the authors' themselves indicated, however, these evaluative efforts are only first steps, and they had serious design problems, such as nonrepresentative sampling and lack of a comparison group.

In the most methodologically advanced study of effectiveness, Solomon and Draine (1995) used a true experimental design to compare the one- and two-year outcomes of clients randomly assigned to receive services from a consumer case management team or from a team of nonconsumer case managers. The sample size was 48 for each group, and the outcomes assessed included subjective quality of life, disposable monthly income, symptomatology, social relationships and functioning, attitudes toward medication compliance, and hospitalization. Results revealed no differences in the one- or two-year outcomes of clients who had been case managed by the consumer team, compared with the nonconsumer team. This finding supported the authors' hypothesis that clients who were case managed by the consumers would fare no differently from those case managed by the nonconsumers. As the authors noted, however, critical methodological issues impeded firm conclusions. In particular, the study lacked sufficient statistical power to detect a difference, if it existed. In addition, it did not contain a control group who received usual services, thus leaving unknown whether either of the case management conditions demonstrated any benefits beyond a services system without case management.

It is important that evaluation efforts of consumer-run programs have begun and that successful models of collaborating with consumers in design, instrumentation, and implementation of such programs have been demonstrated. Now there is a need to go much further in the evaluation of these potentially valuable additions to community care for people with severe and persistent mental illnesses.

## Conclusion

In some parts of the United States, our care system for people with severe mental illnesses approaches being a national shame. Hundreds, even thousands, of such people rotate in and out of hospitals, jails, and homelessness and experience a consistent substandard quality of life. In other places the picture is not horrendous but remains far from optimal. In an era in which we are beginning to find treatments with meaningful demonstrated benefits for people with these illnesses, such interventions are not reaching many people with severe mental illnesses, and their symptoms and marked suffering needlessly persist.

The reasons for our poor mental health care system are many and include broad policy and administrative factors such as the lack of a coherent public health care policy, fragmentation of responsibility, and insufficient funding. These problems will take time to correct and will require persistent and targeted advocacy at the federal, state, and local levels by mental health professionals, consumers, and other citizens.

Yet we need not wait for a uniform national health care policy or more funding to make major improvements in care of people with severe and persistent mental illnesses. We can ensure that available mental health care dollars are funding programs with demonstrated efficacy rather than supporting interventions that have little value for this population. To strengthen the knowledge base of "what works for whom," we also can increase our efforts to evaluate interventions currently being used.

Wider dissemination of PACT will be a helpful step. This model has demonstrated efficacy in terms of marked reductions in hospitalization time, more independent living, more favorable clinical status, and higher satisfaction of clients and their families, which makes it imperative that it be widely implemented. PACT's costs have been found to be similar to or even less than those of traditional models, so it is an attractive alternative to policymakers. Social workers can play a major role in the adoption and implementation of this model. As frequent leaders of social change efforts, they can advocate for its adoption and provide leadership in the development and implementation of PACT teams. My experience is that the model is rewarding for energetic and creative staff because PACT not only supports but requires staff who are flexible; can work independently as well as with team members; can form positive relationships with clients, their families, and community members; and are willing to do whatever is needed to help clients reach their goals.

Much more work is needed in the search for effective and efficient models of community-based care. The PACT model has demonstrated efficacy, and research now needs to address such questions as which clients in the mental health system are most appropriate for PACT, what are its critical ingredients, how long clients need it, how it can be modified for certain special populations, how it can have more powerful effects on social and work functioning, and how it fits with the rest of the services system (Drake & Burns, 1995; Test, 1992). Other effective models of community-based care are needed, especially ones that will substantially affect social supports and social functioning for people with serious mental illness. Two promising models have been presented here, the psychosocial rehabilitation center (clubhouse) approach and consumer-run programs. Both require further evaluation of their effectiveness if they are to survive in this era of cost containment. Social work researchers, with their applied research training and strong consumer-oriented focus, will be ideal participants in this critical work.

# References

Beard, J. H. (1978). The rehabilitation services of Fountain House. In L. I. Stein & M. A. Test (Eds.), *Alternative to mental hospital treatment* (pp. 201–208). New York: Plenum Press.

Beard, J. H., Malamud, T. J., & Rossman, E. (1978). Psychiatric rehabilitation and long-term rehospitalization rates: The findings of two research studies. *Schizophrenia Bulletin, 4*, 622–635.

Beard, J. H., Pitt, R. B., Fisher, S. H., & Goertzel, V. (1963). Evaluating the effectiveness of a psychiatric rehabilitation program. *American Journal of Orthopsychiatry, 33*, 701–712.

Bellack, A. S., & Mueser, K. T. (1993). Psychosocial treatment for schizophrenia. *Schizophrenia Bulletin, 19*, 317–336.

Bond, G. R. (1992). Vocational rehabilitation. In R. P. Liberman (Ed.), *Handbook of psychiatric rehabilitation* (pp. 244–263). New York: Macmillan.

Bond, G. R., Miller, L. D., Krumwied, R. D., & Ward, R. S. (1988). Assertive case management in three CMHCs: A controlled study. *Hospital and Community Psychiatry, 39,* 411–418.

Bond, G. R., Witheridge, T. F., Dincin, J., Wasmer, D., Webb, J., & De Graaf-Kaser, R. (1990). Assertive community treatment for frequent users of psychiatric hospitals in a large city: A controlled study. *American Journal of Community Psychology, 18,* 865–890.

Borkman, T. J. (1991). Introduction to the special issue. *American Journal of Community Psychology, 19,* 643–650.

Brekke, J. S., & Test, M. A. (1987). An empirical analysis of services delivered in a model community support program. *Psychosocial Rehabilitation Journal, 10,* 51–61.

Brekke, J. S., & Test, M. A. (1992). A model for measuring the implementation of community support programs: Results from three sites. *Community Mental Health Journal, 28,* 227–247.

Brown, N. B., & Parrish, J. (1995). CSP: Champion of self-help. *Journal of the California Alliance for the Mentally Ill, 6*(3), 6–7.

Burns, B. J., & Santos, A. B. (1995). Assertive community treatment: An update of randomized trials. *Psychiatric Services, 46,* 669–675.

Chamberlin, J., Rogers, E. S., & Ellison, M. S. (1996). Self-help programs: A description of their characteristics and their members. *Psychiatric Rehabilitation Journal, 19,* 33–42.

Chamberlin, J., Rogers, J. A., & Sneed, C. S. (1989). Consumers, families, and community support systems. *Psychosocial Rehabilitation Journal, 12,* 93–106.

Cook, J. A. (1995). Program evaluation and research at Thresholds. *New Directions for Mental Health Services, 68,* 75–85.

Cook, J. A., & Razzano, L. (1992). Natural vocational supports for persons with severe mental illness: Thresholds supported competitive employment program. *New Directions for Mental Health Services, 56,* 23–41.

Deci, P. A., Santos, A. B., Hiott, W., Schoenwald, S., & Dias, J. K. (1995). Dissemination of assertive community treatment programs. *Psychiatric Services, 46,* 676–678.

Dincin, J. (Ed.). (1995). A pragmatic approach to psychiatric rehabilitation: Lessons from Chicago's Thresholds program. *New Directions for Mental Health Services, 68.*

Dincin, J., & Witheridge, T. F. (1982). Psychiatric rehabilitation as a deterrent to recidivism. *Hospital and Community Psychiatry, 33,* 645–650.

Dixon, L. B., Krauss, N., Kernan, E., Lehman, A. F., & DeForge, B. R. (1995). Modifying the PACT model to serve homeless persons with severe mental illness. *Psychiatric Services, 46,* 684–688.

Drake, R. E., & Burns, B. J. (1995). Special section on Assertive Community Treatment: An introduction. *Psychiatric Services, 46,* 667–668.

Emerick, R. E. (1990). Self-help groups for former patients: Relations with mental health professionals. *Hospital and Community Psychiatry, 41,* 401–407.

Essock, S. M., & Kontos, N. (1995). Implementing assertive community treatment teams. *Psychiatric Services, 466,* 679–683.

Frey, J. L. (1994). Long term support: The critical element to sustaining competitive employment: Where do we begin? *Psychosocial Rehabilitation Journal, 17,* 127–134.

Frey J. L., & Godfrey M. (1991). A comprehensive clinical vocational assessment: The PACT approach. *Journal of Applied Rehabilitation Counseling, 22*(2), 25–28.

Hogarty, G. E., Anderson, C. M., Reiss, D. J., Kornblith, S. J., Greenwald, D. P., Ulrich, R. F., & Carter, M. (1991). Family psychoeducation, social skills training, and maintenance chemotherapy in the aftercare treatment of schizophrenia: II. Two-year effects of a controlled study on relapse and adjustment. *Archives of General Psychiatry, 48,* 340–347.

Hoult, J., Reynolds, I., Charbonneau-Powis, M., Weekes, P., & Briggs, J. (1983). Psychiatric hospital versus community treatment: The results of a randomized trial. *Australian and New Zealand Journal of Psychiatry, 17,* 160–167.

Kaufmann, C. L., Ward-Colasante, M.A.R., & Farmer, J. (1993). Development and evaluation of drop-in centers operated by mental health consumers. *Hospital and Community Psychiatry, 44,* 675–678.

Knapp, M., Beecham, J., Koutsogeorgopoulou, V., Hallam, A., Fenyo, A., Marks, I. M., Connolly, J., Audini, B., & Muijen, M. (1994). Service use and costs of home-based versus hospital-based care for people with serious mental illness. *British Journal of Psychiatry, 165,* 195–203.

Lehman, A. F. (1995). Vocational rehabilitation in schizophrenia. *Schizophrenia Bulletin, 21,* 645–656.

Liberman, R. P. (1982). What is schizophrenia? *Schizophrenia Bulletin, 8,* 435–437.

Lieberman, M. A., Gowdy, E. A., & Knutson, L. C. (1991). The Mental Health Outreach Project: A case study in self-help. *Psychosocial Rehabilitation Journal, 14,* 100–104.

Macias, C., Kinney, R., & Rodican, C. (1995). Transitional employment: An evaluative description of Fountain House practice. *Journal of Vocational Rehabilitation, 5,* 151–158.

Marks, I. M., Connolly, J., Muijen, M., Audini, B., McNamee, G., & Lawrence, R. E. (1994). Home-based versus hospital care for people with serious mental illness. *British Journal of Psychiatry, 165,* 179–194.

Marx, A. J., Test, M. A., & Stein, L. I. (1973). Extrohospital management of severe mental illness. *Archives of General Psychiatry, 29,* 505–511.

McFadden, L., Seidman, E., & Rappaport, J. (1992). A comparison of espoused theories of self- and mutual help: Implications for mental health professionals. *Professional Psychology: Research and Practice, 23,* 515–520.

McFarlane, W. R., Stastny, P., & Deakins, S. (1992). Family-aided assertive community treatment: A comprehensive rehabilitation and intensive case management approach for persons with schizophrenic disorders. *New Directions for Mental Health Services, 53,* 43–54.

McGrew, J., & Bond, G. (1995). Critical ingredients of assertive community treatment: Judgments of the experts. *Journal of Mental Health Administration, 22,* 113–125.

McGrew, J. H., Bond, G. R., Dietzen, L., & Salyers, M. (1994). Measuring the fidelity of implementation of a mental health program model. *Journal of Consulting and Clinical Psychology, 62,* 670–678.

Mechanic, D., & Rochefort, D. A. (1990). Deinstitutionalization: An appraisal of reform. *Annual Review of Sociology, 16,* 301–327.

Morse, G. A., Calsyn, R. J., Allen, G., Tempelhoff, B., & Smith, R. (1992). Experimental comparison of the effects of three treatment programs for homeless mentally ill people. *Hospital and Community Psychiatry, 43,* 1005–1010.

Mowbray, C. T., Chamberlain, P. J., Jennings, M., & Reed, C. (1988). Consumer-run mental health services: Results from five demonstration projects. *Community Mental Health Journal, 24,* 151–156.

Mowbray, C. T., & Tan, C. (1993). Consumer-operated drop-in centers: Evaluation of operations and impact. *Journal of Mental Health Administration, 20,* 8–19.

Mowbray, C. T., Wellwood, R., & Chamberlain, P. J. (1988). Project Stay: A consumer-run support service. *Psychosocial Rehabilitation Journal, 12,* 33–42.

Mulder, R. (1985). *Evaluation of the Harbinger Program, 1982–1985.* Lansing, MI: Department of Mental Health.

Nuechterlein, K., & Dawson, M. (1984). A heuristic vulnerability/stress model of schizophrenic episodes. *Schizophrenia Bulletin, 10,* 300–312.

Olfson, M. (1990). Assertive community treatment: An evaluation of the experimental evidence. *Hospital and Community Psychiatry, 41,* 634–641.

Propst, R. N. (1992). Standards for clubhouse programs: Why and how they were developed. *Psychosocial Rehabilitation Journal, 16,* 25–30.

Rosenheck, R., Neale, M., Leaf, P., Milstein, R., & Frisman, L. (1995). Multisite experimental cost study of intensive psychiatric community care. *Schizophrenia Bulletin, 21,* 129–140.

Russert, G. R., & Frey, J. L. (1991). The PACT vocational model: A step into the future. *Journal of Applied Rehabilitation Counseling, 14,* 7–18.

Santos, A. B., Deci, P. A., Lachance, K. R., Dias, J. K., Sloop, T. B., Hiert, T. G., & Bevilacqua, J. J. (1993). Providing assertive community treatment for severely mentally ill patients in a rural area. *Hospital and Community Psychiatry, 44,* 34–39.

Segal, S. P., Silverman, C., & Temkin, T. (1995). Characteristics and service use of long-term members of self-help agencies for mental health clients. *Psychiatric Services, 46,* 269–274.

Solomon, P., & Draine, J. (1995). The efficacy of a consumer case management team: 2-year outcomes of a randomized trial. *Journal of Mental Health Administration, 22,* 135–146.

Stein, L. I., & Test, M. A. (1980). Alternative to mental hospital treatment. I. Conceptual model, treatment program, and clinical evaluation. *Archives of General Psychiatry, 37,* 392–397.

Stein, L. I., & Test, M. A. (1985). The evolution of the Training in Community Living model. *New Directions for Mental Health Services, 26,* 7–16.

Strauss, J. S., Hafez, H., Lieberman, P., & Harding, C. M. (1985). The course of psychiatric disorder. III: Longitudinal principles. *American Journal of Psychiatry, 142,* 289–296.

Stroul, B. A. (1986). *Models of community support services: Approaches to helping persons with long-term mental illness.* Boston: Center for Psychiatric Rehabilitation.

Teague, G. B., Drake, R. B., & Ackerson, T. H. (1995). Evaluating use of continuous treatment teams for persons with mental illness and substance abuse. *Psychiatric Services, 46,* 689–695.

Test, M. A. (1981). Effective treatment of the chronically mentally ill: What is necessary? *Journal of Social Issues, 37,* 71–86.

Test, M. A. (1992). The Training in Community Living Model. In R. P. Liberman (Ed.), *Handbook of psychiatric rehabilitation* (pp. 153–170). New York: Macmillan.

Test, M. A., Burke, S. S., & Wallisch, L. S. (1990). Gender differences of young adults with schizophrenic disorders in community care. *Schizophrenia Bulletin, 16,* 331–344.

Test, M. A., Knoedler, W. H., & Allness, D. J. (1985). The long-term treatment of young schizophrenics in a community support program. In L. I. Stein & M. A. Test (Eds.), *New directions for mental health services: Vol. 26. The Training in Community Living Model: A decade of experience* (pp. 17–27). San Francisco: Jossey-Bass.

Test, M. A., Knoedler, W. H., Allness, D. J., Burke, S. S., Brown, R. L., & Wallisch, L. S. (1991). Long-term community care through an assertive continuous treatment team. In C. A. Tamminga & S. C. Schultz (Eds.), *Advances in neuropsychiatry and psychopharmacology: Vol. 1. Schizophrenia research* (pp. 239–246). New York: Raven Press.

Test, M. A., & Stein, L. I. (1980). Alternative to mental hospital treatment: III. Social cost. *Archives of General Psychiatry, 37,* 409–412.

The clubhouse model [Special Issue]. (1992). *Psychosocial Rehabilitation Journal.*

Toro, P. A., Reischl, T. M., Zimmerman, M., Rappaport, J., Seidman, E., Luke, D. A., & Roberts, L. J. (1988). Professionals in mutual help groups: Impact on social climate and members' behavior. *Journal of Consulting and Clinical Psychology, 56,* 631–632.

Torrey, E. F. (1986). Continuous treatment teams in the care of the chronically mentally ill. *Hospital and Community Psychiatry, 37,* 1243–1247.

Weisbrod, B. A., Test, M. A., & Stein, L. I. (1980). Alternative to mental hospital treatment: II. Economic benefit–cost analysis. *Archives of General Psychiatry, 37,* 400–405.

Young, J., & Williams, C. L. (1988). Whom do mutual-help groups help? A typology of members. *Hospital and Community Psychiatry, 39,* 1178–1182.

Zinman, S. (1986). Self-help: The wave of the future. *Hospital and Community Psychiatry, 37,* 213.

# Substance Abuse Interventions

Robert F. Schilling and Nabila El-Bassel

For more than a decade, polls have reported that Americans consider drug abuse to be among the nation's most serious problems. If part of this concern is a result of a disproportionate amount of press coverage of illicit drug use, it also reflects a perception that alcohol and other mood-altering substances are in some way related to many of the most pressing contemporary social ills. Most Americans perceive that law enforcement is an important element in containing drug abuse but, perhaps less uniformly, they also believe that chemical dependency is a condition that needs treatment. As most Americans have grown used to high-quality health care, it is no accident that the United States has developed a vast and expensive drug abuse treatment industry, largely funded through private and public health insurance (Gerstein & Harwood, 1990; Weisner & Morgan, 1992).

This chapter begins with a brief description of substance abuse intervention, beginning with efforts based on law enforcement and prevention. Then the changing views of chemical dependency and how the evolving understanding of addictive processes affects approaches to treatment are discussed. The major treatment settings, philosophies, and approaches are examined, with roles of social workers emphasized. Alternative treatments and treatment of selected special populations are described, followed by a discussion of the influence of managed care and other structural changes on the treatment of people with substance abuse disorders. Controversial harm reduction perspectives and substance abuse treatment in the context of socioeconomic disadvantage are then discussed. Finally, some new approaches to treating and reducing the harmful effects of drug and alcohol abuse are offered.

## Law Enforcement

Three major approaches to reducing substance abuse can be delineated: supply reduction; demand reduction, which includes prevention and treatment; and harm reduction. Efforts to reduce the supply of chemical substances are carried out in foreign countries, at the U.S. borders, and within the country. Offshore programs, undertaken with the aid of foreign governments, include various strategies to reduce the agricultural production, processing, and transit of illicit substances—primarily heroin, cocaine, and marijuana—at their source. Border interdiction efforts attempt to stop drugs at the point of entry into the country. Domestic law enforcement, carried out by federal, state, and local entities, attempts to reduce the amount of illicit drugs that are grown, processed, and distributed within the country. Domestic law enforcement also is concerned with the illegal sale and distribution of alcohol and tobacco—substances that account for far more morbidity and mortality than do illicit substances. Finally, the court and correctional systems can potentially reduce the supply of drugs through prosecution, adjudication, and incarceration or supervision.

A decades-old debate centers on the extent to which supply-side efforts can reduce drug abuse, and evidence can be marshaled to support either position. Our own observations bring us to the conclusion that supply-side efforts may reduce levels of drug abuse in the United States. However, it is difficult to demonstrate that our nation's efforts in foreign lands have been successful in a sustained way, and the limits of border interdiction are abundantly clear. With the domestic production of increasingly potent marijuana, phencyclidine (PCP), and methamphetamines, foreign eradication and border surveillance become still less relevant strategies to reduce the supply of illicit substances. Domestically, concentrated police efforts can temporarily reduce drug trafficking in urban neighborhoods, but lasting declines in drug-related arrests appear to be related to many factors, including policing. Tough sentencing policies remove low-level criminals from the streets—most incarcerated people were arrested for drug-related crimes—but there is little evidence to suggest that such laws deter sellers of drugs. The United States now has the dubious distinction of being the country with the largest proportion of its population behind bars, and the rise in public spending for prisons appears to be nearing an end. Some observers believe that drug-related crimes will reach new peaks when the next large birth cohorts enter adolescence in the near future (Clarke, 1996; Siegfried, 1996). In our view, these observations evidence the limits of supply reduction approaches to the problem of drug abuse. Although social workers have important roles in many supply reduction settings (such as prisons and criminal justice diversion programs), their tasks focus more on demand reduction than on reducing the supply of illicit drugs and improperly distributed alcohol.

## Prevention and Social Work

It is wise to prevent the harmful use of mood-altering substances, given the adverse personal and societal consequences of drug and alcohol abuse and the difficulty of treating established addictive disorders (Altman, 1995; Schinke & Cole, 1995). Chemical dependence inflicts the most harm, including possible high-risk behaviors for AIDS, when young people are becoming adults, beginning careers, and rearing families. Thus, even modest reductions in risk behavior among certain age groups and populations may yield substantial and lifelong returns. Aside from a few narrowly disseminated prevention programs (Botvin, Schinke, & Orlandi, 1995; Kolata, 1996; Schinke et al., 1986), it is difficult to find demonstrably effective prevention approaches in use (Kreft & Brown, 1998).

Social workers are ideally prepared to develop and carry out drug abuse prevention strategies by virtue of their experience with the populations at risk, behaviors and attitudes related to drug abuse, and the communitywide implications of prevention practice (Van Wormer, 1995). No other profession has more experience in tailoring services for low-income populations from nondominant ethnic and racial groups, who make up a disproportionate number of people with substance abuse disorders.

Social workers appreciate that successful prevention strategies are likely to be integrated within social structures, including the family and the workplace. They understand that communitywide shifts in values and knowledge must occur if people's intentions and behaviors are to be sustained in the social environment. Social worker practitioners are skilled in collaborating with community leaders, agencies, and groups. As a profession, however, social work cannot claim unique expertise in altering conduct or conditions related to the initiation of drug use.

Relatively few social workers are now in positions with the principal task of prevention of addictive behavior. The prospects for preventive social work suffered in the 1970s as the nation and the profession turned their attention away from community organization, and schools of social work dropped concentrations in this method of practice. Prevention curricula have yet to be adopted in most schools of social work, so beginning social workers have limited backgrounds in prevention. They encounter few role models in academe or the field who are engaged in prevention. Whatever the merits of the profession's person-in-environment perspective, it has not resulted in much interest in well-conceptualized preventive interventions targeted at communities and intact groups. Traditionally, the profession has attracted people who seek to help individuals and families in agency-based, direct practice settings. The majority of social work practitioners feel most useful and comfortable in situations that involve an identified problem and an accessible, ideally voluntary, client or family. In contrast, a community at risk is impersonal and difficult to define, will never directly ask for help, and cannot readily indicate when an intervention has been successful or appreciated.

Consequently, few social workers are involved in carefully delineated efforts to prevent the initiation of drug use or to prevent early use from becoming abuse. It is tempting to address prevention as one aspect of intervention, but the prevention of substance abuse by social workers merits attention on its own (Schilling & McAlister, 1990; Schinke & Cole, 1995). Because treatment and prevention of substance abuse are more dissimilar than alike, we will not attempt to cover the latter in this chapter.

## Treatment and Social Work

The scope of substance abuse is large and is likely to remain a serious threat to the well-being of some parts of society, but the size of the population that could benefit from treatment is a matter of considerable debate. The adherents of various positions can advance arguments based on differing definitions of abuse and dependence, epidemiologic considerations, and moral and philosophical arguments (Alasuutari, 1992; Peele, 1988, 1989). Few informed people would suggest that most substance abusers would avail themselves of treatment offered on any given day. Thus, the number of people who can currently benefit from treatment is some unknown fraction of the chemically dependent population.

As they are in the field of mental health as a whole, social workers are a prominent profession in chemical dependency treatment. Three relatively distinct roles can be identified: (1) case management and referral, (2) clinical practice, and (3) supervision and administration.

### CASE MANAGEMENT AND REFERRAL

In their direct practice roles in schools, child welfare agencies, programs for homeless people, and programs for elderly people, social workers are often responsible for identifying and making referrals for the treatment of substance abuse and for managing caseloads of people receiving chemical dependency treatment. The skills required to carry out these roles include screening, steering, accessing and brokering of services, and advocacy (Hepworth & Larsen, 1990; Ivanoff, Blythe, & Tripodi, 1994; Schilling, Schinke, & Weatherly, 1988).

## CLINICAL PRACTICE

Social workers also counsel rehabilitation inpatients, conduct therapy with selected patients on methadone medication, and monitor the progress of recovering people in outpatient treatment and community settings (Van Wormer, 1995). A brief list of only a few of the skills required, depending on the setting, includes multidimensional assessment (Hepworth & Larsen, 1990), enhancing motivation (Miller, 1989), social skills training (Chaney, 1989; Schilling, El-Bassel, Hadden, & Gilbert, 1995), stress management (Stockwell & Town, 1989), and relapse prevention (Annis & Davis, 1989; Marlatt & Barrett, 1994; Wilson, 1992) as well as marital and family therapy (Kaufman, 1994; O'Farrell & Cowles, 1989; Steinglass, 1994; Zweben & Pearlman, 1983; Zweben, Pearlman, & Li, 1988), group therapy (Golden & Khantzian, 1994), and psychodynamic approaches that draw on insight and transference phenomena (Frances, Franklin, & Borg, 1994; Woody, Mercer, & Luborsky, 1994).

## SUPERVISION AND ADMINISTRATION

Most often, social workers are found in supervisory and administrative capacities in a range of substance abuse treatment settings. For example, social workers supervise counselors in inpatient rehabilitation units, direct program areas within therapeutic communities and methadone maintenance clinics, and manage agencies and program divisions in youth, criminal justice, and employee assistance settings. Social work supervisors in such positions ideally have direct practice experience with chemically dependent people as well as an understanding of several approaches to treating drug and alcohol abuse. In addition, able supervisors model effective treatment interventions, provide the supervisee with opportunities to take measured risks with substance-using clients, and offer constructive feedback on the social worker's performance (Jacobs, David, & Meyer, 1995).

Kadushin (1992) identified six conditions for effective teaching and learning in the supervisory relationship: We learn best if

1. we are highly motivated
2. we can devote most of our energies in the learning situation to learning
3. learning is attended by positive satisfaction—that is, when it is successful and rewarding
4. we are actively involved in the learning process
5. the content is meaningfully presented
6. the supervisor takes into consideration the supervisee's special qualities as a learner.

Although research on supervision per se in the field of drug abuse treatment is scant, most clinical trials testing psychobehavioral interventions with drug-involved clients have developed sophisticated methods for training therapists to carry out prescribed treatment strategies. The most extensive collection of supervision of training manuals available, which set the standard for both researchers and program developers, was produced in the MATCH study, a multisite trial that compared motivational enhancement therapy, cognitive–behavioral coping skills therapy, and 12-step facilitation therapy (Nowinski, Baker, & Carroll, 1992).

Social workers who administer substance abuse treatment programs will face increasingly difficult management choices that require a broad range of skills. Skidmore (1995) listed no less than 18 ways in which competent administrators can act. Among the most salient are creating innovative policies; trusting staff enough to value their opinions; planning (to reach targets and goals); setting priorities (recognizing that some are more important than others); delegating authority; and motivating and even inspiring staff to use their talents to carry out agency functions. Unquestionably, policy changes present daily challenges to even the most adept managers of social services programs, including those in chemical dependency settings (Au, 1994). In the words of Menefee and Thompson (1994),

> No longer are social work managers predominantly concerned with structures, processes and conditions within the agency; they now give equal if not more attention to the entire context of services delivery by actively monitoring and managing the boundary between the external environment and the internal organizational arrangements. . . . No longer are social work managers planning exclusively at the operational or program level; they are now envisioning the future, planning strategically, and promoting innovation. (pp. 14–15)

# Evolving Perceptions of Addiction

Societal views of addiction and our understanding of its nature continue to evolve. A generation from now, researchers and practitioners will perceive our present understanding of addictive processes as flawed, just as we now view as naive the conceptualizations of substance abuse from decades past. Several major changes in our view of addiction have come about in the past 20 years.

## *PRIMARY DISORDER AND PRAGMATIC STRATEGIES*

One important change has been to define addiction as a primary disorder, rather than a result of other psychological problems or events or as a symptom of "underlying pathology" (Chafetz, Blane, & Hill, 1970; Khantzian, 1980; Silber, 1974). Another change is the recognition of addiction as a chronic condition, likely to occur over long periods, which is largely refractive to present forms of treatment (Daley, 1988; Fillmore, 1987; Fillmore & Midanik, 1984; Hermos, LoCastro, Glynn, Bouchard, & De Labry, 1988). Similarly, it appears that at any one time, only a small number of substance-dependent people will take steps to enter available forms of treatment (Gerstein & Harwood, 1990; Institute of Medicine, 1990).

In addition, failure to directly attend to chemical abuse and dependence renders other forms of psychological treatment pointless. When drug abuse has been assessed or is suspected, helping professionals routinely attempt to involve the client in substance abuse treatment, either before or in combination with other treatment approaches or services. In many cases, practitioners may require substance-abusing people to enroll in such treatment as a condition of participation in other services or opportunities, such as family counseling, job training, or housing. For drug users who have been arrested or lost children to child protective authorities, programs that emphasize alternatives to incarceration or return of parental custody may be conditioned on participation in chemical dependency treatment (Davis, 1984).

Paralleling the increasing acceptance of substance abuse as a primary disorder is a shift away from traditional insight-oriented therapy, which focused on latent experiences antecedent to the onset of the substance abuse disorder (Blatt, McDonald, Sugarman, & Wilber, 1984; Brickman, 1988; Vaillant, 1981). Social workers and other practitioners and program developers are turning to pragmatic, empirically derived helping strategies that deal directly with drinking and drug use (Miller & Hester, 1989). The goals of treatment are to help the client reduce and, ideally, to stop using drugs and alcohol as well as to develop new behavior patterns to avoid relapse. Moreover, programs and movements once driven by seemingly disparate ideologies (for example, methadone maintenance, therapeutic communities, Alcoholics Anonymous) have come to use or at least recognize the legitimacy of many of the same interventive elements. These developments came about as a result of the maturation of the field of chemical dependency treatment, accruing findings that demonstrate the difficulty of effecting lasting change in addictive behavior and external system forces that affect many treatment settings. For example, therapeutic communities, rehabilitation centers, and detoxification units are all giving attention to relapse prevention, accepting the reality of increasingly shorter inpatient stays, and demonstrating new interest in outpatient care. There is widespread understanding within the treatment community that existing interventive strategies have limited potency when addictive disorders co-occur with an array of serious personal, interpersonal, and social problems. Unfortunately, only a few examples exist of demonstrably effective (leading to positive outcomes) linkages between the treatment community and the disparate social services and health care networks that serve indigent people.

## DISEASE MODEL

The medicalization of addiction—the "disease model"—has become dominant (Miller, 1991; Stephens, 1991; Williams, 1988), and dependence on alcohol or drugs is now perceived by most helping professionals, and by an increasing proportion of the public, as an illness rather than a moral weakness. Alcoholics Anonymous (AA) and the other 12-step movements that have grown from AA have been influential in advancing the disease concept of addiction. The illness metaphor is not unique to drug and alcohol problems: It is in some ways consistent with other trends in a society that have been far more successful in describing and diagnosing problems than in developing treatments or shaping social agendas to deal with them (for example, child abuse, violence, severe mental illness, and learning or conduct disorders).

An important aspect of the genesis of AA was a reaction to the perceived failure of the established medical community to appropriately respond to alcoholism. The promulgation of the disease concept of addiction is not entirely consistent with the beliefs and practices that characterize 12-step programs and many drug abuse rehabilitation settings. The emphases on individual responsibility and the acceptance of self as an alcoholic (addict) are perspectives that seem more akin to notions of moral righteousness and humanity's powerlessness than to curing an ailment. The disease concept tends to mask the shades of addiction and overlooks the reality that chemical dependency is related to many factors beyond the biological and personal susceptibility of a person. More recently, we have come to understand that addiction is a complex phenomenon that often affects all areas of a person's life and others around him or her, and it cannot be viewed simply as a within-person problem. Its limitations notwithstanding, however, the disease model has been a useful vehicle for moving the locus of addiction away from one of moral weakness.

## Substance Abuse in Relation to Other Human Problems

Alcohol and drug abuse have long been known to contribute to and be associated with many other misfortunes and disabling conditions, such as poverty and dementia. In recent decades, investigators from many fields, including epidemiology, sociology, and the helping professions, have demonstrated that chemical dependence is correlated with social and economic disadvantage, psychiatric disability, and morbidity and mortality. Still more recently, scientists have studied the correlation of drug abuse and injury, crime, family disorganization, and homelessness. Increases in comorbidity are probably due to both an actual increase in some forms of drug abuse (such as crack cocaine use), correlated social phenomena (for example, homelessness, violence), and increased surveillance. Clinicians and services providers are now better trained to consider and assess drug abuse and dependence, and law enforcement and public health officials have installed systems for tracking rates of chemical dependence in households, schools and colleges, and criminal justice and health care settings.

Although media portrayals of drug abuse sometimes reflect the lifestyles of certain entertainers and professional athletes, problems of chemical dependence are more than ever experienced by the most disadvantaged populations. Crime and violence, family disintegration, mental disorder, unemployment, and homelessness are highly correlated with chemical abuse and dependency (Anderson, 1995; Schilling, Ivanoff, El-Bassel, & Soffa, 1997), and in many urban communities, these conditions are now demonstrably worse than in past decades (Danzinger & Gottschalk, 1993; Jencks & Peterson, 1991; Yee et al., 1995).

Impoverished urban neighborhoods have more than their share of both legal and illegal drugs, and drug abuse exacerbates many social ills that have so long visited the inner cities and some suburban and rural communities (Jencks & Peterson, 1991). It would be a mistake, however, to conclude that multigenerational poverty has been created by drug abuse. One explanation of the correlation between poverty and drug abuse is that people who have no stake in society will be vulnerable to drug experimentation and abuse or will have little reason to give up drugs if they begin using them.

A substantial body of evidence from the fields of child development, criminal justice, and poverty have shown that the seeds of adverse social development are sown early in life. Too many children who are raised in adverse familial and environmental circumstances fail to receive the nurturing and guidance that will make them secure and receptive to the learning opportunities in the social environment. Too often, these same children then fail to learn how to get along with peers or respond to adult supervision, and they become involved in a series of unconventional behaviors, including drug experimentation, abuse, and dependence. In most cases, these same youths have learning or educational deficits that distinguish them from their mainstream peers. Without hope and with impoverished emotional and social repertoires, these adolescents may have established decade-long addiction before they experience their first treatment. Even if they are prepared to respond to daily challenges without drugs or alcohol, they will learn that they are unprepared for life in an increasingly Darwinian society. Many chemically dependent people will become abstinent only when they both find a reason to become sober and some prosocial niche that protects them from the inevitable slip and consequent relapse.

If drugs exacerbate the troubles of those who are least privileged, they also provide transitory relief from poverty, joblessness, boredom, and despair. Treatment philosophies assume that drug users will have a better life when they are off drugs, but for most indigent people contemplating detoxification, treatment, or a life of recovery, cessation of drug use portends no change in many of life's abysmal circumstances. Treatment providers are aware of this socioeconomic reality, and therapeutic communities and some other programs have developed employment readiness training, job placement, and housing as program components. In our own view, indigent clients are unlikely to respond well to drug abuse interventions unless their posttreatment life options are expanded.

The relationship between poverty and drug abuse notwithstanding, it would be impractical to attempt to directly address the problem of drug abuse through economic uplifting. First, there is little consensus on how to remedy the problems of the least-privileged populations (although some would argue that our nation lacks will more than knowledge of what to do about poverty and related racism and unemployment). Second, basing efforts to reduce drug abuse on long-term solutions to massive social problems is a high-risk proposition, given the scope of severe drug and alcohol abuse in the United States and the incomplete understanding of poverty and substance misuse. Finally, although the conditions of poverty may render people and communities vulnerable to drug abuse, the use and abuse of drugs and alcohol remain personal choices.

Thus, society and the treatment community are left with a daunting task: how to design and test interventions that somehow deal with the personal and interpersonal facets of addiction, yet not ignore the environmental and economic dimensions of a person's life. The difficulty of this task cannot be underestimated, even if there were jobs ready for every recovering drug user and alcoholic.

By their very nature, addictive processes are highly reinforcing and extremely refractive to treatment, even among people who have many assets and opportunities. The problem of drug abuse can be truly discouraging when the addiction is woven into a fabric of social problems that extend over time and across all life domains. The limited effectiveness of our interventive strategies is readily apparent in the face of such difficult life circumstances. Nonetheless, appreciation of the social context of chemical dependency and confronting the limitations of our present treatments are necessary if more effective interventive approaches are to be found (Friedman, DesJarlais, & Ward, 1994).

## Organizing Treatment

Substance abuse treatment services have developed in ways that reflect the changing epidemiology of substance use, how addictions are perceived by society, preferences of people who experience problems with drugs and alcohol, advances in understanding of addiction treatment, and changes in health care delivery and financing. Drug and alcohol treatment has been organized around target populations (such as families or women), settings (such as work site or prison), program purposes (for example, detoxification, methadone maintenance), ideologies (for example, therapeutic community, AA), or program structures (such as inpatient rehabilitation or halfway house). Treatment may be approached from various philosophical or theoretical perspectives, including those based on self-help and empowerment, brief treatment, psychodynamics, social learning, and the disease model. In turn, these perspectives find application in practical strategies including cognitive–behavioral skills training, empowerment, motivational counseling, and 12-step programs. Despite the differences in population focus, setting, purpose, ideology, and structure, addiction treatment approaches overlap with, borrow from, and coexist with one another.

## SERVICES INTEGRATION

An important aspect of almost all treatment approaches is the transition from more expensive and isolated levels of care to less costly care settings in the community. Better linkages are needed between these two phases. Intensive program settings (rehabilitation, detoxification, therapeutic communities) are designed to provide a safe environment during the initial period of abstinence, separation from harmful influences, assessment and diagnosis, self-appraisal, relapse prevention skills, and planning for a drug-free life. Less intensive aftercare (individual and group therapy, 12-step fellowship meetings) is designed to help substance users maintain abstinence or at least reduced levels of drug and alcohol use.

Integration across levels of care can be accomplished either between or within organizations. Intensive, first-phase programs and aftercare settings can collaboratively develop integrated services networks based on ongoing relationships, shared goals, and parallel interventive strategies. Alternatively, a single organization can offer a spectrum of services or at least inpatient care and aftercare. Cross-provider networks are already developing and expanding through managed care organizations, including health maintenance organizations (HMOs).

Notwithstanding the long overdue advances that integrated services arrangements represent, organizational restructuring alone will address only some of the problems associated with multiple levels of care. If recovering people are to benefit optimally from multilevel care, service providers will need to develop effective strategies for effecting the transition between settings. Many patients who want to be detoxified in a hospital ward or treated in an inpatient rehabilitation center may have little desire to participate in outpatient programs. Those who are motivated to begin aftercare will often lose sight of their objective when they experience familiar environments and personal difficulties.

## DETOXIFICATION, SELF-HELP, AND TREATMENT SETTINGS

As a first step toward rehabilitation, detoxification provides a controlled, safe, and comfortable environment for drug-dependent people to rid their systems of psychoactive substances. (A relatively small number of detoxification patients are methadone program participants, and those contemplating methadone maintenance, who are experiencing or anticipating severe withdrawal from opiates, barbiturates, or alcohol.) Detoxification inpatient stays are rapidly becoming shorter, and it is clear that inpatient detoxification will be used less in the future. Few treatment providers have systematically attempted to improve on the low rates of detoxified patients who make the transition into treatment and self-help (McCusker, Bigelow, Luippold, Zorn, & Lewis, 1995). Detoxification counselors, who are often supervised by social workers, prefer that their clients enter some kind of residential program immediately following their discharge from detoxification. In practice, most counselors focus on three major alternatives for detoxified drug users: inpatient rehabilitation, therapeutic communities, and day treatment. They tend to refer patients to settings where they know the intake personnel. In addition, detoxification staff emphasize the importance of 12-step participation as a necessary rehabilitative element. The critical task of detoxification providers is to find better ways of helping substance users enter treatment and maintain longer periods of sobriety.

## Alcoholics Anonymous and Narcotics Anonymous

Twelve-step groups, by virtue of their number and geographic distribution, must be considered among the more successful approaches to the treatment of chemical dependency (Emrick, 1994; Kurtz, 1990). Yet the very nature of the informal and self-directed help seeking inherent in the AA–NA (Narcotics Anonymous) model may not support the necessary structure, monitoring, and guidance needed to overcome the established substance use patterns evidenced by patients in rehabilitation, detoxification, and therapeutic community settings. Depending on a given person's circumstances, AA or NA may be viewed as an end in itself, as a bridge during the transition to other forms of treatment, or as one element in a plan to seek both immediate and long-term help with chemical dependency. Recovering social workers participate in 12-step groups, and social workers refer many drug users to AA or NA. However, they have no official role in the organizations, which are operated exclusively by local volunteers.

## Inpatient Rehabilitation

Residential rehabilitation programs attempt to alter addictive behavior by isolating the person from his or her drug-using network, environments, and daily routines linked to a drug-using lifestyle. Although specific program elements and the emphasis on various program aspects vary across organizations, virtually all programs include educational groups on addiction as a disease, health aspects of drug and alcohol abuse, and 12-step fellowship groups. Individual and group counseling, often provided by social workers, may include family therapy; behavioral strategies to cope with anger, rejection, and boredom; and insight therapy concerned with the antecedents of the present dysfunction. Many programs attempt to prepare patients for the inevitable temptations that usually result in relapse. Clients participate in various recreational activities, such as writing, games, and sports. All these program elements are potentially useful, and empirical support can be found for some components, such as certain motivational strategies (Miller, 1989), self-control training (Hester & Miller, 1989), and skills training (Chaney, 1989; Daley & Marlatt, 1992). Nevertheless, it remains difficult to specify what treatment elements are associated with lasting behavior change.

Many rehabilitation units are affiliated with hospitals, and an increasing proportion are part of large corporate enterprises. Most inpatient rehabilitation programs charge high fees, although some of the least expensive nonprofit organizations are among the most highly respected. The managed care revolution has forced programs to drastically shorten lengths of stay. Programs that once had a minimum stay of 120 days may now "rehabilitate" people whose insurance so dictates in as few as 10. Some treatment units are operating under capacity, and rehabilitation programs are rapidly developing new mixtures of services in response to constraints imposed by managed care and emerging regulations for publicly funded patients.

## Therapeutic Communities

Therapeutic communities (TCs) cost considerably less than rehabilitation units (Hubbard et al., 1989). They employ many professional helping agents, and social workers have roles as counselors, supervisors, and administrators. The forerunners of today's TCs were small groups of heroin addicts who lived together under shared rules and norms. Strictly enforced codes included complete abstinence from drugs (although not necessarily alcohol), confrontational group sessions, and a hierarchy of privileges and governance not unlike some aspects of the military (De Leon, 1994).

Like AA and NA, therapeutic communities expend considerable effort reaching out to prospective recruits. Modern TCs may take the form of large national and international organizations with dozens of living units, fleets of vehicles, and their own commercial enterprises. They are less rigidly operated than in the past, and group sessions have become less confrontational. Still, rigorous program requirements preclude many potential applicants from considering therapeutic communities, and attrition rates are high, even among the self-selected group who enter (De Leon & Schwartz, 1984). Until recently, nearly all TCs required prospective participants to commit to at least a 12-month stay. However, with declining enrollments and cost containment pressures, some therapeutic communities have begun to offer stays as short as six months. As with inpatient rehabilitation, it is difficult to know what program elements are associated with completion or favorable outcomes in TCs.

## Halfway Houses

The term "halfway house" derives from the field of alcoholism treatment and refers to a residence that is less restrictive and expensive than residential rehabilitation but more structured than living independently in the community. Participants are usually in transition from rehabilitation units, but they also may enter through other referral sources if the person is deemed to be an acceptable risk. Employment is usually a prerequisite, and participants engage in daily living tasks and individual and group therapeutics that are similar to some TC activities (Geller, 1992). Trained to help clients move across different levels of care, social workers are often responsible for maintaining the linkages between halfway houses and employers, family, other informal supports, and aftercare.

## Outpatient Treatment

*Outpatient care* is defined here as individual or group counseling delivered by social workers or other professionals with expertise in chemical dependency. Day treatment is an intensive form of outpatient care that occupies at least four hours per day of the recovering person's time for at least three days per week (Institute of Medicine, 1990). Program activities may include groups, individual sessions, recreation, and education. Evening programs, which are restricted to employed people, may require 10 to 20 hours of weekly participation for several months (Schilling & Sachs, 1993). Faced with declining revenues due to managed care restrictions, many inpatient rehabilitation programs and therapeutic communities have begun their own outpatient programs.

In the past, outpatient programs were designed for recovering people who had already passed through more intensive inpatient programs or for people who were functioning successfully in work or other life domains despite their chemical dependence. Outpatient treatment is characterized by high attrition and uneven participation rates. These attrition rates may increase even more in the future, when the client mix will include people who in the past would have first gone through inpatient rehabilitation. Given the high rates of attrition and relapse across all forms of treatment, however, it may be that over a period of months, such people will fare no worse than their peers who experienced inpatient care.

## PHARMACOTHERAPY

In this context, the term "pharmacotherapy" refers to the use of prescription drugs to maintain drug or alcohol abstinence (Moss, 1990; Washton, 1988). Pharmacotherapeutic management may be achieved through the reduction of craving, the creation of aversive associations, or the management of withdrawal symptoms. Pharmacotherapy is usually considered a "second-line" form of treatment beginning after sociobehavioral treatment approaches (individual and group therapy and self-help groups) have been tried (Schuckit, 1995; Washton, 1988).

### Methadone Treatment of Heroin Abuse

The most common drug used in treating drug abuse is methadone, a synthetic narcotic used primarily for opiate detoxification. Methadone is a long-acting opiate that shares most properties of heroin, including addiction, sedation, and respiratory depression (Schuckit, 1995). It has relatively few side effects and is administered orally in a liquid, once a day—usually under clinical supervision. When a maintenance level dose is reached, it almost completely blocks the effects of a heroin "high" and thus controls craving. After a period of maintenance, the clinician and patient may work out a program to decrease the dosage incrementally. However, program compliance and positive outcomes are associated with moderately high dosage, and it appears that programs routinely prescribe dosages that are too low to provide optimal benefit (Ball & Ross, 1991).

Methadone maintenance is strictly controlled by federal regulation. Virtually all patients must submit urine samples that are screened for the presence of opiates and other illicit substances. This testing is not announced in advance by program staff. Patients found to be using such substances are supposed to be removed from methadone maintenance, but in practice, positive urine screens invoke warnings, suggestions for counseling, and more frequent screening schedules. Only infrequently are they the sole cause of patients' being removed from methadone maintenance treatment programs.

Methadone provides people with opiate dependency an opportunity for life stabilization and linkages with medical and social resources (Lowinson, Marion, Joseph, & Dole, 1992). It also appears to decrease criminal activity and needle use associated with heroin addiction (Ball & Ross, 1991; DesJarlais & Friedman, 1988). Hence methadone reduces health risks such as hepatitis and HIV infection (Caplehorn & Ross, 1995; Hartgers, Van Den Hoek, Krijnen, & Coutinho, 1990; Vanichseni,

Wongsuwan, Staff of BMA Narcotics Clinic No. 6, Choopanya, & Wongpanich, 1991).

Methadone is not without its detractors. Evidence suggests that the drug is difficult to give up (Kosten, 1992; O'Brien, 1996; Witters & Venturelli, 1988). Most patients receiving methadone lead lives characterized by poverty and, by conventional standards, ineffectual participation in work, family, and community (Ball & Ross, 1991; El-Bassel, Schilling, Turnbull, & Su, 1993; Schilling, El-Bassel, Schinke, Nichols, et al., 1991). Most methadone patients considered this form of treatment only after long periods of opiate use and repeated failure to abstain and came from impoverished backgrounds even before they became addicted to opiates. It is perhaps unfair to expect that methadone alone could remedy problems that developed over many years. Nevertheless, about one-third of patients drop out in the first year, and as many as half use cocaine and often heroin while in a methadone maintenance treatment program (MMTP) (Ball & Ross, 1991; Cushman, 1988; National Institute on Drug Abuse & National Institute on Alcohol Abuse and Alcoholism, 1990).

MMTP patients require supportive, often crisis-oriented services to help them function effectively in personal, social, and economic realms (Stark, 1989). In many MMTP settings, social workers provide such services, supplementing the work of less-trained drug counselors. They may teach patients interpersonal, parental, or recreational skills; organize support networks; and provide linkages to housing, health care, legal services, and vocational and educational services.

## Disulfiram Treatment for Alcohol Abuse

Disulfiram (Antabuse) is widely used in the treatment of alcohol abuse. Administered in pill form over extended periods, disulfiram is an aversive agent that interferes with the normal metabolism of alcohol in the body. Although disulfiram does not decrease the desire to drink, patients abstain because they wish to avoid a severe physiological reaction after ingestion of alcohol. A patient on disulfiram who drinks alcohol will experience a variety of symptoms including nausea, irregular heartbeat, headache, sweating, weakness, and confusion (Fuller, 1989).

Several studies that compared disulfiram with no medication have shown a higher rate of abstinence with disulfiram (Schuckit, 1995), but the more rigorously designed studies found no impact beyond placebo effects (Chick et al., 1992; Johnsen et al., 1987). Disulfiram is not an ideal agent for aversive conditioning because of the time lag between ingestion of alcohol and the reaction as well as the unpredictable intensity of the reaction (Schuckit, 1995). In addition, compliance is a major problem in disulfiram therapy (Fuller et al., 1986); an effective strategy is a contract stipulating that a spouse or significant other observe when the patient takes the drug each day (O'Farrell & Bayog, 1986). Because many social workers are trained in contracting and routinely intervene with social network members, such procedures can be accomplished by social workers in collaboration with physicians.

## Pharmacotherapeutic Treatment of Cocaine Abuse

Pharmacotherapeutic agents may block some effects of cocaine, treat cocaine-induced states such as withdrawal and craving, or produce an aversive reaction if taken with cocaine (Tutton & Crayton, 1993). Bromocriptine (Parlodel) is the most popular cocaine antagonist and is used to prevent the euphoric effects of cocaine. It has been shown to have some effectiveness in reducing craving, improving mood, and increasing energy among detoxification patients, most productively in the first two weeks of treatment (Clow & Hammer, 1991; Dackis & Gold, 1985; Giannini, Folts, Feather, & Sullivan, 1989). Antidepressants, particularly desipramine (Norpramin), also have been evaluated for the treatment of cocaine craving and withdrawal symptoms (Arndt, Dorozynsky, Woody, McLellan, & O'Brien, 1992; Herring & Gold, 1988; Johnson & Vocci, 1993). Antidepressants may reverse cocaine-induced supersensitivity of dopamine receptors (Gawin et al., 1989; Vaughan, 1990; Zedonis & Kosten, 1991). However, several studies do not support the efficacy of desipramine over a placebo (Carroll, Rounsaville, Gordon, et al., 1994; Carroll, Rounsaville, Nich, et al., 1994). A relatively new drug, buprenorphine (Buprenex), acts as a mixed opiate agonist and antagonist and is used to treat cocaine abuse in opiate users. Buprenorphine has been shown to significantly diminish cocaine use if used instead of methadone (Kosten, Kleber, & Morgan, 1989; Mello, Mendelson, Bree, & Lukas, 1989; Rosen & Kosten, 1991). As yet, no medication has produced consistently positive results in improving the relapse rate for cocaine dependence (Schuckit, 1996).

## PSYCHOTHERAPEUTIC AND SOCIOBEHAVIORAL STRATEGIES

Sociobehavioral intervention strategies have been shown to increase the effectiveness of pharmacologic treatments (Carroll & Rounsaville, 1993; Kosten et al., 1992; McLellan, Arndt, Metzger, Woody, & O'Brien, 1993; O'Malley et al., 1992). Psychosocial counseling may serve a supportive role by enhancing medication compliance, altering cognition and behavior associated with drug abuse, and helping the client adjust to a drug-free state (Calsyn, Saxon, Freeman, & Whittaker, 1990; Childress, McLellan, Woody, & O'Brien, 1991).

Apart from their concomitant use with pharmacotherapeutic agents, numerous psychotherapeutic approaches have been used in the long search to treat chemical dependence and abuse. As ever, psychoanalytic therapy is rich in theory (Leeds & Morgenstern, 1996), but its utility remains open to question because of its cost, inappropriateness for most substance-dependent patients, and the difficulty of reliably determining the actual intervention elements for empirical scrutiny (Woody et al., 1994).

Psychotherapy also may be applied in a more eclectic manner to a large proportion of clients—that is, the therapist helps the client gain access to both latent unconscious meaning and applicable conscious realms (Galanter & Castaneda, 1990; Gallant, 1994; Zimberg, 1994). Although some psychotherapists who base their approaches on the tenets and methods of psychoanalysis, ego psychology, and personal psychology will continue to work with drug-involved clients, mentalistic approaches to the treatment of addictive disorders have lost favor over the past two decades. First, drug abuse treatment has for the most part been characterized by pragmatic approaches that rely on informational and confrontational means of bringing the user to seek the paths of recovery. Second, in recent decades the addiction field has de-emphasized approaches that cannot specify both the intervention elements and the intended outcomes of the treatment. Third, although most professionals in the field of addiction treatment consider early life experiences to be contributing factors to drug abuse disorders, only a small and diminishing number of them believe that drug abuse treatment should attempt to deal with historical events as a way of reducing drug use and maintaining abstinence. Finally, the increasing focus on outcomes and short-term treatment in addiction treatment will further restrict the application of insight-oriented therapy. Although social workers trained in these methods may conduct insight-oriented therapy with people who have been in recovery for long periods, it appears that the new order in health care priorities will preclude such therapy, except for those relative few who can pay on their own.

## Approaches Based on Principles of Reinforcement and Social Learning

Across an increasing proportion of chemical dependence treatment settings, psychodynamic counseling has been largely replaced by strategies to alter environmental contingencies, cognitions, and behavior related to drug use. For example, contingency management can be used with methadone patients, increasing or decreasing their medication depending on the presence of drugs in their urine samples. Contingent use of methadone is sometimes used with patients who have not responded well to traditional methadone maintenance protocols (Carroll, 1996), with both favorable (McCarthy & Borders, 1985; Noliman & Crowley, 1990; Saxon, Wells, Fleming, Jackson, & Calsyn, 1996) and unfavorable results (Dolan, Black, Penk, Robinowitz, & DeFord, 1985). However, because positive effects of contingency management may diminish over time, it may be most appropriate to use such strategies only for short periods (Noliman & Crowley, 1990).

A token economy system is another form of contingency management. In one study, tokens could be earned through supplying clean urine samples, attending counseling sessions, and promptly obtaining daily methadone. Patients could raise their doses by earning extra tokens, but doses would decrease if tokens were not given to the staff. When compared with the control group, patients using the token economy showed significantly lower rates of drug-positive urine samples (Glosser, 1983).

Cognitively, people who are recovering need to become aware of the social cues, environmental determinants, and internal thoughts that draw them toward alcohol and other psychoactive substances (Monti, Abrams, Kadden, & Cooney, 1989). Successful recovery is associated with the establishment of new thinking patterns that enable a person to anticipate and avoid high-risk circumstances (Sobell, Toneatto, & Sobell, 1990). Behaviorally, people in recovery will be more likely to achieve sustained periods of sobriety if they learn and practice a repertoire of new behaviors—that is, actions that follow or complement the newly learned cognitions (El-Bassel, Ivanoff, Schilling, Borne, & Gilbert, 1997; Schilling, El-Bassel, Serrano, & Wallace, 1992). Cognitions and behaviors may be linked in a series of self-instructions that guide the person across the shoals of craving and habit. For example, a recovering heroin user has learned to recognize feelings of loneliness and boredom as emotions that weaken his intentions to avoid opiates. He fears that his walk to the nearby convenience store may take him past an abandoned building where dealers sell heroin and other drugs. Talking to himself, as he has practiced in the rehabilitation center, he names his feelings ("Uh-oh, I'm starting to feel really down"), states the risks at hand ("Man, I could be easy for any dope dealer"), specifies an avoidance tactic ("I'm not going to that store—I'll go to the 'One Stop' instead"), and remembers to call his brother who has promised to help in these circumstances ("I'll drop a quarter at the corner"). He walks to the alternate store and calls his brother, who then meets him there.

Cognitive–behavioral strategies also may include skills that enable the recovering person to seek help, turn down requests from former drug-use associates, and manage internal anger and interpersonal conflict. Recovering drug users also may participate in contracts with spouses, family members, friends, or treatment providers.

## Social Support and Social Networks in Addiction Treatment

The concept of social support has become an increasingly popular focus of inquiry for both researchers and practitioners, including those who cite its potential contribution to chemical dependency treatment. Arguably traceable to Mary Richmond's work (1917), the utility and value of social support approaches have been recognized by social workers of many theoretical perspectives, who have incorporated the approaches into assessments and interventions with diverse client populations.

The addiction literature offers complex and conflicting indications about whether social support discourages or promotes substance abuse. In terms of its positive role, social support has been found to be associated with commitment to and maintenance of behavior change as well as successful alcohol and drug treatment outcomes (Cronkite & Moos, 1980; Gordon & Zrull, 1991; MacDonald, 1987; Tucker, 1982; Ward, Bendel, & Lange, 1983). Conversely, social networks are associated with use of illicit drugs (Kandel, Kessler, & Margulies, 1978; Mermelstein, Cohen, Lichtenstein, Baer, & Kamarck, 1986; Pakier, 1990), high-risk drug use (Tucker, 1985), and relapse (Hawkins & Fraser, 1984). Naturally occurring partner support encourages early maintenance of abstinence from smoking among women, and studies have shown that success in quitting is associated with telephone contacts with fellow quitters and having partners who were former smokers or who successfully quit concurrently (Coppotelli & Orleans, 1985). According to Cohen and colleagues (1988), social support facilitates change in addictive behavior through four processes: (1) buffering stress, (2) influencing the ability to initiate or maintain behavior change, (3) influencing the availability of cues to addictive behavior in the environment, and (4) applying social influence in treatment.

A recently completed study provides a clarification of the social networks of African American and Latina women on methadone (El-Bassel, Cooper, Chen, & Schilling, in press). Respondents reported an average kin network of 3.3 people and an average nonkin network of 2.6. Of their kin, women most often mentioned as network members their children (29 percent), their siblings (26 percent), other relatives (21 percent), parents (15 percent), and spouses (9 percent). Among nonkin relationships, the women most often noted friends (50 percent), neighbors (27 percent), sex partners (14 percent), and professional helpers (7 percent). Women sought out 63 percent of network members to talk about important concerns, speaking with nonkin more often than with kin. The findings suggest that the social networks of drug users are similar to those of non–drug users in terms of structure and function but consist inordinately of people who use and approve of the use of illegal drugs.

Social networks of alcohol and drug abusers can be assessed and joined in treatment and aftercare. Potentially useful modalities include peer support, which is a central aspect of 12-step and therapeutic approaches, social diffusion (Friedman et al., 1994; McCrady & Irvine, 1989), and communication and help-seeking skills (Schilling, El-Bassel, Schinke, Gordon, & Nichols, 1991). In peer support, clients can be recruited to provide support to one another that promotes a sense of mutuality and a goal of abstinence among them. Under the leadership of the abstinent clients, participants come to understand that recovery is in their own hands. Applying social diffusion approaches, drug treatment counselors may train recovering drug users to disseminate messages that lead to change in drug-use norms among their peers and maintenance of behavior change.

Network intervention can include modalities that teach clients interpersonal and communications skills to assist them in identifying non-drug-using network members and obtaining informal support from these people. Significant others (kin and nonkin) also can be taught communication and help-seeking skills to enable them to assist drug-using clients with accessing support and connecting to non-drug-using networks. Thus, interventions to alter network structures can enhance social supports and insulate recovering clients from harmful network influences.

We have tested the feasibility of some of these treatment modalities with incarcerated women and detoxification and methadone patients. While they were in jail, female offenders were taught how to identify people in their networks who would be willing to assist them in their recovery process after release. They also were taught specific communication skills that would empower them to turn to these people for help (El-Bassel et al., 1995). In a current study with detoxification patients, we are using a skills-building approach to teach clients how to identify a significant other in their network who would help them in their recovery process after they leave the program. In another continuing study with patients in a methadone maintenance program, women are taught help-seeking and communication skills to encourage them to connect and interact with non-drug-using networks. They are learning how to identify and avoid people who may harm their recovery process, mobilize network members who may enhance their recovery process, identify the types of support they need (emotional, instrumental, financial), and match these types of support with the resources available within their networks.

Drug treatment programs can develop systematic ways of mobilizing clients' social networks. Social workers and counselors at these programs might be trained to assess social networks and involve kin and nonkin in the treatment process. Despite the increased interest in social support among social workers, there is still insufficient understanding of how to best capitalize on social relationships in initiating treatment and sustaining recovery.

## Employment

Vocational strategies also are useful in helping drug users adapt to new life-role expectations. New welfare regulations instituted in 1996 stipulate limits on family assistance and require most parents to work within a specified period. New legislation provides sanctions for drug-using parents who are receiving public assistance and requires drug users who are receiving Supplemental Security Income insurance to participate in chemical dependency treatment and seek work. Most treatment providers hold that the convention of work is desirable for recovering drug users, and successful addiction recovery is associated with steady employment. However, it may not be practical to include work-based elements in drug treatment programs, and many people who participate in methadone programs, AA, and NA do not have jobs. In an increasingly demanding job market, social workers will be challenged to help recovering drug users obtain and maintain jobs or, assuming that their living expenses are otherwise supported, find nonremunerative ways of occupying their time productively. "Job jeopardy" is used as a lever to persuade impaired workers to engage in treatment but, at least for blue-collar workers, there is no clear evidence that this motivator enhances treatment effectiveness (Gerstein & Harwood, 1990; Schilling & Sachs, 1993). The difficulty and salience of such prosocial involvement should not be underestimated, because studies have found that chemically dependent people become attracted to unconventional lifestyles early in life (Donovan & Jessor, 1985; Oetting, Edwards, & Beauvais, 1988; Schilling, Schinke, & El-Bassel, in press) and unstructured daily patterns have become ingrained over long periods of addiction.

## ALTERNATIVE TREATMENTS

Given the intractable nature of chemical dependence, it is not surprising that unconventional treatments are sought by treatment providers, drug users, and family members. Two interesting approaches are reduced environmental stimulation therapy (REST) and acupuncture.

### Reduced Environmental Stimulation Therapy

REST is based on an understanding of brain wave activity. In the REST procedure, a person is exposed to a setting with restricted stimulation, such as a light-proof, soundproof, dark room or flotation tank. Over one to two hours, the person's brain wave activity slows, pulse and blood pressure are decreased, and production of natural endorphins increases (Fine & Turner, 1985). This relaxed state also may bring about improvement in intellectual functioning (Kammerman, 1977).

According to REST's proponents, such "stimulus hunger" expedites a highly efficient learning process called "superlearning." Verbal messages, factual information, and motor skills acquired in superlearning are more likely to be retained under REST conditions (Cooper & Adams, 1988). In the treatment of drug and alcohol addiction, informational messages are provided after a period of REST when the client is receptive to such information (Cooper, Adams, & Scott, 1988; Suedfeld, 1980). Despite promising outcomes with alcohol users (Cooper et al., 1988), REST remains a largely experimental approach. However, its procedures appear to have possibilities for enhancing the potency of clinician–client interaction, and social workers and other professionals in substance abuse treatment might profitably explore REST approaches.

### Acupuncture

Acupuncture is an ancient Chinese method of treating medical and psychological ailments by use of strategically placed needles to redirect and balance the body's energy flow. Across a range of settings, auricular acupuncture is being used with patients in detoxification from alcohol, cocaine, and heroin; to ease the severity of acute withdrawal symptoms; to suppress cravings for drugs; and to enhance mental and physical functioning (Brumbaugh, 1993; Smith & Khan, 1988). Acupuncture may promote the production of beta-endorphins, but the precise mechanisms through which it might work are unknown (Brumbaugh, 1993; McLellan, Grossman, Blaine, & Haverkos, 1993).

The demonstrated efficacy of acupuncture as a treatment for substance abuse is mixed. Two placebo-design studies using acupuncture as a detoxification treatment with alcoholics showed favorable results (Bullock, Culliton, & Olander, 1989; Bullock, Umen, Culliton, & Olander, 1987; Worner, Zeller, Schwarz, Zwas, & Lyon,

1992). At their two-month follow-up, experimental subjects reported fewer drinking episodes and expressed less need for alcohol than did control subjects. In a single-blind study of heroin users, one group found that attendance varied inversely with self-reports of the frequency of drug use, thus suggesting that those with lighter use patterns found the treatment modality more helpful, or simply that addiction severity is inversely correlated with participation in any treatment (Washburn et al., 1993). Two studies comparing acupuncture to methadone found that acupuncture produced outcomes superior to those of methadone regimens (Newmeyer, Johnson, & Klot, 1984; Washburn, Keenan, & Nazareno, 1990).

At least three acupuncture studies, however, found no significant differences between experimental and control groups (Avants, Margolin, Chang, Kosten, & Birch, 1995; Lipton, Brewington, & Smith, 1990; Worner et al., 1992). Because consensus has not yet been reached on the efficacy of acupuncture alone as a treatment method, researchers have suggested using acupuncture in conjunction with traditional substance abuse modalities (Brumbaugh, 1993; Geijer, 1987; Smith & Khan, 1988). Plausibly, a degree of the "success" or, surely, much of the popularity of acupuncture may have to do with its novelty, low demand on patients, and generalized placebo effects. Acupuncture appears to have few risks, and social workers and other helping agents might consider ways in which demonstrably useful sociobehavioral strategies could be combined with this interesting treatment approach.

## SPECIAL POPULATIONS

A special population focus is essential to understanding substance abuse intervention. Some of the groups meriting attention include homeless people, women, elderly men and women, people with co-occurring mental disorders, and people in prison.

### Homeless People

Social workers' training is especially useful in work with homeless people who use substances because they have skills in advocacy, outreach, referral, tracking, and managing transitions between systems. Many drug and alcohol treatment facilities are reluctant to serve homeless people because their instability predicts poor treatment outcomes. What is more, homeless people have medical, mental health, and other problems that tax services and treatment providers. Even treatment facilities specifically geared for chemically dependent homeless people often do not have the capacity to address the interrelated needs of addiction and mental health treatment, housing, health care, and employment services (Lubran, 1990). Most such programs are locally based and are driven more by specific community needs than by treatment philosophy (McCarty, Argeriou, Huebner, & Lubran, 1991).

In 1987, the National Institute on Alcohol Abuse and Alcoholism (NIAAA) and the National Institute on Drug Abuse (NIDA) established a series of demonstration projects to provide drug treatment for homeless people and assess and evaluate new strategies for this population. Several of the projects sought to improve physical and psychological access to care through low-demand services settings, or "sobering up stations" (Bonham, Hague, Abel, Cummings, & Deutsch, 1990; Dexter, 1990), and intensive outreach (Blankertz & White, 1990; Ridlen, Asamoah, Edwards, & Zimmer, 1990). Coordination of care across systems was accomplished primarily through case management, including outreach, assessment, treatment planning, linkage, monitoring and evaluation, client advocacy, crisis intervention, resource development, aftercare services, system advocacy, supportive counseling, and practical support (Willenbring, Whelan, Dahlquist, & O'Neal, 1990). One project promoted a continuum of care by building interorganizational linkages (McCarty, Argeriou, Krakow, & Mulvey, 1990), and all demonstration sites linked treatment with structured transitional housing (Cox, Meijer, Carr, & Freng, 1993; Pope et al., 1993; Wright, Mora, & Hughes, 1990). Some programs offered parenting and child care services within residential substance abuse treatment facilities (Conrad, Hultman, & Lyons, 1993; Nyamathi & Flaskerud, 1992); others sought to increase treatment motivation for female drug users by attending to their health care and family issues (Leipman, Wolper, & Vazquez, 1992).

It is neither necessary nor realistic to expect that homeless people be drug free before they can be placed in housing. However, it is now clear that the behavior patterns associated with drug and alcohol abuse can undermine individual housing placements and program efforts to create housing for the homeless. The comprehensiveness of many integrated programs (Miescher & Galanter, 1996) notwithstanding, few programs have as yet developed models that can effectively address the housing, addiction, mental health, and other needs of chemically dependent homeless people.

## Women

Most drug and alcohol treatment programs were first designed by and for men, and as a result, many have not been sensitive to the needs of women (Goldberg, 1995; Mondanaro, 1989; Wald, Harvey, & Hibbard, 1995). Women who are substance abusers often face additional societal stigma because they are seen as sexually promiscuous, weak willed, and negligent of their children (Finkelstein, 1993; Kumpfer, 1991; Nelson-Zlupko, Dore, Kauffman, & Kaltenbach, 1996). The rejection, stigma, and blame experienced by drug-involved women results in poor self-esteem, guilt, depression, and increased isolation (Kumpfer, 1991; Zuckerman & Bresnahan, 1991). Other barriers to treatment include transportation difficulties and lack of child care, family treatment, and outreach to women (Colorado Women's Task Force on Substance Abuse Services, 1990; Michaels, Noonan, Hoffman, & Brennan, 1988).

Gender-sensitive program models are beginning to address the gender and economic barriers that inhibit women from seeking and entering treatment. Such programs acknowledge the gender differences in the causes and consequences of substance abuse (Beckman, 1994) and deliver services in settings compatible with women's interactional styles and gender roles (Reed, 1987). Such programs also attend to the sequelae of emotional, sexual, and physical abuse, whether past or current, because these traumas often relate to drug or alcohol use (El-Bassel, Schilling, et al., 1997; Gilbert, El-Bassel, Schilling, & Friedman, 1997; Irwin et al., 1995; Miller et al., 1993).

An increasing number of treatment programs have been specifically designed for drug-involved women and their children (Chang, Carroll, Behr, & Kosten, 1992; Mackie-Ramos & Rice, 1988). These programs recognize women's roles as mothers and provide child care, parenting skills classes, and peer support groups (Luthar & Walsh, 1995). Additional services, such as onsite gynecological and reproductive health care, self-esteem workshops, women-only therapy groups, assertiveness training, and life-planning skills training, have been found to be relevant to women's recovery (Blume, 1990; Nelson-Zlupko et al., 1996; Nelson-Zlupko, Kauffman, & Dore, 1995).

Research has suggested that successful treatment for female substance abusers acknowledges the importance of interpersonal relationships in women's lives (Sumners, 1991; Travis, 1988). If family members are involved and supportive, the effectiveness of treatment is improved (Beckman, 1994; Ettorre, 1992; Hser, Anglin, & McGlothlin, 1987; Lisansky, 1989). Group treatment appears to be particularly useful for female substance abusers because it provides an opportunity for sharing experiences, building communication skills, interpersonal learning, and gathering resources (Greif & Drechsler, 1993; Kauffman, Dore, & Nelson-Zlupko, 1995). Ideally, treatment programs would address the complex socioemotional, educational, vocational, parental, health, and mental health needs of drug-dependent women and their families. Unfortunately, the rhetoric of "holistic" treatment belies the reality that as yet there is little sound evidence to indicate that such enriched programming, even if it were affordable, would necessarily lead to intended outcomes.

## Elderly Populations

Substance abuse among elderly populations has only recently begun to receive attention from treatment providers and researchers. The paucity of research on drug abuse among aged people appears to be associated with underreporting, social isolation of elderly people, inadequate screening instruments, and misdiagnosis (Miller, Belkin, & Gold, 1991; Widner & Zeichner, 1991). Elderly men and women may misuse alcohol or prescription or illicit drugs because of loneliness, social inactivity, multiple losses, health problems, or economic stresses (Crawley, 1993; Kostyk, Lindblom, Fuchs, & Tabisz, 1994). Such self-medication may serve as a way to gain control over one's life because the person self-diagnoses, evaluates, and determines the ailment and its remedy (Crawley, 1993). Elderly substance abusers have been found to be less likely than younger people to seek treatment, so identification and assessment are critical (Crawley, 1993; King, Van Hasselt, Segal, & Hersen, 1994).

Programs for chemically dependent elderly people have claimed success by use of peer groups (Kofoed, Tolson, Atkinson, Toth, & Turner, 1987; Kostyk et al., 1994) or social support networks (Atkinson, Tolson, & Turner, 1993; Lindblom, Kostyk, Tabisz, Jacyk, & Fuchs, 1992; Rathbone-McCuan, Schiff, & Resch, 1984; Zimberg, 1984) to encourage attendance and facilitate recovery. Elderly alcoholics benefit from age-specific programs. Because older alcoholics typically consume smaller amounts of alcohol, they tend not to require detoxification or treatment for withdrawal symptoms. Also, they appear to respond positively to supportive social intervention without confrontation (Zimberg, 1984).

Social workers have important roles in outreach to elderly substance abusers, identification of support systems, creation of peer guidance programs, and planning treatment. Intervention may take place in hospitals, nursing homes, day programs, or home health programs, and they may include traditional drug treatment approaches such as 12-step programs, individual and family therapy, recreational therapy, and linkages with health and community services. As with most areas of chemical dependency treatment, intervention strategies that are demonstrably and robustly effective with elderly populations have yet to be developed.

## People with Co-occurring Mental Disorders

Dually diagnosed people are those diagnosed with a serious Axis I mental disorder (such as schizophrenia or bipolar disorder) in addition to an Axis I substance abuse or dependence disorder (American Psychiatric Association, 1994). These people are often isolated and mistrusting, and their problems challenge the most dedicated mental health workers in coordination of care. Comprehensive treatment should include accurate diagnostic assessment, supportive psychotherapy, pharmacotherapy, group therapy, and an integrated treatment plan (Beeder & Millman, 1995; Director, 1995). Studies have found a correlation between dual diagnosis and homelessness (Belcher, 1989; Center for Mental Health Services and Mental Health Services Administration, 1994; Drake, Osher, & Wallach, 1991), and social work intervention with dually diagnosed patients should include outreach efforts and concrete services, such as housing, and assistance in obtaining entitlements, training in daily living skills, and help with building social support systems (Drake, McHugo, & Noordsky, 1993; Evans & Sullivan, 1990). Understandably, it has been difficult to specify and test treatment strategies for people with such disparate needs and who do not readily or predictably respond to even intensive efforts by social workers and others from the fields of mental health and chemical dependency.

## People in Prison

In 1991, the percentage of male prisoners who tested positive for drugs at the time of arrest varied regionally, from 36 percent in Omaha to 75 percent in San Diego. Comparable rates were found for arrests in Chicago (74 percent, 61 percent, and 21 percent) and Los Angeles (62 percent, 44 percent, and 10 percent) (Maguire, Pastore, & Flanagan, 1993). Among female prisoners, 70 percent to 80 percent have alcohol and drug dependence problems (El-Bassel, Ivanoff, et al., 1997; National Commission on AIDS, 1991). These rates, substantially above those of a decade earlier, are in part attributable to new mandatory sentencing procedures for many felony drug offenses and increased enforcement of drug-related laws. Aware of the association between drug and alcohol abuse and criminal activity, legislators, judges, lawyers, correctional officials, and treatment providers expanded the range of treatment services for drug-involved offenders. Social workers frequently administer programs based within jails and prisons, which tend to have positive (but eventually vanishing) outcomes over time (Inciardi, 1993; Leukefeld & Tims, 1988).

One result of prison and jail overcrowding has been an increased use of sentencing and incarceration alternatives, alternative correctional facilities, and early entry into work-release programs or parole (Koehler & Lindner, 1992; Schilling et al., 1997). Martin and Inciardi (1993) observed that case management is one of the essential activities involved in the supervision and provision of treatment for drug-involved offenders. One potentially useful form of case management, developed in community work with people with severe mental illness, is Assertive Community Treatment (ACT) (Test, Knoedler, & Allness, 1985). ACT staff are continuously available to monitor their clients' well-being as well as anticipate or attend to crises that threaten the patient's ability to remain outside the hospital. ACT staff know the patients well, have considerable latitude in decision making, and either take direct action on their own or assertively effect needed referrals. The linking, monitoring, and advocacy functions of case management are particularly useful in overseeing the daily progress of clients as they negotiate a world that offers many opportunities for returning to previous levels of dysfunction. Although no rigorous studies have shown case management to be effective with drug-involved offenders, there is much to be said for approaches that attend to the ongoing nature of addictive behavior and nonconforming lifestyles. As with many domains within substance abuse treatment, social workers could rationally opt for expanded roles in developing and evaluating innovative strategies for monitoring and treating drug-involved offenders.

## MANAGED CARE

New forces within the health care field have questioned many established practices, including existing approaches to the treatment of substance abuse. Managed care and other cost-containment efforts have reduced expenditures of large sums on supposedly high-impact treatments that appear to have had little lasting benefit. These actions have been buttressed by results from several recent studies (Bengen-Selzer, 1995; Horvath & Kaye, 1995; Human Organization Science Institute, 1995; "Mental Health," 1995; Seligman, 1995) as well as earlier investigations (Hayashida et al., 1989; McCrady et al., 1986). Proponents of brief therapy are finding receptive listeners in the managed care industry. Considerable evidence has indicated that brief and less costly treatment is often at least as effective as longer-term and costlier substance abuse interventions (Babor, 1994; Holder, Longabaugh, Miller, & Rubonis, 1991; Miller & Rollnick, 1991). Providers of managed care now require that briefer, less costly treatments be tried first, and they have limited inpatient stays and capped annual and lifetime substance abuse treatment benefits.

In this economic climate, low-cost programs, such as brief outpatient detoxification, short-term rehabilitation, outpatient counseling, group therapy, and day treatment, are receiving considerable attention. It is not surprising that entrepreneurial rehabilitation programs, which used to depend on AA and other 12-step groups for aftercare, are rapidly developing their own outpatient programs. With more stringent limits on coverage for inpatient rehabilitation services, rehabilitation centers increasingly provide outpatient services for new patients and people discharged from their own detoxification and short-term inpatient facilities.

In the recent past, health insurance coverage for substance abuse treatment was generous, allowing payment for periods as long as two weeks for detoxification and many months for inpatient rehabilitation, but coverage for aftercare was minimal or even absent. Efficacy was not considered in either the fees charged or the reimbursement formulas of insurers and governmental payers. Within a few years, a new set of priorities will be in place, emphasizing outpatient treatment and short patient stays as well as rigid goal setting, outcome determination, and oversight that many clinicians fear will be almost entirely driven by cost considerations.

Convenience, choice, and provider autonomy appear to be the early casualties of the cost-driven changes in health care delivery. In the area of chemical dependency treatment, however, it will be difficult to charge that patient care outcomes have been adversely affected by cost containment. First, the overall efficacy of any single treatment is low. Second, it is not clear which kinds of treatments lead to better outcomes, let alone which treatments are best for which patients (Gerstein, 1994). Finally, it appears that brief, low-cost interventions are generally at least as effective as costlier long-term treatments (Epstein, 1992; Heather, 1989; Miller & Rollnick, 1991).

Although such system changes may be threatening to substance abuse treatment providers at all levels, they have brought about a much-needed awakening in the field. For example, in the past, inpatient detoxification was never questioned, even though there was often no medical need for such high-cost services and surely no evidence that such placements led to beneficial outcomes. Similarly, the need for follow-up was always clear, but the system provided no fees or incentives for services providers to make even passive inquiries about patients who had left care during the previous week, month, or year.

The cost-driven changes in substance abuse treatment are likely to have many consequences, some of which will be positive. As in other areas of mental health care, increasing attention to outcomes is potentially good for clients who receive treatment for substance abuse disorders. No longer will third-party payers (and patients, family members, and referring professionals) assume that all forms of intervention are efficacious, and no more will costlier and longer treatments be accepted as necessarily better for the patient.

### BARRIERS TO TREATMENT

Until recently, many advocates claimed that long waiting lists were proof of a shortage of treatment slots across most forms of treatment. Reductions in health insurance coverage, the managed care environment, and changing drug use patterns have sharply decreased waiting periods in many settings. The actual insufficiency of treatment slots was always open to debate, because many mitigating factors determine whether a substance abuser would enter a treatment program if a space were available. Some drug and alcohol abusers will take initial steps to enter treatment but will nevertheless be unable to navigate a difficult and, until recently, often overcrowded treatment system. The extent to which drug and alcohol abusers encounter system barriers after making bona fide efforts to enter treatment settings is unknown (Marlatt, Tucker, Donovan, & Vuchinich, 1997). Their professional expertise in social and organizational systems notwithstanding, social workers have devoted little research or even systematic analysis to understanding or improving treatment entry and referral.

## Harm Reduction Model

The harm reduction model differs from present drug control policies and treatment philosophies focused on abstinence. According to the proponents of harm reduction, drug use is a public health issue that requires incremental, pragmatic, nonjudgmental interventions and policies. Harm reduction is grounded in the perspectives of law and community attitudes rather than treatment, and its objective is to reduce the broader medical, social, and economic costs of drug use to both users and society at large. The harm reduction model acknowledges that drugs are present in our communities, that users may not always use drugs safely (DesJarlais, 1995), and that drug abuse is a relapsing condition (Brettle, 1991). Although abstinence is not rejected as a desirable objective for many drug users, it is viewed as only one way in which individuals and society can reduce problems associated with chemical dependence.

Practitioners who subscribe to the harm reduction model may encourage behavior changes across several dimensions. These might include an adjustment in dosage (quantity), potency (toxicity), frequency of drug use, access (legal or illegal methods of acquisition), preparation (such as filtering adulterants out of injectable drugs), route of administration (nasal or injection), polydrug use patterns, use of safer equipment (new syringes) or disinfection and care of paraphernalia, attitudinal state when using drugs, or setting (where, when, and with whom drugs are taken). Any of these behavioral and environmental factors may be monitored to reduce risk to the person and to public health (Newcombe, 1995).

One harm reduction strategy is to discourage use of drugs deemed more harmful in favor of less harmful substances. Drug policy in the Netherlands, for example, makes a distinction between "soft drugs" (such as marijuana) and "hard drugs" (such as heroin, cocaine, and amphetamines) (Marlatt & Tapert, 1993). Users and sellers of soft drugs are treated more leniently by law enforcement, in the belief that users will tend to select safer substances and avoid elements of the hard-drug markets associated with violence and organized crime. In contrast, American drug policy treats all drug use as dangerous and illegal, with a "zero tolerance" approach that often does not distinguish between degrees of use or potential harm.

The harm reduction model evolved in Great Britain in recent decades partly as a natural extension of that nation's historically nonpunitive attitudes toward opiate use and partly as a response to an epidemic of drug use, particularly heroin. The initial goals were to prevent the transmission of HIV through the distribution of clean needles and reduce crime associated with illegal drug distribution and use (Stimson, 1996). Interest in this model spread to the Netherlands, where drug users themselves organized an effort to implement needle exchange programs to prevent hepatitis B transmission. Dutch drug policies evolved to include outreach and education as well as wide and easy availability of condoms, drug treatment programs, access to methadone, and zoned public areas of tolerance (Brettle, 1991; O'Hare, 1992). In Bern, Switzerland, harm reduction took the form of an experiment, a café-style "shooting room" staffed by social workers who provide clean needles, syringes, condoms, and referrals to drug and medical treatment (Haemmig, 1995).

The Dutch also have led the way in low-threshold substance abuse treatment. Programs do not insist on total abstinence as a requirement or even a necessary goal of treatment. Treatment providers and outreach staff recognize that for most drug users, overcoming addiction is a process characterized by ambivalence, trial and error, and relapse. Treatment is conceptualized as a range of services and experiences, which may include clients' determined and regular participation in inpatient or outpatient care but also may include outreach, education, and harm reduction suggestions and supplies provided by substance abuse treatment staff. User-friendly services such as roving methadone buses build trust between drug users and helping professionals and facilitate referrals to formal treatment, health care, or other services. By consistently implementing this nonjudgmental philosophy of access, the Dutch claim to be in contact with 60 percent to 80 percent of the drug-using population (Engelsman, 1989).

Although much less developed in the United States, harm reduction trends are observable in this country. Law enforcement and community groups have sought to reduce the harm caused by drunken driving through bartender education and the creation of "free ride" programs on New Year's Eve and other holidays. Public health campaigns, in the form of public service announcements and legally mandated signs in bars and restaurants, have been used to inform the public about the effects of drugs and alcohol on a fetus. Some communities have passed local laws (often conflicting with state and federal laws) decriminalizing marijuana or allowing distribution of new needles and syringes to drug users. Underlying these policies is the belief is that in many cases, it is not possible to control or stop a person's drinking or drug use, but untoward consequences of drug and alcohol use can be prevented or minimized.

Unfortunately, American attitudes toward drug use, reflected in legislation and treatment policies, are often driven by symbolism and morality rather than pragmatic problem solving (Klingemann, Takala, & Hunt, 1992). For example, most treatment programs require abstinence as a prerequisite to admission (Marlatt & Tapert, 1993). Public funding, official support for, and public acceptance of needle distribution programs and methadone maintenance clinics have been limited by a strong sentiment that drug use should not be excused or accommodated in any way. This sentiment is reflected in laws, regulations, and street-level policies of police officers and treatment providers. Thus, even though injection drug use may now account for the majority of new HIV infections in the United States (Centers for Disease Control and Prevention, 1997; Holmberg, 1994, 1996), the criminal justice and treatment systems have until recently resisted new responses to the problems of drug abuse.

To reduce individual and public health risks associated with drug abuse, including AIDS, policymakers and treatment providers should consider a range of harm reduction strategies. Options include more varied treatments for alcohol and drug abuse; low-threshold treatment entry; widespread access to needles and syringes through pharmacies and distribution programs; street outreach, including active referral for services; and targeted public education campaigns. Although harm reduction has been framed in terms of policy, meaningful change will require not only new laws and regulations, but also attitudinal shifts by treatment providers and all branches of the criminal justice system.

## Improving Substance Abuse Treatment

Along with the deeper understanding of the chronic and relapsing nature of substance abuse disorders has come an inescapable realization that even the best available treatments result in modest outcomes that rapidly diminish over time. Unfortunately, changes in the field of chemical dependency treatment appear to have been driven more by modifications in the financing of care than by efforts to develop innovative interventions that address the chronicity and relapsing nature of addictive behavior. Nevertheless, with treatment providers being forced to consider new treatment approaches, the next few years may be an optimal time to consider, develop, and test new treatment strategies.

### TREATMENT ENTRY

With "one-shot" recovery now shown to be an outmoded perspective, it is appropriate to consider treatment as a series of therapeutic experiences that the substance abuser will undergo over a period of years or even decades. Most people in treatment at any given time have received treatment before, and successive treatment episodes generally predict longer periods of abstinence. Understanding the phenomenon of treatment entry is an obvious and pragmatic approach to reducing the long and damaging periods before initial treatment and between subsequent treatment episodes.

AA and many treatment providers depict the entry into treatment as following an event or realization referred to as "hitting bottom." Although such scenarios may be authentic in some cases, the beginnings of recovery are more accurately described as opportunities marked by ambivalence. Intake staff correctly perceive that clients' interest in treatment often wanes—and more so when the waiting period is long. Both intake staff and clients may perceive that there is little connection between their efforts and the likelihood of a successful entry into the treatment setting. Theories of self-efficacy and outcome expectancy suggest that neither group has reason to believe that their efforts will be fruitful. Program developers and treatment specialists have given little attention to how and under what circumstances people enter treatment and even less thought to how treatment intake processes may discourage clients (Marlatt et al., 1997).

Whether in HMOs or other managed care networks, treatment providers need to find better and more direct pathways into treatment, both initially and after relapse. For example, inpatient and outpatient treatment providers could give informational talks in worksite, criminal justice, and other settings, as representatives of 12-step programs do.

Referral agents, who are quite knowledgeable about available treatment resources, also merit attention. By virtue of their position, they may have access to information about the substance abuser's problem and can often determine whether a person might profit from work with a particular treatment provider. Referral agents also can draw on their personal connections to treatment providers. Marketers of treatment services target referral agents, and those efforts will surely increase as the competition for patients increases. Treatment providers and referral agents have common objectives, and they should explore ways of going beyond the essentially passive system of referral that now exists.

Treatment providers tend to discount the importance of the preliminary intake process, in part because until recently, inquiring applicants far outnumbered available treatment slots. Intake personnel often treat callers or in-person applicants with indifference, if not disrespect. They have been trained to believe, with some justification, that expressions of initial interest often are not followed by steps toward treatment entry on the part of the client. In turn, prospective clients have high ambivalence about treatment and low estimations of their own ability to endure or profit from treatment. Treatment providers need to re-examine their intake processes and consider how their intake personnel can make the prospect of treatment attractive, yet screen out applicants who demonstrate no motivation for treatment. Social workers, more than members of any other profession, are trained in the process of making referrals and should be concerned with these issues.

## TREATMENT MATCHING

If the wide range of treatment approaches attests to the failure to develop robustly effective interventions, this variety also speaks to the needs of differing clients. Over the past decade, many observers have called for an end to the question "Does chemical dependency treatment work?" The better question is "For whom and under what circumstances does a given treatment work?" Despite the promise of matching specific treatments to people who would most likely benefit from them (Marlatt, 1988; Miller & Hester, 1989), its therapeutic utility has proven elusive (Hester, 1994). Although some client characteristics, such as years of substance use, social class, and presence of a supportive social network, appear to reliably predict treatment outcome, variables predicting success in a given treatment approach have generally been more difficult to discern. Nonetheless, the increased understanding of the heterogeneity of addictive processes would surely lend credence to the treatment-matching hypothesis. Most attempts to find predictors of success in specific treatment have focused on variables at the personal level. Social workers might expand these explorations to include phenomena that capture the person in his or her environment as well as concern themselves with system issues such as funding and reimbursement, referral processes, and community support systems.

## SPECIFYING TREATMENT

More than in the past, treatment providers need to be open to participating in appropriately measured outreach innovations. Cost-driven managed care has forced treatment providers to justify, and to some extent specify, program elements. Treatment providers now are dealing with such global parameters as length of stay, inpatient versus outpatient care, and the need for medical supervision. In the future, more efficacious and cost-effective treatments will evolve if providers regularly ask themselves "Why is this intervention component included, and what evidence is there to indicate that it influences patient outcomes?" For example, many detoxification and rehabilitation settings provide patients with information about the physical ailments associated with drug abuse, yet programs have no way of knowing whether the information they provide is understood and acted on by the client or is in any way related to reduced drug and alcohol use. Treatment providers need not be researchers, but they should consider the underlying basis for and evidence supporting the use of their chosen intervention strategies (Gambrill, 1990; Thyer, 1991).

## ATTENTION TO OUTCOME AND FOLLOW-UP

Managed care networks will make it possible and desirable for treatment providers to track patient outcomes over time. As treatment providers are ever more becoming part of HMOs or managed care networks, it will be logical to develop procedures by which each discharge would invoke standard protocols for referral or transfer and by which follow-up would be carried out for clinical and evaluative purposes. Treatment providers understand that patterns of recovery will be variable and unpredictable, usually characterized by relapse and repeated attempts to avoid or reduce drug and alcohol use. Accordingly, simplistic categorical indicators of treatment outcome are losing favor to more complex determinations of posttreatment status. Outcome assessments need to capture alternating periods of abstinence and recovery, appraise quantities and circumstances of use, and measure personal and social functioning (Curry, Marlatt, Peterson, & Lutton, 1993; Institute of Medicine, 1990; Schneider, Kviz, Isola, & Filstead, 1995).

## ENHANCING POSTDETOXIFICATION OUTCOMES

Improved postdetoxification outcomes would be possible if more dynamic intervention within detoxification units, improved follow-up, and coordination with treatment settings were carried out. Treatment providers must recognize that information is a necessary but not sufficient element in the process of change in effective interventions. Patients going through detoxification not only must learn about treatment alternatives but also must actively participate in a decision to choose, for example, a therapeutic community or a day treatment center.

Motivational interviewing, with its brief time frame and attention to the ambivalence associated with recovery, may be a particularly useful approach applicable in detoxification settings (Allsop & Saunders, 1991; Bell & Rollnick, 1996; Rollnick & Morgan, 1995). In addition, patients could learn about and prepare for the challenges of the journey from detoxification to treatment through discussion, modeling, guided practice, and "homework" extending to the postdetoxification period. Programs might systematically apply role induction strategies to prepare the patient for the roles of treatment seeker and self-help participant as well as provide social support structures to ease the transition from detoxification to treatment and aftercare.

## COMMUNITY REINFORCEMENT

Although professionals in the field of chemical dependency treatment have come to understand that addiction is a chronic and relapsing condition, most treatment approaches still do not reflect this understanding. An exception is the community reinforcement approach (CRA) developed by Azrin and colleagues (Azrin, 1976; Azrin, Sisson, Meyers, & Godley, 1982; Hunt & Azrin, 1973). CRA is a "broad spectrum behavioral treatment . . . developed to utilize recreational, familial, and vocational reinforcers to aid clients in the recovery process" (Meyers & Smith, 1995, p. 1). Combining operant and social systems perspectives, CRA uses the community to reward nondrinking and other prosocial behavior (Sisson & Azrin, 1989).

Although most of the research on CRA has been conducted with people with severe alcohol dependence, the approach is being applied in studies with heroin and cocaine users. In addition, CRA may be integrated with disulfiram and methadone treatment. Critical elements of the approach include

- an initial assessment and functional analysis
- sobriety sampling, to enable the client to experience sobriety without first having to make a lifelong commitment to abstinence
- a detailed treatment plan based on the 10 sections of the Happiness Scale, which serves as a baseline and indicates areas needing immediate attention, motivates the client by pinpointing specific areas that require change, evaluates ongoing progress, and helps the client discriminate problem areas from nonproblem areas
- skills training, including interpersonal skills, problem solving, and drink refusal
- goal setting
- social and recreational counseling
- relapse prevention.

CRA proponents also have developed employment and marital strategies in recognition of the importance of jobs and adaptive relationships in maintaining drug- and alcohol-free lives (Meyers & Smith, 1995).

Most recently trained social workers have had courses that draw on principles of reinforcement. Moreover, social work's person-in-environment perspective is entirely compatible with the community and social systems aspects of CRA. The comprehensiveness and community focus of CRA recognize that addictive processes exist only in the context of a person's daily living environment. It seems unlikely that the comprehensive and sophisticated strategies tested in federally funded studies will be broadly disseminated among treatment providers in the near future. Nevertheless, it appears that better and longer-lasting treatments will not occur unless the principles akin to those in community reinforcement are adopted in existing or new treatment settings.

## BELATED ARRIVAL OF HARM REDUCTION

Because many aspects of harm reduction are antithetical to moral beliefs held by a large number of Americans, the United States has been slow in adopting the kinds of policies that some European countries have embraced. The AIDS pandemic and obvious limitations of existing drug abuse treatments and criminal justice sanctions lend strength to arguments for new drug policies guided by the harm reduction perspective. The social structures in this country also are influenced by pragmatism, however, so it is not unreasonable to predict that this force will bring about change in drug control policies.

The growing recognition of the failure of our past conceptualizations of drug control and treatment is stimulating changes consonant with harm reduction trends. Although cost driven, the shift away from "curative" long-term treatment to short-term intervention is consistent with the understanding of addiction as a long-term, refractive problem that does not respond to one-time, expensive remedies. Rehabilitation centers and even therapeutic communities now espouse the desirability of stays that are a fraction of the minimum offered in the recent past. Having experienced numerous "wars" on drugs, many law enforcement officials acknowledge the limits of criminal justice approaches to drug abuse. Official posture aside, methadone maintenance clinics have come to accept that a substantial number of patients will continue to use cocaine and opiates. Psychopharmacologic treatment and other "magic bullets" have proven elusive, and there is increasing recognition that for now, even the best treatments effect changes that are difficult to discern one year later. All these realizations may result in attitudinal shifts among those who deal daily with chemically dependent people.

Efforts to deal with the harmful effects of drugs and alcohol will necessarily be seen as incremental, limited, and continuing. The United States is beginning an uncontrolled experiment, admittedly with some changes occurring at a very slow pace. Nonetheless, because harm reduction remains a largely untested notion in the United States, it is imperative that the effects of these changes be monitored. Social work researchers and other social scientists should now be designing studies to evaluate the effectiveness and possible unintended consequences of newly instituted changes in treatment policy, deregulation, and resource allocation.

## Conclusion

No profession is better prepared than social work to grapple with the rapid changes occurring in the field of chemical dependency treatment. Many treatment providers are understandably having difficulty accepting the many changes driven by cost that show little concern for the well-being of the substance-dependent person. Our controversial viewpoint is that many of these changes were inevitable, given the decades of escalating costs with little evidence to show that large expenditures were necessarily related to positive addiction treatment outcomes. It is unfortunate that the changes in health care delivery, including drug abuse treatment, came about almost solely from the consideration of cost. Nevertheless, within a few short years, a revolution has occurred in chemical dependency treatment. In this new treatment environment, there will be many opportunities for forward-thinking social workers, including those trained in organizational systems issues, evaluation technology, and empirically based clinical decision making. Social workers will need to find ways of demonstrating that the outcomes associated with quality treatment elements merit additional expenditures. More than ever, there is a need for social workers and other addiction specialists to develop and test innovative treatment strategies that are integrated with broader approaches aimed at the adverse socioeconomic conditions that give rise to drug abuse.

# References

Alasuutari, P. (1992). *Desire and craving: A cultural theory of alcoholism.* Albany: State University of New York Press.

Allsop, S., & Saunders, B. (1991). Reinforcing robust resolutions: Motivation in relapse prevention with severely dependent problem drinkers. In W. Miller & S. Rollnick (Eds.), *Motivational interviewing* (pp. 236–247). New York: Guilford Press.

Altman, D. (1995). Strategies for community health intervention: Promises, paradoxes, pitfalls. *Psychosomatic Medicine, 57,* 226–233.

American Psychiatric Association. (1994). *Diagnostic and statistical manual of mental disorders* (4th ed.). Washington, DC: Author.

Anderson, N. (1995). Toward understanding the association of socioeconomic status and health: A new challenge for the biopsychosocial approach. *Psychosomatic Medicine, 58,* 213–225.

Annis, H., & Davis, C. (1989). Relapse prevention. In R. Hester & W. Miller (Eds.), *Handbook of alcoholism treatment approaches: Effective alternatives* (pp. 170–182). Needham Heights, MA: Allyn & Bacon.

Arndt, I., Dorozynsky, L., Woody, G., McLellan, A., & O'Brien, C. (1992). Desipramine treatment of cocaine dependence in methadone-maintained patients. *Archives of General Psychiatry, 49,* 888–893.

Atkinson, R., Tolson, R., & Turner, J. (1993). Factors affecting outpatient treatment compliance of older male problem drinkers. *Journal of Studies on Alcohol, 54,* 102–106.

Au, C. (1994). The status of theory and knowledge development in social welfare administration. *Administration in Social Work, 18*(3), 27–57.

Avants, S., Margolin, A., Chang, R., Kosten, T., & Birch, S. (1995). Acupuncture for the treatment of cocaine addiction: Investigation of a needle puncture control. *Journal of Substance Abuse Treatment, 12,* 195–205.

Azrin, N. (1976). Improvements in the community reinforcement approach to alcoholism. *Behaviour Research and Therapy, 14,* 339–348.

Azrin, N., Sisson, W., Meyers, R., & Godley, M. (1982). Alcoholism treatment by disulfiram and community reinforcement therapy. *Journal of Behavior Therapy and Experimental Psychiatry, 13,* 105–112.

Babor, T. (1994). Avoiding the horrid and beastly sin of drunkenness: Does dissuasion make a difference? *Journal of Consulting and Clinical Psychology, 62,* 1127–1140.

Ball, J., & Ross, A. (1991). *The effectiveness of methadone maintenance treatment: Patients, programs, services, and outcome.* New York: Springer-Verlag.

Beckman, L. (1994). Treatment needs of women with alcohol problems. *Alcohol Health & Research World, 18,* 206–211.

Beeder, A., & Millman, R. (1995). Treatment strategies for comorbid disorders: Psychopathology and substance abuse. In A. Washton (Ed.), *Psychotherapy and substance abuse: A practitioner's handbook* (pp. 76–102). New York: Guilford Press.

Belcher, J. (1989). On becoming homeless: A study of chronically mentally ill persons. *Journal of Community Psychology, 17,* 173–185.

Bell, A., & Rollnick, S. (1996). Motivational interviewing in practice: A structured approach. In F. Rotgers, D. Keller, & J. Morgenstern (Eds.), *Treating substance abuse: Theory and technique* (pp. 266–285). New York: Guilford Press.

Bengen-Selzer, B. (1995). *Fourth generation managed behavioral health: What does it look like? Part one: Managed Medicaid, outcomes and integrated services delivery.* Providence, RI: Manisses Communications Group.

Blankertz, L., & White, K. (1990). Implementation of a rehabilitation program for dual-ly diagnosed homeless. Treating alcoholism and drug abuse among homeless men and women: Nine community demonstration grants [Special Issue]. *Alcoholism Treatment Quarterly, 7,* 149–164.

Blatt, S., McDonald, C., Sugarman, A., & Wilber, C. (1984). Psychodynamic theories of opiate addiction: New directions for research. *Clinical Psychology Review, 4,* 1–34.

Blume, S. (1990). Chemical dependency in women: Important issues. *American Journal of Drug and Alcohol Abuse, 16,* 297–307.

Bonham, G., Hague, D., Abel, M., Cummings, P., & Deutsch, R. (1990). Louisville's Project Connect for the homeless alcohol and drug abuser. Treating alcoholism and drug abuse among homeless men and women: Nine community demonstration grants. *Alcoholism Treatment Quarterly, 7,* 57–78.

Botvin, G., Schinke, S., & Orlandi, M. (1995). *Drug abuse prevention with multiethnic youth.* Thousand Oaks, CA: Sage Publications.

Brettle, R. (1991). HIV and harm reduction for injection drug users. *AIDS, 5,* 125–136.

Brickman, B. (1988). Psychoanalysis and substance abuse: Toward a more effective approach. *Journal of the American Academy of Psychoanalysis, 16,* 359–379.

Brumbaugh, A. (1993). Acupuncture: New perspectives in chemical dependency treatment. *Journal of Substance Abuse Treatment, 10,* 35–43.

Bullock, M., Culliton, P., & Olander, R. (1989). Controlled trial of acupuncture for severe recidivist alcoholism. *Lancet, 1,* 1435–1439.

Bullock, M., Umen, A., Culliton, P., & Olander, R. (1987). Acupuncture treatment of alcoholic recidivism: A pilot study. *Alcoholism: Clinical and Experimental Research, 11,* 292–295.

Calsyn, D., Saxon, A., Freeman, G., Jr., & Whittaker, S. (1990). Effects of education on high risk HIV transmission behaviors. *NIDA Research Monograph, 105,* 482–483.

Caplehorn, J., & Ross, M. (1995). Methadone maintenance and the likelihood of risky needle-sharing. *International Journal of the Addictions, 30,* 685–698.

Carroll, K. (1996). Integrating psychotherapy and pharmacotherapy in substance abuse treatment. In F. Rotgers, D. Keller, & J. Morgenstern (Eds.), *Treating substance abuse: Theory and technique* (pp. 286–318). New York: Guilford Press.

Carroll, K., & Rounsaville, B. (1993). Implications of recent research on psychotherapy for drug abuse. In G. Edwards, J. Strang, & J. Jaffe (Eds.), *Drugs, alcohol, and tobacco: Making the science and policy connections* (pp. 211–221). New York: Oxford University Press.

Carroll, K., Rounsaville, B., Gordon, L., Nich, C., Jatlow, P., Bisighini, R., & Gawin, F. (1994). Psychotherapy and pharmacotherapy for ambulatory cocaine abusers. *Archives of General Psychiatry, 51,* 177–187.

Carroll, K., Rounsaville, B., Nich, C., Gordon, L., Wirtz, P., & Gawin, F. (1994). One-year follow-up of psychotherapy and pharmacotherapy for cocaine dependence. *Archives of General Psychiatry, 51,* 989–997.

Center for Mental Health Services, Mental Health Services Administration. (1994). *Making a difference: Interim status report of the McKinney research demonstration program for homeless mentally ill adults.* Rockville, MD: U.S. Department of Health and Human Services.

Centers for Disease Control and Prevention. (1997). *HIV/AIDS surveillance report: U.S. HIV and AIDS cases reported through June, 1997. 9*(1).

Chafetz, M., Blane, H., & Hill, M. (1970). *Frontiers of alcoholism.* New York: Science House.

Chaney, E. (1989). Social skills training. In R. Hester & W. Miller (Eds.), *Handbook of alcoholism treatment approaches: Effective alternatives* (pp. 206–221). Needham Heights, MA: Allyn & Bacon.

Chang, G., Carroll, K., Behr, H., & Kosten, T. (1992). Improving treatment outcome in pregnant opiate-dependent women. *Journal of Substance Abuse Treatment, 9,* 327–330.

Chick, J., Gough, K., Falkowski, W., Kershaw, P., Hore, B., Mehta, B., Ritson, B., Ropner, R., & Totley, D. (1992). Disulfiram treatment of alcoholism. *British Journal of Psychiatry, 161,* 84–89.

Childress, A., McLellan, A., Woody, G., & O'Brien, C. (1991). Are there minimum conditions necessary for methadone maintenance to reduce intravenous drug use and AIDS risk behaviors? *NIDA Research Monograph, 106,* 167–177.

Clarke, J. W. (1996). Black-on-black violence. *Society, 33,* 46–50.

Clow, D., & Hammer, R. J. (1991). Cocaine abstinence following chronic treatment alters cerebral metabolism in dopaminergic reward regions: Bromocriptine enhances recovery. *Neuropsychopharmacology, 4,* 71–75.

Cohen, S., Lichtenstein, E., Mermelstein, R., Kingsolvers, K., Baer, J., & Kamarck, T. (1988). Social support interventions for smoking cessation. In B. Gottlieb (Ed.), *Marshaling social support: Formats, processes, and effects* (pp. 211–240). Newbury Park, CA: Sage Publications.

Colorado Women's Task Force on Substance Abuse Services. (1990, August). *Barriers to substance abuse treatment for women.* Boulder, CO: Prevention Center.

Conrad, K., Hultman, C., & Lyons, J. (1993). Treatment of the chemically dependent homeless: A synthesis. *Alcoholism Treatment Quarterly, 10,* 235–246.

Cooper, G., & Adams, H. (1988). An overview of REST technology. *Journal of Substance Abuse Treatment, 5,* 69–75.

Cooper, G., Adams, H., & Scott, J. (1988). Reduced environmental stimulation therapy (REST) and reduced alcohol consumption. *Journal of Substance Abuse Treatment, 5,* 61–68.

Coppotelli, H., & Orleans, C. (1985). Partner support and other determinants of smoking cessation maintenance among women. *Journal of Consulting and Clinical Psychology, 53,* 455–460.

Cox, G., Meijer, L., Carr, D., & Freng, S. (1993). Systems Alliance and Support (SAS): A program of intensive case management for chronic public inebriates: Seattle. *Alcoholism Treatment Quarterly, 10,* 125–138.

Crawley, B. (1993). Self-medication and the elderly. In E. Freeman (Ed.), *Substance abuse treatment: A family systems perspective* (pp. 217–238). Newbury Park, CA: Sage Publications.

Cronkite, R., & Moos, R. (1980). Determinants of the posttreatment functioning of alcoholic patients: A conceptual framework. *Journal of Consulting and Clinical Psychology, 48,* 305–316.

Curry, S., Marlatt, G., Peterson, A., & Lutton, J. (1993). Survival analysis and assessment of relapse rates. In D. Donovan & G. Marlatt (Eds.), *Assessment of addictive behaviors* (pp. 454–473). New York: Guilford Press.

Cushman, P. (1988). Cocaine use in a population of drug abusers on methadone. *Hospital and Community Psychiatry, 39,* 1205–1207.

Dackis, C., & Gold, M. (1985). Bromocriptine as treatment of cocaine abuse. *Lancet, 1,* 1151–1152.

Daley, D. (1988). Five perspectives on relapse in chemical dependency. In D. Daley (Ed.), *Relapse: Conceptual, research and clinical perspectives* (pp. 3–26). Binghamton, NY: Haworth Press.

Daley, D., & Marlatt, G. (1992). Relapse prevention: Cognitive and behavioral interventions. In J. Lowinson, P. Ruiz, R. Millman, & J. Langrod (Eds.), *Substance abuse: A comprehensive textbook* (pp. 533–542). Baltimore: Williams & Wilkins.

Danziger, S., & Gottschalk, P. (1993). *Uneven tides: Rising inequality in America.* New York: Russell Sage Foundation.

Davis, S. (1984). Effects of chemical dependency in parenting women. In R. Watson (Ed.), *Drug and alcohol abuse reviews, Vol. 5: Addictive behaviors in women.* Totowa, NJ: Humana Press.

De Leon, G. (1994). Therapeutic communities. In M. Galanter & H. Kleber (Eds.), *The American Psychiatric Press textbook of substance abuse treatment* (pp. 391–414). Washington, DC: American Psychiatric Press.

De Leon, G., & Schwartz, S. (1984). Therapeutic communities: What are the retention rates? *American Journal of Drug and Alcohol Abuse, 10,* 267–284.

DesJarlais, D. (1995). Harm reduction: A framework for incorporating science into drug policy. *American Journal of Public Health, 85,* 10–12.

DesJarlais, D., & Friedman, S. (1988). The psychology of preventing AIDS among intravenous drug users. *American Psychologist, 43,* 865–870.

Dexter, R. (1990). Treating homeless and mentally ill substance abusers in Alaska. In M. Argeriou & D. McCarty (Eds.), *Treating alcoholism and drug abuse among the homeless: Nine community demonstration grants* (pp. 25–30). Binghamton, NY: Haworth Press.

Director, L. (1995). Dual diagnoses: Outpatient treatment of substance abusers with co-existing psychiatric disorders. In A. Washton (Ed.), *Psychotherapy and substance abuse: A practitioner's handbook* (pp. 375–393). New York: Guilford Press.

Dolan, M., Black, J., Penk, W., Robinowitz, R., & DeFord, H. (1985). Contracting for treatment termination to reduce illicit drug use among methadone maintenance treatment failures. *Journal of Consulting and Clinical Psychology, 53,* 549–551.

Donovan, J., & Jessor, R. (1985). Structure of problem behavior in adolescence and young adulthood. *Journal of Consulting and Clinical Psychology, 53,* 890–904.

Drake, R., McHugo, G., & Noordsky, D. (1993). Treatment of alcoholism among schizophrenia outpatients: 4-year outcomes. *American Journal of Psychiatry, 150,* 328–329.

Drake, R., Osher, F., & Wallach, M. (1991). Homelessness and dual diagnoses. *American Psychologist, 46,* 1149–1158.

El-Bassel, N., Cooper, D., Chen, D. R., & Schilling, R. F. (in press). Personal social networks and HIV status among women on methadone. *AIDS Care.*

El-Bassel, N., Ivanoff, A., Schilling, R., Borne, D., & Gilbert, L. (1997). Skills-building and social support enhancement to reduce HIV risk among women in jail. *Criminal Justice and Behavior, 24,* 205–223.

El-Bassel, N., Ivanoff, A., Schilling, R., Gilbert, L., Borne, D., & Chen, D. (1995). Preventing AIDS/HIV in drug-abusing incarcerated women through skills building and social support enhancement: Preliminary outcomes. *Social Work Research, 19,* 131–141.

El-Bassel, N., Schilling, R., Irwin, K., Faruque, S., Gilbert, L., Chu, K. T., Serrano, Y., & Edlin, B. R. (1997). Sex trading and psychological distress among women recruited from the streets of Harlem. *American Journal of Public Health, 87,* 66–70.

El-Bassel, N., Schilling, R., Turnbull, J., & Su, K. (1993). Correlates of alcohol use among methadone patients. *Alcoholism: Clinical and Experimental Research, 17,* 681–686.

Emrick, C. (1994). Alcoholics Anonymous and other 12-step groups. In M. Galanter & H. Kleber (Eds.), *The American Psychiatric Press textbook of substance abuse treatment* (pp. 351–358). Washington, DC: American Psychiatric Press.

Engelsman, E. (1989). Dutch policy on the management of drug-related problems. *British Journal of Addiction, 84,* 211–218.

Epstein, L. (1992). *Brief treatment and a new look at the task-centered approach.* New York: Macmillan.

Ettorre, E. (1992). *Women and substance use.* New Brunswick, NJ: Rutgers University Press.

Evans, K., & Sullivan, J. (1990). *Dual diagnosis: Counseling the mentally ill substance abuser.* New York: Guilford Press.

Fillmore, K. (1987). Prevalence, incidence and chronicity of drinking patterns and problems among men as a function of age: A longitudinal and cohort analysis. *British Journal of Addiction, 82,* 77–83.

Fillmore, K., & Midanik, L. (1984). Chronicity of drinking problems among men: A longitudinal study. *Journal of Studies on Alcohol, 45,* 228–236.

Fine, T., & Turner, J. (Eds.). (1985). *Proceedings of the First International Conference on REST and self-regulation.* Toledo, OH: IRIS Publications.

Finkelstein, N. (1993). Treatment programming for alcohol and drug dependent pregnant women. *International Journal of Addictions, 28,* 1275–1310.

Frances, R., Franklin, J., & Borg, L. (1994). Psychodynamics. In M. Galanter & H. Kleber (Eds.), *The American Psychiatric Press textbook of substance abuse treatment* (pp. 239–252). Washington, DC: American Psychiatric Press.

Friedman, S., DesJarlais, D., & Ward, T. (1994). Social models for changing health-relevant behavior. In R. DiClemente & J. Peterson (Eds.), *Preventing AIDS: Theories and methods of behavioral interventions* (pp. 95–116). New York: Plenum Press.

Fuller, R. (1989). Antidipsotropic medications. In R. Hester & W. Miller (Eds.), *Handbook of alcoholism treatment approaches: Effective alternatives* (pp. 117–127). Needham Heights, MA: Allyn & Bacon.

Fuller, R., Branchey, L., Brightwell, D., Derman, R., Emrick, C., Iber, F., James, K., Lacoursiere, R., Lee, K., Lowenstam, I., Maany, I., Neiderhiser, D., Nocks, J., & Shaw, S. (1986). Disulfiram treatment for alcoholism: A Veterans Administration cooperative study. *JAMA, 256,* 1449–1455.

Galanter, M., & Castaneda, R. (1990). Psychotherapy. In A. Bellack & M. Hersen (Eds.), *Handbook of comparative treatments for adult disorders* (pp. 463–478). New York: John Wiley & Sons.

Gallant, D. (1994). Alcohol. In M. Galanter & H. Kleber (Eds.), *The American Psychiatric Press textbook of substance abuse treatment* (pp. 67–90). Washington, DC: American Psychiatric Press.

Gambrill, E. (1990). *Critical thinking in clinical practice: Improving the accuracy of judgments and decisions about clients.* San Francisco: Jossey-Bass.

Gawin, F., Kleber, H., Byck, R., Rounsaville, B., Kosten, T., Jatlow, P., & Morgan, L. (1989). Desipramine facilitation of initial cocaine abstinence. *Archives of General Psychiatry, 46,* 117–121.

Geijer, R. (1987). Heroine-verslaving en acupunctuur [Heroin addiction and acupuncture]. Unpublished manuscript, Rotterdam Public Health Service, the Netherlands.

Geller, A. (1992). Rehabilitation programs and halfway houses. In J. Lowinson, P. Ruiz, R. Millman, & J. Langrod (Eds.), *Substance abuse: A comprehensive textbook* (pp. 458–466). Baltimore: Williams & Wilkins.

Gerstein, D. (1994). Outcome research: Drug abuse. In M. Galanter & H. Kleber (Eds.), *The American Psychiatric Press textbook of substance abuse treatment* (pp. 45–64). Washington, DC: American Psychiatric Press.

Gerstein, D., & Harwood, H. (1990). *Treating drug problems* (Vol. 1). Washington, DC: National Academy Press.

Giannini, A., Folts, D., Feather, J., & Sullivan, B. (1989). Bromocriptine and amantadine in cocaine detoxification. *Psychiatry Research, 29,* 11–16.

Gilbert, L., El-Bassel, N., Schilling, R. F., & Friedman, E. (1997). Childhood abuse as a risk for partner abuse among women on methadone maintenance. *American Journal of Drug and Alcohol Abuse, 23,* 581–595.

Glosser, D. (1983). The use of a token economy to reduce illicit drug use among methadone maintenance clients. *Addictive Behaviors, 8,* 93–104.

Goldberg, M. (1995). Substance-abusing women: False stereotypes and real needs. *Social Work, 40,* 789–798.

Golden, S., & Khantzian, E. (1994). Group therapy. In M. Galanter & H. Kleber (Eds.), *The American Psychiatric Press textbook of substance abuse treatment* (pp. 303–314). Washington, DC: American Psychiatric Press.

Gordon, A., & Zrull, M. (1991). Social networks and recovery: One year after inpatient treatment. *Journal of Substance Abuse Treatment, 8,* 143–152.

Greif, G., & Drechsler, M. (1993). Common issues for parents in a methadone maintenance group. *Journal of Substance Abuse Treatment, 10,* 339–343.

Haemmig, R. (1995). The streetcorner agency with shooting room ("Fixerstuebli"). In P. O'Hare, R. Newcombe, A. Matthews, E. Buning, & E. Drucker (Eds.), *The reduction of drug-related harm* (pp. 181–185). New York: Routledge.

Hartgers, C., Van Den Hoek, J., Krijnen, P., & Coutinho, R. (1990, June). *Risk factors and heroin and cocaine use trends among injection drug users (IDUs) in low threshold methadone programs, Amsterdam 1985–1989.* Paper presented at the Sixth International Conference on AIDS, San Francisco.

Hawkins, J., & Fraser, M. (1984). Social network analysis and drug misuse. *Social Service Review, 58,* 81–97.

Hayashida, M., Alterman, A., McLellan, A., O'Brien, C., Purtill, J., Volpicelli, J., Raphaelson, A., & Hall, C. (1989). Comparative effectiveness and costs of inpatient and outpatient detoxification of patients with mild-to-moderate alcohol withdrawal syndrome. *New England Journal of Medicine, 320,* 358–365.

Heather, N. (1989). Brief intervention strategies. In R. Hester & W. Miller (Eds.), *Handbook of alcoholism treatment approaches: Effective alternatives* (pp. 93–116). Needham Heights, MA: Allyn & Bacon.

Hepworth, D., & Larsen, J. (1990). *Direct social work practice.* Belmont, CA: Wadsworth.

Hermos, J., LoCastro, J., Glynn, R., Bouchard, G., & De Labry, L. (1988). Predictors of reduction and cessation of drinking in community-dwelling men: Results from the normative aging study. *Journal of Studies on Alcohol, 49,* 363–368.

Herring, P., & Gold, M. (1988). Pharmacological adjuncts in the treatment of opioid and cocaine addicts. *Journal of Psychoactive Drugs, 20,* 233–242.

Hester, R. (1994). Outcome research: Alcoholism. In M. Galanter & H. Kleber (Eds.), *The American Psychiatric Press textbook of substance abuse treatment* (pp. 35–44). Washington, DC: American Psychiatric Press.

Hester, R., & Miller, W. (1989). Self-control training. In R. Hester & W. Miller (Eds.), *Handbook of alcoholism treatment approaches: Effective alternatives* (pp. 141–150). Needham Heights, MA: Allyn & Bacon.

Holder, H., Longabaugh, R., Miller, W., & Rubonis, A. (1991). The cost effectiveness of treatment for alcoholism: A first approximation. *Journal of Studies on Alcohol, 52,* 517–540.

Holmberg, S. (1994). Emerging epidemiologic patterns of HIV in the United States. *AIDS Research and Human Retroviruses, 10*(Suppl. 2), 51.

Holmberg, S. (1996). The estimated prevalence and incidence of HIV in 96 large US metropolitan areas. *American Journal of Public Health, 86,* 642–654.

Horvath, J., & Kaye, N. (1995). *Medicaid managed care: A guide for states.* Portland, ME: National Academy for State Health Policy.

Hser, Y., Anglin, M., & McGlothlin, W. (1987). Sex differences in addict careers: I. Initiation of use. *American Journal of Drug and Alcohol Abuse, 13,* 33–57.

Hubbard, R., Marsden, M., Rachal, J., Harwood, H., Cavanaugh, E., & Ginzburg, H. (1989). *Drug abuse treatment: A national study of effectiveness.* Chapel Hill: University of North Carolina Press.

Human Organization Science Institute. (1995). *Evaluation of the implementation of Pennsylvania's Act 152 (1988): The quantitative findings (including a reprint of the qualitative perspective).* Philadelphia: Villanova University.

Hunt, G., & Azrin, N. (1973). A community-reinforcement approach to alcoholism. *Behaviour Research and Therapy, 11,* 91–104.

Inciardi, J. A. (Ed.). (1993). *Drug treatment and criminal justice.* Newbury Park, CA: Sage Publications

Institute of Medicine. (1990). *Broadening the base of treatment for alcohol problems.* Washington, DC: National Academy Press.

Irwin, K., Edlin, B., Wong, L., Faruque, S., McCoy, H., Word, C., Schilling, R., McCoy, C., Evans, P., & Holmberg, S. (1995). Urban rape survivors: Characteristics and prevalence of human immunodeficiency virus and other sexually transmitted infections. *Obstetrics and Gynecology, 85,* 330–336.

Ivanoff, A., Blythe, B., & Tripodi, T. (1994). *Involuntary clients in social work practice.* New York: Aldine de Gruyter.

Jacobs, D., David, P., & Meyer, D. (1995). *The supervisory encounter.* New Haven, CT: Yale University Press.

Jencks, C., & Peterson, P. (1991). *The urban underclass.* Washington, DC: Brookings Institution.

Johnsen, J., Stowell, A., Bache-Wiig, J., Strensrud, T., Ripel, A., & Morland, J. (1987). A double-blind placebo controlled study of male alcoholics given a subcutaneous disulfiram implantation. *British Journal of Addiction, 82,* 607–613.

Johnson, D., & Vocci, F. (1993). Medications development at the National Institute on Drug Abuse: Focus on cocaine. *NIDA Research Monograph, 135,* 57–70.

Kadushin, A. (1992). *Supervision in social work.* New York: Columbia University Press.

Kammerman, M. (1977). *Sensory isolation and personality change.* Springfield, IL: Charles C Thomas.

Kandel, D., Kessler, R., & Margulies, R. (1978). Antecedents of adolescent initiation into stages of drug use: A developmental analysis. *Journal of Youth and Adolescence, 7,* 13–40.

Kaufman, E. (1994). Family therapy: Other drugs. In M. Galanter & H. Kleber (Eds.), *The American Psychiatric Press textbook of substance abuse treatment* (pp. 331–348). Washington, DC: American Psychiatric Press.

Kauffman, E., Dore, M., & Nelson-Zlupko, L. (1995). The role of women's therapy groups in the treatment of chemical dependence. *American Journal of Orthopsychiatry, 65*, 355–363.

Khantzian, E. (1980). The alcoholic patient: An overview and perspective. *American Journal of Psychotherapy, 34*, 4–19.

King, C., Van Hasselt, V., Segal, D., & Hersen, M. (1994). Diagnosis and assessment of substance abuse in older adults: Current strategies and issues. *Addictive Behaviors, 19*, 41–55.

Klingemann, H., Takala, J., & Hunt, G. (1992). *Cure, care, or control.* Albany: State University of New York Press.

Koehler, R., & Lindner, C. (1992). Alternative incarceration: An inevitable response to institutional overcrowding. *Federal Probation, 56*(3), 12–18.

Kofoed, L., Tolson, R., Atkinson, R., Toth, R., & Turner, J. (1987). Treatment compliance of older alcoholics: An elder-specific approach is superior to "mainstreaming." *Journal of Studies on Alcohol, 48*, 47–51.

Kolata, G. (1996, September 18). Experts are at odds on how to best tackle rise in teenagers' drug use. *New York Times,* p. B7.

Kosten, T. (1992). Pharmacotherapies. In T. Kosten & H. Kleber (Eds.), *Clinician's guide to cocaine addiction: Theory, research, and treatment* (pp. 273–289). New York: Guilford Press.

Kosten, T., Gawin, F., Kosten, T., Morgan, C., Rounsaville, B., Schottenfeld, R., & Kleber, H. (1992). Six-month follow-up of short-term pharmacotherapy for cocaine dependence. *American Journal of the Addictions, 1*, 40–49.

Kosten, T., Kleber, H., & Morgan, C. (1989). Treatment of cocaine abuse with buprenorphine. *Biological Psychiatry, 26*, 637–639.

Kostyk, D., Lindblom, L., Fuchs, D., & Tabisz, E. (1994). Chemical dependency in the elderly: Treatment phase. *Journal of Gerontological Social Work, 22*, 175–191.

Kreft, I.G.G., & Brown, J. H. (1998). Zero effects of drug prevention programs: Issues and solutions. *Evaluation Review, 22*, 3–14.

Kumpfer, K. (1991). Treatment programs for drug abusing women. *Future of Children, 1*, 50–59.

Kurtz, L. (1990). Twelve-step programs. In T. Powell (Ed.), *Working with self-help* (pp. 93–119). Silver Spring, MD: National Association of Social Workers.

Leeds, J., & Morgenstern, J. (1996). Psychoanalytical theories of substance abuse. In F. Rotgers, D. Keller, & J. Morgenstern (Eds.), *Treating substance abuse: Theory and technique* (pp. 68–83). New York: Guilford Press.

Leipman, M. R., Wolper, B., & Vazqez, J. (1982). An ecological approach for motivating women to accept treatment for drug dependency. In B. G. Reed, G. M. Beschner, & J. Mondanaro (Eds.), *Treatment services for drug dependent women* (Vol. 2, pp. 1–61, Treatment Research Monograph Series, DHHS Publication No. [ADM]82-1219). Washington, DC: U.S. Government Printing Office.

Leukefeld, C., & Tims, F. (1988). Compulsory treatment: A review of findings. *Compulsory treatment of drug abuse: Research and clinical practice, NIDA Research Monograph, 86*, 236–251.

Lindblom, L., Kostyk, D., Tabisz, E., Jacyk, W., & Fuchs, D. (1992). Chemical abuse. An intervention program for the elderly. *Journal of Gerontological Nursing, 18*(4), 6–14.

Lipton, D., Brewington, V., & Smith, M. (1990, August). *Acupuncture and crack addicts: A single-blind placebo test of efficacy.* Paper presented at Advances in Cocaine Treatment, NIDA Technical Review Meeting, Rockville, MD.

Lisansky, E. (1989). Special issues of women. *Journal of Drug and Alcohol Dependence, 13,* 9–12.

Lowinson, J., Marion, I., Joseph, H., & Dole, V. (1992). Methadone maintenance. In J. Lowinson, P. Ruiz, R. Millman, & J. Langrod (Eds.), *Substance abuse: A comprehensive textbook* (pp. 550–561). Baltimore: Williams & Wilkins.

Lubran, B. (1990). Alcohol and drug abuse among the homeless population: A national response. In M. Argeriou & D. McCarty (Eds.), *Treating alcoholism and drug abuse among the homeless: Nine community demonstration grants* (pp. 11–23). Binghamton, NY: Haworth Press.

Luthar, S., & Walsh, K. (1995). Treatment needs of drug-addicted mothers. *Journal of Substance Abuse Treatment, 12,* 341–348.

MacDonald, J. (1987). Predictors of treatment outcome for alcoholic women. *International Journal of the Addictions, 22,* 235–248.

Mackie-Ramos, R., & Rice, J. (1988). Group psychotherapy with methadone maintained pregnant women. *Journal of Substance Abuse Treatment, 5,* 151–161.

Maguire, K., Pastore, A., & Flanagan, T. (1993). *Sourcebook of criminal justice statistics, 1992.* Washington, DC: U.S. Government Printing Office.

Marlatt, G. (1988). Matching clients to treatment: Treatment models and stages of change. In D. Donovan & G. Marlatt (Eds.), *Assessment of addictive behaviors* (pp. 474–484). New York: Guilford Press.

Marlatt, G., & Barrett, K. (1994). Relapse prevention. In M. Galanter & H. Kleber (Eds.), *The American Psychiatric Press textbook of substance abuse treatment* (pp. 285–299). Washington, DC: American Psychiatric Press.

Marlatt, G., & Tapert, S. (1993). Harm reduction: Reducing the risks of addictive behaviors. In J. Baer, G. Marlatt, & R. McMahon (Eds.), *Addictive behaviors across the life span* (pp. 243–273). Newbury Park, CA: Sage Publications.

Marlatt, G., Tucker, J. A., Donovan, D. M., & Vuchinich, R. (1997). *Help-seeking by substance abusers: The role of harm reduction and behavioral–economic approaches to facilitate treatment entry and intention* (NIDA Research Monograph 165). Washington, DC: U.S. Department of Health and Human Services.

Martin, S., & Inciardi, J. A. (1993). Case management approaches for criminal justice clients. In J. A. Inciardi (Ed.), *Drug treatment and criminal justice* (pp. 81–96). Newbury Park, CA: Sage Publications.

McCarthy, J., & Borders, O. (1985). Limit setting on drug abuse in methadone maintenance patients. *American Journal of Psychiatry, 142,* 1419–1423.

McCarty, D., Argeriou, M., Huebner, R., & Lubran, B. (1991). Alcoholism, drug abuse, and the homeless. *American Psychologist, 46,* 1139–1148.

McCarty, D., Argeriou, M., Krakow, M., & Mulvey, K. (1990). Stabilization services for homeless alcoholics and drug abusers. In M. Argeriou & D. McCarty (Eds.), *Treating alcoholism and drug abuse among the homeless: Nine community demonstration grants* (pp. 31–46). Binghamton, NY: Haworth Press.

McCrady, B., & Irvine, S. (1989). Self-help groups. In R. Hester & W. Miller (Eds.), *Handbook of alcoholism treatment approaches: Effective alternatives* (pp. 153–169). Needham Heights, MA: Allyn & Bacon.

McCrady, B., Longabaugh, R., Fink, E., Stout, R., Beattie, M., & Ruggieri-Authelet, A. (1986). Cost-effectiveness of alcoholism treatment in partial hospital versus inpatient settings after brief inpatient treatment. *Journal of Consulting and Clinical Psychology, 54,* 708–713.

McCusker, J., Bigelow, C., Luippold, R., Zorn, M., & Lewis, B. (1995). Outcomes of a 21-day drug detoxification program: Retention, transfer to further treatment, and HIV risk reduction. *American Journal of Alcohol and Drug Abuse, 21*, 1–16.

McLellan, A., Arndt, I., Metzger, D., Woody, G., & O'Brien, C. (1993). The effects of psychosocial services in substance abuse treatment. *JAMA, 269*, 1953–1959.

McLellan, A., Grossman, D., Blaine, J., & Haverkos, H. (1993). Acupuncture treatment for drug abuse: A technical review. *Journal of Substance Abuse Treatment, 10*, 569–576.

Mello, N., Mendelson, J., Bree, M., & Lukas, S. (1989). Buprenorphine suppresses cocaine self-administration by rhesus monkeys. *Science, 245*, 859–862.

Menefee, D., & Thompson, J. (1994). Identifying and comparing competencies for social work management: A practice driven approach. *Administration in Social Work, 18*(3), 1–25.

Mental health: Does therapy help? (1995, November). *Consumer Reports,* pp. 734–739.

Mermelstein, R., Cohen, S., Lichtenstein, E., Baer, J., & Kamarck, T. (1986). Social support and smoking cessation and maintenance. *Journal of Consulting and Clinical Psychology, 54*, 447–453.

Meyers, R., & Smith, J. (1995). *Clinical guide to alcohol treatment: The community reinforcement approach.* New York: Guilford Press.

Michaels, B., Noonan, M., Hoffman, S., & Brennan, R. (1988). A treatment model of nursing care for pregnant chemical abusers. In I. Chasnoff (Ed.), *Drugs, alcohol, and parenting* (pp. 47–57). Boston: Kluwer Academic Press.

Miescher, A., & Galanter, M. (1996). Shelter-based treatment of the homeless alcoholic. *Journal of Substance Abuse Treatment, 13*, 135–140.

Miller, B., Downs, W., & Testa, M. (1993). Interrelationships between victimization experiences and women's alcohol use. *Journal of Studies on Alcohol, 11*(Suppl.), 109–117.

Miller, N. (1991). Drug and alcohol addiction as a disease. *Alcohol Treatment Quarterly, 8*(4), 43–55.

Miller, N., Belkin, B., & Gold, M. (1991). Alcohol and drug dependence among the elderly: Epidemiology, diagnosis, and treatment. *Comprehensive Psychiatry, 32*, 153–165.

Miller, W. (1989). Increasing motivation for change. In R. Hester & W. Miller (Eds.), *Handbook of alcoholism treatment approaches: Effective alternatives* (pp. 67–80). Needham Heights, MA: Allyn & Bacon.

Miller, W., & Hester, R. (1989). Treating alcohol problems: Toward an informed eclecticism. In R. Hester & W. Miller (Eds.), *Handbook of alcoholism treatment approaches: Effective alternatives* (pp. 3–14). Needham Heights, MA: Allyn & Bacon.

Miller, W., & Rollnick, S. (1991). Brief intervention: More pieces of the puzzle. In W. Miller & S. Rollnick (Eds.), *Motivational interviewing* (pp. 30–35). New York: Guilford Press.

Mondanaro, J. (1989). *Chemically dependent women.* Lexington, MA: Lexington Books.

Monti, P., Abrams, D., Kadden, R., & Cooney, N. (1989). *Treating alcohol dependence: A coping skills training guide.* New York: Guilford Press.

Moss, H. (1990). Pharmacotherapy. In A. Bellack & M. Hersen (Eds.), *Handbook of comparative treatments for adult disorders* (pp. 506–520). New York: John Wiley & Sons.

National Commission on AIDS. (1991, March). *Report on HIV disease in correctional facilities.* Washington, DC: Author.

National Institute on Drug Abuse & National Institute on Alcohol Abuse and Alcoholism. (1990). *Highlights from the 1989 National Drug and Alcoholism Treatment Unit Survey (NDATUS).* Rockville, MD: Author.

Nelson-Zlupko, L., Dore, M., Kauffman, E., & Kaltenbach, K. (1996). Women in recovery: Their perceptions of treatment effectiveness. *Journal of Substance Abuse Treatment, 13,* 51–59.

Nelson-Zlupko, L., Kauffman, E., & Dore, M. (1995). Gender differences in drug addiction and treatment: Implications for social work intervention with substance-abusing women. *Social Work, 40,* 45–54.

Newcombe, R. (1995). The reduction of drug-related harm: A conceptual framework for theory, practice and research. In P. O'Hare, R. Newcombe, A. Matthews, E. Buning, & E. Drucker (Eds.), *The reduction of drug-related harm* (pp. 1–14). New York: Routledge.

Newmeyer, J., Johnson, G., & Klot, S. (1984). Acupuncture as a detoxification modality. *Journal of Psychoactive Drugs, 16,* 241–261.

Noliman, D., & Crowley, T. (1990). Difficulties in a clinical application of methadone dose contingency contracting. *Journal of Substance Abuse Treatment, 7,* 291–224.

Nowinski, J., Baker, S., & Carroll, K. (1992). *Twelve-step facilitation therapy manual.* Washington, DC: U.S. Department of Health and Human Services, National Institute on Alcohol Abuse and Alcoholism.

Nyamathi, A., & Flaskerud, J. (1992). A community-based inventory of current concerns of impoverished homeless and drug-addicted minority women. *Research in Nursing and Health, 15,* 121–129.

O'Brien, C. (1996). Recent developments in the pharmacotherapy of substance abuse. *Journal of Consulting and Clinical Psychology, 64,* 677–686.

Oetting, E., Edwards, R., & Beauvais, F. (1988). Social and psychological factors underlying inhalant abuse. In R. Crider & B. Rouse (Eds.), *Epidemiology of inhalant abuse: An update* (pp. 172–203). Rockville, MD: National Institute on Drug Abuse.

O'Farrell, T., & Bayog, R. (1986). Antabuse contracts for married alcoholics and their spouses: A method to insure Antabuse taking and decrease conflict about alcohol. *Journal of Substance Abuse Treatment, 3,* 1–8.

O'Farrell, T., & Cowles, K. (1989). Marital and family therapy. In R. Hester & W. Miller (Eds.), *Handbook of alcoholism treatment approaches: Effective alternatives* (pp. 183–205). Needham Heights, MA: Allyn & Bacon.

O'Hare, P. (1992). Preface: A note on the concept of harm reduction. In P. O'Hare, R. Newcombe, A. Matthews, E. Buning, & E. Drucker (Eds.), *The reduction of drug-related harm* (pp. ix–x). New York: Routledge.

O'Malley, S., Jaffe, A., Chang, G., Schottenfeld, R., Meyer, R., & Rounsaville, B. (1992). Naltrexone and coping skills therapy for alcohol dependence: A controlled study. *Archives of General Psychiatry, 49,* 881–887.

Pakier, A. (1990). Predictors of substance abuse in a methadone maintained sample. *Dissertation Abstracts International, 51*(2-B), 1020.

Peele, S. (1988). A moral vision of addiction: How people's values determine whether they become and remain addicts. In S. Peele (Ed.), *Visions of addiction* (pp. 201–233). Lexington, MA: Lexington Books.

Peele, S. (1989). *Diseasing of America: Addiction treatment out of control.* Lexington, MA: Lexington Books.

Pope, A., Conrad, K., Baxter, W., Elbaum, P., Lisiccki, J., Daghestani, A., Hultman, C., & Lyons, J. (1993). Case managed residential care for homeless addicted veterans: Evanston VA Hospital. *Alcoholism Treatment Quarterly, 10,* 155–170.

Rathbone-McCuan, E., Schiff, S., & Resch, J. (1984). The aging alcoholic: A summary of the Michigan experiment as a model of outreach and intervention. In G. Lesnoff-

Caravaglia (Ed.), *Handbook of applied gerontology* (pp. 297–309). New York: Human Sciences Press.

Reed, B. (1987). Developing women-sensitive drug dependence treatment services: Why so difficult? *Journal of Psychoactive Drugs, 19,* 151–164.

Richmond, M. (1917). *Social diagnosis.* New York: Russell Sage Foundation.

Ridlen, S., Asamoah, Y., Edwards, H., & Zimmer, R. (1990). Outreach and engagement for homeless women at risk of alcoholism. In M. Argeriou & D. McCarty (Eds.), *Treating alcoholism and drug abuse among the homeless: Nine community demonstration grants* (pp. 99–109). Binghamton, NY: Haworth Press.

Rollnick, S., & Morgan, M. (1995). Motivational interviewing: Increasing readiness for change. In A. Washton (Ed.), *Psychotherapy and substance abuse: A practitioner's handbook* (pp. 179–191). New York: Guilford Press.

Rosen, M., & Kosten, T. (1991). Buprenorphine: Beyond methadone? *Hospital and Community Psychiatry, 42,* 347–349.

Saxon, A., Wells, E., Fleming, C., Jackson, T., & Calsyn, D. (1996). Pre-treatment characteristics, program philosophy, and level of ancillary services as predictors of methadone maintenance treatment outcome. *Addiction, 91,* 1197–1209.

Schilling, R., El-Bassel, N., Hadden, B., & Gilbert, L. (1995). Skills-training groups to reduce HIV transmission and drug use among methadone patients. *Social Work, 40,* 91–101.

Schilling, R., El-Bassel, N., Schinke, S., Gordon, K., & Nichols, S. (1991). Building skills of recovering women drug users to reduce heterosexual AIDS transmission. *Public Health Reports, 106,* 297–304.

Schilling, R., El-Bassel, N., Schinke, S., Nichols, S., Botvin, G., & Orlandi, M. (1991). Sexual behavior, attitudes towards safer sex, and gender among a cohort of 244 recovering IV drug users. *International Journal of the Addictions, 26,* 865–883.

Schilling, R., El-Bassel, N., Serrano, Y., & Wallace, B. (1992). AIDS prevention strategies for ethnic-racial minority substance users. *Journal of Psychology of Addictive Behaviors, 6,* 81–90.

Schilling, R. F., Ivanoff, A., El-Bassel, N., & Soffa, F. (1997). Research on HIV-related behavior in transitional correctional settings. *Criminal Justice, 24,* 256–277.

Schilling, R., & McAlister, A. (1990). Preventing drug use in adolescents through media interventions. *Journal of Consulting and Clinical Psychology, 58,* 416–424.

Schilling, R., & Sachs, C. (1993). Attrition from an evening alcohol rehabilitation program. *American Journal of Drug and Alcohol Abuse, 19,* 239–248.

Schilling, R., Schinke, S., & El-Bassel, N. (in press). Substance abuse. In A. Bellack & M. Hersen (Eds.), *Psychopathology in adulthood* (rev. ed.). Needham Heights, MA: Allyn & Bacon.

Schilling, R., Schinke, S., & Weatherly, R. (1988). Service trends in a conservative era: Social workers rediscover the past. *Social Work, 33,* 5–9.

Schinke, S., & Cole, K. (1995). Prevention in community settings. In G. Botvin, S. Schinke, & M. Orlandi (Eds.), *Drug abuse prevention with multiethnic youth* (pp. 215–232). Thousand Oaks, CA: Sage Publications.

Schinke, S., Schilling, R., Gilchrist, L., Whittaker, J., Kirkham, M., Senechal, V., Snow, W., & Maxwell, J. (1986). Definitions and methods for prevention research with youth and families. *Children and Youth Services Review, 8,* 257–266.

Schneider, K., Kviz, F., Isola, M., & Filstead, W. (1995). Evaluating multiple outcomes and gender in alcoholism treatment. *Addictive Behaviors, 20,* 1–21.

Schuckit, M. (1995). *Drug and alcohol abuse.* New York: Plenum Press.

Schuckit, M. (1996). Recent developments in the pharmacotherapy of alcohol dependence. *Journal of Consulting and Clinical Psychology, 64,* 669–676.

Seligman, M. (1995). The effectiveness of psychotherapy. *American Psychologist, 50,* 965–974.

Siegfried, M. L. (1996). The inner city in the 21st century: Huxley's *Brave New World* revisited? *Journal of Interdisciplinary Studies, 8,* 19–30.

Silber, A. (1974). Rationale for the technique of psychotherapy with alcoholics. *International Journal of Psychoanalytic Psychotherapy, 3,* 28–47.

Sisson, R., & Azrin, N. (1989). The community reinforcement approach. In R. Hester & W. Miller (Eds.), *Handbook of alcoholism treatment approaches: Effective alternatives* (pp. 242–258). Needham Heights, MA: Allyn & Bacon.

Skidmore, R. (1995). *Social work administration: Dynamic management and human relationships.* Needham Heights, MA: Allyn & Bacon.

Smith, M., & Khan, I. (1988). An acupuncture programme for the treatment of drug-addicted persons. *Bulletin on Narcotics, 40,* 35–41.

Sobell, L., Toneatto, T., & Sobell, M. (1990). Behavior therapy. In A. Bellack & M. Hersen (Eds.), *Handbook of comparative treatments for adult disorders* (pp. 479–504). New York: John Wiley & Sons.

Stark, M. (1989). A psychoeducational approach to methadone maintenance treatment. *Journal of Substance Abuse Treatment, 6,* 169–181.

Steinglass, P. (1994). Family therapy: Alcohol. In M. Galanter & H. Kleber (Eds.), *The American Psychiatric Press textbook of substance abuse treatment* (pp. 315–330). Washington, DC: American Psychiatric Press.

Stephens, R. (1991). *The street addict role: A theory of heroin addiction.* Albany: State University of New York Press.

Stimson, G. (1996). Has the United Kingdom averted an epidemic of HIV-1 infection among drug injectors? *Addiction, 91,* 1085–1088.

Stockwell, T., & Town, C. (1989). Anxiety and stress management. In R. Hester & W. Miller (Eds.), *Handbook of alcoholism treatment approaches: Effective alternatives* (pp. 222–230). Needham Heights, MA: Allyn & Bacon.

Suedfeld, P. (1980). *Restricted environmental stimulation.* New York: Wiley-Interscience.

Sumners, A. (1991). Women in recovery. In E. Bennett & D. Woolf (Eds.), *Substance abuse: Pharmacologic, developmental, and clinical perspectives* (pp. 280–292). Albany, NY: Delmar.

Test, M. A., Knoedler, W. H., & Allness, D. J. (1985). The long-term treatment of young schizophrenics in a community support program. In L. I. Stein & M. A. Test (Eds.), *New directions for mental health services: Vol. 26. The Training in Community Model: A decade of experience* (pp. 17–27). San Francisco: Jossey-Bass.

Thyer, B. (1991). Guidelines for evaluating outcome studies on social work practice. *Research on Social Work Practice, 1,* 76–91.

Travis, C. (1988). *Women and health psychology.* Hillsdale, NJ: Erlbaum.

Tucker, M. (1982). Social support and coping: Applications for the study of female drug abuse. *Journal of Social Issues, 38,* 117–137.

Tucker, M. (1985). Coping and drug use among heroin-addicted women and men. In S. Shiffman & T. Wills (Eds.), *Coping and substance abuse* (pp. 147–170). Orlando, FL: Academic Press.

Tutton, C., & Crayton, J. (1993). Current pharmacotherapies for cocaine abuse: A review. *Journal of Addictive Diseases, 12,* 109–127.

Vaillant, G. (1981). Dangers of psychotherapy in the treatment of alcoholism. In M. Bean, E. Khantzian, J. Mack, G. Vaillant, & N. Zinberg (Eds.), *Dynamic approaches to the understanding and treatment of alcoholism* (pp. 36–54). New York: Free Press.

Vanichseni, S., Wongsuwan, B., Staff of BMA Narcotics Clinic No. 6, Choopanya, K., & Wongpanich, K. (1991). A controlled trial of methadone maintenance in a population of intravenous drug users in Bangkok: Implications for prevention of HIV. *International Journal of the Addictions, 26,* 1313–1320.

Van Wormer, K. (1995). *Alcoholism treatment: A social work perspective.* Chicago: Nelson-Hall.

Vaughan, A. (1990). Frontiers in pharmacologic treatment of alcohol, cocaine, and nicotine dependence. *Psychiatric Annals, 20,* 695–709.

Wald, R., Harvey, S., & Hibbard, J. (1995). A treatment model for women substance users. *International Journal of the Addictions, 30,* 881–888.

Ward, D., Bendel, R., & Lange, D. (1983). A reconsideration of environmental resources and the posttreatment functioning of alcoholic patients. *Journal of Health and Social Behavior, 23,* 310–317.

Washburn, A., Keenan, P., & Nazareno, J. (1990). Preliminary findings: Study of acupuncture-assisted heroin detoxification. *Multicultural Inquiry and Research on AIDS Quarterly Newsletter, 4,* 3–6.

Washburn, A., Fullilove, R., Fullilove, M., Keenan, P., McGee, B., Morris, K., Sorensen, J., & Clark, W. (1993). Acupuncture heroin detoxification: A single-blind clinical trial. *Journal of Substance Abuse Treatment, 10,* 345–351.

Washton, A. (1988). Preventing relapse to cocaine. APT Foundation North American Conference: Cocaine abuse and its treatment. *Journal of Clinical Psychiatry, 49,* 34–38.

Weisner, C., & Morgan, P. (1992). Rapid growth and bifurcation: Public and private alcohol treatment in the United States. In H. Klingemann, J. Takala, & G. Hunt (Eds.), *Cure, care, or control* (pp. 223–252). Albany: State University of New York Press.

Widner, S., & Zeichner, A. (1991). Alcohol abuse in the elderly: Review of epidemiology research and treatment. *Clinical Gerontologist, 11,* 3–18.

Willenbring, M., Whelan, J., Dahlquist, J., & O'Neal, M. (1990). Community treatment of the chronic public inebriate: I. Implementation. In M. Argeriou & D. McCarty (Eds.), *Treating alcoholism and drug abuse among the homeless: Nine community demonstration grants* (pp. 79–98). Binghamton, NY: Haworth Press.

Williams, R. (1988). Nature, nurture, and family. *New England Journal of Medicine, 318,* 770–771.

Wilson, P. (1992). Relapse prevention: Conceptual and methodological issues. In P. Wilson (Ed.), *Principles and practice of relapse prevention* (pp. 1–22). New York: Guilford Press.

Witters, W., & Venturelli, P. (1988). *Drugs and society* (2nd ed.). Boston: Jones & Bartlett.

Woody, G., Mercer, D., & Luborsky, L. (1994). Individual psychotherapy: Other drugs. In M. Galanter & H. Kleber (Eds.), *The American Psychiatric Press textbook of substance abuse treatment* (pp. 275–284). Washington, DC: American Psychiatric Press.

Worner, T., Zeller, B., Schwarz, H., Zwas, F., & Lyon, D. (1992). Acupuncture fails to improve treatment outcome in alcoholics. *Drug and Alcohol Dependence, 30,* 169–173.

Wright, A., Mora, J., & Hughes, L. (1990). The Sober Transitional Housing and Employment Project (STHEP): Strategies for long-term sobriety, employment and housing. In M. Argeriou & D. McCarty (Eds.), *Treating alcoholism and drug abuse among the homeless: Nine community demonstration grants* (pp. 47–56). Binghamton, NY: Haworth Press.

Yee, B., Castro, F., Hammond, W., John, R., Wyatt, G., & Yung, B. (1995). Panel IV: Risk-taking and abusive behaviors among ethnic minorities. *Health Psychology, 14,* 622–631.

Zedonis, D., & Kosten, T. (1991). Depression as prognostic factor for pharmacological treatment of cocaine dependence. *Psychopharmacological Bulletin, 27,* 337–343.

Zimberg, S. (1984). Diagnosis and management of the elderly alcoholic. In R. Atkinson (Ed.), *Alcohol and drug abuse in old age* (pp. 24–32). Washington, DC: American Psychiatric Press.

Zimberg, S. (1994). Individual psychotherapy: Alcohol. In M. Galanter & H. Kleber (Eds.), *The American Psychiatric Press textbook of substance abuse treatment* (pp. 263–274). Washington, DC: American Psychiatric Press.

Zuckerman, B., & Bresnahan, K. (1991). Developmental and behavioral consequences of prenatal drug and alcohol exposure. *Very Young Child, 38*(6), 1–20.

Zweben, A., & Pearlman, S. (1983). Evaluating the effectiveness of conjoint treatment of alcohol-complicated marriages: Clinical and methodological issues. *Journal of Marital and Family Therapy, 9,* 61–72.

Zweben, A., Pearlman, S., & Li, S. (1988). A comparison of brief advice and conjoint therapy in the treatment of alcohol abuse: The results of the marital systems study. *British Journal of Addiction, 83,* 899–916.

# The Conceptual and Empirical Base of Case Management for Adults with Severe Mental Illness

Phyllis Solomon

Over the past 15 years, case management has emerged as the dominant mode for serving the most vulnerable populations, be they frail elderly clients, people with mental disabilities, people with AIDS, seriously emotionally disturbed children, or severely mentally ill adults (Austin, 1990; Friesen & Poertner, 1995). Case management has been promoted as the major strategy for public services system integration for clients with multiple problems who have difficulty navigating fragmented and uncoordinated service delivery systems (Austin, 1990; Johnson & Rubin, 1983; Lurie, 1978; Mechanic, 1991). Much of this enthusiasm for case management has been based on limited research evidence, but recently there has been a burgeoning of pertinent research focused on adults with severe mental illness. This research has resulted from both the critical importance of case management for this target group and the priority that the National Institute of Mental Health (NIMH) placed on services research for this population. This chapter explores the theoretical, empirical, and practical base of case management for people with severe mental illness. This grounding is essential for social workers to both understand the service implications for those they treat and have an impact on the changing role of case management in this era of behavioral health care reform.

## Case Management

### HISTORICAL ROOTS

Case management was developed in response to the consequences of deinstitutionalization. When clients with major psychiatric illnesses lived in state hospitals, all their basic human needs and their medical care were provided within the confines of the institution. On discharge from the hospital, the diversity of social, welfare, and psychiatric services they needed were provided by a multiplicity of agencies and institutions. Extensive efforts were required to coordinate appropriate services packages for people who often lacked the skills to make their way through an uncoordinated, complex, and fragmented public services delivery system. The optimal way to establish a coordinated, continuous, flexible, and comprehensive array of needed services for these discharged clients was to locate responsibility in one accountable services provider or agency with a range of available backup support and emergency services (Borland, McRae, & Lycan, 1989; Ozarin, 1978). Therefore, the initial impetus for case management was to ensure that clients with serious mental illness would efficiently receive needed services. Case management thus became the linchpin of the community support system conceived by NIMH (Turner & Tenhor, 1978). With time it became apparent to many professionals working with seriously mentally ill clients that case managers had to "maintain intimate contact" with them to achieve these objectives effectively (Sledge, Astrachan, Thompson, Rakfeldt, & Leaf, 1995). Thus, case managers became providers as well as coordinators of services (Lamb, 1980).

In contrast to the public sector, the private sector has recently come to use case management as a strategy to control rising health care costs. In this system, case managers do not provide service but function as utilization reviewers to control allocation of scarce resources by attempting to substitute lower-cost treatment alternatives (Sledge et al., 1995).

The State Comprehensive Mental Health Services Plan Act of 1986 and its subsequent amendments require every state and all U.S. territories to provide case management services to all seriously mentally ill adults who receive substantial amounts of public funds. The nature of the specific services is left to the state to decide.

## THEORETICAL BASIS

Case management is theoretically consistent with social work. To determine the services and support requirements, case managers need to understand clients in the context of the clients' environments. This parallels systems theory or, more specifically, the person-in-environment conceptualization of social work (Roberts-DeGennaro, 1987). To assess client needs case managers use a biopsychosocial framework. Preventing hospitalization is a major objective of case management. Psychiatrically vulnerable clients need assistance, supports, and services from the three domains of medical care, psychological supports, and social welfare to reduce their vulnerability to psychiatric decompensation and possible resulting hospitalization (Solomon & Meyerson, 1997). The vulnerability of clients to hospitalization is mediated by enhanced supports in their social environment, a strategy that is consistent with the "vulnerability, stress, coping and competence model of mental disorders" (Anthony & Liberman, 1986, p. 547).

## DEFINITION

Case management is a ubiquitous term used to describe a variety of activities (Sledge et al., 1995), and "even when clear and operational definitions are offered, they are at great variance" (Bachrach, 1989, p. 883). This multiplicity of empirical referents results in no clear conceptual definition. Sledge and his colleagues (1995) said that "case management" is a composite term derived from "case," a clinical modality, and "management," an administrative function. Combining these two terms evokes the importance of providing care in the context of managing limited resources.

Intagliata (1982) defined *case management* as "a process or method of ensuring that consumers are provided with whatever services they need in a coordinated, effective, and efficient manner" (p. 657). Solomon (1992) elaborated on this definition by noting that "case management is a coordinated strategy on behalf of clients to obtain the services that they need, when they need them and for as long as they need these services" (p. 164), which implies the necessity of continuity of care. These

definitions provide a rather ambiguous indication of outcomes, but they do not clarify the precise meaning of "case management" per se. A more specific understanding
of case management can be obtained from the functional roles of case managers
and their activities (Bachrach, 1992). The *NASW Standards for Social Work Case Manage-*
*ment* (NASW, 1992) focuses on the activities engaged in by social workers who are
case managers. The standards supply a definition that applies to the diverse populations served by social workers and therefore also is applicable to those with severe
mental illness: "Social work case management is a method of providing services
whereby a professional social worker assesses the needs of the client and the client's
family, when appropriate, and arranges, coordinates, monitors, evaluates, and advocates for a package of multiple services to meet the specific client's complex needs"
(p. 5). The standards noted that case management addresses "both the individual
client's biopsychosocial status as well as the state of the social system in which case
management operates" (p. 5). This is comparable to much case management provided for those with severe mental illness.

## ACTIVITIES AND FEATURES

Although there are many case management models and programs, a range of tasks
is relatively common to most. Generally, there are five basic functions of case management: assessment, planning, linking, monitoring, and advocacy. Case managers
work both on the individual level and the system level. The case manager first conducts an intake assessment that determines if the client is appropriate for the services offered. Thus, the case manager controls access to services either by limiting
or by increasing the client's access. For example, for people who are homeless as
well as seriously mentally ill, case mangers engage in outreach efforts. Assertive outreach also is used to engage clients who miss appointments or are resistant to receiving needed services. Identification and intake are followed by assessment to identify
and clarify the client's problems. People from several mental health care disciplines
may be involved in this assessment, and various sources of information (for example,
the clients themselves and psychiatric hospital records) may be used. Case management emphasizes strengths rather than deficits, and all models involve history, diagnosis, strengths, problems, deficits, and available environmental resources. This assessment usually concludes with stating services goals (Rothman, 1991; Sledge et al.,
1995; Solomon & Meyerson, 1997). The client's input is usually sought in the development of these goals, but some models are more client driven than others. Services
planning is contingent on the resources available both in the services system and in
the client's informal system, so an assessment of formal and informal environmental
resources also is required (Rothman, 1991).

A major function of all models of case management is linkage with agencies, services, and resources, which may include assistance in obtaining entitlements or informal linkage with family members or other natural supports, if appropriate. The
"brokering" function goes beyond linkage in that it may take some negotiating to
have the services provider accept a client or to obtain a priority rating for a client.
The "advocacy" function goes even further; for example, it may include changing a
policy so that certain clients have access to needed services for which they may not
be eligible or may not be a priority population. To increase available benefits and resources, case managers negotiate for their clients with agencies and policymakers to
gain additional resources and change policies. Linkage, brokering, and advocacy also
involve coordination of services and resources to ensure an integrated and consistent

delivery plan. In addition, case managers monitor services and supports to be sure that they are received by and appropriate to their clients. Evaluation and reassessment are done if there is a need to alter the objectives or to change resources to meet the planned objectives. All case managers engage to some degree in providing direct services. At a minimum, case managers have to establish a relationship with their clients and provide supportive counseling. The clinical model of case management is distinctive because psychotherapy is a central component (Rothman, 1991; Sledge et al., 1995; Solomon & Meyerson, 1997). Some mental health professionals believe that case management is an integral part of the job of a good therapist— that is, without therapeutic involvement, a comprehensive assessment of client needs and means to meeting them cannot be developed (Harris & Bergman, 1993; Lamb, 1980).

Regardless of the model of case management used, there is a relatively high degree of consensus on certain features of case management when serving adults with severe and persistent mental illness, particularly those diagnosed with schizophrenia and major affective disorders. These features include low client–staff ratios; delivery of services in the client's own environment rather than in the service provider's office or a hospital office; crisis intervention available 24 hours a day, seven days a week; no limitation on service provision; and assertive outreach to clients (Solomon & Meyerson, 1997).

## QUALIFICATIONS OF CASE MANAGERS

Case managers do not have to be affiliated with any particular profession or discipline (Bachrach, 1992; Sands, 1991). Some case managers are neither college educated nor members of a particular profession (Cnaan, 1994; Sands, 1991). There also is a question of the actual necessity of professional skills for the effective implementation of case management (Johnson & Rubin, 1983). However, case managers without professional training still must have the requisite skills, which may be obtained through in-service training, and may need increased clinical supervision.

Consumers of mental health services also can function as case management aides or as full-fledged case managers. Studies have shown that consumers of mental health services can deliver nonclinical case management services as effectively as can nonconsumers (Solomon & Draine, 1995b, 1995c). Family members also often function as de facto case managers for a seriously mentally ill relative (Intagliata, Willer, & Egri, 1986; Lurie, 1978; Ozarin, 1978), filling in where the services system has failed.

Social workers are particularly well suited to perform many case management functions because of their training in social orientation to the person in the environment (Johnson & Rubin, 1983; Sledge et al., 1995). The profession historically has conducted these same activities under the rubric of casework (Netting, 1992). However, social workers often prefer not to work with clients who are seriously mentally ill, and they do not want to participate in some of the required activities of case management, which they feel do not use their professional skills effectively. Thus, there appears to be a gap between social work orientation and practice (Johnson & Rubin, 1983). Dill (1987) has promoted the use of paraprofessionals for linkage and monitoring, particularly for accompanying clients to services. The cost-effectiveness of this option is appealing. In Great Britain there has been a movement toward the use of nurses, who can address the medical and psychiatric functions of this work, to fill these case management roles (Sledge et al., 1995).

## MODELS

Six case management models are currently in practice. Although they may differ in their theoretical and philosophical orientations, in actual practice the distinctions among the models are frequently blurred.

### Assertive Community Treatment

This model was developed by Stein and Test (1980) as an alternative to inpatient treatment at a psychiatric hospital in Madison, Wisconsin. The original program was called Training in Community Living (TLC), and the name was later changed to Program of Assertive Community Treatment (PACT). As discussed in detail in chapter 15, this program is a comprehensive system of care for those with severe psychiatric disorders, and case management serves as the coordinating function for this community-based system of care. The original intention of PACT was to transfer all the functions served by the long-term psychiatric hospital into the community. Its goals were to increase clients' community integration and psychosocial functioning, improve their quality of life, and decrease their symptomatic behaviors. The major strategy used to achieve these goals was the teaching of social and behavioral skills in the client's own environment. The intention was to eliminate the need to generalize skills from a learning environment to the one in which those skills are used. It was further expected that these techniques would increase the likelihood of maintaining clients in treatment (Solomon & Meyerson, 1997; Test, 1992).

This model has been the impetus for much of the case management that is in practice today with clients who have severe psychiatric disorders. The Assertive Community Treatment (ACT) model is an adaptation of the original PACT, with less direct services provision and greater emphasis on services coordination. The case manager functions as an "assertive resource coordinator" (Test, 1992). The ACT model still calls for the provision of the full range of medical, psychosocial, and rehabilitation services to be delivered by the team (Burns & Santos, 1995). The basic goals and tenets of the original model are retained (Solomon, 1992; Solomon & Meyerson, 1997). ACT maintains

- an interdisciplinary treatment team, often including a psychiatrist, a nurse, and at least two case managers
- assertive outreach for the delivery of services in the client's own environment
- continuous services provision and crisis availability
- skill training in the client's community that includes daily living skills, budgeting, and symptom management
- small caseloads
- supportive counseling
- educational support for families and significant others
- assertive outreach.

The ACT team shares responsibility for the care of all clients in the program. Depending on the number of team members, the number of clients served can vary from 50 to 120, usually with a staff–client ratio of one to 10 or 12. The team provides medication management and clinical care for the clients, but for other services clients are dependent on the services environment. In some cases, specialists in vocational or substance abuse services or other areas may be included in the team, and family members also have been included. The team usually meets daily to keep all team members up to date on the status of each client.

## Rehabilitation Model

The rehabilitation model is based on the principles developed by the Boston University Psychiatric Rehabilitation Center. Within this model, case managers assist clients with obtaining the skills and resources they need to overcome environmental barriers and achieve their personal goals. Ultimately, these efforts can improve the clients' social functioning in their environments of choice. The goals are self-selected by the client with help from the case manager. They focus on the development of specific skills to achieve the working, living, or recreational environment of choice with the least amount of professional assistance (Hodge & Draine, 1993; Robinson & Toff-Bergman, 1990; Solomon, 1992; Solomon & Meyerson, 1997).

The rehabilitation model process begins with a functional assessment that includes identifying the client's strengths, deficits, and abilities and the available resources to assist in supporting the necessary skills development. The assessment focuses on the client's specific environment because different environments require different skills. For example, an employment environment requires time punctuality and appropriate dress, whereas an independent-living arrangement requires meal preparation, house cleaning, and shopping. The case manager also ensures that the client receives appropriate support in times of crisis, in coping with the environment, and in developing the needed personal and social skills. Case managers continue to work with clients until they can assume responsibility for their own care (Goering, Wasylenki, Farkas, & Ballantyne, 1988).

## Strengths Model

In the strengths model, the case manager assists clients with the environmental supports needed to develop and achieve their identified goals. This model is based on two assumptions regarding human behavior. First, people who can be successfully self-sustaining in the community have the ability to use and to develop their own potential, and second, they have access to needed resources to accomplish this goal (Rapp, 1995). The case manager assesses the client's strengths and helps create personal and environmental opportunities so that clients can achieve successes and enhance their strengths. The community in general, not the mental health system per se, is viewed as the network of available resources rather than as an obstacle. Because people with severe psychiatric disorders frequently have functional impairments that hinder their ability to obtain resources for human growth and development, case managers assist clients in obtaining needed resources from the community at large. They act as mentors, teaching clients resource acquisition skills through modeling behaviors and having the clients practice these skills. This model uses group supervision to foster creative brainstorming in development of strategies for acquiring resources and resolving problems (Rapp, 1995; Solomon & Meyerson, 1997).

## Clinical Model

The clinical model incorporates both the administrative functions of case management and direct clinical care. Case managers not only assist clients in obtaining needed services, resources, and skills training; they also provide support and psychotherapy (Kanter, 1989; Lamb, 1980; Roach, 1993). This model emphasizes both linkages to formal and informal resources and clients' development of internal resources for purposes of survival, growth, and adaptation to their psychiatric disorder and social environment (Kanter, 1989). Consequently, case managers aid clients in functional skills acquisition and in increasing psychological capacity. This model is based on the premise that the functions of case management are consistent with those of a therapist, and that only psychotherapeutic involvement with clients can help case managers obtain the information needed to make an adequate and comprehensive assessment of needs (Lamb, 1980; Solomon & Meyerson, 1997).

## Expanded Broker (Generalist) Model

This model is most closely akin to traditional casework. As a broker of services, the case manager's primary role is to provide clients with needed information, resources, and services—that is, the major tasks are brokering and linking clients with services. This model is more often based in the office than are other models of case management. Because caseloads are generally high in this model, case managers may be more responsive to clients who are more demanding or in crisis. This model sometimes is expanded to provide limited skills training and enhancement of problem-solving and coping skills (Johnson & Rubin, 1983; Solomon & Meyerson, 1997).

## Intensive Model

Some states, such as New York and Pennsylvania, have instituted an intensive case management (ICM) model to meet the needs of clients who frequently use services (Bachrach, 1989; Shern, Surles, & Waizer, 1989). The intensive model integrates many of the features of ACT and the strengths and rehabilitation models. It may be delivered either individually or by a team, although, unlike ACT, a team usually does not maintain shared responsibility for clients. Case managers use assertive outreach in maintaining contact with clients and engaging them in treatment by delivering services in the clients' own environments. To ensure continuity of care, the services are available 24 hours a day, seven days a week. Emergency services are coordinated with ICM—for example, if a client contacts a hospital emergency room, the case manager is notified immediately. Services are rehabilitative in orientation: Case managers help clients identify their goals and provide skills training to achieve them. In addition, case managers act as agents of system change by advocating for needed services on behalf of clients. "Case managers are expected to increase clients' community tenure through a more effective use of services, and ultimately by enhancing natural supports and better community integration" (Shern et al., 1989, p. 111).

## *EFFICACY*

Since the late 1980s, research has markedly increased on case management for people with severe psychiatric diagnoses. These studies include a number of research reviews (Bond, McGrew, & Fekete, 1995; Chamberlain & Rapp, 1991; Draine, 1997; Mueser, Bond, Drake, & Resnick, in press; Olfson, 1990; Rubin, 1992; Scott & Dixon, 1995; Solomon, 1992; Test, 1992). Most of this research studied the ACT model. There has been no research on the clinical model, and only one study of the rehabilitation model, which found increases in vocational functioning, recreational activities, and independence in living but no difference in hospitalization (Goering et al., 1988). The study of the rehabilitation model used a matched group design, which is relatively weak. Consequently, no conclusions can be made regarding the efficacy of those two models. For the broker model, there has been a limited number of studies (Rapp, 1995), including two rigorous studies employing experimental designs that showed an increase in hospitalizations and no statistically significant increase in quality of life (Curtis, Millman, & Struening, 1992; Dozier, Lee, Keir, Toprac, & Mason, 1993; Franklin, Solovitz, Mason, Clemons, & Miller, 1987). The increase in hospitalizations was attributed to case managers being knowledgeable and able to obtain access to resources (Dozier et al., 1993; Franklin, et al., 1987). Other studies with weaker designs found somewhat more positive results, such as fewer unmet needs (Bigelow & Young, 1991; Hornstra, Brice-Wolfe, Sagluyu, & Riffle, 1993). Two relatively rigorous studies have been conducted on the strengths model: One found no difference in the rates of hospitalizations, and the other found no reduction in subsequent use of inpatient services (Macias, Kinney, Farley, Jackson, & Vos, 1994; Modrcin, Rapp, & Poertner, 1988). These two studies did find improvement in social functioning and behavior symptomatology, but the sample sizes were small, and the study by Modrcin and colleagues had high attrition rates (Draine, 1997). Scott and Dixon (1995) reviewed case management studies and noted that there was wide variability of program characteristics that fall within the category of intensive case management. The rigor of the research designs also varied (Mueser et al., in press). The evidence has suggested that these programs reduce the use of hospitalization, but in some studies the results were not statistically significant. In addition, ICM has been found to increase other use of mental health services (Scott & Dixon, 1995).

As discussed in chapter 15, the most research has been done on ACT, much of it by use of experimental designs, so more specific conclusions can be drawn with regard to this model. The early studies of the PACT program found decreases in hospitalization for members of the experimental group compared with those clients in the control group who received hospitalization plus standard aftercare services, as well as some improvement in social adjustment and quality of life for clients in the experimental group (Hoult, Reynolds, Charbonneau-Powis, Weekes, & Briggs, 1983; Mulder, 1982; Stein & Test, 1980; Test & Stein, 1980).

The studies in the various research reviews of ACT programs varied greatly with regard to design, setting, sample characteristics, measures, service domains assessed, and nature of services environments; however, the conclusions were relatively consistent. The ACT model was found to be effective in reducing hospitalization rates and increasing rates of retention in community-based mental health services, but clinical outcomes, such as social adjustment, symptomatology, quality of life, and employment status, were more inconsistent and moderate at best when positive (Bond et al., 1995; Rapp, 1995; Rubin, 1992; Scott & Dixon, 1995; Solomon, 1992). The reduction in hospitalization was noted particularly for clients with histories of numerous hospitalizations. Audini, Marks, Lawrence, Connolly, and Watts (1994) found that the positive outcomes were difficult to sustain when clients left the program.

In addition, the effectiveness of ACT programs was found to be linked to greater fidelity to the model (McGrew, Bond, Dietzen, & Salyers, 1994). Thus, this program model shows promise for being highly effective if its implementation remains faithful to major components of the program. Lack of fidelity to the model was exemplified in the study by Solomon and Draine (1995a), which found that for homeless people with severe mental illness who were being released from jail, there was a nonsignificant trend for clients receiving ACT services to be more likely to return to jail than those receiving intensive forensic case management or the usual care of the system. Solomon and Draine (1995a) explained this finding by noting that intensive services easily may evolve to more monitoring services, which results in the observance of violation of probation or parole, and consequently, a return to jail. Furthermore, it appears that to obtain beneficial effects in specific areas of functioning, such as a vocational rehabilitation program, services need to be directed toward those objectives, with specialists in those areas included as team members. For example, ACT has shown positive effects in housing stability for seriously mentally ill people who have been homeless as well as a reduction in substance use among dually diagnosed, mentally ill substance abusers, when the services were directed at these objectives and such specialists were included on the team (Mueser et al., in press). Satisfaction of family members and clients in ACT programs has been high when this factor was assessed (Hoult, Reynolds, Charbonneau-Powis, Coles, & Briggs, 1981; Solomon & Draine, 1994). Families feel a sense of security for their ill relative within the ACT program (Burns & Santos, 1995).

## COST ANALYSES

In this era of managed care, cost of services is a major concern. Cost-effectiveness and cost–benefit analysis of case management are closely related to the efficacy of the service. One of the most comprehensive cost–benefit analyses examined the original PACT program. Although the experimental program had higher direct costs than did standard care, these costs were offset by increased benefits from work productivity (Weisbrod, Test, & Stein, 1980). Similarly, Hoult, Reynolds, and colleagues (1983, 1984) found that the annual direct and indirect costs were substantially less for the experimental PACT model than for the standard care. Knapp and colleagues (1994) found similar results for PACT in London, and there were no greater costs to communities in terms of increased arrests or to families with regard to burden for PACT treatment. The results found for the ACT programs were more inconsistent, with some studies finding cost savings and others not (Bond, 1984; Bond, Miller, Krumwied, & Ward, 1988). Again, fidelity to the model was found to be important for cost savings to accrue (Bond et al., 1988).

Evidence of cost savings also has been found for ICM (Jerrel & Hu, 1989; Quinlaven et al., 1995; Scott & Dixon, 1995). However, these results were modified somewhat when more costly, highly structured residential options were substituted for hospitalization (Borland et al., 1989). No cost analyses have been conducted on the strengths, rehabilitation, and broker models. Rapp (1995) noted that the precepts of the strengths model suggest the potential for reduced cost—for example, use of paraprofessionals as case managers, use of community resources instead of professional mental health services, and outcomes of reduced hospitalization and increased vocational functioning. In contrast, the broker model is likely to be more costly because it usually involves an increase in use of inpatient services.

## PROCESS ASSESSMENT

Process assessment in case management is difficult because established models are adapted to location and frequently are not specified with enough detail for replication (Bachrach, 1980; Brekke & Wolkon, 1988; Rapp, 1995). Also, as models become well accepted, a number of their elements become a part of standard treatment. (It appears that ICM evolved through just such a process.) What is of importance is the determination of those services elements that are effective in producing positive outcomes for clients (Rapp, 1995). McGrew and Bond (1995) conducted a study of the critical components of the ACT model according to the judgments of experts on ACT programs and found high agreement for ratings of importance for 73 program elements. Based on that research, McGrew and colleagues developed a measure of fidelity that included ratings in areas such as form structure, engagement process, service coordinating, treatment goals, and client characteristics for ACT and later found that programs with the highest fidelity showed the greatest reduction in days of hospitalization (McGrew et al., 1994).

Rapp (1995) analyzed the effective elements of case management based on empirical research and commentary by experts in the mental health field. Although the team approach is the hallmark of ACT, he concluded that team-delivered case management is no more effective than individual case management. This finding was modified somewhat by the research of McGrew et al. (1994), which found that shared caseloads were important in reducing days of hospitalization. Furthermore, consensus has been reached that teams are needed for backup, support, services planning, reduced burnout, and improved creativity but that teams of two or three members are likely to be inefficient, and that inefficiency may reduce the amount of direct service delivered (McGrew & Bond, in press). The evidence is equivocal for assertive outreach in services delivery in the client's environment, but it does seem to favor outreach, particularly in reference to increased retention rates and satisfaction with services. Rapp (1995) noted that the lack of efficacy in the broker model, which is largely based in the office, also argues for the importance of teams in case management. Furthermore, given the lack of effectiveness of broker case management (Franklin et al., 1987) and often the lack of available services (Dozier et al., 1993; Stein, 1992), it appears that improved client outcomes are produced when case managers deliver the greatest part of services rather than use referrals to services elsewhere. Case management services with caseloads of fewer than 20 clients appear to produce more positive outcomes. There are some data to indicate that case management may produce positive effects in a short time, but without continued services, researchers have found that the gains clients achieve will deteriorate (Audini et al., 1994; McRae, Higgins, Lycan, & Sherman, 1990; Stein & Test, 1980). Therefore, it appears that services need to be long term or of indefinite duration.

Evidence has been increasing on the importance of the therapeutic relationship between the case manager and the client in producing positive clinical and psychosocial outcomes (Gehrs & Goering, 1995; Neale & Rosenheck, 1995; Solomon, Draine, & Delaney, 1995). Until recently, this area of research was neglected because people with severe mental disorders, particularly schizophrenia, were not considered capable of developing an alliance—undoubtedly an important component of all case management services.

## Future Directions for Research

Research on case management has greatly advanced in recent years, but the findings have remained somewhat limited. Case management appears to have had the most impact on system-level outcomes and only minimal effects on clinical and psychosocial outcomes. Several factors have likely contributed to these limited outcomes. Methodological weaknesses include brief duration of the studies, small sample sizes, biased comparison groups, enhanced comparison or control groups who receive some aspects of case management, problems in establishing the experimental model, lack of retention of subjects, and inadequate outcome measures (Burns & Santos, 1995; Orwin, Sonnefeld, Garrison-Mogren, & Smith, 1994; Solomon, 1997). Differences in outcomes also may be attributable to "differences in the definition of case management, the types of systems of care within which case management is embedded, the types of clients served," as well as design issues (Mechanic, Schlesinger, & McAlpine, 1995, p. 42). Santos, Henggeler, Burns, Arana, and Meisler (1995) also noted that differences in outcomes may be a result of differences in the level of acuity of the sample at intake. Future studies can be designed to correct for some of these methodological deficiencies, for example, by increasing the study duration so that severely disabled clients have an opportunity to obtain new skills and change their ways of living. Research also needs to focus on the implementation of the study, as well as the outcomes, by improved monitoring of the intervention. Examining the effectiveness of different services elements is essential in beginning to understand those aspects of case management that produce favorable outcomes. Given the paucity of research on the clinical, rehabilitation, and broker models of case management, more controlled trials are needed.

Research emphasis also should be placed on assessing the quality of the relationship between the case manager and the client. Outcomes such as social functioning and quality of life may be more responsive to the quality of that relationship (Mechanic et al., 1995). Studies are needed to determine which service elements— such as home-based services, teaching daily living skills, or assertive follow-up—are essential to producing positive outcomes (Marks et al., 1994). In the current environment of managed care, assessing the quality of services is critical. Environmental factors, including case manager and organizational characteristics, should be assessed and measured in future research. The efficacy of case management frequently depends on referrals for services. In some cases, it seems to be expected that use of case management will fix an uncoordinated and fragmented mental health services system and provide needed but unavailable support and services. Often such a solution may not be possible (Stein, 1992). Managed care will have an impact on the way case management is delivered, and little is known about the effectiveness of case management in the private sector (Mechanic et al., 1995). Future research needs to consider these environmental dimensions. The effectiveness of case management also needs to be examined with regard to client subgroups, such as people with personality disorders, because questions have been raised about the appropriateness of case management for these clients (Harris, 1990). Determining which models of case management are effective for which client groups is important to delivering the most cost-effective services.

## Conclusion

Social workers can use the diversity of their knowledge and skills to provide the most effective case management to adults with severe mental illness. Practitioners must be flexible and responsive to meet the needs of this vulnerable population in the changing health care environment. Given the multiplicity of problems of the population, multidisciplinary teams appear to be essential for the planning and delivery of services, even if the responsibility for care remains with only one person. It is further evident that case management practice with clients with severe mental illness occurs on both the macro and the micro level. Building relationships with clients is as important as building relationships with other professionals and providers. Keeping abreast of the changing health care policies and how they affect the availability of services, resources, and entitlements is paramount in ensuring effective services for social work clients now and in the future.

# References

Anthony, W., & Liberman, R. (1986). The practice of psychiatric rehabilitation: Historical, conceptual, and research base. *Schizophrenia Bulletin, 12,* 542–559.

Audini, B., Marks, I., Lawrence, R., Connolly, J., & Watts, V. (1994). Home-based versus out-patient/in-patient care for people with serious mental illness: Phase II of a controlled study. *British Journal of Psychiatry, 165,* 204–210.

Austin, C. (1990). Case management: Myths and realities. *Families in Society, 71,* 398–405.

Bachrach, L. (1980). Overview: Model programs for chronic mental patients. *American Journal of Psychiatry, 137,* 1023–1031.

Bachrach, L. (1989). Case management: Toward a shared definition. *Hospital and Community Psychiatry, 40,* 883–884.

Bachrach, L. (1992). Case management revisited. *Hospital and Community Psychiatry, 43,* 209–210.

Bigelow, D., & Young, D. (1991). Effectiveness of a case management program. *Community Mental Health Journal, 27,* 115–123.

Bond, G. (1984). An economic analysis of psychosocial rehabilitation. *Hospital and Community Psychiatry, 35,* 356–362.

Bond, G., McGrew, J. H., & Fekete, D. (1995). Assertive outreach for frequent users of psychiatric hospitals: A meta-analysis. *Journal of Mental Health Administration, 22,* 4–16.

Bond, G., Miller, L., Krumwied, R., & Ward, R. (1988). Assertive case management in three CMHC: A controlled study. *Hospital and Community Psychiatry, 39,* 411–418.

Borland, A., McRae, J., & Lycan, C. (1989). Outcomes of five years of continuous intensive case management. *Hospital and Community Psychiatry, 40,* 369–376.

Brekke, J., & Wolkon, G. (1988). Monitoring program implementation in community mental health settings. *Evaluation and the Health Professions, 11,* 425–440.

Burns, B., & Santos, A. (1995). Assertive community treatment: An update of randomized trials. *Psychiatric Services, 46,* 669–675.

Chamberlain, R., & Rapp, C. (1991). A decade of case management: A methodological review of outcome research. *Community Mental Health Journal, 27,* 171–188.

Cnaan, R. (1994). The new American social work gospel: Case management of the chronically mentally ill. *British Journal of Social Work, 24,* 533–557.

Curtis, J., Millman, E. J., & Struening, E. (1992). Effect of case management on rehospitalization and utilization of ambulatory care services. *Hospital and Community Psychiatry, 43,* 895–899.

Dill, A. (1987). Issues in case management for the chronically mentally ill. In D. Mechanic (Ed.), *Improving mental health services: What the social sciences can tell us* (pp. 61–70). San Francisco: Jossey-Bass.

Dozier, M., Lee, S., Keir, S., Toprac, M., & Mason, M. (1993). A case management program in Texas revisited. *Psychosocial Rehabilitation Journal, 17,* 183–188.

Draine, J. (1997). A critical review of randomized field trials of case management for individuals with serious and persistent mental illness. *Research on Social Work Practice, 7,* 32–52.

Franklin, J., Solovitz, B., Mason, M., Clemons, J., & Miller, G. (1987). An evaluation of case management. *American Journal of Public Health, 77,* 674–678.

Friesen, B., & Poertner, J. (Eds.). (1995). *From case management to service coordination for children with emotional, behavioral or mental disorders: Building on family strengths.* Baltimore: Paul H. Brookes.

Gehrs, M., & Goering, P. (1995). The relationship between the working alliance and rehabilitation outcomes of schizophrenia. *Psychosocial Rehabilitation Journal, 18,* 43–54.

Goering, P., Wasylenki, D., Farkas, M., & Ballantyne, R. (1988). What difference does case management make? *Hospital and Community Psychiatry, 38,* 272–276.

Harris, M. (1990). Redesigning case-management services for work with character-disordered young adult patients. In N. Cohen (Ed.), *Psychiatry takes to the streets* (pp. 156– 176). New York: Guilford Press.

Harris, M., & Bergman, H. (Eds.). (1993). *Case management for mentally ill patients.* Langhorne, PA: Harwood.

Hodge, M., & Draine, J. (1993). Development of support through case management. In R. Flexer & P. Solomon (Eds.), *Psychiatric rehabilitation in practice* (pp. 155–169). Boston: Andover Medical.

Hornstra, R. K., Brice-Wolfe, V., Sagluyu, K., & Riffle, D. (1993). The effect of intensive case management on hospitalization of patients with schizophrenia. *Hospital and Community Psychiatry, 44,* 844–853.

Hoult, J., & Reynolds, I. (1984). Schizophrenia: A comparative trial of community-oriented and hospital-oriented psychiatric care. *Acta Psychiatrica Scandinavica, 69,* 359–372.

Hoult, J., Reynolds, I., Charbonneau-Powis, M., Coles, P., & Briggs, J. (1981). A controlled study of psychiatric hospital versus community treatment: The effect on relatives. *Australian and New Zealand Journal of Psychiatry, 15,* 323–328.

Hoult, J., Reynolds, I., Charbonneau-Powis, M., Weekes, P., & Briggs, J. (1983). Psychiatric hospital versus community treatment: The results of a randomized trial. *Australian and New Zealand Journal of Psychiatry, 17,* 160–167.

Intagliata, J. (1982). Improving the quality of community care for the chronically mentally disabled: The role of case management. *Schizophrenia Bulletin, 8,* 655–673.

Intagliata, J., Willer, B., & Egri, G. (1986). Role of the family in case management of the mentally ill. *Schizophrenia Bulletin, 12,* 699–708.

Jerrel, J., & Hu, T. (1989). Cost-effectiveness of intensive clinical and case management compared with an existing system. *Inquiry, 26,* 224–234.

Johnson, P., & Rubin, A. (1983). Case management in mental health: A social work domain? *Social Work, 28,* 49–55.

Kanter, J. (1989). Clinical case management: Definition, principles, components. *Hospital and Community Psychiatry, 40,* 361–368.

Knapp, M., Beecham, J., Koutsogeorgopoulou, V., Hallam, A., Fenyo, A., Marks, I. M., Connolly, J., Audini, B., & Muijen, M. (1994). Service use and costs of home-based versus hospital-based care for people with serious mental illness. *British Journal of Psychiatry, 165,* 195–203.

Lamb, H. R. (1980). Therapist-case managers: More than brokers of service. *Hospital and Community Psychiatry, 31,* 762–764.

Lurie, N. (1978). Case management. In J. Talbott (Ed.), *The chronic patient* (pp. 159–164). Washington, DC: American Psychiatric Association.

Macias, C., Kinney, R., Farley, O. W., Jackson, R., & Vos, B. (1994). The role of case management within a community support system: Partnership with psychosocial rehabilitation. *Community Mental Health Journal, 30,* 323–339.

Marks, I., Connolly, J., Muijen, M., Audini, B., McNamee, G., & Lawrence, R. (1994). Home-based versus hospital-based care for people with serious mental illness. *British Journal of Psychiatry, 165,* 179–194.

McGrew, J., & Bond, G. (1995). Critical ingredients of Assertive Community Treatment: Judgments of the experts. *Journal of Mental Health Administration, 22,* 113–125.

McGrew, J., & Bond, G. (in press). The association between program characteristics and service delivery in Assertive Community Treatment. *Administration and Policy in Mental Health.*

McGrew, J., Bond, G., Dietzen, L., & Salyers, M. (1994). Measuring the fidelity of implementation of a mental health program model. *Journal of Consulting and Clinical Psychology, 62,* 670–678.

McRae, J., Higgins, M., Lycan, C., & Sherman, W. (1990). What happens to patients after five years of intensive case management stops? *Hospital and Community Psychiatry, 41,* 175–179.

Mechanic, D. (1991). Strategies for integrating mental health services. *Hospital and Community Psychiatry, 42,* 797–801.

Mechanic, D., Schlesinger, M., & McAlpine, D. (1995). Management of mental health and substance abuse services: State of the art and early results. *Milbank Quarterly, 73,* 19–55.

Modrcin, M., Rapp, C., & Poertner, J. (1988). The evaluation of case management services with the chronically mentally ill. *Evaluation and Program Planning, 11,* 307–314.

Mueser, K., Bond, G., Drake, R., & Resnick, S. (in press). Case management for the severely mentally ill: A review of the research. *Schizophrenia Bulletin.*

Mulder, R. (1982). *Evaluation of the Harbinger Program.* Unpublished manuscript.

National Association of Social Workers. (1992). *NASW standards for social work case management.* Washington, DC: Author.

Neale, M. S., & Rosenheck, R. A. (1995). Therapeutic alliance and outcome in a VA intensive case management program. *Psychiatric Services, 46,* 719–721.

Netting, F. E. (1992). Case management: Service or symptom? *Social Work, 37,* 160–164.

Olfson, M. (1990). Assertive community treatment: An evaluation of the experimental evidence. *Hospital and Community Psychiatry, 41,* 634–641.

Orwin, R., Sonnefeld, L., Garrison-Mogren, R., & Smith, N. (1994). Pitfalls in evaluating the effectiveness of case management program for homeless persons. *Evaluation Review, 18,* 153–207.

Ozarin, L. (1978). The pros and cons of case management. In J. Talbott (Ed.), *The chronic patient* (pp. 165–170). Washington, DC: American Psychiatric Association.

Quinlaven, R., Hough, R., Crowell, A., Beach, C., Hofstetter, R., & Kenworthy, K. (1995). Service utilization and cost of care for severely mentally ill clients in an intensive case management program. *Psychiatric Services, 46,* 365–371.

Rapp, C. (1995). *The active ingredients of effective case management: A research synthesis.* Unpublished, manuscript, University of Kansas School of Social Welfare.

Roach, J. (1993). Clinical case management with severely mentally ill adults. In M. Harris & H. Bergman (Eds.), *Case management for mentally ill patients* (pp. 17–40). Langhorne, PA: Harwood.

Roberts-DeGennaro, M. (1987). Developing case management as a practice model. *Social Case Work, 68*, 466–470.

Robinson, G. K., & Toff-Bergman, G. (1990). *Choices in case management: Current knowledge and practice for mental health programs.* Washington, DC: Mental Health Policy Resource Center.

Rothman, J. (1991). A model of case management: Toward empirically based practice. *Social Work, 36*, 520–528.

Rubin, A. (1992). Is case management effective for people with serious mental illness? A research review. *Health & Social Work, 17*, 138–150.

Sands, R. (1991). *Clinical social work practice in community mental health.* New York: Macmillan.

Santos, A., Henggeler, S., Burns, B., Arana, G., & Meisler, N. (1995). Research on field-based services: Models for reform in the delivery of mental health care to populations with complex clinical problems. *American Journal of Psychiatry, 152*, 1111–1123.

Scott, J., & Dixon, L. (1995). Assertive Community Treatment and case management for schizophrenia. *Schizophrenia Bulletin, 21*, 657–668.

Shern, D., Surles, R., & Waizer, J. (1989). Designing community treatment systems for the most seriously mentally ill: A state administrative perspective. *Journal of Social Issues, 45*, 105–117.

Sledge, W., Astrachan, B., Thompson, K., Rakfeldt, J., & Leaf, P. (1995). Case management in psychiatry: An analysis of tasks. *American Journal of Psychiatry, 152*, 1259–1265.

Solomon, P. (1992). The efficacy of case management services for severely mentally disabled clients. *Community Mental Health Journal, 28*, 163–180.

Solomon, P. (1997). Issues in designing and conducting randomized human service trials: Lessons from the field. *Journal of Social Service Research.*

Solomon, P., & Draine, J. (1994). Family perceptions of consumers as case managers. *Community Mental Health Journal, 30*, 165–176.

Solomon, P., & Draine, J. (1995a). One-year outcomes of a randomized trial of case management with seriously mentally ill clients leaving jail. *Evaluation Review, 19*, 256–273.

Solomon, P., & Draine, J. (1995b). One-year outcomes of a randomized trial of consumer case management. *Evaluation and Program Planning, 18*, 117–127.

Solomon, P., & Draine, J. (1995c). The efficacy of a consumer case management team: 2-year outcomes of a randomized trial. *Journal of Mental Health Administration, 22*, 135–146.

Solomon, P., Draine, J., & Delaney, M. A. (1995). The working alliance and consumer case management. *Journal of Mental Health Administration, 22*, 126–134.

Solomon, P., & Meyerson, A. (1997). Social stabilization: Achieving satisfactory community adaptation for the disabled mentally ill. In A. Tasman, J. Kay, & J. Lieberman (Eds.), *Psychiatry* (pp. 1727–1750). Philadelphia: W. B. Saunders.

State Comprehensive Mental Health Services Plan Act of 1986, P.L. 99-660, 100 Stat. 3794.

Stein, L. (1992). On the abolishment of the case manager. *Health Affairs, 11*, 172–177.

Stein, L., & Test, M. A. (1980). Alternative to mental hospital treatment. I. Conceptual model, treatment program, and clinical evaluation. *Archives of General Psychiatry, 37*, 392–397.

Test, M. A. (1992). The Training in Community Living model. In R. P. Liberman (Ed.), *Handbook of psychiatric rehabilitation* (pp. 153–170). New York: Macmillan.

Test, M. A., & Stein, L. (1980). Alternative to mental hospital treatment. III. Social cost. *Archives of General Psychiatry, 37,* 409–412.

Turner, J., & Tenhor, W. (1978). The NIMH Community Support Program: Pilot approach to a needed social reform. *Schizophrenia Bulletin, 4,* 319–349.

Weisbrod, B. A., Test, M. A., & Stein, L. I. (1980). Alternative to mental hospital treatment. II. Economic benefit-cost analysis. *Archives of General Psychiatry, 37,* 400–405.

# Index

# About the Editors

**Janet B.W. Williams, DSW,** is a research scientist and deputy director of the Biometrics Research Department at the New York State Psychiatric Institute and professor of clinical psychiatric social work in the Departments of Psychiatry and Neurology at Columbia University College of Physicians and Surgeons, New York City. In 1994 Dr. Williams founded the Society for Social Work and Research and served for two years as its first president. She sits on the Scientific Advisory Committee of the Institute for the Advancement of Social Work Research. She is well known for her work on DSM-III, DSM III-R, and DSM-IV and has authored many rating instruments, interview guides, and more than 200 publications.

**Kathleen Ell, DSW,** is professor in the School of Social Work at the University of Southern California, Los Angeles. She has conducted extensive research on psychological distress, morbidity, and mortality resulting from life-threatening illness and on health care–seeking behavior. A hallmark of her research and numerous publications has been their focus on low-income and ethnically diverse populations. She is currently engaged in studies on translating effective interventions to improve follow-up of abnormal cancer screens among low-income women and to improve the detection and treatment of depression among medically underserved populations within real world health service systems. She has authored more than 50 publications and serves on the editorial board of *Social Work Research.*

# About the Contributors

**Jamie M. Abelson, MSW, ACSW,** is an adjunct lecturer at the School of Social Work and a research associate at the Institute for Social Research, both at the University of Michigan, Ann Arbor. He has worked for 10 years on the National Comorbidity Survey overseeing a series of diagnostic validation studies. He serves as lead trainer for the World Health Organization Composite International Diagnostic Interview Training and Research Center at the University of Michigan.

**Eugene Aisenberg, MSW,** a Council on Social Work Education Research Fellow, is a doctoral student in the School of Social Work at the University of Southern California, Los Angeles. His research focus is on children's exposure to community violence and its psychological and emotional effects. He also works as a therapist in the Child Abuse Treatment Program of Drew Child Development Corporation, Los Angeles.

**Lee W. Badger, MSW, PhD,** is a professor of social work at the School of Social Work, University of Alabama, Tuscaloosa, and in 1998 will become a professor at the Graduate School of Social Service, Fordham University, New York City. For almost 20 years she has engaged in research focused on mental health services, with a particular emphasis on the recognition and management of mood disorders in the primary care sector.

**Kia J. Bentley, PhD, LCSW,** is an associate professor of social work at Virginia Commonwealth University, Richmond, where she teaches mental health practice and policy, research methods, and practice theory. In 1996 she worked with Joseph Walsh to produce the book *The Social Worker and Psychotropic Medication* (Brooks/Cole). She is currently studying the meaning of medication for consumers and practitioners' role dilemmas in medication management. A longtime member of NASW and a consulting editor for *Social Work,* she also serves on the board of directors for the Virginia Alliance for the Mentally Ill.

**Nancee Blum, MSW, LISW,** is a social work specialist in the Department of Psychiatry at the University of Iowa, Iowa City, and an adjunct instructor in the College of Medicine and the School of Social Work there. Her primary interest is research in and treatment of personality disorders. She is coauthor of *The Structured Interview for DSM Personality* (American Psychiatric Press).

**John S. Brekke, PhD,** has been on the faculty of the School of Social Work at the University of Southern California, Los Angeles, since 1984. With funding from the National Institute of Mental Health, he is currently studying how psychobiological factors can be integrated with psychosocial factors in a biosocial model of rehabilitation in schizophrenia, and the generalization of family-based interventions to ethnic minorities with severe and persistent mental disorders.

**Laura Clary** is completing her undergraduate major in psychology at Smith College, Northampton, MA.

**Iris Cohen, MSW,** is a doctoral student in the interdisciplinary PhD program in social work and sociology at Boston University and has been a research assistant at that university's School of Social Work. Previous degree work was completed at Cornell University and New York University. She specializes in oncology social work.

**Sophia F. Dziegielewski, PhD, LCSW,** is a visiting associate professor in the School of Social Work, University of Central Florida, Orlando. She has held faculty appointments at the University of Alabama, the departments of family and preventive medicine and psychiatry at Meharry Medical College, the University of Tennessee, and the U.S. Army Military College at Ft. Benning, GA. Her practice interest centers on establishing time-limited, outcome-based treatments.

**Nabila El-Bassel, DSW,** is an associate professor at the School of Social Work, Columbia University, New York City, and the associate director of the Social Intervention Group there. Her research interests include drug abuse, HIV prevention, women's health, family violence, social supports, and social problems of recent immigrants.

**Pat Fobair, MPH, LCSW,** is a clinical social worker, group therapist, research coordinator, and intervention specialist in psychosocial research projects in radiation oncology at the University of California–San Francisco Stanford Health Services. She initiated her first hospital-based patient group in 1970. In addition to leading five weekly groups at the medical center, she coleads a group in a study concerned with the effectiveness of groups in improving quality of life and longevity among patients with metastatic breast cancer.

**Ronald C. Kessler, PhD,** is a professor of health care policy at Harvard Medical School. He is the recipient of Research Scientist and MERIT awards from the National Institute of Mental Health. He is the principal investigator of the National Comorbidity Survey and director of the World Health Organization's International Consortium in Psychiatric Epidemiology, a cross-national collaborative effort to foster comparative studies of psychological disorders.

**Carl G. Leukefeld, DSW,** is a professor of psychiatry and the director of the Center on Drug and Alcohol Abuse Research at the University of Kentucky, Lexington. Before beginning his appointment there, he worked for 20 years with the National Institute on Drug Abuse and the U.S. Public Health Service. He has coedited several books and currently writes on criminal justice and AIDS prevention and treatment.

**Ellen P. Lukens, MSW, PhD,** is an assistant professor of social work at the School of Social Work, Columbia University, and a research scientist at New York State Psychiatric Institute, New York City. As both a clinician and a researcher she has a long-standing interest in the impact of schizophrenia on family members and the value of collaboration among family members and professionals in the monitoring and care of that severe mental illness.

**Bruce Pfohl, MD,** is a professor of psychiatry in the College of Medicine at the University of Iowa. He is an active clinician and the director of the Psychiatry Outpatient Clinic at University Hospitals, Iowa City. He was a member of the DSM-IV Personality Disorders Work Group and is author of *The Structured Interview for DSM-IV Personality Disorders.*

**Enola K. Proctor, PhD,** is the Frank J. Bruno professor of social work research at the George Warren Brown School of Social Work, Washington University, St. Louis. She is the director of the Center for Mental Health Services Research there, supported by a National Institute of Mental Health grant. She has been principal or coprincipal investigator on several funded studies of health and mental health services use among vulnerable populations.

**Elizabeth H. Rand, MD,** is an associate professor and the chair of the Department of Psychiatry and Neurology at the School of Medicine, Tuscaloosa Program, University of Alabama. Psychiatry in the primary care sector of the health care system has been a major focus of her research.

**Mary Carmel Ruffolo, PhD,** is an associate professor at the School of Social Work, Syracuse University, New York, teaching social work practice with a special focus on child mental health services, case management, and health system issues. She is the principal investigator for a National Institute of Mental Health five-year study focusing on developing and evaluating a multiple family group psychoeducational intervention model for parents of children with serious emotional disturbances enrolled in several of New York State's intensive case management programs.

**Robert F. Schilling, PhD, ACSW,** is a professor in the School of Social Work, Columbia University, New York City, and he directs that institution's Social Intervention Group. His research concerns prevention of HIV/AIDS, substance abuse, and related social problems, and he has a particular interest in the design, development, and testing of interventions in low-income urban communities.

**John P. Shields, MSW,** is the program evaluation manager for the Northeast Georgia Regional Board for Mental Health, Mental Retardation, and Substance Abuse Services. He manages the quantitative and qualitative program evaluation efforts of contracted public-sector services providers across a 23-county region in northeast Georgia. He is also a doctoral student at the School of Social Work, University of Georgia, Athens.

**Elizabeth S. Slade, MSW,** is a PhD candidate at the School of Social Work, University of Southern California, Los Angeles. Her research focuses on community-based methods of psychosocial rehabilitation for people with schizophrenia. She has published on the relationships between service factors and functional outcomes in community-based care and on subjective experience in schizophrenia.

**Phyllis Solomon, PhD,** is a professor of social work in psychiatry, School of Social Work, University of Pennsylvania, Philadelphia. She has conducted a number of research studies on service interventions and services delivery for adults with severe mental illness and their families. She has published and presented extensively on case management services, consumer-delivered services, and psychiatric rehabilitation services.

**Gail Steketee, PhD,** is a professor and the associate dean of academic affairs at the School of Social Work, Boston University. She completed earlier degree work at Harvard University and Bryn Mawr Graduate School of Social Work and Social Research. Currently she collaborates on several research projects studying the treatment of obsessive–compulsive disorder (OCD) and the family roles in behavioral treatment for OCD and agoraphobia. Her list of publications includes two books,

*When Once Is Not Enough* (New Harbinger Press) and *Treatment of Obsessive–Compulsive Disorder* (Guilford Press).

**Arlene Rubin Stiffman, PhD,** is a professor at the George Warren Brown School of Social Work, Washington University, St. Louis, where she is the associate director of their National Institute of Mental Health–funded Center for Mental Health Services Research. She has been the principal investigator for several funded studies of adolescent mental health and behavioral problems. Her publications have centered on multisector services and on the person-in-environment relationship.

**Mary Ann Test, PhD,** is a professor at the School of Social Work and an affiliate professor in the Department of Psychiatry at the University of Wisconsin, Madison. Previously she was the director of research and psychology at the Mendota Mental Health Institute, Madison. With Leonard Stein she codeveloped the Program of Assertive Community Treatment. For 25 years her work has concentrated on creating and evaluating effective models for community care.

**Helle Thorning, MSW, CSW,** is the director of social work at the New York State Psychiatric Institute; an assistant clinical professor of psychiatric social work at the College of Physicians and Surgeons, Columbia University; and a doctoral candidate in clinical social work at New York University, New York City. Her long-standing commitment is to studying the impact of mental illness on families and family life.

**Bruce A. Thyer, PhD, LCSW,** is a research professor of social work and an adjunct professor of psychology at the University of Georgia, Athens, and an associate clinical professor of psychiatry and health behavior at the Medical College of Georgia. He is editor of the journal *Research on Social Work Practice*. His most recent book is the *Handbook of Empirical Social Work Practice*, coedited with John Wodarski (John Wiley & Sons).

**Barbara L. Van Noppen, MSW,** is a clinical social worker in the OCD Clinic at Butler Hospital, Providence, RI, and conducts a private practice. She is a research associate in the Department of Psychiatry and Human Behavior, Division of Biology and Medicine, at Brown University, Providence. She is internationally recognized for her expertise in treating families with obsessive–compulsive disorder.

**Robert Walker, MSW, LCSW, BCD,** is the director of the Bluegrass East Comprehensive Care Center in Lexington, KY, a private, nonprofit mental health center. He is an assistant professor in the College of Social Work, University of Kentucky, Lexington. He has published on substance abuse, personality disorders, and domestic violence, and he serves on the Examination Committee of the American Association of State Social Work Boards, developing examinations for social work certification and licensure.

**Joseph Walsh, PhD, LCSW,** is an assistant professor in the School of Social Work, Virginia Commonwealth University, Richmond, where he teaches courses in clinical practice, generalist practice, and research methods. For 19 years he worked in psychiatric hospitals and community mental health centers and comanaged a clinic pharmacy. With Kia J. Bentley he coauthored *The Social Worker and Psychotropic Medication* (Brooks/Cole).

**Shanyang Zhao, PhD,** is an assistant professor of sociology at Temple University, Philadelphia. His research interests include the study of social risk factors for mental illness, with a special focus on anxiety disorder. He is also interested in the evaluation of survey-based mental health diagnostic instruments.

**Advances in Mental Health Research**

Cover design by **The Watermark Design Office**

Book design and composition by **Christine Cotting, UpperCase Publication Services**

Printed by **Boyd Printing Company**

# RESEARCH TOOLS FOR SOCIAL WORKERS FROM NASW PRESS

**Advances in Mental Health Research:** *Implications for Practice,* Janet B. W. Williams and Kathleen Ell, Editors, cofunded by the National Institute of Mental Health. This book provides the latest scientific knowledge for treating the wide range of conditions and issues encountered in social work practice. Today, public policy deliberations and the health care reimbursement system are creating an urgent need to prove that social work mental health practice is based on scientific knowledge. *Advances in Mental Health Research* will help you work toward that goal.

*ISBN: 0-87101-291-X. Item #291X. $27.95.*

**New Directions for Social Work Practice Research,** *edited by Miriam Potocky-Tripodi and Tony Tripodi.* This timely and provocative book helps you put your finger on the pulse of research in social work practice—past, present, and future. Contributors from the United States and the United Kingdom, all prominent social work researchers, offer a variety of critical assessments of practice research, provide a wealth of new data on the current status of research, and clearly lay down their own visions of the agenda for future studies.

*ISBN: 0-87101-305-3. Item #3053. $28.95.*

**Social Work Research Methods:** *Building Knowledge for Practice,* edited by Stuart A. Kirk. In this unique supplementary text, students will learn different approaches to conducting social work research in their required research courses. Filled with recent examples taken from NASW Press and other research journals, *Social Work Research Methods* illustrates the latest approaches for diverse fields of practice, populations, levels of intervention, and methodologies. Designed to supplement all of the current major social work research textbooks, *Social Work Research Methods* is a valuable teaching aid for all levels of research courses.

*ISBN: 0-87101-300-2. Item #3002a. $41.95.*

**A Primer on Single-Subject Design for Clinical Social Workers,** *by Tony Tripodi.* This practical guide demonstrates how to build the single-subject design model into your practice without disruption and then use it easily—to make key clinical decisions, monitor the effectiveness of treatment, promote client understanding, and demonstrate accountability in clinical practice.

*ISBN: 0-87101-238-3. Item #2383. $31.95.*

**Encyclopedia of Social Work, 19th Edition,** *Richard L. Edwards, Editor-in-Chief.* Three volumes provide nearly 3,000 pages of information on virtually every aspect of social work. Expanded content areas include new technologies, research, global changes, U.S. policy developments, and evolving roles for social workers. EXTRA VALUE—the *1997 Supplement* is included with the set!

*Casebound—ISBN: 0-87101-255-3. Item #2553. $159.00.*
*Softcover version—ISBN: 0-87101-256-1. Item #2561. $129.00*

**Encyclopedia of Social Work, 19th Edition, 1997 Supplement,** *Richard L. Edwards, Editor-in-Chief.* The publication of the *Supplement* brings the *Encyclopedia* up to date with the most current concerns in social work. Over 400 pages of new information. A total of 30 all new entries and 15 new biographies.

*ISBN: 0-87101-277-4. Item #2774. $37.95.*

**Social Work Research.** The *Social Work Research* journal publishes exemplary research to advance the development of knowledge and inform social work practice. The journal includes analytic reviews of research, theoretical articles pertaining to social work research, evaluation studies, and diverse research studies that contribute to knowledge about social work issues.

*ISSN: 1070-5309. Published quarterly: March, June, September, December. Pricing on next page.*

**(Order form and information on reverse side)**

# ORDER FORM

| Qty. | Title | Item # | Price | Total |
|------|-------|--------|-------|-------|
| __ | Advances in Mental Health Research | 291X | $27.95 | _____ |
| __ | New Directions for SW Practice Research | 3053 | $28.95 | _____ |
| __ | Social Work Research Methods | 3002a | $41.95 | _____ |
| __ | A Primer on Single-Subject Design | 2383 | $31.95 | _____ |
| __ | Encyclopedia of Social Work, 19th Edition | | | |
| __ |    (Casebound version) | 2553 | $159.00 | _____ |
| __ |    (Softcover version) | 2561 | $129.00 | _____ |
| __ | Encyclopedia of Social Work, 19th Edition, 1997 Supplement | 2774 | $37.95 | _____ |
| __ | Social Work Research (Member) | 7001 | $40.00 | _____ |
| __ | Social Work Research (Student Member) | 7101 | $28.00 | _____ |
| __ | Social Work Research (Individual Nonmember) | 7201 | $69.95 | _____ |
| __ | Social Work Research (Library/Institution) | 7301 | $99.95 | _____ |

**POSTAGE AND HANDLING**

Minimum postage and handling fee is $4.95. Orders that do not include appropriate postage and handling will be returned.

DOMESTIC: Please add 12% to orders under $100 for postage and handling. For orders over $100 add 7% of order.

CANADA: Please add 17% postage and handling.

OTHER INTERNATIONAL: Please add 22% postage and handling.

| | |
|---|---|
| Subtotal | _____ |
| Postage and Handling | _____ |
| DC residents add 6% sales tax | _____ |
| MD residents add 5% sales tax | _____ |
| Total | _____ |

❏ **Check or money order** (payable to NASW Press) for $ _____.

❏ **Credit card**
  ❏ NASW Visa* | ❏ Visa | ❏ NASW MasterCard* | ❏ MasterCard | ❏ Amex

_____      _____
Credit Card Number                        Expiration Date

Signature _____

*Use of these cards generates funds in support of the social work profession.*

Name _____

Address _____

City _____ State/Province _____

Country _____ Zip _____

Phone _____ E-mail _____

NASW Member # (if applicable) _____

*(Please make checks payable to NASW Press. Prices are subject to change.)*

NASW PRESS
P. O. Box 431
Annapolis JCT, MD 20701
USA

**Credit card orders call
1-800-227-3590**
(In the Metro Wash., DC, area, call 301-317-8688)
**Or fax your order to 301-206-7989**
**Or order online at http://www.naswpress.org**

*Visit our Web site at http://www.naswpress.org.*     AMHR101

3407